AMERICAN ACADEMY
OF OPHTHALMOLOGY®
Protecting Sight. Empowering Lives.

MW01701677

8 External Disease and Cornea

Last major revision 2021–2022

2022–2023
BCSC
Basic and Clinical Science Course™

Published after collaborative review with the European Board of Ophthalmology subcommittee

The American Academy of Ophthalmology is accredited by the Accreditation Council for Continuing Medical Education (ACCME) to provide continuing medical education for physicians.

The American Academy of Ophthalmology designates this enduring material for a maximum of 15 *AMA PRA Category 1 Credits*™. Physicians should claim only the credit commensurate with the extent of their participation in the activity.

CME expiration date: June 1, 2024. *AMA PRA Category 1 Credits*™ may be claimed only once between June 1, 2021, and the expiration date.

BCSC® volumes are designed to increase the physician's ophthalmic knowledge through study and review. Users of this activity are encouraged to read the text and then answer the study questions provided at the back of the book.

To claim *AMA PRA Category 1 Credits*™ upon completion of this activity, learners must demonstrate appropriate knowledge and participation in the activity by taking the posttest for Section 8 and achieving a score of 80% or higher. For further details, please see the instructions for requesting CME credit at the back of the book.

Cover image: From BCSC Section 12, *Retina and Vitreous*. Confocal scanning laser ophthalmoscopy multicolor fundus image (30° field of view) of a healthy eye. *(Courtesy of Lucia Sobrin, MD.)*

FSC www.fsc.org MIX Paper from responsible sources FSC® C001701

Printed in China.

Basic and Clinical Science Course

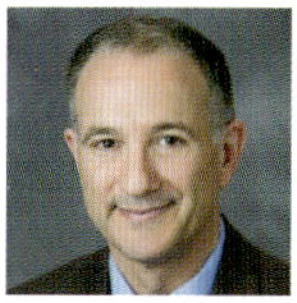

Christopher J. Rapuano, MD, Philadelphia, Pennsylvania
Senior Secretary for Clinical Education

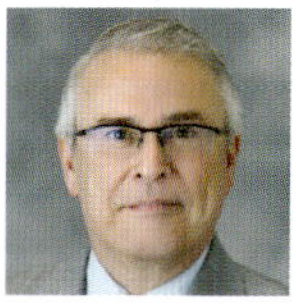

J. Timothy Stout, MD, PhD, MBA, Houston, Texas
Secretary for Lifelong Learning and Assessment

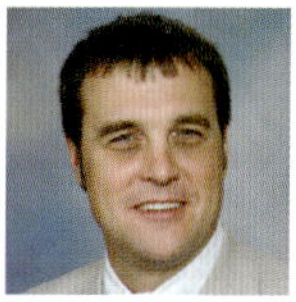

Colin A. McCannel, MD, Los Angeles, California
BCSC Course Chair

Section 8

Faculty for the Major Revision

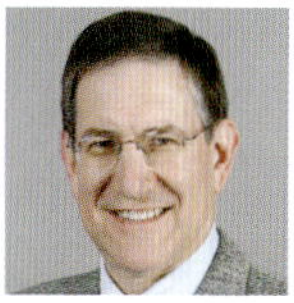

Robert S. Feder, MD
Chair
Chicago, Illinois

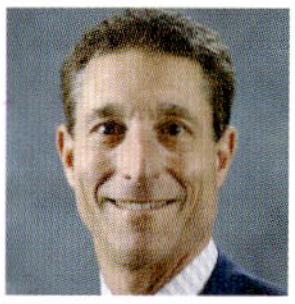

Gregg J. Berdy, MD
Saint Louis, Missouri

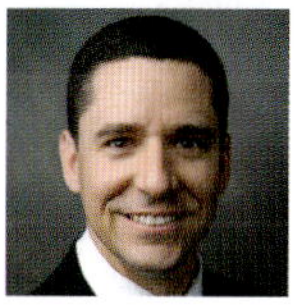

Joseph D. Iuorno, MD
Richmond, Virginia

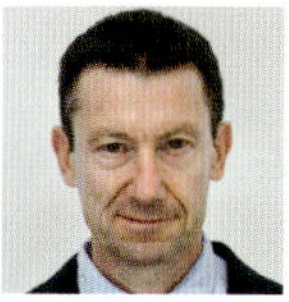

Arie L. Marcovich, MD, PhD
Rehovot, Israel

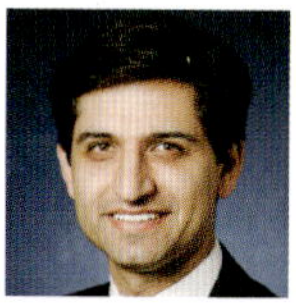

Shahzad I. Mian, MD
Ann Arbor, Michigan

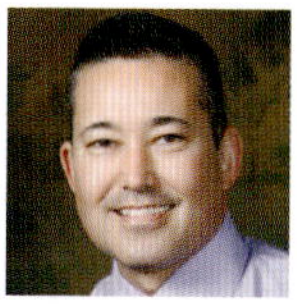

Charles D. Reilly, MD
San Antonio, Texas

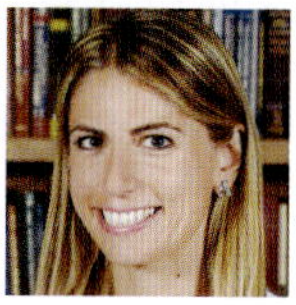

Danielle Trief, MD, MSc
New York, New York

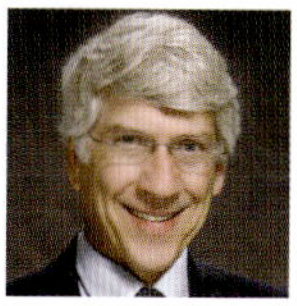

David D. Verdier, MD
Grand Rapids, Michigan

The Academy acknowledges the following committees for review of this edition:

Vision Rehabilitation Committee: Mary Lou Jackson, MD, Vancouver, Canada

BCSC Resident/Fellow Reviewers: Sharon L. Jick, MD, *Chair,* St. Louis, Missouri; Amar K. Bhat, MD; Adam Rothman, MD; Mark P. Breazzano, MD; Shawn Lin, MD; Daniel M. Vu, MD; Brittni A. Scruggs, MD

Practicing Ophthalmologists Advisory Committee for Education: Bradley D. Fouraker, MD, *Chair, Primary Reviewer*; Tampa, Florida; Cynthia S. Chiu, MD, Oakland, California; George S. Ellis Jr, MD, New Orleans, Louisiana; Stephen R. Klapper, MD, Carmel, Indiana; Gaurav K. Shah, MD, Town and Country, Missouri; Rosa A. Tang, MD, MPH, MBA, Houston, Texas; Troy M. Tanji, MD, Waipahu, Hawaii; Michelle S. Ying, MD, Ladson, South Carolina

The Academy also acknowledges the following committee for assistance in developing Study Questions and Answers for this BCSC Section:

Resident Self-Assessment Committee: Evan L. Waxman, MD, PhD, *Chair,* Pittsburgh, Pennsylvania; Robert A. Beaulieu, MD, Royal Oak, Michigan; Benjamin W. Botsford, MD, New York, New York; Olga M. Ceron, MD, Grafton, Massachusetts; Eva DeVience, MD, Windsor Mill, Maryland; Kevin Halenda, MD, Cleveland, Ohio; Amanda D. Henderson, MD, Baltimore, Maryland; Andrew M. Hendrick, MD, Atlanta, Georgia; Joshua Hendrix, MD, Dalton, Georgia; Matthew B. Kaufman, MD, Portland, Oregon; Zachary A. Koretz, MD, MPH, Pittsburgh, Pennsylvania; Kevin E. Lai, MD, Indianapolis, Indiana; Kenneth C. Lao, MD, Temple, Texas; Yasha S. Modi, MD, New York, New York; Mark E. Robinson, MD, MPH, Columbia, South Carolina; Jamie B. Rosenberg, MD, New York, New York; Tahira Scholle, MD, Houston, Texas; Syed Mahmood Shah, MD, Pittsburgh, Pennsylvania; Ann Shue, MD, Sunnyvale, California; Jeong-Hyeon Sohn, MD, Shavano Park, Texas; Misha F. Syed, MD, League City, Texas; Parisa Taravati, MD, Seattle, Washington; Tanu O. Thomas, MD, El Paso, Texas; Sarah Van Tassel, MD, New York, New York; Matthew S. Wieder, MD, Scarsdale, New York; Jules A. Winokur, MD, Great Neck, New York

EB

European Board of Ophthalmology: Lotte Welinder, MD, *Liaison,* Aalborg, Denmark; Christina Grupcheva, MD, Varna, Bulgaria

Financial Disclosures

Academy staff members who contributed to the development of this product state that within the 24 months prior to their contributions to this CME activity and for the duration of development, they have had no financial interest in or other relationship with any entity that produces, markets, resells, or distributes health care goods or services consumed by or used in patients, or with any competing commercial product or service.

The authors and reviewers state that within the 24 months prior to their contributions to this CME activity and for the duration of development, they have had the following financial relationships:*

Dr Berdy: Aerie Pharmaceuticals (C), Alcon (C, L), Allergan (C, L), Bausch + Lomb (C, L), Bio-Tissue (L), ImprimisRx (C), Novartis (C,L), Ocular Science (C, L), Shire/Takeda (C, L), Sun Pharma (C, L), TearScience/Johnson & Johnson (C)

Dr Fouraker: Addition Technology (C, L), AJL Ophthalmic (C, L), Alcon (C, L), OASIS Medical (C, L)

Dr Jackson: Astellas Pharma (C)

Dr Klapper: AdOM Advanced Optical Technologies (O)

Dr Marcovich: EyeYon Medical (C, P), Johnson & Johnson Vision (C, L), Mor Isum (P), Shire/Takeda (C), Steba Biotech (P), Yeda (P)

Dr Mian: CentraSight (S), Shire/Takeda (S), VisionCare/Samsara Vision (S)

Dr Modi: Alimera Sciences (C), Allergan (C), Genentech (C), Théa (C), ZEISS (C)

Dr Reilly: Abbott (S), Alcon (S), Allergan (S), Bausch + Lomb (S), Glaukos (S), Merck (S), Senju Pharmaceutical Co. (S)

Dr Robinson: Horizon Therapeutics (O)

Dr Shah: Allergan (C, S), Bausch + Lomb (L), DORC International/Dutch Ophthalmic, USA (S), Regeneron Pharmaceuticals (C, L)

Dr Tang: EMD Serono (L), Horizon Therapeutics (C, S), Immunovant (S), Novartis (S), Quark Pharmaceuticals (C, S), Regenera Pharma (S), Sanofi (L), ZEISS (L)

Dr Van Tassel: Aerie Pharmaceuticals (C), Allergan (C), Equinox (C), New World Medical (C)

The other authors and reviewers state that within the 24 months prior to their contributions to this CME activity and for the duration of development, they have had no financial interest in or other relationship with any entity that produces, markets, resells, or distributes health care goods or services consumed by or used in patients, or with any competing commercial product or service.

* C = consultant fee, paid advisory boards, or fees for attending a meeting; E = employed by or received a W2 from a commercial company; L = lecture fees or honoraria, travel fees or reimbursements when speaking at the invitation of a commercial company; O = equity ownership/stock options in publicly or privately traded firms, excluding mutual funds; P = patents and/or royalties for intellectual property; S = grant support or other financial support to the investigator from all sources, including research support from government agencies, foundations, device manufacturers, and/or pharmaceutical companies

Recent Past Faculty

Mary K. Daly, MD
Denise de Freitas, MD
Stephen E. Orlin, MD
Elmer Y. Tu, MD
Woodford S. Van Meter, MD
Robert W. Weisenthal, MD

In addition, the Academy gratefully acknowledges the contributions of numerous past faculty and advisory committee members who have played an important role in the development of previous editions of the Basic and Clinical Science Course.

American Academy of Ophthalmology Staff

Dale E. Fajardo, EdD, MBA, *Vice President, Education*
Beth Wilson, *Director, Continuing Professional Development*
Denise Evenson, *Director, Brand & Creative*
Susan Malloy, *Acquisitions and Development Manager*
Stephanie Tanaka, *Publications Manager*
Rayna Ungersma, *Manager, Curriculum Development*
Jasmine Chen, *Manager, E-Learning*
Sarah Page, *Online Education and Licensing Manager*
Lana Ip, *Senior Designer*
Beth Collins, *Medical Editor*
Eric Gerdes, *Interactive Designer*
Lynda Hanwella, *Publications Specialist*
Debra Marchi, *Permissions Assistant*

American Academy of Ophthalmology
655 Beach Street
Box 7424
San Francisco, CA 94120-7424

Contents

Introduction to the BCSC xv
Introduction to Section 8 xvii

Objectives 1

1 Structure and Function of the External Eye and Cornea. 3
Highlights 3
Eyelids 3
Lacrimal Functional Unit 5
Tear Film 6
Conjunctiva 7
Sclera 8
Cornea 8
Zones of the Cornea 9
Corneal Epithelium 10
Bowman Layer 10
Corneal Stroma 11
Descemet Membrane 12
Corneal Endothelium 13
Limbus 14
Defense Mechanisms of the External Eye and Cornea 14

2 The Approach, Techniques, and Devices for Examination of the External Eye and Cornea 19
Highlights 19
External Eye Exam 19
General Appearance 19
The Eyelids. 20
Corneal Sensation. 20
Slit-Lamp Biomicroscopy 21
Illumination Techniques 22
Clinical Use 26
Ocular Surface Staining and Evaluation of Tear Function. 26
Ocular Surface Staining 27
Evaluation of Tear Production 30
Evaluation of Corneal Contour 32
Keratometry 32
Keratoscopy 33
Corneal Topography. 33
Corneal Tomography 36

Corneal Biomechanics. 40
Corneal Resistance Factor 40
Newer Technologies 40
Endothelial Appearance and Function 40
Specular Microscopy 40
Pachymetry 41
Other Imaging Modalities 42
Confocal Microscopy 42
Anterior Segment Optical Coherence Tomography 44
Ultrasound Biomicroscopy 45

3 Clinical Approach to Ocular Surface Disease 47
Highlights 47
Common Clinical Findings in Ocular Surface Disease 47
Conjunctival Signs of Inflammation 47
Corneal Signs of Inflammation 52
Clinical Approach to Dry Eye. 54
Mechanisms of Dry Eye 57
Aqueous Tear Deficiency. 59
Evaporative Dry Eye 63
Treatment of Dry Eye 66
Eyelid Conditions Associated With Ocular Surface Disease. 76
Rosacea 76
Seborrheic Blepharitis 78
Staphylococcal Blepharitis 80
Staphylococcal Blepharoconjunctivitis 81
Marginal Keratitis. 82
Phlyctenular Keratoconjunctivitis (Phlyctenulosis). 83
Hordeola and Chalazia. 84

4 Eyelid, Conjunctival, and Corneal Conditions Associated With Ocular Surface Disorders. 87
Highlights 87
Introduction 87
Eyelid Disease 88
Floppy Eyelid Syndrome 88
Distichiasis and Trichiasis 89
Conjunctival Disease 90
Superior Limbic Keratoconjunctivitis 90
Conjunctivochalasis 92
Surface Disorders of the Cornea 93
Exposure Keratopathy 93
Neurotrophic Keratopathy 94
Recurrent Corneal Erosion 97
Dellen 100
Limbal Stem Cell Deficiency 100

Toxic Corneal Epithelial Cell Reactions to Topical Ophthalmic Medications 102
Self-Induced Ocular Surface Disorders 105

5 Therapeutic Interventions for Ocular Surface Disorders 107
Highlights 107
Introduction 107
Conjunctival Interventions for Ocular Surface Disorders 107
Pterygium Excision 107
Autologous Conjunctival Transplantation 114
Conjunctival Flap for Corneal Disease 114
Conjunctival Biopsy 118
Treatment of Conjunctivochalasis 119
Limbal Stem Cell Transplantation 120
Mucous Membrane Grafts 123
Corneal Interventions for Ocular Surface Disorders 125
Superficial Keratectomy and Corneal Biopsy 125
Surgical Management of Recurrent Corneal Erosion 126
Management of Persistent Corneal Epithelial Defects, Thinning, and Perforation 128
Tarsorrhaphy 132
Corneal Tattooing 134

6 Congenital Anomalies of the Cornea and Sclera 137
Highlights 137
Developmental Anomalies of the Anterior Segment 137
Anomalies of Size and Shape of the Cornea 137
Corneal Dystrophies 145
Developmental Anomalies of the Cornea and Associated Anterior Segment Structures 145
Secondary Abnormalities Affecting the Infant Cornea 151
Intrauterine Keratitis: Bacterial and Syphilitic 151
Congenital Corneal Keloid 152
Limbal Dermoid 152
Congenital Corneal Anesthesia 153
Congenital Glaucoma 154
Birth Trauma 154
Metabolic Disorders 155

7 Clinical Approach to Degenerations and Depositions of the Conjunctiva, Cornea, and Sclera 157
Highlights 157
Degenerations and Depositions of the Conjunctiva 157
Age-Related Changes 157
Pinguecula 158
Pterygium 158

Conjunctival Concretions 160
Conjunctival Epithelial Inclusion Cysts. 160
Conjunctivochalasis 162
Conjunctival Vascular Tortuosity and Hyperemia 162
Degenerations and Depositions of the Cornea 162
Age-Related Changes 162
Epithelial and Subepithelial Degenerations and Depositions. 162
Mid- and Deep Stromal Degenerations and Depositions 170
Endothelium 175
Degenerations and Depositions in the Sclera 178
Drug-Induced Depositions and Pigmentations 179
Cornea Verticillata 179
Other Drug-Induced Corneal Deposits. 181

8 Diagnosis and Management of Corneal Dystrophies . . 183
Highlights 183
General Considerations 183
Major Corneal Dystrophies 187
Epithelial and Subepithelial Dystrophies 187
Epithelial–Stromal *TGFBI* Dystrophies 192
Stromal Dystrophies. 202
Endothelial Dystrophies 210

9 Clinical Approach to Corneal Ectatic Disease 217
Highlights 217
Keratoconus 217
Pellucid Marginal Degeneration 229
Keratoglobus. 232
Appendix 9.1. 235
Intrastromal Corneal Ring Segments for Treatment of Ectasia 235
Appendix 9.2. 241
Corneal Crosslinking for Corneal Ectasia. 241

10 Systemic Disorders With Corneal and Other Anterior Segment Manifestations. 247
Highlights 247
Introduction 247
Inherited Metabolic Diseases 248
Lysosomal Storage Diseases. 248
Disorders of Amino Acid, Nucleic Acid, Protein, and Mineral Metabolism 257
Skeletal and Connective Tissue Disorders 266
Ehlers-Danlos Syndrome. 266
Marfan Syndrome. 269
Osteogenesis Imperfecta 270
Goldenhar-Gorlin Syndrome 270
Nutritional Disorder: Vitamin A Deficiency 272

Hematologic Disorders . . . 273
Endocrine Diseases . . . 275
Diabetes . . . 275
Multiple Endocrine Neoplasia . . . 276
Parathyroid Disease . . . 276
Dermatologic Diseases . . . 277
Ichthyosis . . . 277
Ectodermal Dysplasia . . . 278
Xeroderma Pigmentosum . . . 278

11 Infectious Diseases of the Cornea and External Eye: Viral Infections . . . 281
Highlights . . . 281
Virology . . . 281
DNA Viruses: Herpesviruses . . . 284
Herpes Simplex Virus Eye Diseases . . . 284
Varicella-Zoster Virus Dermatoblepharitis, Conjunctivitis, and Keratitis . . . 298
Epstein-Barr Virus Dacryoadenitis, Conjunctivitis, and Keratitis . . . 303
Cytomegalovirus Keratitis and Anterior Uveitis . . . 304
Other DNA Viruses . . . 306
Adenoviruses . . . 306
Poxviruses . . . 310
Papillomaviruses . . . 312
RNA Viruses . . . 313
Coronaviruses . . . 313
Paramyxoviruses . . . 314
Picornaviruses . . . 315
Retroviruses . . . 315
Rhabdoviruses . . . 315

12 Infectious Diseases of the Cornea and External Eye: Bacterial, Fungal, and Parasitic Infections . . . 317
Highlights . . . 317
Normal Ocular Flora . . . 317
Pathogenesis of Ocular Infections . . . 318
Diagnostic Laboratory Techniques . . . 320
Specimen Collection . . . 321
Infections of the Eyelid Margin and Conjunctiva . . . 322
Staphylococcal Blepharitis . . . 322
Fungal and Parasitic Infections of the Eyelid Margin . . . 322
Bacterial Conjunctivitis in Children and Adults . . . 323
Parinaud Oculoglandular Syndrome . . . 333
Infections of the Cornea and Sclera . . . 334
Bacterial Keratitis . . . 334
Fungal Keratitis . . . 341
Corneal Stromal Inflammation Associated With Systemic Infection . . . 347

Loiasis . . . 349
Microbial Scleritis . . . 349

13 Diagnosis and Management of Immune-Related Disorders of the Cornea and External Eye . . . 353
Highlights . . . 353
Definition . . . 353
Immune-Mediated Diseases of the Eyelid . . . 354
Contact Dermatoblepharitis . . . 354
Atopic Dermatitis . . . 355
Immune-Mediated Disorders of the Conjunctiva . . . 356
Seasonal Allergic Conjunctivitis and Perennial Allergic Conjunctivitis . . . 356
Vernal Keratoconjunctivitis . . . 358
Atopic Keratoconjunctivitis . . . 361
Ligneous Conjunctivitis . . . 364
Stevens-Johnson Syndrome, Stevens-Johnson Syndrome/Toxic Epidermal Necrolysis Overlap, and Toxic Epidermal Necrolysis . . . 365
Mucous Membrane Pemphigoid . . . 368
Ocular Graft-vs-Host Disease . . . 374
Conjunctivitis/Episcleritis Associated With Reactive Arthritis . . . 375
Immune-Mediated Diseases of the Cornea . . . 376
Thygeson Superficial Punctate Keratitis . . . 376
Interstitial Keratitis Associated With Infectious Diseases . . . 377
Cogan Syndrome . . . 379
Marginal Keratitis . . . 380
Peripheral Ulcerative Keratitis Associated With Systemic Immune-Mediated Diseases . . . 382
Mooren Ulcer . . . 385
Immune-Mediated Diseases of the Episclera and Sclera . . . 387
Episcleritis . . . 387
Scleritis . . . 388

14 Clinical Approach to Neoplastic Disorders of the Conjunctiva and Cornea . . . 395
Highlights . . . 395
Introduction . . . 395
Approach to the Patient With a Neoplastic Ocular Surface Lesion . . . 396
Management of Patients With Ocular Surface Tumors . . . 397
Observation . . . 397
Surgery . . . 397
Topical Chemotherapy . . . 398
Other Treatment Options . . . 399
Treatment Follow-Up . . . 400
Tumors of Epithelial Origin . . . 400
Benign Epithelial Tumors . . . 400
Ocular Surface Squamous Neoplasia . . . 402

Glandular Tumors of the Conjunctiva 407
Oncocytoma 407
Sebaceous Carcinoma 407
Tumors of Neuroectodermal Origin 408
Benign Pigmented Lesions 409
Preinvasive Pigmented Lesions 412
Malignant Pigmented Lesions. 414
Neurogenic and Smooth-Muscle Tumors 416
Vascular and Mesenchymal Tumors 416
Benign Tumors 416
Malignant Tumors. 418
Lymphocytic Tumors 419
Lymphoid Hyperplasia 419
Lymphoma 420
Metastatic Tumors 421

15 Clinical Aspects of Toxic and Traumatic Injuries of the Anterior Segment 423
Highlights 423
Chemical Injuries. 423
Alkali Burns 424
Acid Burns 425
Management 429
Thermal and Radiation Injuries. 432
Thermal Burns 432
Ultraviolet Radiation 433
Ionizing Radiation 434
Injuries Caused by Animal and Plant Substances 435
Insect and Arachnid Injuries 435
Plant Injuries 436
Blunt Trauma 436
Subconjunctival Hemorrhage 436
Corneal Involvement 437
Traumatic Anterior Uveitis 439
Traumatic Mydriasis and Miosis. 439
Iridodialysis and Cyclodialysis 440
Traumatic Hyphema. 440
Penetrating and Perforating Ocular Trauma 446
Conjunctival Laceration 446
Conjunctival Foreign Bodies 447
Corneal Foreign Bodies 448
Evaluation and Management of Perforating Ocular Trauma. 450
Evaluation 450
Nonsurgical Management 451
Surgical Management 452

16 Clinical Approach to Corneal Transplantation 463
Highlights . . . 463
Corneal Transplantation . . . 463
Corneal Transplant Procedures and Trends . . . 465
Keratoplasty and Eye Banking . . . 465
Tissue Processing and Preservation . . . 465
Donor-Cornea Selection . . . 467
Transplantation for the Treatment of Corneal Disease . . . 469
Preoperative Evaluation and Preparation of the Transplant Patient . . . 470
Penetrating Keratoplasty . . . 472
Intraoperative Complications . . . 476
Postoperative Care and Complications . . . 476
Control of Postoperative Corneal Astigmatism and Refractive Error . . . 485
Lamellar Keratoplasty . . . 488
Anterior Lamellar Keratoplasty and Deep Anterior Lamellar Keratoplasty . . . 488
Complications . . . 490
Endothelial Keratoplasty . . . 491
Advantages . . . 495
Disadvantages . . . 495
Intraoperative Complications . . . 496
Postoperative Care and Complications . . . 497
Emerging Methods for Treatment of Endothelial Dysfunction . . . 506
Pediatric Corneal Transplantation . . . 507
Corneal Autograft Procedures . . . 509
Keratoprosthesis . . . 510

Additional Materials and Resources . . . 513
Requesting Continuing Medical Education Credit . . . 515
Study Questions . . . 517
Answers . . . 525
Index . . . 533

Introduction to the BCSC

The Basic and Clinical Science Course (BCSC) is designed to meet the needs of residents and practitioners for a comprehensive yet concise curriculum of the field of ophthalmology. The BCSC has developed from its original brief outline format, which relied heavily on outside readings, to a more convenient and educationally useful self-contained text. The Academy updates and revises the course annually, with the goals of integrating the basic science and clinical practice of ophthalmology and of keeping ophthalmologists current with new developments in the various subspecialties.

The BCSC incorporates the effort and expertise of more than 100 ophthalmologists, organized into 13 Section faculties, working with Academy editorial staff. In addition, the course continues to benefit from many lasting contributions made by the faculties of previous editions. Members of the Academy Practicing Ophthalmologists Advisory Committee for Education, Committee on Aging, and Vision Rehabilitation Committee review every volume before major revisions, as does a group of select residents and fellows. Members of the European Board of Ophthalmology, organized into Section faculties, also review volumes before major revisions, focusing primarily on differences between American and European ophthalmology practice.

Organization of the Course

The Basic and Clinical Science Course comprises 13 volumes, incorporating fundamental ophthalmic knowledge, subspecialty areas, and special topics:

1 Update on General Medicine
2 Fundamentals and Principles of Ophthalmology
3 Clinical Optics and Vision Rehabilitation
4 Ophthalmic Pathology and Intraocular Tumors
5 Neuro-Ophthalmology
6 Pediatric Ophthalmology and Strabismus
7 Oculofacial Plastic and Orbital Surgery
8 External Disease and Cornea
9 Uveitis and Ocular Inflammation
10 Glaucoma
11 Lens and Cataract
12 Retina and Vitreous
13 Refractive Surgery

References

Readers who wish to explore specific topics in greater detail may consult the references cited within each chapter and listed in the Additional Materials and Resources section at the back of the book. These references are intended to be selective rather than exhaustive, chosen by the BCSC faculty as being important, current, and readily available to residents and practitioners.

Multimedia

This edition of Section 8, *External Disease and Cornea*, includes multimedia related to topics covered in the book: videos, activities, and case studies developed by members of the BCSC faculty. The content is available to readers of the print and electronic versions of Section 8 (www.aao.org/bcscvideo_section08, www.aao.org/bcscactivity_section08, and www.aao.org/bcsccasestudy_section08). Mobile-device users can scan the QR codes below (a QR-code reader may need to be installed on the device) to access the multimedia.

Videos Activities Case Studies

Self-Assessment and CME Credit

Each volume of the BCSC is designed as an independent study activity for ophthalmology residents and practitioners. The learning objectives for this volume are given on page 1. The text, illustrations, and references provide the information necessary to achieve the objectives; the study questions allow readers to test their understanding of the material and their mastery of the objectives. Physicians who wish to claim CME credit for this educational activity may do so by following the instructions given at the end of the book.*

Conclusion

The Basic and Clinical Science Course has expanded greatly over the years, with the addition of much new text, numerous illustrations, and video content. Recent editions have sought to place a greater emphasis on clinical applicability while maintaining a solid foundation in basic science. As with any educational program, it reflects the experience of its authors. As its faculties change and medicine progresses, new viewpoints emerge on controversial subjects and techniques. Not all alternate approaches can be included in this series; as with any educational endeavor, the learner should seek additional sources, including Academy Preferred Practice Pattern Guidelines.

The BCSC faculty and staff continually strive to improve the educational usefulness of the course; you, the reader, can contribute to this ongoing process. If you have any suggestions or questions about the series, please do not hesitate to contact the faculty or the editors.

The authors, editors, and reviewers hope that your study of the BCSC will be of lasting value and that each Section will serve as a practical resource for quality patient care.

* This activity meets the Self-Assessment CME requirements defined by the American Board of Ophthalmology (ABO). Please be advised that the ABO is not an accrediting body for purposes of any CME program. ABO does not sponsor this or any outside activity, and ABO does not endorse any particular CME activity. Complete information regarding the ABO Self-Assessment CME Maintenance of Certification requirements is available at https://abop.org/maintain-certification/cme-self-assessment/.

Introduction to Section 8

For the 2021–2022 major revision of Section 8, *External Disease and Cornea,* the committee listened carefully to readers and made a number of important changes and added new features, the most significant of which are discussed below.

Online Case Studies

A new feature, the online case studies explore corneal ectasia and ocular surface lesions, supporting and enhancing the material presented in the text. These case studies are easily accessed via QR codes in the chapters.

CASE STUDY 9-1 Corneal ectasia.
Courtesy of Robert S. Feder, MD.

Key Points

This new feature identifies information throughout the chapters that should not be missed. Their subtle presentation allows readers to add their own highlights to the pages as well.

a minimal risk of malignant transformation but should be followed more closely. PAM with moderate to severe atypia carries a 30% risk of progression to melanoma. Every effort

Clinical Pearls

The "Clinical Pearl" boxes throughout the book present information that has direct impact on the diagnosis and management of corneal disease and can be quickly incorporated into clinical practice.

CLINICAL PEARL

In patients with visually significant cataract and pterygium, a staged surgical approach is indicated. After the pterygium is excised and the corneal contour has stabilized, cataract surgery can be planned; this approach can lead to improved long-term refractive results (Fig 7-5).

New and Revised Images

All the images were carefully reviewed, and many new, high-quality images were added to help illustrate clinical points. Existing images were edited to make them more informative, and poor-quality images were removed.

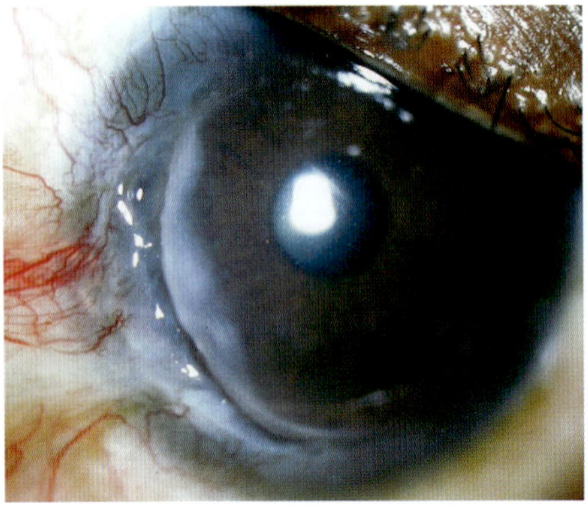

Figure 13-25 Mooren ulcer. Temporal cornea in the right eye demonstrates severe peripheral corneal ulceration. *(Courtesy of Arie L. Marcovich, MD, PhD.)*

Multimedia

Over 30 new videos were added; many of these videos provide excellent demonstrations of surgical procedures. Three new animations illustrate complex processes to aid viewer understanding.

Online Appendix

This major revision includes access to an online appendix (www.aao.org/bcscappendix_section08), a microbiology primer that serves as a refresher for readers who may wish to refamiliarize themselves with topics covered in this volume.

Organizational Changes and Readability

Content has been reorganized for a more logical flow and easier readability, with emphasis on teaching the information senior residents need to know. The chapter on therapeutic interventions for ocular surface disorders was moved to follow the 2 chapters on ocular surface disorders. In addition, the coverage of corneal dystrophies and corneal ectasia was split into 2 chapters. Long paragraphs of text have been split into smaller subsections and bulleted lists. Tables that clarify material in the text and present related differential diagnoses in a comparative way have been added.

Many thanks to the BCSC Section 8 committee for their diligent work and commitment to improving an already excellent cornea and external disease text.

Objectives

Upon completion of BCSC Section 8, *External Disease and Cornea,* the reader should be able to

- describe the anatomy of the external eye and cornea
- explain the overall strategy, examination, and technology used for systematic evaluation of the cornea and the external eye
- identify the distinctive clinical signs and treatment of specific diseases of the ocular surface
- identify the most common underlying causes of dry eye and the appropriate approach to management
- name the distinguishing clinical features of congenital diseases of the cornea and sclera
- identify unique clinical features that help differentiate the more common corneal dystrophies and describe an appropriate management strategy for each
- list the risk factors, clinical signs, and breadth of management options of corneal ectasia
- describe the basic principles and the clinical approach to the diagnosis and treatment of viral, bacterial, fungal, and parasitic keratitis
- identify the common corneal manifestations of systemic disease and describe their treatments
- define an approach to the evaluation, diagnosis, and management of immune-related diseases of the external eye and cornea
- list the risk factors, diagnosis, and treatment of neoplastic disease of the cornea and the external eye
- describe the indications for and techniques of surgical procedures used in the management of corneal disease and trauma

- discuss common surgical interventions for ocular surface disorders such as pterygium and corneal melts
- explain the role of full-thickness and contemporary partial-thickness keratoplasty in the treatment of corneal disease

CHAPTER 1

Structure and Function of the External Eye and Cornea

This chapter includes a related video. Go to www.aao.org/bcscvideo_section08 or scan the QR code in the text to access this content.

This chapter includes a related activity. Go to www.aao.org/bcscactivity_section08 or scan the QR code in the text to access this content.

Indicates selected key points within the chapter.

Highlights

- The external eye has both anatomical and immunologic defense mechanisms for protection against infection and other ocular conditions.
- Knowledge of corneal anatomy is vital for an understanding of corneal disease classifications and mastery of evolving keratoplasty techniques.
- The cornea is a transparent and avascular tissue. Transparency results from the organization of keratocytes, fibers, and the extracellular matrix within the corneal stroma as well as the delicate balance of forces controlling stromal water content.

Eyelids

The functions of the eyelid include eye protection, tear distribution, ocular surface cleaning, regulation of light exposure, and contribution to the tear film. Except for fine vellus hairs, the eyelashes (cilia) are the only hairs of the eyelid. Eyelashes catch small particles and work as sensors to stimulate reflex eyelid closure. Blinking stimulates the lacrimal pump to release tears, which are then spread across the cornea, flushing away foreign material. Most individuals blink an average of 10–15 times per minute at rest, 20 times per minute or more during a conversation, and as few as 5 times per minute when concentrating (eg, reading). Blink frequency also changes in different positions of gaze. The orbicularis oculi muscle, which is innervated by cranial nerve (CN) VII, closes the upper and lower eyelids (Fig 1-1). The levator palpebrae muscle, innervated by CN III, inserts into the tarsal plate and skin and elevates the upper eyelid. The Müller muscle, innervated by sympathetic nerves, also contributes to the elevation of the upper eyelid. The inferior tarsal muscle helps retract the lower eyelid.

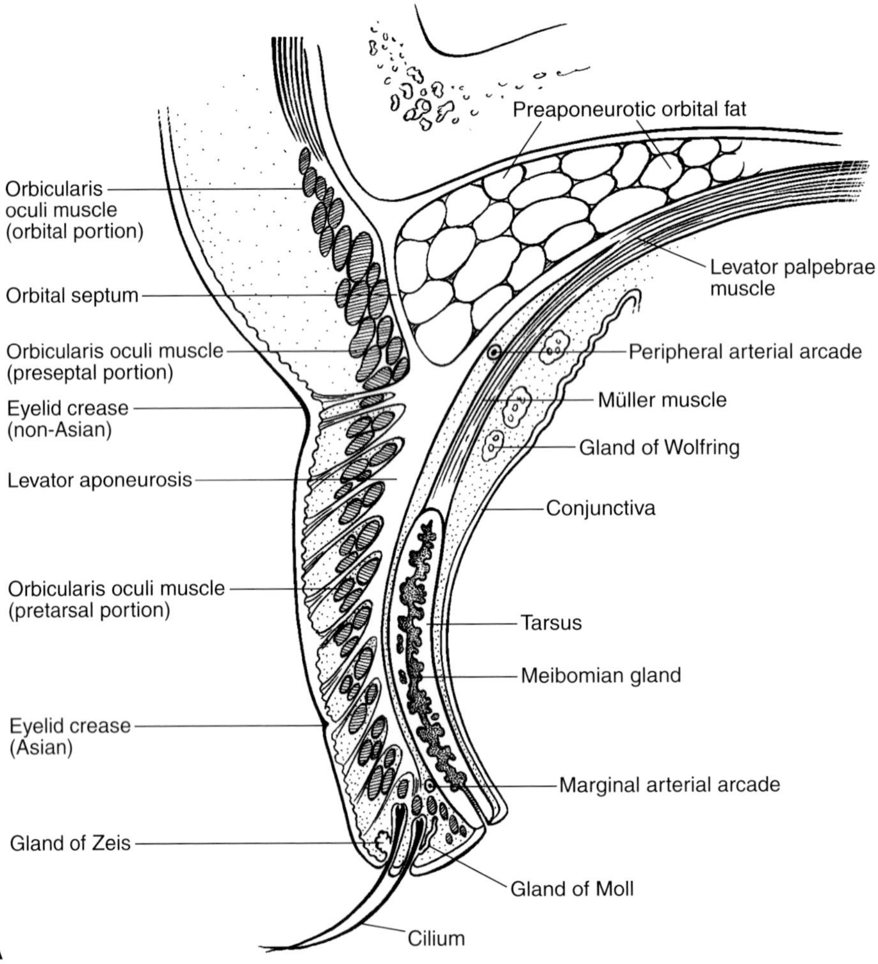

Figure 1-1 The eyelid. **A,** Illustration of a cross section of the upper eyelid.

(Continued)

The epidermis of the eyelids abruptly changes from keratinized to nonkeratinized stratified squamous epithelium at the mucocutaneous junction of the eyelid margin, along the row of *meibomian gland* orifices. Holocrine sebaceous glands and eccrine sweat glands are present in the eyelid skin. Near the eyelid margin are apocrine sweat glands (the *glands of Moll*) and numerous modified sebaceous glands (the *glands of Zeis*).

For additional discussion of eyelid anatomy, see BCSC Section 2, *Fundamentals and Principles of Ophthalmology,* and Section 7, *Oculofacial Plastic and Orbital Surgery.*

Argilés M, Cardona G, Pérez-Cabré E, Rodríguez M. Blink rate and incomplete blinks in six different controlled hard-copy and electronic reading conditions. *Invest Ophthalmol Vis Sci.* 2015;56(11):6679–6685.

Lin LK, Gokoffski KK. Eyelids and the corneal surface. In: Mannis MJ, Holland EJ, eds. *Cornea.* Vol 1. 4th ed. Elsevier; 2017:40–45.

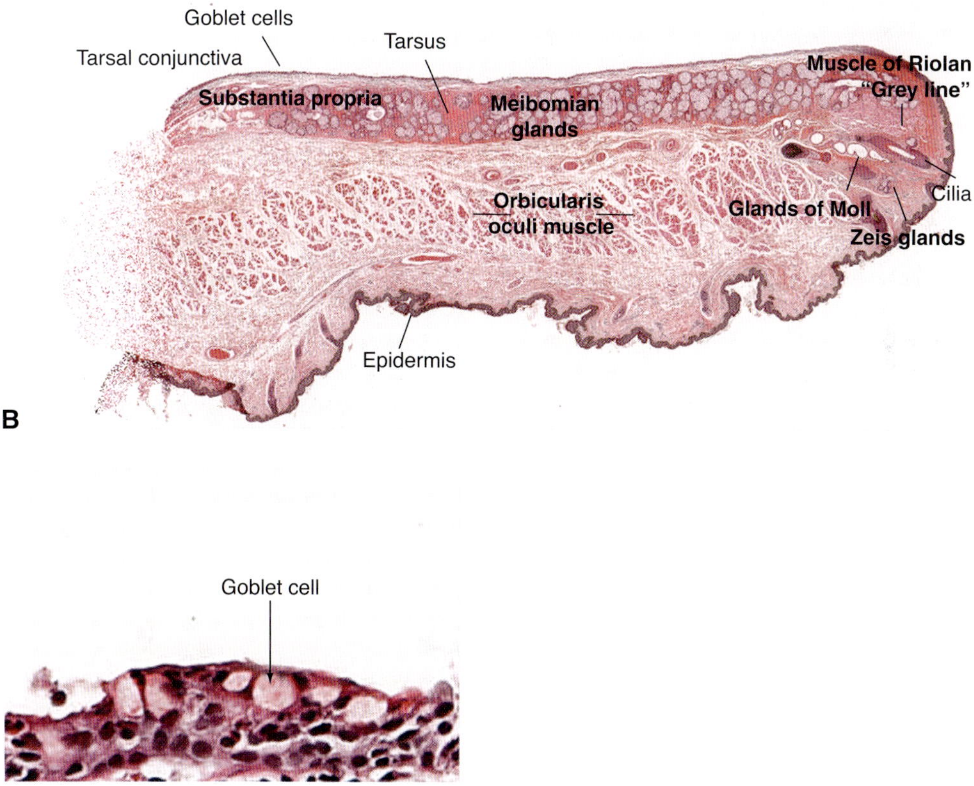

Figure 1-1 *(continued)* **B,** Hematoxylin-eosin (H&E) stained section of the normal eyelid. *(Part A illustration by Christine Gralapp, part B © American Academy of Ophthalmology 2020.)*

Lacrimal Functional Unit

The lacrimal functional unit (LFU) comprises the lacrimal glands, ocular surface, and eyelids, as well as the sensory and motor nerves that connect these components (Video 1-1; Fig 1-2). The LFU is responsible for the following:

- regulation, production, health, and integrity of the tear film (carrying out lubricating, antimicrobial, and nutritional roles)
- health of the ocular surface (maintaining corneal transparency and the surface stem cell population)
- quality of the image projected onto the retina

VIDEO 1-1 Perception of touch and innervation of the lacrimal functional unit.
Modified with permission from Pflugfelder SC, Beuerman RW, Stern ME, eds. Dry Eye and Ocular Surface Disorders. *Published by CRC Press. © Marcel Dekker; 2004, reproduced by arrangement with Taylor & Francis Books UK.*

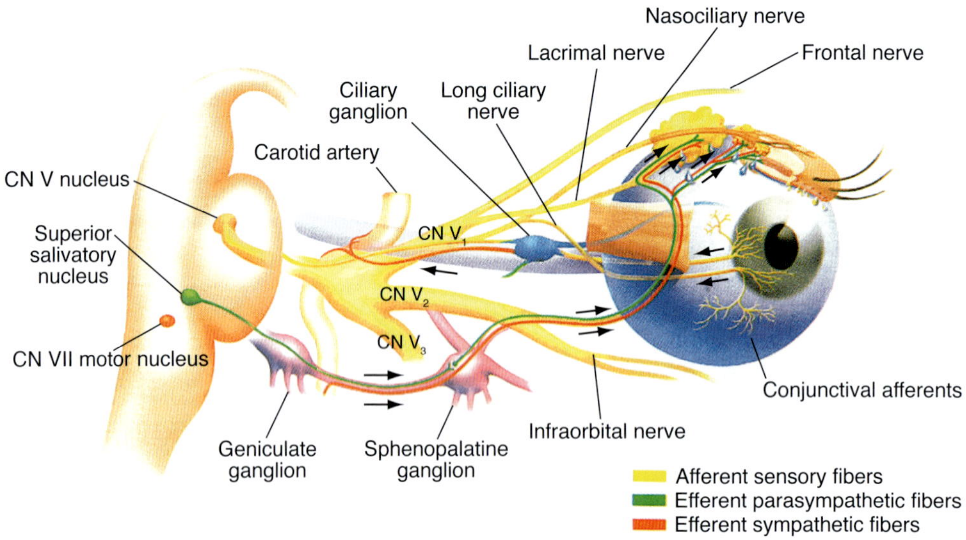

Figure 1-2 The sensory and motor nerves connecting the components of the lacrimal functional unit. CN = cranial nerve. *(Modified with permission from Pflugfelder SC, Beuerman RW, Stern ME, eds.* Dry Eye and Ocular Surface Disorders. *Published by CRC Press. © Marcel Dekker; 2004, reproduced by arrangement with Taylor & Francis Books UK.)*

The LFU responds to environmental, endocrinologic, and cortical influences. The afferent component of the LFU is mediated through ocular surface and trigeminal nociceptors, which synapse with the efferent nerves (autonomic and motor nerves) in the brainstem. The autonomic nerve fibers innervate the meibomian glands, conjunctival goblet cells, and lacrimal glands. The motor nerve fibers innervate the orbicularis muscle to initiate blinking. During blinking, the meibomian glands express lipid, and the tears are replenished from the inferior tear meniscus and spread across the cornea while excess tears are directed into the lacrimal puncta.

Pflugfelder SC, Beuerman RW, Stern ME, eds. *Dry Eye and Ocular Surface Disorders.* CRC Press/Taylor & Francis; 2004.

Tear Film

The tear film is currently thought to be a mixed gel consisting of soluble mucus, fluids, and proteins that are contributed by the lacrimal gland, conjunctival goblet cells, and surface epithelium (Fig 1-3). This hydrophilic gel moves over the glycocalyx of the superficial corneal epithelial cells and is topped by a lipid layer produced by the meibomian glands.

A healthy tear film is critical for both good vision and a healthy eye. Functions of the tear film include

- maintaining a smooth optical surface between blinks
- contributing to refractive power of the eye through the air–tear film interface
- removing irritants, pathogens, toxins, allergens, and debris

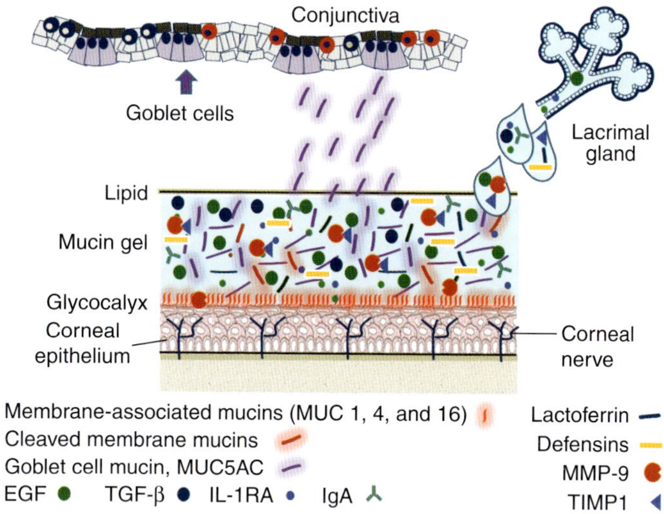

Figure 1-3 The tear film consists of a mixed mucin/aqueous layer produced by the lacrimal glands, conjunctival goblet cells, and surface epithelium. It is topped by a lipid layer produced by the meibomian glands. Its functions include lubrication (mucins), healing (epidermal growth factor [EGF]), and protection of the cornea against infection (lactoferrin, defensins, immunoglobulin A [IgA]). When the tear film is inflamed, it produces interleukin 1 receptor antagonist (IL-1RA), transforming growth factor β (TGF-β), and tissue inhibitor of matrix metalloproteinase 1 (TIMP 1). MMP-9 = matrix metalloproteinase 9. *(Modified with permission from Pflugfelder SC. Tear dysfunction and the cornea: LXVIII Edward Jackson Memorial Lecture.* Am J Ophthalmol. *2011;152(6):902, with permission from Elsevier.)*

- facilitating the diffusion of oxygen and other nutrients to the cornea and conjunctiva
- maintaining homeostasis of the normal ocular flora
- contributing to the antimicrobial defense of the ocular surface

Maintenance of the tear film is thus critical to normal corneal function.

Pflugfelder SC. Tear dysfunction and the cornea: LXVIII Edward Jackson Memorial Lecture. *Am J Ophthalmol.* 2011;152(6):900–909.

Conjunctiva

The conjunctiva can be broadly divided into 3 geographic zones as follows:

- *palpebral, or tarsal:* starts at the mucocutaneous junction of the upper and lower eyelids and covers the inner eyelid; it is tightly adherent to the underlying tarsus
- *bulbar:* covers the ocular surface and is loosely attached to the Tenon capsule; it inserts into the limbus
- *forniceal:* covers the superior and inferior fornices

The *plica semilunaris* is a crescent-shaped vertical fold of conjunctiva, located at the medial angle of the eye. The *caruncle*—a fleshy, ovoid mass approximately 5 mm high and 3 mm wide—is attached to the inferomedial side of the plica semilunaris and contains goblet cells and lacrimal tissue, as well as hairs, sebaceous glands, and sweat glands. This area also contains the lacus lacrimalis (lacrimal lake), a small triangular space where tears accumulate after bathing the ocular surface.

The cell morphology of the conjunctival epithelium varies from stratified cuboidal over the tarsus and columnar in the fornices to squamous on the globe. Goblet cells account for up to 10% of basal cells of the conjunctival epithelium and are most numerous in the palpebral conjunctiva, the inferonasal bulbar conjunctiva, and the area of the plica semilunaris.

The *substantia propria* of the conjunctiva consists of loose connective tissue. Conjunctiva-associated lymphoid tissue (CALT), which consists of lymphocytes and other leukocytes, is present, especially in the fornices. Lymphocytes interact with mucosal epithelial cells through reciprocal regulatory signals mediated by growth factors, cytokines, and neuropeptides.

The palpebral conjunctiva shares its blood supply with the eyelids. The bulbar conjunctiva is supplied by the anterior ciliary arteries, which arise from muscular branches of the ophthalmic artery. These capillaries are fenestrated and leak fluid, producing chemosis (conjunctival swelling), as a response to allergies or other inflammatory events.

Sclera

The sclera is the opaque, white, fibrous tissue that extends from the corneal limbus to the optic nerve, where it merges to form the dural sheath of the optic nerve. It is divided into 3 layers (from outermost inward): episclera, stroma, and lamina fusca. The scleral stroma is composed of collagen fibers, which have varied orientation, separation, and diameter, resulting in the sclera's opaque appearance in contrast to the cornea. The sclera receives its vascular supply from the anterior and posterior ciliary arteries and drains through the vortex veins. The thickness of the sclera ranges from 0.3 mm to 1 mm; it is thinnest behind the insertions of the rectus muscles. It is innervated by the ciliary nerves of cranial nerve V_1.

For additional discussion of the sclera, see BCSC Section 2, *Fundamentals and Principles of Ophthalmology,* and Section 4, *Ophthalmic Pathology and Intraocular Tumors.*

Cornea

The cornea is a transparent, avascular tissue that consists of 5 layers (Activity 1-1; Fig 1-4): epithelium, Bowman layer, stroma, Descemet membrane, and endothelium; these are discussed in the subsections that follow.

In adults, the cornea measures approximately 11–12 mm horizontally and 10–11 mm vertically. It is 500–600 µm thick at its center, gradually increasing in thickness toward the periphery.

ACTIVITY 1-1 Corneal layers and corresponding confocal images.
Confocal images courtesy of Danielle Trief, MD, and David D. Verdier, MD.

For nutrition, the cornea depends on diffusion of glucose from the aqueous humor and diffusion of oxygen through the tear film. The peripheral cornea is supplied with oxygen

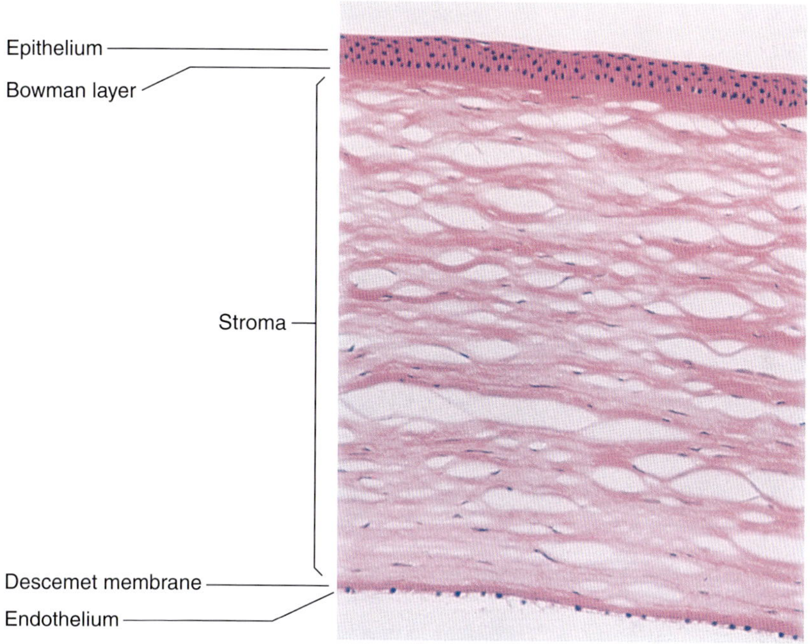

Figure 1-4 The layers of the normal cornea. The epithelium is composed of 4–6 cell layers, but it can increase in thickness to maintain a smooth surface (H&E, x32).

from the limbal circulation. The density of nerve endings in the cornea is among the highest in the body, and the sensitivity of the cornea is 100 times that of the conjunctiva. Sensory nerve fibers extend from the long ciliary nerves, penetrating the cornea in the deep peripheral stroma near the limbus and coursing anteriorly to form a subepithelial plexus.

Zones of the Cornea

The cornea is aspheric, although the central portion of the anterior corneal surface has been described as a spherocylindrical convex mirror. The central cornea is typically 3.00 diopters (D) steeper than the periphery, a positive shape factor *(prolate)*.

Clinically, the cornea can be divided into 5 zones (Fig 1-5) as follows:

- *central zone:* 1–3 mm in diameter; closely resembles a spherical surface
- *paracentral zone:* a 3–4 mm "doughnut" surrounding the central zone; has an outer diameter of 7–8 mm and progressively flattens out from the center
- *apical zone:* comprises the paracentral and central zones, used in contact lens fitting; is primarily responsible for the refractive power of the cornea
- *peripheral* or *transitional zone:* adjacent to the paracentral zone, has an outer diameter of approximately 11 mm; is the area of greatest flattening and asphericity in the normal cornea
- *limbal zone* (limbus): where the cornea steepens prior to joining the sclera at the limbal sulcus; outer diameter averages 12 mm

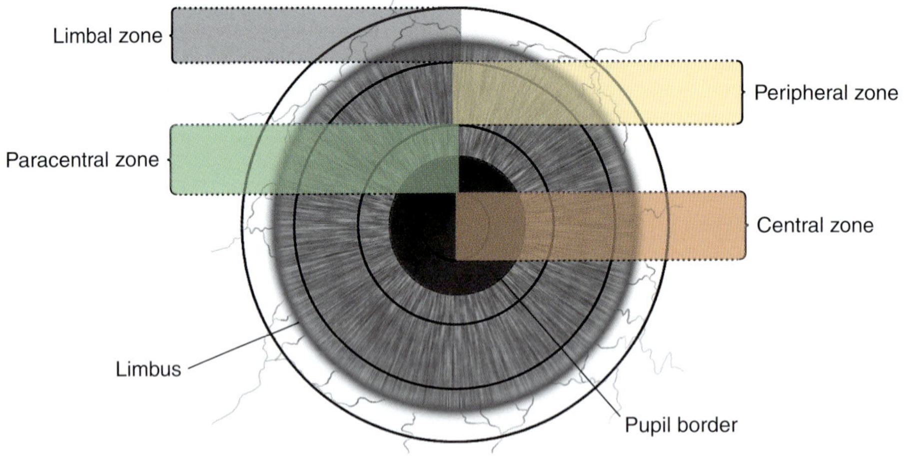

Figure 1-5 Topographic zones of the cornea. *(Illustration by Christine Gralapp.)*

Other corneal reference definitions include the following:

- *optical zone:* the portion of the cornea that overlies the entrance pupil of the iris
- *corneal apex:* the point of maximum curvature, typically temporal to the center of the pupil
- *corneal vertex:* the point located at the intersection of the line of fixation and the corneal surface; represented by the corneal light reflex when illuminated coaxially with fixation. It is the center of the keratoscopic image and does not necessarily correspond to the point of maximum curvature at the corneal apex (Fig 1-6)

Corneal Epithelium

The hydrophobic corneal epithelium is composed of 4–6 layers, which include 1–2 layers of superficial squamous cells, 2–3 layers of broad wing cells, and an innermost layer of columnar basal cells. It is 40–50 µm thick (see Fig 1-4; also see the Pachymetry section in Chapter 2). The epithelium and tear film form an optically smooth surface. Tight junctions between superficial epithelial cells prevent penetration of tear fluid into the stroma. Continuous proliferation of limbal stem cells gives rise to the other layers, which subsequently differentiate into superficial cells. With maturation, these differentiated cells become coated with microvilli on their outermost surface (glycocalyx) and then desquamate into the tears. The process of differentiation takes approximately 7–14 days. Basal epithelial cells secrete a continuous, 50-nm-thick basement membrane, which is composed of type IV collagen, laminin, and other proteins. Corneal clarity depends on the tight packing of epithelial cells, which results in a layer with a nearly uniform refractive index and minimal light scattering.

Bowman Layer

Bowman layer lies anterior to the corneal stroma. Previously considered a membrane, Bowman layer is rather the acellular condensate of irregularly arranged collagen fibrils at

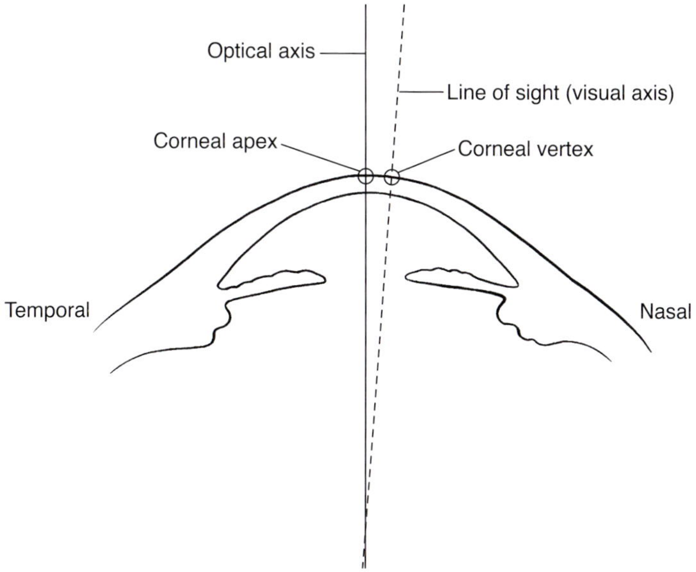

Figure 1-6 Corneal vertex and apex. *(Illustration by Christine Gralapp.)*

the most anterior portion of the stroma (see Fig 1-4). This layer is 15 µm thick and helps maintain the shape of the cornea. If disrupted, it will not regenerate.

Corneal Stroma

The corneal stroma accounts for roughly 90% of total corneal thickness (see Fig 1-4). It is composed of stromal cells (keratocytes), fibers, and an extracellular matrix. The anterior stroma is denser than the posterior stroma due to an increased number of keratocytes and greater interweaving of collagen lamellae. The anterior 40% of the corneal stroma has twice the tensile strength of the posterior 60%. This difference between the anterior and posterior stroma may play a role in the occurrence of corneal ectasia following deep excimer laser ablation.

Keratocytes vary in size and density throughout the stroma and form a 3-dimensional network throughout the cornea. These cells, which are flattened fibroblasts, are located between the stromal collagen lamellae (Fig 1-7) and continually digest and manufacture stromal molecules. Keratocyte density declines with age and also following laser refractive surgery.

The extracellular matrix of the corneal stroma is formed from collagens and proteoglycans. Type I and type V fibrillar collagens are intertwined with filaments of type VI collagen. The major corneal proteoglycans are decorin (associated with dermatan sulfate) and lumican (associated with keratan sulfate).

The even distribution of keratocytes, fibers, and the extracellular matrix in the corneal stroma is necessary for a clear cornea. Corneal transparency also depends on maintaining the water content of the corneal stroma at 78%. Corneal hydration is largely controlled by intact epithelial and endothelial barriers and the functioning of the endothelial pump, which is linked to an ion-transport system controlled by temperature-dependent enzymes

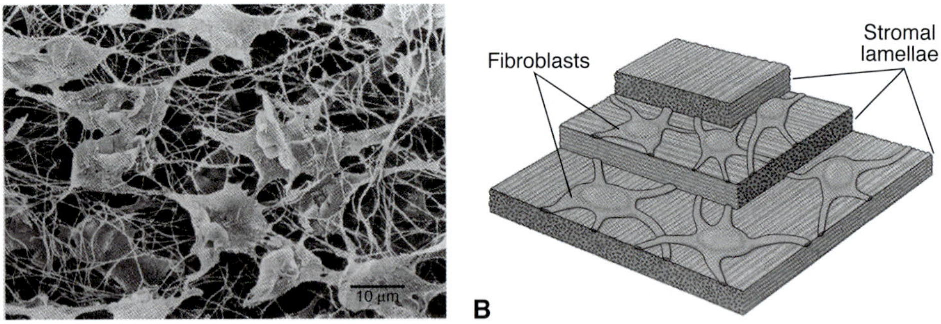

A B

Figure 1-7 Keratocytes **(A)** are flattened fibroblasts **(B)** that are situated between the stromal collagen lamellae. *(Part A courtesy of Nishida T, Yasumoto K, Otori T, Desaki J. The network structure of corneal fibroblasts in the rat as revealed by scanning electron microscopy.* Invest Ophthalmol Vis Sci. *1988;29(12):1887–1890. Part B reproduced with permission from Oyster CW.* The Human Eye: Structure and Function. *Oxford University Press; 1999:331. Reproduced with permission of the Licensor through PLSclear.)*

such as Na^+,K^+-ATPase. In addition, negatively charged stromal glycosaminoglycans tend to repel each other, producing a *swelling pressure (SP)*. Because intraocular pressure (IOP) tends to compress the cornea, the overall imbibition pressure of the corneal stroma is calculated as IOP—SP. Corneal hydration varies from anterior to posterior and increases closer to the endothelium.

The most posterior aspect of the stroma forms a thin, acellular layer (15-µm thick) that is tightly adherent to Descemet membrane. This novel layer is called pre-Descemet layer, or *Dua layer*, and is important in deep anterior lamellar keratoplasty (DALK). Dua layer is strong and resists air dissection from Descemet membrane. During DALK, air is injected on the stromal side of Dua layer to create a big-bubble stromal dissection, forming a type I bubble. This bubble is sturdier and less likely to tear or burst, in contrast to an air dissection between Dua layer and Descemet membrane (a type II bubble).

Dua HS, Faraj LA, Said DG, Gray T, Lowe J. Human corneal anatomy redefined: a novel pre-Descemet's layer (Dua's layer). *Ophthalmology.* 2013;120(9):1778–1785.

Randleman JB, Dawson DG, Grossniklaus HE, McCarey BE, Edelhauser HF. Depth-dependent cohesive tensile strength in human donor corneas: implications for refractive surgery. *J Refract Surg.* 2008;24(1):S85–S89.

Schlötzer-Schrehardt U, Bachmann BO, Tourtas T, et al. Ultrastructure of the posterior corneal stroma. *Ophthalmology.* 2015;122(4):693–699.

Sridhar M. Anatomy of the cornea and ocular surface. *Indian J Ophthalmol.* 2018; 66(2): 190–194.

Descemet Membrane

Descemet membrane is the basement membrane of the corneal endothelium (see Fig 1-4). Its thickness increases with age; at birth, it is 3 µm, increasing to 10–12 µm by adulthood. It is composed of an anterior banded zone that develops in utero and a posterior amorphous, nonbanded zone that is laid down throughout life. The *Schwalbe line* is a gonioscopic landmark that defines the end of the Descemet membrane and the beginning of the trabecular meshwork.

Corneal Endothelium

Corneal endothelial cells lie on the posterior surface of the cornea (see Fig 1-4), composing a monolayer of closely interdigitated cells arranged in a mosaic pattern of mostly hexagonal shapes. If cell loss occurs, especially as a result of trauma or surgery, the defective area is initially covered through a process of cell enlargement and spread of surrounding cells or perhaps peripheral stem cells. These cell findings can be observed by specular or confocal microscopy as polymegethism (variability in cell size) and polymorphism (variability in cell shape). It was previously thought that the corneal endothelial cells were unable to replicate. Scientists are now investigating whether these cells have some mitotic ability, particularly the cells in the corneal periphery. Migration of these cells may be augmented by pharmacological agents such as Rho kinase inhibitors.

Cell density varies throughout the endothelial surface; the concentration is typically highest in the periphery. Central endothelial cell density decreases with age at an average rate of approximately 0.6% per year, diminishing from a count of about 3400 cells/mm^2 at age 15 years to about 2300 cells/mm^2 at age 85 years. The normal central endothelial cell count is between 2000 and 3000 cells/mm^2. It has been observed that eyes with an endothelial cell count below 500 cells/mm^2 may be at risk for development of corneal edema.

As mentioned earlier, the corneal endothelium helps maintain corneal transparency by controlling corneal hydration and maintaining stromal deturgescence. It does so through its functions as a barrier to the aqueous humor and as a metabolic pump that moves ions, and draws water osmotically, from the stroma into the aqueous humor. The barrier and pump functions of the endothelium can be measured clinically by fluorophotometry and pachymetry. The endothelium must also be permeable to nutrients and other molecules from the aqueous humor. Increased permeability and insufficient pump sites occur with reduced endothelial cell density, although the cell density at which clinically evident edema occurs is not an absolute.

For more detailed information on the histology and physiology of the cornea, see BCSC Section 2, *Fundamentals and Principles of Ophthalmology,* Chapter 8.

Amann J, Holley GP, Lee SB, Edelhauser HF. Increased endothelial cell density in the paracentral and peripheral regions of the human cornea. *Am J Ophthalmol.* 2003; 135(5): 584–590.

Bourne WM. Biology of the corneal endothelium in health and disease. *Eye (Lond).* 2003; 17(8): 912–918.

DelMonte DW, Kim T. Anatomy and physiology of the cornea. *J Cataract Refract Surg.* 2011; 37(3):588–598.

Gambato C, Longhin E, Catania AG, Lazzarini D, Parrozzani R, Midena E. Aging and corneal layers: an in vivo corneal confocal microscopy study. *Graefes Arch Clin Exp Ophthalmol.* 2015;253(2):267–275.

Koizumi N, Okumura N, Ueno M, Kinoshita S. New therapeutic modality for corneal endothelial disease using Rho-associated kinase inhibitor eye drops. *Cornea.* 2014;33(11):S25–31.

Nishida T, Saika S, Morishige N. Cornea and sclera: anatomy and physiology. In: Mannis MJ, Holland EJ, eds. *Cornea.* Vol 1. 4th ed. Elsevier; 2017:1–22.

Whikehart DR, Parikh CH, Vaughn AV, Mishler K, Edelhauser HF. Evidence suggesting the existence of stem cells for the human corneal endothelium. *Mol Vis.* 2005;11: 816–824.

Limbus

The limbus is the transition zone between the transparent cornea and the opaque sclera. This area harbors corneal epithelial stem cells, which are responsible for the normal homeostasis and wound repair of the corneal epithelium. The *palisades of Vogt,* which are concentrated in the superior and inferior limbus, are thought to be the site of the limbal stem cells' niche and can be observed biomicroscopically as radially oriented fibrovascular ridges concentrated along the corneoscleral limbus (Fig 1-8). The posterior limbus appears to be responsible for stem cell maintenance, while the function of the anterior limbus may be to prompt regeneration of corneal epithelium.

Stem cells have an unlimited capacity for self-renewal and are slow cycling (ie, they have low mitotic activity). Once stem cell differentiation begins, it is irreversible. Renewal occurs from basal cells, with centripetal migration of stem cells from the periphery. This is known as the *XYZ hypothesis,* where *X* represents proliferation and stratification of limbal basal cells; *Y,* centripetal migration of basal cells; and *Z,* desquamation of superficial cells. The health of the cornea depends on the sum of *X* and *Y* being equal to *Z.* Damage to epithelial stem cells impairs long-term regeneration of corneal epithelial cells. Damage to the limbus leads to loss of the barrier that prevents invasion of the conjunctiva and neovascularization of the ocular surface.

Singh V, Shukla S, Ramachandran C, et al. Science and art of cell-based ocular surface regeneration. *Int Rev Cell Mol Biol.* 2015;319:45–106.

Yoon JJ, Ismail S, Sherwin T. Limbal stem cells: central concepts of corneal epithelial homeostasis. *World J Stem Cells.* 2014;6(4):391–403.

Defense Mechanisms of the External Eye and Cornea

The external eye and cornea comprise complexly integrated tissues that, along with the tear film, help protect the eye against infection. For an in-depth discussion of the immune system, see BCSC Section 9, *Uveitis and Ocular Inflammation.* BCSC Section 2,

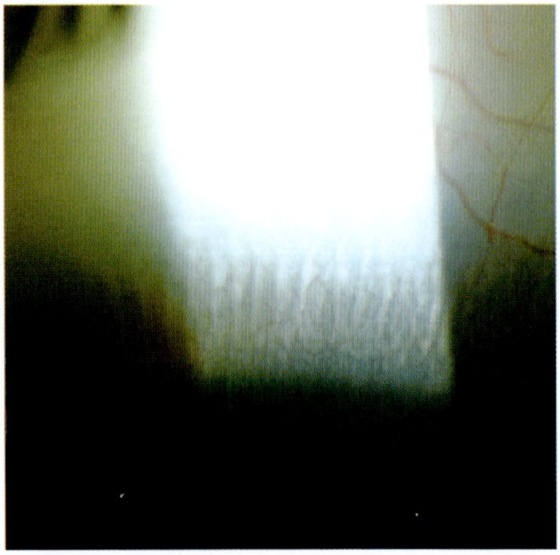

Figure 1-8 Slit-lamp photograph showing the corneoscleral limbus with radially oriented fibrovascular ridges (palisades of Vogt). *(Courtesy of Cornea Service, Paulista School of Medicine, Federal University of São Paulo.)*

Fundamentals and Principles of Ophthalmology, discusses the biochemistry and metabolism of the tear film and cornea.

As discussed earlier, the tear film serves as a protective layer, washing away irritants and pathogens and diluting toxins and allergens. Each functional blink promotes tear turnover. Tears are secreted from the lacrimal gland and spread across the cornea while excess tears are directed into the lacrimal puncta; all of these actions reduce the contact time of microbes and irritants with the ocular surface.

Immunoregulation of the ocular surface occurs through tolerance and regulation of the innate and adaptive arms of the ocular immune response (Fig 1-9). The normal tear

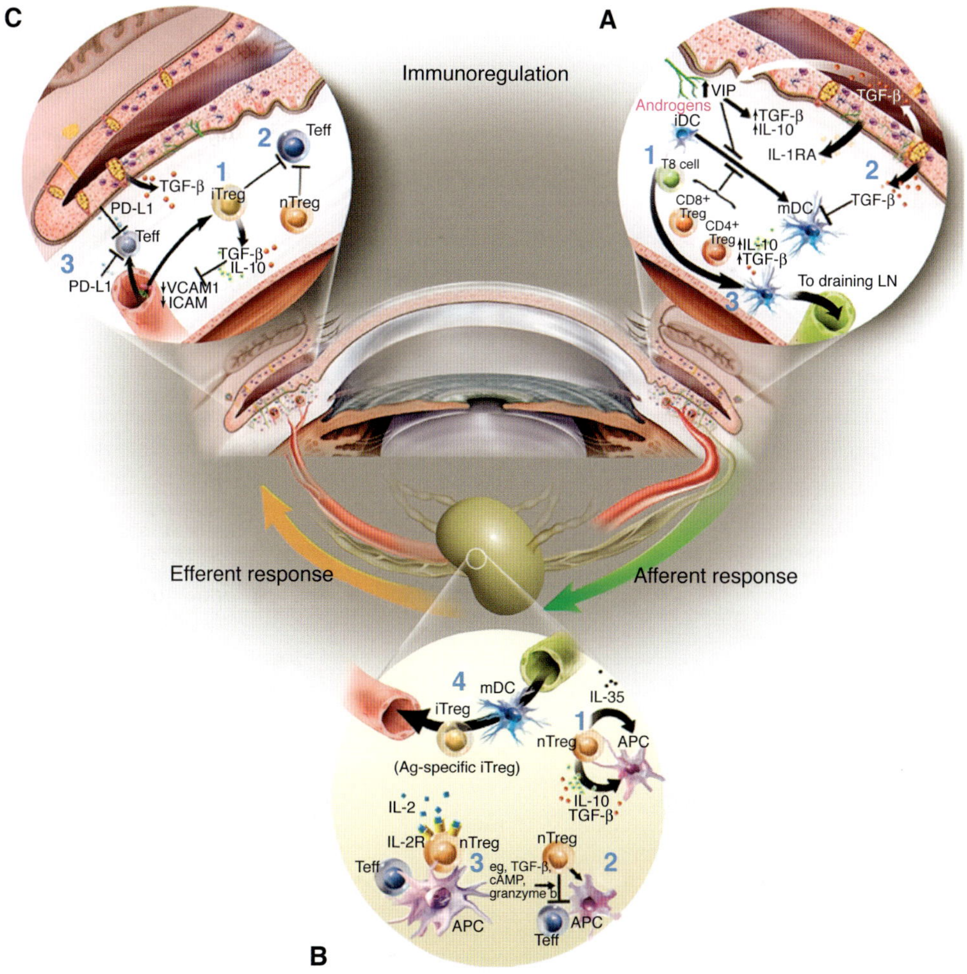

Figure 1-9 Reducing inflammation on the ocular surface. **A,** The following soluble and cellular factors on the ocular surface lead to a reduction in inflammation: (1) Natural regulatory T cells (nTreg cells, which include CD4, CD8, and natural killer cells). (2) The anti-inflammatory cytokine transforming growth factor β (TGF-β), IL-1 receptor antagonist (IL-1RA, which dampens the

(Continued)

Figure 1-9 *(continued)* pro-inflammatory cytokine IL-1), and vasoactive intestinal peptide (VIP). (3) Hormones such as androgen. Together, these factors suppress maturation of the mature dendritic cell (mDC) and survival of autoreactive T cells. **B,** In the lymphoid organs, nTreg cells continue to suppress inflammation by (1) releasing anti-inflammatory cytokines (TGF-β, IL-10); (2) directly disabling pathogenic effector T cells (Teff cells) through cell contact; (3) competing for soluble factors (eg, IL-2); (4) inhibiting cells bearing or responding to autoantigens. **C,** Back on the ocular surface, autoreactive lymphocytes (Teff) are suppressed by TGF-β and nTreg and iTreg cells. Activated T cells are also negatively regulated by programmed death ligand-1 (PD-L1), coupled with integrins on endothelial cells. *(Modified with permission from Springer Nature. Stern ME, Schaumburg CS, Dana R, Calonge M, Niederkorn JY, Pflugfelder SC. Autoimmunity at the ocular surface: pathogenesis and regulation.* Mucosal Immunol. *2010;3(5):425–442.)*

film contains components of the complement cascade, proteins, growth factors, and an array of cytokines. Cytokines such as interleukin 1 and tumor necrosis factor α are significantly upregulated in a variety of corneal inflammatory diseases, such as corneal graft rejection and dry eye disease. Increased expression of growth factors, prostaglandins, neuropeptides, and proteases has been observed in a wide array of immune disorders of the ocular surface.

The normal, uninflamed conjunctiva contains neutrophils, lymphocytes (including regulatory T cells, which dampen the immune response), macrophages, plasma cells, and mast cells. The conjunctival stroma contains dendritic antigen-presenting cells (APCs). The conjunctival epithelium has a special subpopulation of dendritic APCs known as *Langerhans cells,* which are capable of both uptake of antigens and sensitizing of antigen-inexperienced (naïve) T lymphocytes. Hence, these dendritic cells serve as the sentinel cells of the immune system of the ocular surface.

In addition to containing immune cells, the conjunctiva is supplied with blood vessels and lymphatic vessels, which facilitate the trafficking of immune cells and antigens to the draining lymph nodes, where the adaptive immune response is generated. This occurs

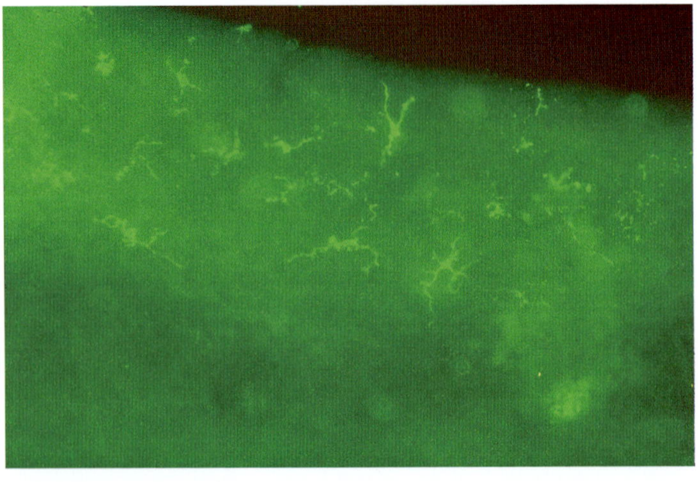

Figure 1-10 Langerhans cells. Langerhans cells are a subclass of dendritic antigen presenting cells (APCs) found on the cornea and conjunctival epithelium. This micrograph shows the predominance of major histocompatibility complex class II⁺ Langerhans cells in the limbus of the uninflamed eye. *(Courtesy of the laboratory of M. Reza Dana, MD.)*

through the recruitment of regulatory T cells, which return to the ocular surface to modulate and suppress the local immune response.

Like the conjunctiva, the normal, uninflamed cornea is endowed with dendritic cells. These dendritic APCs in the corneal epithelium are also Langerhans cells. They are located primarily in the corneal periphery and limbus (Fig 1-10). These APCs are in an activated, mature state (expressing class II major histocompatibility complex [MHC] antigens and costimulatory molecules) and hence are capable of efficiently stimulating T cells. In addition to these dendritic cells, small numbers of lymphocytes are present in the peripheral epithelium and anterior stroma of the cornea. A highly regulated process, mediated by vascular endothelial adhesion molecules and cytokines, controls the recruitment of the various leukocyte subsets from the intravascular compartment into the limbal matrix. Immune responses are also mediated by regulatory T cells in the regional lymph nodes and perhaps at the local level as well. See Chapter 13 for discussion of immune-related disorders and corneal graft rejection.

Ecoiffier T, Yuen D, Chen L. Differential distribution of blood and lymphatic vessels in the murine cornea. *Invest Ophthalmol Vis Sci.* 2010;51(5):2436–2440.

Niederkorn JY. Cornea: window to ocular immunology. *Curr Immunol Rev.* 2011;7(3): 328–335.

Stern ME, Schaumburg CS, Dana R, Calonge M, Niederkorn JY, Pflugfelder SC. Autoimmunity at the ocular surface: pathogenesis and regulation. *Mucosal Immunol.* 2010;3(5):425–442.

CHAPTER 2

The Approach, Techniques, and Devices for Examination of the External Eye and Cornea

This chapter includes a related video. Go to www.aao.org/bcscvideo_section08 or scan the QR code in the text to access this content.

Indicates selected key points within the chapter.

Highlights

- Ocular surface staining (eg, with fluorescein) can yield information on tear film stability, epithelial lesions, and corneal perforation.
- Dysfunction in tear production can be ascertained by Schirmer testing.
- Evaluation of the mires projected onto the cornea during keratometry and Placido disk–based topography can help distinguish irregular astigmatism (distorted mires) due to ocular surface irregularity from regular corneal astigmatism.
- Corneal topography and tomography can give the clinician accurate data on corneal power, elevation, and thickness that are useful in diagnosis, surgical planning, and management of corneal disease.
- An understanding of corneal biomechanics and measurement of corneal thickness can aid in assessment of postrefractive surgery ectasia risk and in proper interpretation of intraocular pressure measurement.
- The health and function of the corneal endothelial cell mosaic can be inferred from pachymetry, specular microscopy, and confocal microscopy.

External Eye Exam

General Appearance

The external eye examination begins with observing the patient upon entering the exam room. The patient's general appearance, body habitus, physical difficulties, personal hygiene, and ease of interaction provide the clinician with valuable information that aids in establishing rapport, determining examination challenges, developing a differential diagnosis, and preparing a treatment plan. The condition of the patient's skin, including the presence and distribution of rashes or lesions, signs of acne rosacea, and the degree of pigmentation can provide clues to diagnosis. External eye conditions, such as proptosis, enophthalmos, malposition, asymmetry, diminished retropulsion, and orbital rim step-off, can also guide the clinician toward diagnosis and a plan for treatment.

The Eyelids

Assessment of the eyelid surface is recommended to identify signs of inflammation, eyelid lesions, or the absence of lashes as well as conditions associated with eyelid position, including eyelid retraction, lagophthalmos, scleral show, ptosis, entropion, and ectropion. Evaluation of the frequency and completeness of blinking may yield crucial information about eyelid function. The eyelid can be everted so that presenting concerns of foreign body sensation or hemorrhage or unusual results of corneal staining can be further investigated.

Corneal Sensation

Corneal sensation is supplied by the ophthalmic branch of the nasociliary branch (V1) of the fifth (trigeminal) cranial nerve. Corneal sensation and the blink response can be assessed by means of a wisp of cotton from a cotton-tipped applicator in the absence of topical anesthesia and before measuring intraocular pressure (IOP). Approaching the patient from the side helps avoid a reflexive flinch from the patient. Corneal sensation findings may be classified as normal, reduced, or absent. The cotton swab can disturb the corneal surface; therefore, it is important to evaluate the cornea prior to checking sensation.

CLINICAL PEARL

An evaluation of corneal sensation with a cotton-tipped applicator is recommended in patients with suspected neurotrophic disease, particularly in the presence of exposure.

Handheld esthesiometer

Quantitative methods for measuring corneal sensation typically are reserved for research or complex cases. The most common quantitative device is the handheld (Cochet-Bonnet) esthesiometer. The Cochet-Bonnet esthesiometer contains a thin, retractable nylon monofilament. The pressure applied by the device is a function of the length of this monofilament. As the length decreases from 60 mm to 5 mm, the pressure increases from 11 mm/gm to a maximum of 200 mm/gm.

STEPS FOR USING THE HANDHELD ESTHESIOMETER

1. Extend the filament to the full length of 60 mm.
2. Retract the filament in 5-mm increments until the patient can feel its contact.
3. Record the length. (The shorter the length, the more reduced the sensation.)

4. Repeat steps 1–3 in the fellow cornea.
5. Repeat steps 1–4 in each quadrant: superior, temporal, inferior, and nasal.
6. Clean the filament and retract it into the device.

Greiner MA, Faulkner WJ, Vislisel JM, Varley GA, Goins KM. Corneal diagnostic techniques. In: Mannis MJ, Holland EJ, eds. *Cornea.* Vol. 1. 4th ed. Elsevier; 2017:116–122.

Slit-Lamp Biomicroscopy

The slit lamp is a fundamental ophthalmic tool. It is capable of producing various types of illumination at different angles, which are used to highlight various lesions and opacities, and it is indispensable for examining the anterior segment. Mastering the slit-lamp examination is crucial for accurate identification of corneal pathology and thus for making the proper diagnosis and therapeutic plan. See the sidebar for tips on using the slit lamp effectively. Figure 2-1 depicts an algorithm for differential diagnosis based on slit-lamp findings.

SLIT LAMP—POINTS TO REMEMBER

- Adjust the oculars for *your* eyes; otherwise, you will miss a great deal of pathology.
- Observe what is there, not what you think should be there.
- Observe what is different, not what is the same.
- Describe your findings in terms of multiple parameters.
- Do not be too quick to label (name) what you see.
- Use bright illumination.
- Use the full range of slit-lamp magnification.
- Ask the patient to blink. Be attentive to what does not move; opacities that move are in the tear film.
- Use various illumination techniques to identify and characterize findings.
- Be sure that the thin slit beam is focused directly on an object for which you are determining depth.
- Paint with light the way an artist uses a paintbrush.
- Always focus on the tissue you want to examine.
- Enjoy examining the cornea. It is a privilege.

Data from Krachmer J, Palay DA. Cornea Atlas. *3rd ed. Saunders; 2014.*

The slit-lamp biomicroscope has 2 rotating arms—1 for the slit illuminator and 1 for the biomicroscope—mounted on a common axis. The illumination unit is essentially a light projector with a beam that is adjustable in width, height, direction, intensity, and color. On examination, reflections of light are visible from the anterior and posterior surfaces of the cornea and lens; these are known as Purkinje images or reflexes. The magnification power of the biomicroscope is adjustable, and the illumination and microscope

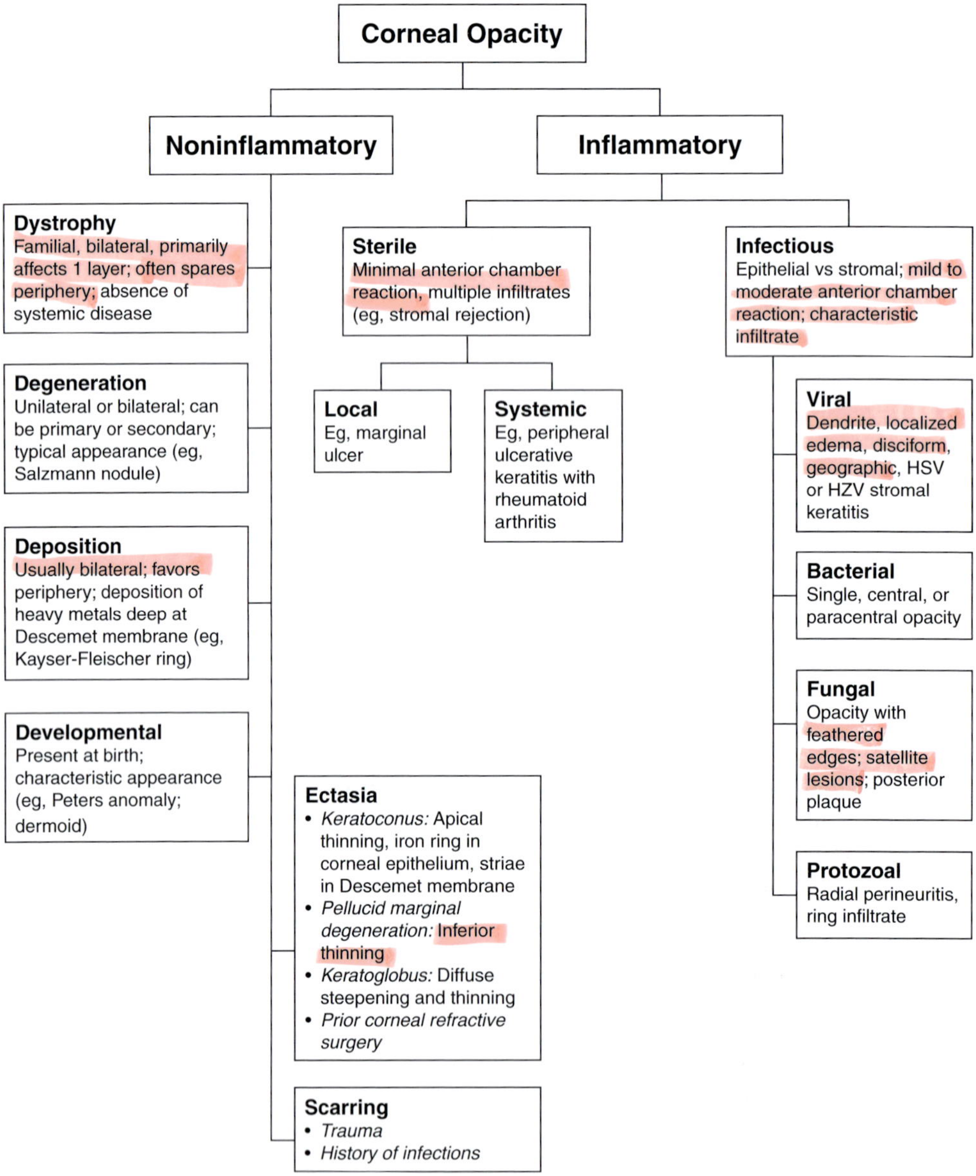

Figure 2-1 Diagnostic algorithm of the corneal opacity. HSV = herpes simplex virus; HZV = herpes zoster virus.

arms are parfocal, arranged so that both focus onto the same spot, with the slit beam centered on the field of view. This setup accommodates various forms of illumination.

Illumination Techniques

At the slit lamp, the target can be illuminated directly or indirectly.

Direct illumination

Direct illumination techniques include diffuse, focal, and specular illumination.

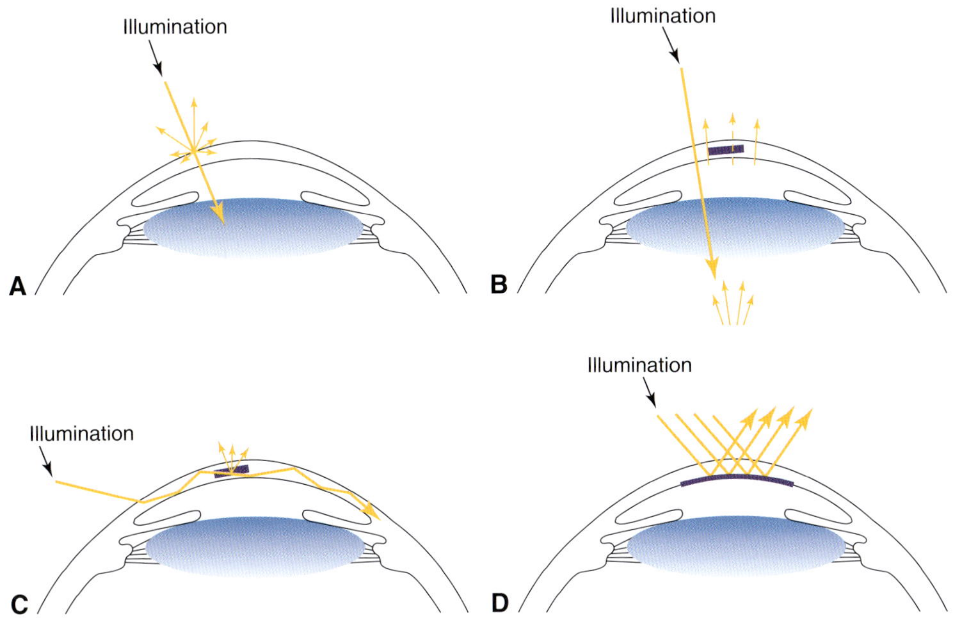

Figure 2-2 Interaction of light rays with the eye in slit-lamp biomicroscopic examination. **A,** Direct illumination. **B,** Retroillumination. **C,** Sclerotic scatter. **D,** Specular reflection. *(Illustration by Kristina Irsch, MD, PhD.)*

Diffuse illumination In diffuse illumination, the light beam is broadened, reduced in intensity, and directed obliquely at the eye. By swinging the illuminator arm to produce highlights and shadows, the visibility of irregularities of the ocular surface (eg, epithelial basement membrane dystrophy) and iris lesions can be improved (Fig 2-2).

Focal illumination In focal illumination, the light beam and the microscope are directed to the same spot, and the slit aperture is narrowed. Focal illumination is achieved with a broad beam or a slit beam:

- Broad-beam illumination, which uses a beam width of about 3 mm, is optimal for visualizing eyelid lesions and opacities associated with corneal dystrophies or scarring.
- Slit-beam illumination, which uses a beam width of about 1 mm or less, yields an optical section of the cornea (Fig 2-3) for evaluation of corneal thinning, edema, stromal infiltrates, and endothelial abnormalities. Reducing the height of the beam facilitates assessment of cell and flare in the anterior chamber. (For more information on cell and flare grading, see BCSC Section 9, *Uveitis and Ocular Inflammation.*)

Specular reflection Another direct illumination technique is based on *specular reflection*, which are normal light reflexes bouncing off a surface (see Fig 2-2D). A faint reflection also comes from the posterior corneal surface. Specular reflection improves visualization of the corneal endothelium. At a magnification power of 25× to 40×, cell density and morphology are clearly visible (Fig 2-4); guttae and keratic precipitates appear as nonreflective dark areas.

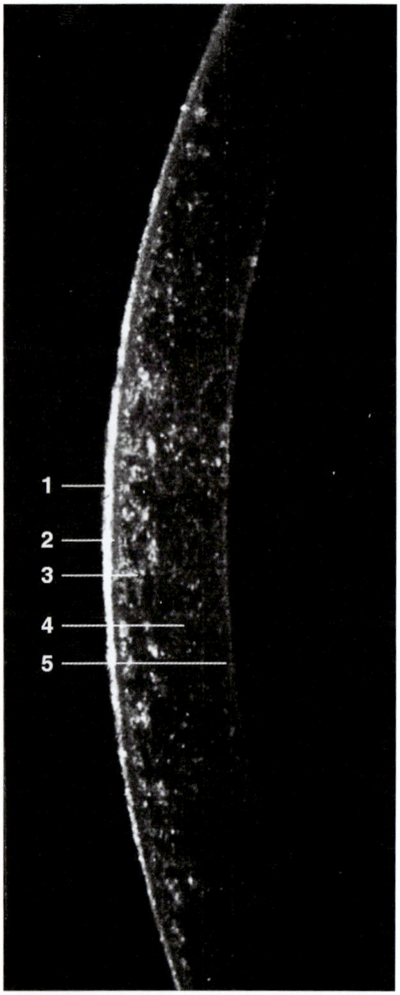

Figure 2-3 Slit section of normal cornea. *1,* Tear film. *2,* Epithelium. *3,* Anterior stroma with a high density of keratocytes. *4,* Posterior stroma with a lower density of keratocytes. *5,* Descemet membrane and endothelium. *(Reproduced with permission from Krachmer JH, Mannis MJ, Holland EJ, eds.* Cornea. *2nd ed. Vol 1. Elsevier/Mosby; 2005:201. © CL Mártonyi, WK Kellogg Eye Center, University of Michigan.)*

STEPS TO VIEWING THE ENDOTHELIAL CELL MOSAIC WITH THE SLIT LAMP (SPECULAR REFLECTION)

1. Position the slit-beam arm 60° from the viewing arm, illuminating with a short slit or 0.2-mm spot.
2. Identify the bright mirror image of the lightbulb filament and the paired epithelial and endothelial Purkinje light reflexes.
3. Superimpose the corneal endothelial light reflex onto the filament mirror image to produce a bright glare.
4. Use the joystick to move the biomicroscope slightly forward to focus on the endothelium just to the right of the bright glare.

Indirect illumination

For indirect illumination, the slit beam is shined on the iris or is used to create a red reflex in order to backlight the cornea. There are 3 types of indirect illumination: proximal illumination, sclerotic scatter, and retroillumination.

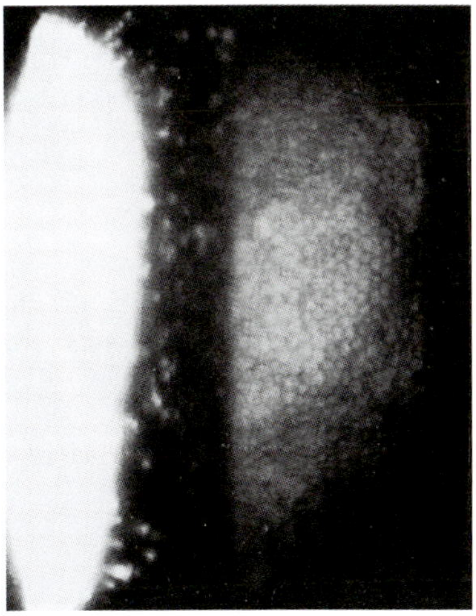

Figure 2-4 Corneal endothelium as visualized with specular reflection using a slit-lamp biomicroscope at 40× magnification. *(Reproduced with permission from Krachmer JH, Mannis MJ, Holland EJ, eds. Cornea. 2nd ed. Vol 1. Elsevier/Mosby; 2005:208. © CL Mártonyi, WK Kellogg Eye Center, University of Michigan.)*

Proximal illumination In proximal illumination, the knob on the illumination arm is turned slightly, decentering the light beam from its isocentric position and causing the light beam and the microscope to be focused on adjacent spots. This method enables visualization of small irregularities with a refractive index similar to that of the surroundings by taking advantage of the opacity of deep tissue layers. By slightly oscillating the light beam, small 3-dimensional lesions, such as corneal foreign bodies, can be detected.

Sclerotic scatter Total internal reflection in the cornea makes *sclerotic scatter* possible. (See BCSC Section 3, *Clinical Optics and Vision Rehabilitation,* for a discussion of total internal reflection.) When the isocentric light beam is decentered, an intense beam shines on the limbus and scatters off the sclera, causing the cornea to glow faintly (see Fig 2-2C). Reflective opacities stand out against the dark field, whereas areas of reduced light transmission in the cornea appear as shades of gray. This technique enables identification of epithelial edema, mild stromal infiltration, nebulae, and cornea verticillata.

Retroillumination Retroillumination can be used to examine more than 1 area of the eye. Crystalline opacities, neovascularization, fingerprint lines, and transillumination of iris defects are best appreciated with this technique. Retroillumination from the iris is achieved by displacing the beam tangentially while examining the cornea (see Fig 2-2B). In the zone between light and dark backgrounds, the visibility of subtle corneal abnormalities is enhanced. Retroillumination from the fundus is performed by aligning the light beam nearly parallel with the examiner's visual axis and rotating the light so that it shines through the edge of the pupil. Corneal surface irregularities (see Figs 8-1 and 8-4A in this volume) and other corneal opacities, phakic and pseudophakic lenses, and a posterior capsule (Fig 2-5) are readily visible against the red reflex.

Mártonyi CL, Maio M. Slit lamp examination and photography. In: Mannis MJ, Holland EJ, eds. *Cornea.* Vol. 1. 4th ed. Elsevier; 2017:79–109.

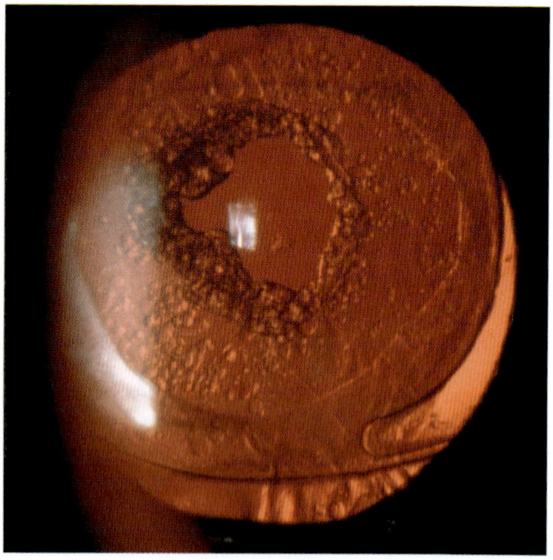

Figure 2-5 Retroillumination reflex from the fundus, highlighting an Nd:YAG laser opening in the posterior capsule with Elschnig pearl formation. *(Courtesy of Stephen E. Orlin, MD.)*

Clinical Use

Direct illumination of the eyelid structures (eyelashes, margin, and meibomian glands), the conjunctiva, and the sclera is recommended as the first step of the slit-lamp examination, with a broad beam applied to illuminate the cornea and overlying tear film in the optical section. Having the patient blink can help the examiner distinguish corneal pathology from debris in the tear film. After the initial low-power screening, much of the examination is performed at higher magnification, and details are examined with a narrow beam. The height of the tear meniscus and discrete lesions in the cornea can be examined with the slit-beam micrometer or an eyepiece reticule. The slit beam is then used to estimate the thickness of the cornea and the depth of the anterior chamber. Early signs of corneal edema on slit-lamp examination include patchy or diffuse haze within the epithelium, mild stromal thickening, faint but deep stromal wrinkles, and folds in Descemet membrane and a patchy or diffuse posterior collagenous layer. A short beam or spot will show anterior chamber flare or cell. Direct and indirect illumination and retroillumination techniques are used to identify abnormalities of the iris and lens. Visualization of more posterior and peripheral intraocular structures usually requires special lenses. Noncontact lenses and contact lenses with angled mirrors extend the slit lamp examination to the angle, peripheral retina, and posterior pole (Video 2-1).

VIDEO 2-1 Slit-lamp techniques.
Used with permission from Mannis MJ, Holland EJ, eds. Cornea. *2nd ed. Elsevier; 2005.*

Ocular Surface Staining and Evaluation of Tear Function

Special testing modalities for evaluation of the external eye and cornea include ocular surface staining by means of fluorescein, rose bengal, or lissamine green (Table 2-1) and examination of tear production and the tear film with Schirmer testing, commercially available microassays, or meibography.

Table 2-1 Ocular Surface Stains

Dye	Fluorescein	Rose Bengal	Lissamine Green
Stains	Precorneal tear film and disrupted cell junctions, erosions	Devitalized cells, healthy cells	Devitalized cells
Toxicity	None	Direct toxicity to epithelial cells, viruses, bacteria, and protozoa	None

Data from Kim J. The use of vital dyes in corneal disease. *Curr Opin Ophthalmol.* 2000;11(4):241–247.

Ocular Surface Staining

Positive and negative staining

Fluorescein, a nontoxic, water-soluble, synthetic dye, is a popular choice for ocular surface staining. Topical fluorescein is available as a preserved 0.25% solution combined with an anesthetic (benoxinate or proparacaine), a nonpreserved 2% unit-dose eye drop, and impregnated paper strips. Fluorexon, a related compound, is available as a 0.35% nonpreserved solution that does not stain most contact lenses. The fluorescein-stained surface is examined at the slit lamp with a cobalt-blue filter; a yellow filter may be employed for improved observation. Fluorescein is also commonly used in applanation tonometry.

Fluorescein stain binds to areas of intercellular junction disruption and epithelial loss, and manifests as punctate erosions, macroerosions, and ulcerative epithelial defects. Sites of fluorescein binding are referred to as *fluorescein-positive*; areas that are not stained are called *fluorescein-negative* and include lesions that project through the tear film, as in epithelial basement membrane dystrophy (see Fig 8-4B) and Thygeson superficial punctate keratitis. Certain disease states produce characteristic punctate staining patterns (Fig 2-6).

When fluorescein collects in an epithelial defect, it diffuses into the corneal stroma, yielding a green flare in the anterior chamber. For this reason, it is important to check the anterior chamber for flare before instilling fluorescein. In the presence of corneal edema, an epithelial defect may not stain as intensely.

> **CLINICAL PEARL**
>
> Care should be given to avoid misclassifying an area containing pooled dye (eg, in an indentation or thinning of the cornea) as an epithelial defect. To absorb any pooled dye, the eye can be anesthetized, and a wisp of cotton can be applied to the area of concern. If the epithelium is intact, the dye will be removed, with no staining noted at the base. Alternatively, an area of pooling can be revealed by irrigating the fluorescein from the surface.

Special fluorescein testing

Tear breakup time (TBUT) is measured by instilling fluorescein and asking the patient to hold the eyelids open after 1 or 2 blinks. The tear film is then evaluated using a broad slit

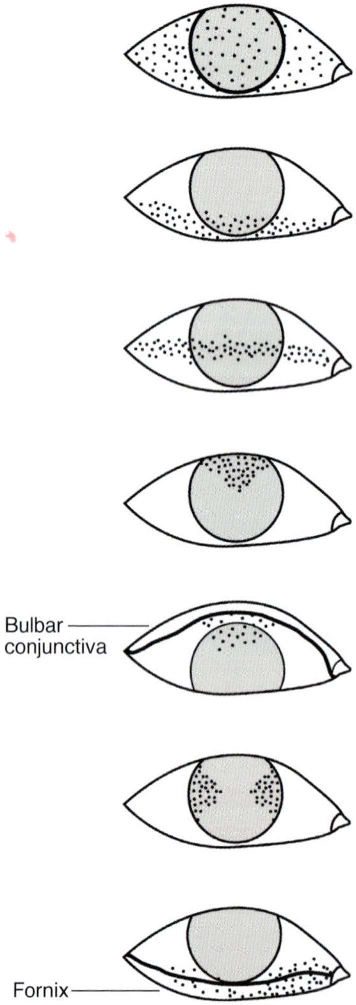

Pattern	Example
Diffuse	Viral conjunctivitis Trauma Toxicity
Inferior	Blepharoconjunctivitis Lagophthalmos Trichiasis
Interpalpebral	Dry eye disease Exposure Neurotrophic keratopathy
Superior	Superior limbic keratoconjunctivitis Foreign body under eyelid Trichiasis Localized limbal stem cell deficiency
Superior conjunctivitis	Superior limbic keratoconjunctivitis
3 and 9 o'clock	Contact lens
Lower conjunctivitis	Mechanical Meibomian gland dysfunction

Figure 2-6 Punctate staining patterns of the ocular surface. *(Illustration by Joyce Zavarro.)*

beam with cobalt blue illumination and counting the seconds until a dry spot appears. The appearance of dry spots in less than 10 seconds is considered an abnormal result. It is important to measure TBUT before any manipulation of the eyelids or instillation of other drops. Fluorescein-anesthetic combination drops are not recommended for this purpose, because excessive fluorescein is typically instilled, and the anesthetic may affect the ocular surface.

In the *dye disappearance test,* fluorescein is applied, and the tear meniscus is observed. Persistence of the dye suggests that the tear drainage system is blocked. The *Seidel test* is performed to detect leakage of aqueous humor through a corneal perforation (Fig 2-7) or leaking trabeculectomy bleb. Fluorescein is instilled at the site of suspected leakage using a moistened strip or concentrated drop, and the presence or absence of clear fluid flowing through the orange dye is determined with cobalt-blue light. Seidel test results in a leaking eye may be negative if the eye is hypotonous.

Rose bengal and lissamine green

Rose bengal and lissamine green (both available as a 1% solution or in impregnated strips) are water-soluble dyes that stain devitalized epithelial cells. These dyes are routinely used for evaluating tear-deficient states and for detecting and assessing various epithelial lesions, such as ocular surface squamous neoplasia (Fig 2-8). Rose bengal is toxic to the epithelium and commonly causes irritation upon instillation. Lissamine green is better tolerated. It has few toxic effects in cultured human corneal epithelial cells and is useful for assessing conjunctival abnormalities.

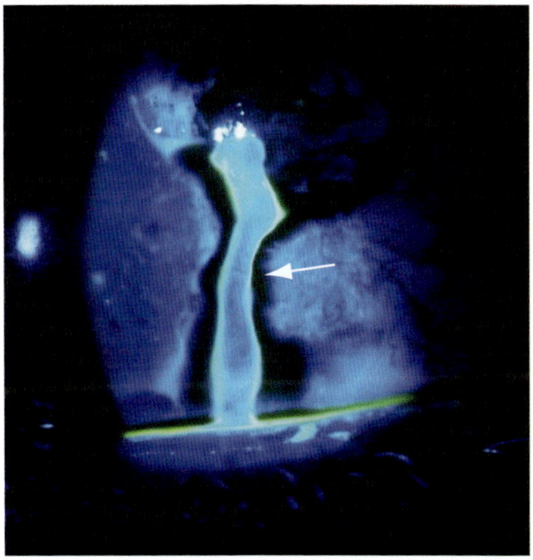

Figure 2-7 Leakage of fluid from the anterior chamber *(arrow)* following a corneal perforation, indicating a positive Seidel test result. *(Courtesy of Stephen E. Orlin, MD.)*

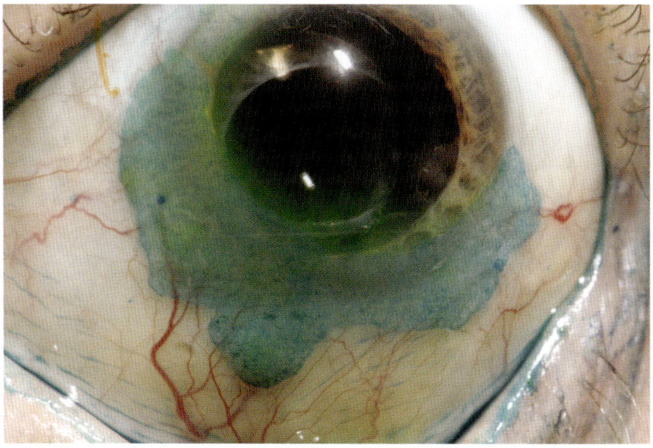

Figure 2-8 Slit-lamp photograph from a patient with conjunctival intraepithelial neoplasia showing staining with lissamine green dye. *(Courtesy of Stephen E. Orlin, MD.)*

Evaluation of Tear Production

Tear production can be assessed with the basic secretion test or by Schirmer testing:

- The *basic secretion test* is performed after instillation of a topical anesthetic and blotting of residual fluid from the inferior fornix. A thin strip of filter paper (5 mm wide, 30 mm long) is placed at the junction of the middle and lateral thirds of the lower eyelid, with 5 mm of the paper length folded over the lid margin posteriorly and the remaining 25 mm projecting anteriorly to the lower-eyelid margin. The test can be performed with the eyes open or closed. Although variations in tear secretion are normal, repeated measurements of less than 3 mm of wetting after 5 minutes are highly suggestive of aqueous tear deficiency (ATD), whereas 3 mm to 10 mm of wetting is an equivocal finding. (See Chapter 3 for a discussion of ATD.)
- The *Schirmer I test* is similar to the basic secretion test but is performed without anesthesia and addresses both basic and reflex tearing. Less than 5 mm of wetting after 5 minutes is diagnostic of ATD. Although this test is relatively specific, its sensitivity is low.
- The *Schirmer II test* addresses reflex secretion under topical anesthesia. After the filter-paper strips have been inserted into the inferior fornices, a cotton-tipped applicator is used to irritate the nasal mucosa. Wetting of less than 15 mm after 2 minutes is suggestive of a defect in reflex secretion. Consistent longitudinal results of these tests are highly suggestive of ATD.

Quantitative tear film tests

Several commercial assays are available to measure components of the tear film, but the objectivity and reproducibility of these tests have not yet been confirmed. Whether results of these tests alter diagnosis and management of dry eye is uncertain. Tear-film osmolarity can be assessed from microliter volumes of tears. Assay results exceeding 308 mOsm/L are considered highly indicative of ATD, but some study findings have shown no correlation between tear osmolarity and signs and symptoms of dry eye.

Lactoferrin is an iron-binding protein secreted by the lacrimal gland that serves an antibacterial function in the tear film. Lactoferrin levels are correlated with aqueous production. Results of microassays of lactoferrin provide an indirect measure of lacrimal gland function; low lactoferrin levels are associated with dry eye. Microassays of immunoglobulin E (IgE) in the tear film can be employed to distinguish between aqueous tear deficiency and ocular allergies. Lactoferrin and IgE can be measured concurrently from 0.5 μL of tears using a commercially available test.

Matrix metalloproteinase 9 (MMP-9) is an inflammatory cytokine secreted by distressed epithelial cells. Dry eye etiology is multifactorial and may involve inflammation of the ocular surface and eyelids (eg, blepharitis), with release of MMP-9. Elevated MMP-9 values (>40 ng/mL) are suggestive of evaporative dry eye (see Chapter 3). However, elevated MMP-9 also occurs in allergy, infection, and peripheral ulcerative keratitis. Assays also are available for biomarkers associated with Sjögren syndrome, an autoimmune disease associated with dry eye, dry mouth, and joint pain. The test is more sensitive than other blood assays, such as those for SS-A and SS-B antibody and rheumatoid factor.

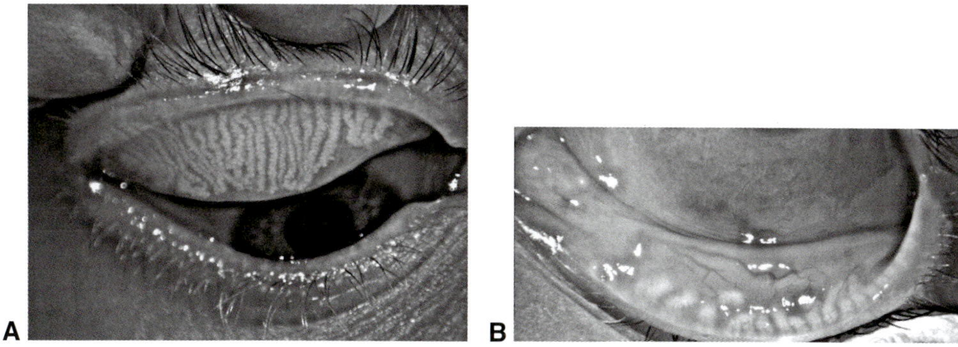

Figure 2-9 Meibography findings in normal and atrophic states. **A,** Upper-eyelid infrared meibograph depicting normal meibomian gland architecture. Note the long, straight glands with very little tortuosity. **B,** Lower eyelid meibograph showing severe gland truncation and atrophy. *(Courtesy of Mina Massaro-Giordano, MD.)*

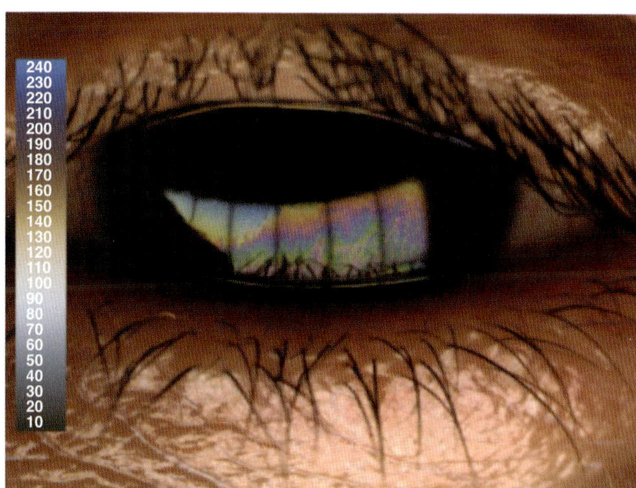

Figure 2-10 Interferometry image shows the normal "rainbow" pattern of the lipid layer in the tear film. *(Courtesy of Mina Massaro-Giordano, MD.)*

Interferometry and infrared meibography enable objective recordings of meibomian gland dropout (Fig 2-9), precise quantification of the height of the tear film meniscus, and measurement of the thickness and structure of the lipid layer with submicrometer accuracy (Fig 2-10).

Qualitative tear film tests

Meibomian gland dysfunction (MGD) is a major cause of evaporative dry eye (see Chapter 3). Slit-lamp examination of the eyelid margin and meibomian gland orifices is helpful in the evaluation of MGD. However, interferometry and infrared meibography are vital for examining meibomian gland structure and pathology. They also allow for real-time evaluation of the blink rate, the completeness of blink patterns, and TBUT, in a noninvasive manner.

American Academy of Ophthalmology Cornea/External Disease Committee, Hoskins Center for Quality Eye Care. Preferred Practice Pattern Guidelines. *Dry Eye Syndrome.* American Academy of Ophthalmology; 2018. www.aao.org/ppp

Bunya VY, Langelier N, Chen S, Pistilli M, Vivino FB, Massaro-Giordano G. Tear osmolarity in Sjögren syndrome. *Cornea.* 2013;3(32):922–927.

Craig JP, Nichols KK, Akpek EK, et al. TFOS DEWS II definition and classification report. *Ocul Surf.* 2017;15(3):276–283.

Evaluation of Corneal Contour

The shape and curvature of the cornea are structural elements that determine its refractive power, a functional property. With the advent of specialty contact lens fitting, premium intraocular lens (IOL) implantation, and refractive surgery, knowledge about the shape, curvature, and power of the cornea has become increasingly important.

The refractive power of the cornea is determined by *Snell's law of refraction*: the difference between 2 refractive indices (eg, air and the tear film) divided by the radius of curvature. The refractive index of air is 1.000; aqueous and tears, 1.336; and corneal stroma, 1.376. The air–tear film interface is the most powerful refractive element of the eye.

BCSC Section 3, *Clinical Optics and Vision Rehabilitation,* covers these topics in greater depth.

Dawson DG, Ubels JL, Edelhauser HF. Cornea and sclera. In: Alm A, Kaufman PL, eds. *Adler's Physiology of the Eye.* 11th ed. Elsevier; 2011:71–130.

Keratometry

CLINICAL PEARL

The keratometer is helpful for detecting corneal surface irregularities in and around the visual axis, evident as distortion of the keratometry mires (see Fig 8-4C).

The most common types of manual keratometers are the Helmholtz type (more frequently used by ophthalmologists) and the Javal-Schiøtz type (discussed in BCSC Section 3, *Clinical Optics and Vision Rehabilitation*). The Helmholtz keratometer is a 1-position device with adjustable image size. The examiner aligns "plus sign" and "minus sign" mires (Fig 2-11).

The manual keratometer has certain limitations. It allows for visualization of only a 4-mm region of the cornea at a time; the patient must alter his or her gaze for other areas to be seen. Keratometry is based on the assumption that the cornea has a symmetric spherocylindrical shape with major and minor axes separated by 90°; it does not account for spherical aberrations, and it is susceptible to focusing and misalignment errors. If the cornea is irregular, distortion of the mires reduces the accuracy of the measurement.

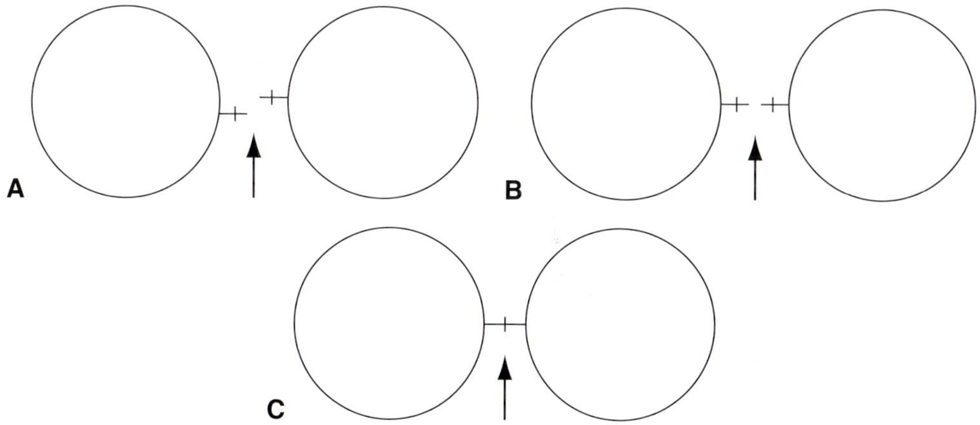

Figure 2-11 Keratometry. **A,** Misalignment of the keratometry mires (plus sign). **B,** Correct alignment of the mires prior to correcting power. **C,** Alignment of the keratometry mires and power in the 180° meridian.

Despite these drawbacks, the manual keratometer does allow for accurate measurement of central-anterior corneal astigmatism. Clinicians can also use the keratometer dynamically by comparing measurements in primary gaze with those in upgaze. Steepening of the inferior cornea is an early sign of keratoconus. Newer technology is supplanting the keratometer for contact lens fitting, corneal refractive surgical planning, and IOL selection (see also BCSC Section 11, *Lens and Cataract*).

Keratoscopy

Unlike keratometry, which yields quantitative data limited to a central 4.0-mm area, keratoscopy provides qualitative results over a larger area. Keratoscopy findings include the shape and quality of the projected rings as well as the distance between the rings. The mires appear closer together in the steeper part of the cornea, and the short axis depicts the steeper meridian. Along the flat (long) axis, the mires appear farther apart (Fig 2-12). This information can be helpful for detection of paracentral and peripheral disorders of corneal contour, such as keratoconus, pellucid marginal degeneration, and astigmatism following penetrating keratoplasty.

Corneal Topography

Corneal topography is a noninvasive imaging modality for mapping the curvature of the corneal surface. Placido disk–based corneal topography involves the projection of keratoscopic rings (ie, mires) onto the cornea. Irregularities of the mires signify irregularities of the corneal surface, which can be associated with vision loss.

The keratoscopic images reflected from the corneal surface are digitally captured and analyzed by computer. Computerized topography systems allow for analyses of pupil size and location, regular and irregular astigmatism, keratoconus risk, simulated corneal curvature measurements, wavefront analysis, dry eye screening, meibomian gland imagery,

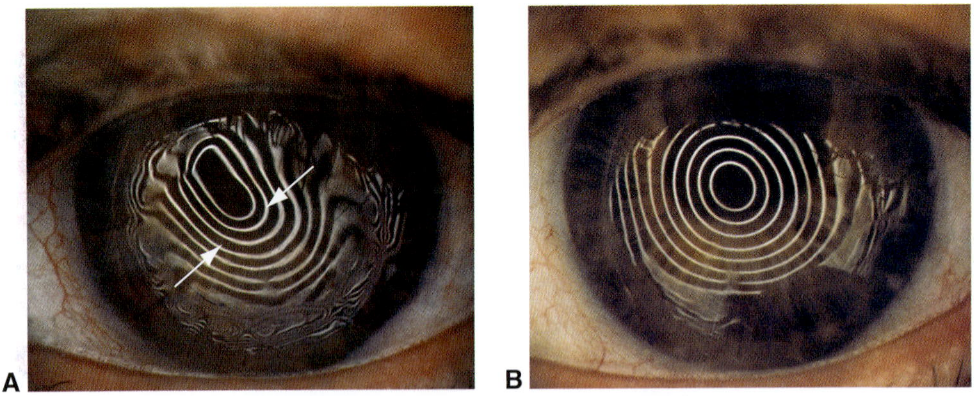

Figure 2-12 Keratoscopy findings before and after suture removal in a postkeratoplasty patient. **A,** With sutures in place, keratoscopic mires are closer together in the axis of steep curvature *(arrows)* and farther apart in the flat axis. **B,** Keratoscopic mires round out after sutures are cut. *(Courtesy of Stephen E. Orlin, MD.)*

and angle kappa. Measurements are made at thousands of points, and color-coded *power maps* are generated from these data. Notably, these devices can assess only the anterior corneal surface and tear film. There are 3 types of anterior power maps:

- *The axial curvature map* closely approximates the power of the central 1 mm to 2 mm of the cornea but fails to depict the true shape and power of the peripheral cornea (Fig 2-13).
- The *tangential map* typically shows better sensitivity to peripheral changes, as it applies less "smoothing" of the curvature than does the axial map (Fig 2-14). (In these maps, diopters are relative units of curvature and do not equal diopters of corneal power.)
- *The mean curvature map* uses an infinite number of spheres to assess curvature. The algorithm yields a minimum- and maximum-size best-fit sphere; from the radius of each of these, the mean curvature (ie, the arithmetic mean of the principal curvatures) is displayed. These powers are mapped with colors representing diopter changes, allowing for more sensitivity to peripheral changes in curvature (Fig 2-15).

Before any topographic maps are interpreted, the Placido disk images should be checked for centration and image quality. The color scale must be reviewed to determine the type of map being studied. The scale can dramatically influence the interpretation of the map.

CLINICAL PEARL

Smaller increments of the color scale increase sensitivity but exaggerate small changes, whereas larger increments decrease sensitivity but can mask meaningful variations.

The absolute scale is constant for all examinations and is useful for comparisons over time and among patients. The normalized, or relative, scale adjusts to the range of powers

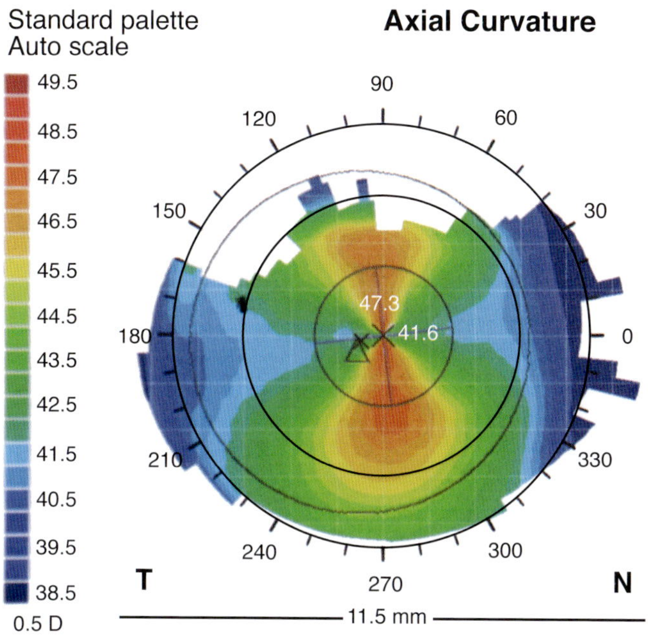

Figure 2-13 Topography of a patient with regular "with-the-rule" astigmatism depicted by a symmetric bow-tie pattern. *(Courtesy of Stephen E. Orlin, MD.)*

on the corneal surface and differs for each cornea. Thus, the power range and step size may be narrow or broad. In addition to the limitations of the algorithms, the accuracy of corneal topography mapping is susceptible to the following issues:

- misalignment
- limited stability (test-to-test variation)
- focus errors
- tear-film effects
- distortions
- limited coverage area (central and limbal)
- a lack of standardized data maps
- colors that may be absolute or varied (normalized)

Nevertheless, corneal topography maps allow clinicians to detect keratoconus early, identify subclinical and frank keratoconus during refractive surgery screenings, and recognize and predict corneal ectasia after refractive surgery. (Refer to Chapter 9 for a more complete discussion of keratoconus and corneal ectasia.) Corneal mapping is also useful in managing congenital and postoperative astigmatism, particularly following penetrating keratoplasty, and in monitoring pterygia, scarring, and degenerative changes in the cornea. Complex peripheral corneal pathology may result in an axis of astigmatism in spectacles that is not aligned with the axis of the power map.

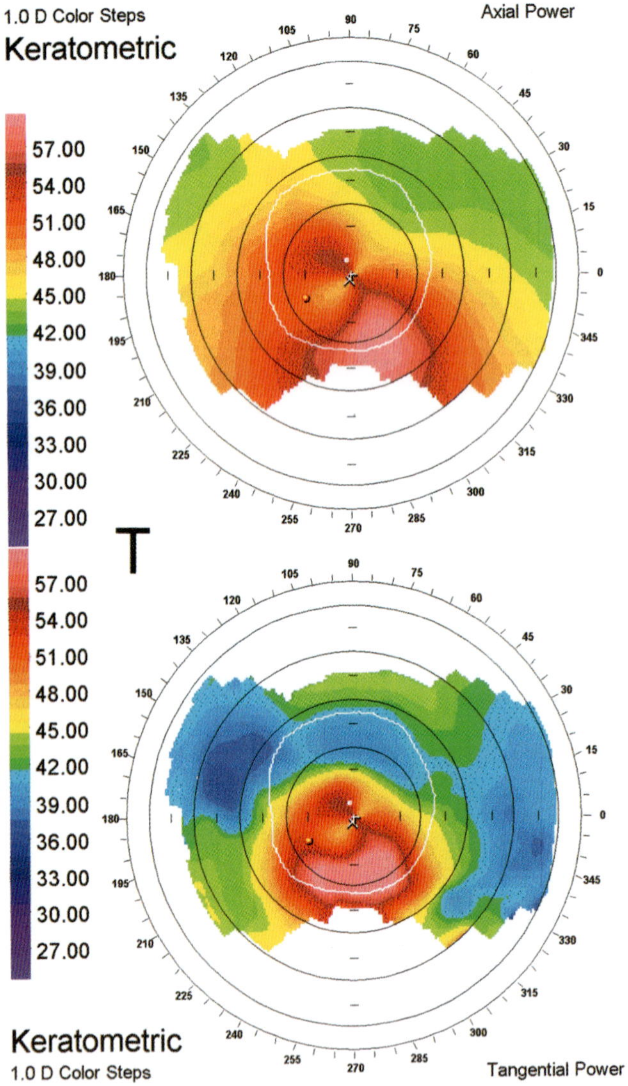

Figure 2-14 Corneal topography in a patient with keratoconus. The top image shows axial curvature; the bottom shows tangential curvature. Note that the steeper curve at the bottom is more closely aligned with the cone. *(Courtesy of John E. Sutphin, MD.)*

Corneal Tomography

In corneal tomography, a 3-dimensional image of the cornea is generated. This approach is useful for evaluating anterior and posterior corneal curvature and elevation, corneal thickness, and anterior-chamber depth, as well as for imaging the iris and lens. Corneal tomography systems can be utilized for ectasia risk detection (Fig 2-16) prior to refractive surgery and for monitoring keratoconus progression and determining need for corneal crosslinking. (See Chapter 9 and Appendix 9.2 on corneal crosslinking.)

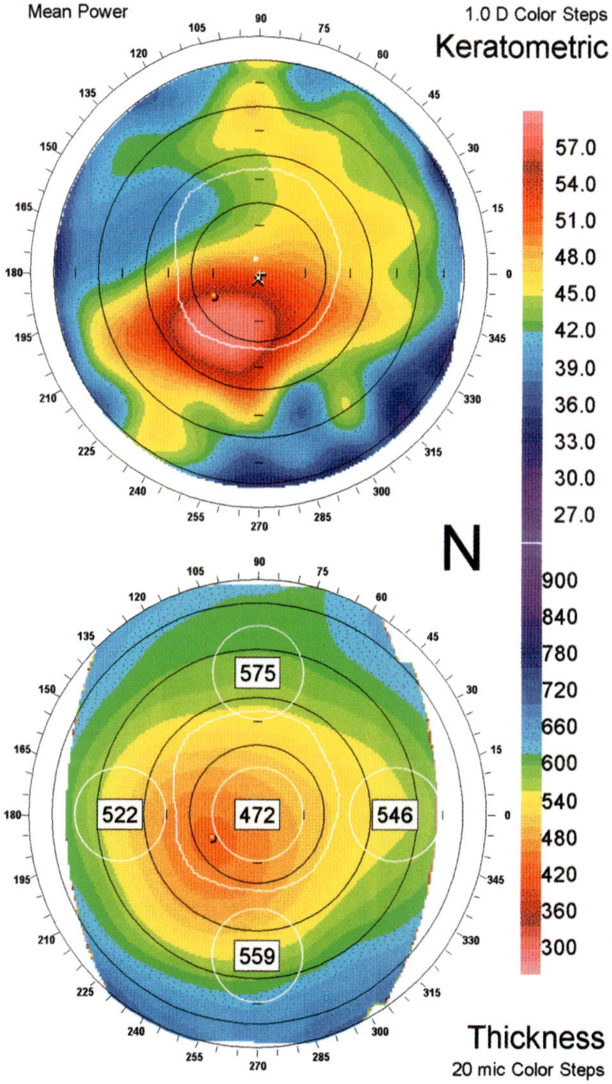

Figure 2-15 Power and pachymetry maps in a patient with keratoconus (also depicted in Fig 2-14). The top image shows mean curvature. The steepest part of the cornea in the top image is coincident with the thinnest part of the cornea in the bottom image. The pachymetry map below also shows decentration of the corneal thinning. In a normal cornea, the thinnest part is more centrally located. *(Courtesy of John E. Sutphin, MD.)*

Table 2-2 provides an overview of methods and instruments for corneal topography and tomography.

Corneal tomographic data are obtained with various instruments, including scanning-slit technology and Scheimpflug-based corneal tomography. Corneal tomographic data and imaging can also be obtained with anterior segment optical coherence tomography (AS-OCT), which is discussed later in this chapter.

Table 2-2 Methods and Instruments for Corneal Topography and Tomography

Method(s)	Instruments
Keratoscopy or Placido disk–based topography	Atlas (Carl Zeiss Meditec) Topographic Modeling System (TMS-5; Tomey) OPD-Scan III (Nidek)
Horizontal scanning-slit	Orbscan IIz (Bausch + Lomb)
Scheimpflug imaging	Pentacam (Oculus Optikgeräte) TMS-5 (Tomey) Oculyzer (WaveLight Laser Technologie AG)
Scheimpflug imaging with Placido disk–based topography	Galilei (Ziemer Ophthalmic Systems AG) Sirius (Costruzione Strumenti Oftalmici)
Rotating optical coherence tomography integrated into the Atlas topography system	Visante (Carl Zeiss Meditec) SS-1000 Casia (Tomey)
Arc scanning with very-high-frequency ultrasound	Artemis II (ArcScan)

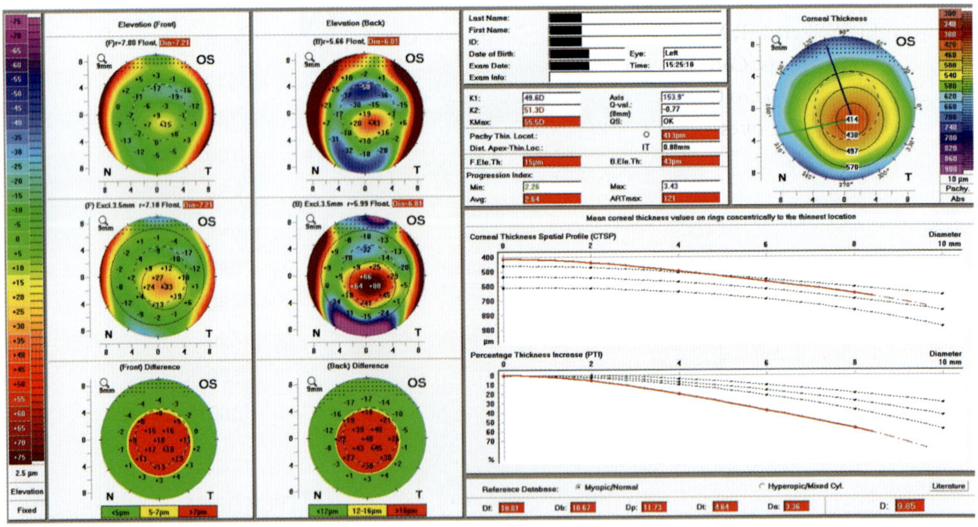

Figure 2-16 Ectasia risk can be assessed using Scheimpflug tomography. Anterior and posterior elevations are determined, modifying the best-fit sphere to accentuate elevation *(left side)*. Pachymetric data are examined for progression of thinning from the thinnest cornea to the limbus (curvilinear graphs, *middle right*). *(Courtesy of Robert W. Weisenthal, MD.)*

Scanning-slit technology In combination with Placido disk–based topography, scanning-slit technology provides elevation mapping and pachymetric data. The posterior elevation map is mathematically derived and tends to overestimate posterior corneal curvature, especially in patients who have undergone laser in situ keratomileusis (LASIK). This technology can be used to screen for ectasia risk by comparing posterior and anterior elevation. Relative pachymetric data can help with identifying thinning decentration but are less reliable for planning excimer laser ablation.

Scheimpflug-based corneal tomography A Scheimpflug system images the anterior segment with dual cameras perpendicular to a slit beam, creating an optical section of the cornea and lens. Scheimpflug-based systems generate reliable information on anterior curvature, corneal thickness, anterior-chamber depth, anterior and posterior elevation, and pupil diameter. As a result, the thickness and topography of the entire anterior and posterior surface of the cornea can be displayed (Fig 2-17). In addition, a densitometry function addresses opacification of the cornea or lens. Several devices have employed the Scheimpflug principle with rotational scanning, dual-rotational scanning, and Placido disk–based topography.

Ambrósio R Jr, Belin MW. Imaging of the cornea: topography vs tomography. *J Refract Surg.* 2010;26(11):847–849.

Belin MW, Asota IM, Ambrósio R Jr, Khachikian SS. What's in a name: keratoconus, pellucid marginal degeneration, and related thinning disorders. *Am J Ophthalmol.* 2011;152(2):157–162.

Dharwadkar S, Nayak BK. Corneal topography and tomography. *J Clin Ophthalmol Res.* 2015;3(1):45–62.

Kim EJ, Weikert MP, Martinez CE, Klyce SD. Keratometry and topography. In: Mannis MJ, Holland EJ, eds. *Cornea.* Vol. 1. 4th ed. Elsevier; 2017:144–153.

Oliveira CM, Ribeiro C, Franco S. Corneal imaging with slit-scanning and Scheimpflug imaging techniques. *Clin Exp Optom.* 2011;94(1):33–42.

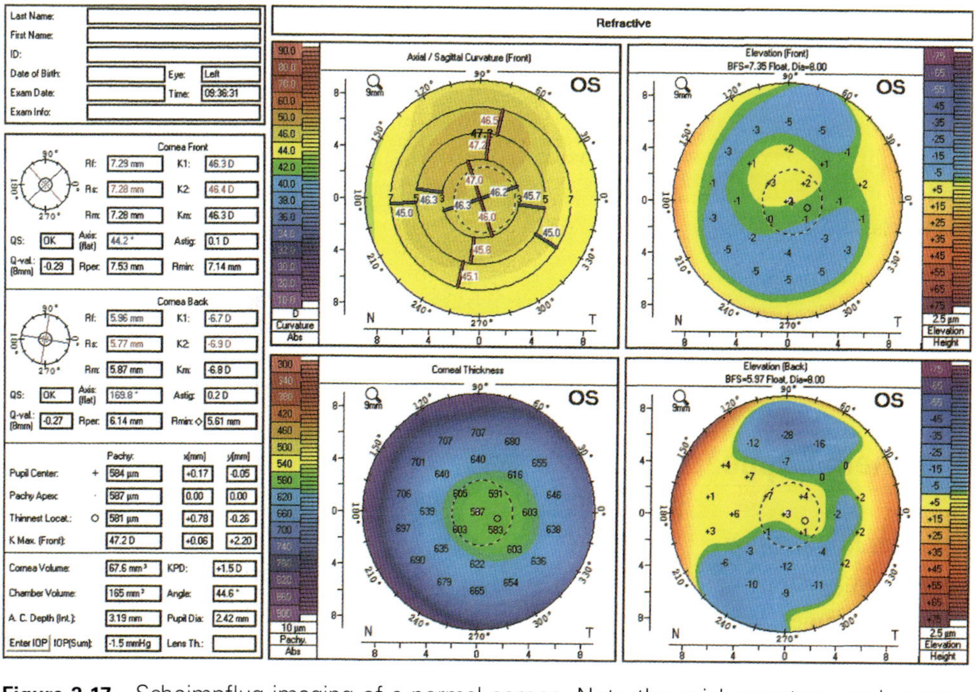

Figure 2-17 Scheimpflug imaging of a normal cornea. Note the axial curvature, pachymetry, and anterior elevation and posterior elevation maps. *(Courtesy of Stephen E. Orlin, MD.)*

Corneal Biomechanics

The biomechanical properties of the cornea affect corneal function, and consequently, visual function. For example, the elastic and viscous elements of the cornea are implicated in keratoconus and ectasia. These properties can be evaluated in the clinic using commercially available instruments. One measure of elasticity, *corneal hysteresis*, is defined as the difference (in mm Hg) between the pressure at which the cornea bends inward during air-jet applanation and the pressure at which it bends out again. Corneal hysteresis may provide clues about ectasia risk prior to corneal refractive surgery.

Corneal Resistance Factor

The corneal resistance factor (CRF) is calculated from the correlation between hysteresis and corneal thickness. CRF values are normally distributed within the general population. Patients who have undergone LASIK or photorefractive keratectomy or whose corneas have an inherent biomechanical weakness (eg, keratoconus) tend to have lower CRF values, as do patients with edema secondary to Fuchs endothelial corneal dystrophy. Knowledge of the CRF may help contextualize IOP values, which are affected by corneal thickness. The CRF is less informative for screening refractive surgery patients for risk of ectasia or in documenting corneal stiffness associated with corneal crosslinking, aging, and diabetes.

Newer Technologies

Recently developed technologies for evaluating corneal biomechanics integrate dynamic corneal imaging with Placido disk–based technology, Scheimpflug imaging, or optical coherence tomography (OCT) and yield accurate measurements of corneal deformation induced by air puffs. These devices can be applied to differentiate normal corneas from ectatic corneas or corneas treated with crosslinking from untreated ones. Using these devices, investigators have shown that corneal deformation is influenced by IOP, corneal thickness, and elastic biomechanical properties.

Dawson DG, Ubels JL, Edelhauser HF. Cornea and sclera. In: Alm A, Kaufman PL, eds. *Adler's Physiology of the Eye.* 11th ed. Elsevier; 2011:71–130.

Piñero DP, Alcón N. In vivo characterization of corneal biomechanics. *J Cataract Refract Surg.* 2014;40(6):870–887.

Endothelial Appearance and Function

Specular Microscopy

Specular microscopy (contact or noncontact techniques) and confocal microscopy can be performed to measure certain parameters of the corneal endothelial cell mosaic, including density, the coefficient of variation (CV), and the percentage of hexagonal cells.

Density The central endothelial cell density typically exceeds 3500 cells/mm^2 in children and gradually decreases with age to approximately 2000 cells/mm^2 in older adults. An average

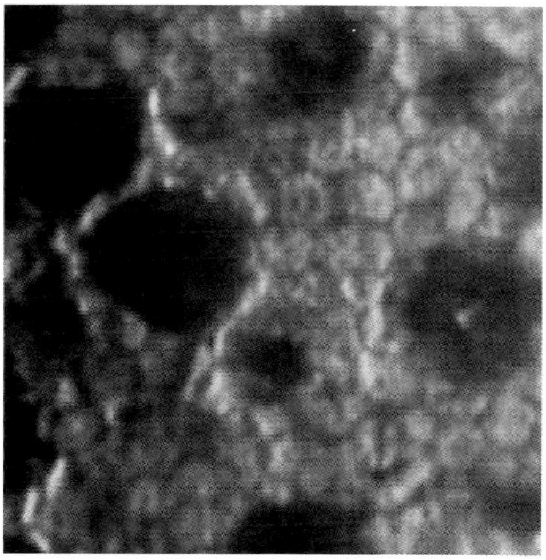

Figure 2-18 Specular microscopy showing Fuchs endothelial corneal dystrophy with guttae, dark shadows. *(Courtesy of John E. Sutphin, MD.)*

density for adults is 2400 cells/mm^2 (range, 1500–3500 cells/mm^2), with cell sizes ranging from 150 µm^2 to 350 µm^2. Low cell density (ie, fewer than 1000 cells/mm^2) may yield a transparent cornea, but such corneas are at risk of corneal decompensation following intraocular surgery. Dark areas on microscopy are suggestive of guttae on the cornea (Fig 2-18).

Coefficient of variation The standard deviation of the mean cell area is divided by the mean cell area and is a unitless number, typically <0.30. *Polymegethism* is a condition characterized by increased variation in cell area that is associated with contact lens wear. Patients with significant polymegethism (CV, >0.40) may develop corneal edema following intraocular surgery.

Percentage of hexagonal cells The percentage of cells with 6 apices is approximately 100% in normal eyes. Lower percentages of hexagonal cells indicate poorer endothelial health. *Pleomorphism* refers to variability in cell shape. Patients with high pleomorphism (<50% hexagonal cells) may be at greater risk of endothelial decompensation after intraocular surgery.

American Academy of Ophthalmology. *Corneal Endothelial Photography: Three-Year Revision OTA*. Ophthalmic Technology Assessment. American Academy of Ophthalmology; 1997. (Reviewed for currency 2019.)

American Academy of Ophthalmology Cornea/External Disease Committee, Hoskins Center for Quality Eye Care. Preferred Practice Pattern Guidelines. *Corneal Edema and Opacification*. American Academy of Ophthalmology; 2018. www.aao.org/ppp

Sayegh RR, Benetz BA, Lass JH. Specular microscopy. In: Mannis MJ, Holland EJ, eds. *Cornea*. Vol. 1. 4th ed. Elsevier; 2017:160–179.

Pachymetry

Corneal thickness is a sensitive indicator of endothelial function and is measured with a pachymeter. Ultrasonic pachymetry is a simple technique based on the speed of sound in the normal cornea (1640 m/sec). The applanating tip of the pachymeter is set perpendicular to the ocular surface to avoid tilting errors. The thinnest zone of the normal cornea is approximately 1.5 mm temporal to the geographic center, and the cornea thickens in the paracentral and peripheral zones. The typical central thickness is 540–550 μm. Knowledge of corneal thickness provides context for interpreting the IOP. Thicker corneas are associated with artificially higher IOP measurements, while thin corneas cause IOP readings to be lower than the actual IOP. Low pachymetry findings (indicating a thin cornea) are an independent risk factor for glaucoma, even after adjusting for factitious lowering of the IOP.

Pachymetry can be used to assess the corneal endothelium, which has dual roles as a barrier and as a metabolic pump. The endothelial pump balances the leak rate to maintain corneal thickness and a corneal stromal water content of 78%. Acute corneal edema often results from an altered barrier effect of the endothelium or epithelium. Folds in Descemet membrane are first seen when corneal thickness increases by 10% or more; epithelial edema secondary to endothelial decompensation occurs when corneal thickness exceeds 700 μm. Stromal edema alters corneal transparency, but vision loss is most severe when epithelial microcysts or bullae occur. Patients at risk of symptomatic corneal edema following intraocular surgery include those with central corneal thickness greater than 640 μm, bilaterally asymmetric corneal thickening, or greater thickness of the central cornea than the inferior cornea unilaterally.

CLINICAL PEARL

Increased corneal thickness lasting several hours after waking compared with pachymetry measurements in the afternoon may indicate endothelial dysfunction. The absence of evaporation during overnight sleep may also result in blurred vision in the morning.

Pachymetry has largely been supplanted by technologies that generate precise maps of corneal thickness and curvature, such as scanning-slit technology, Scheimpflug-based anterior segment imaging, optical low coherence reflectometry, AS-OCT, and high-resolution ultrasonography.

Brandt JD, Beiser JA, Kass MA, Gordon MO. Central corneal thickness in the Ocular Hypertension Treatment Study (OHTS). *Ophthalmology.* 2001;108(10):1779–1788.

Khaja WA, Grover S, Kelmenson AT, Ferguson LR, Sambhav K, Chalam KV. Comparison of central corneal thickness: ultrasound pachymetry versus slit-lamp optical coherence tomography, specular microscopy, and Orbscan. *Clin Ophthalmol.* 2015;12(9):1065–1070.

Liu J, Roberts CJ. Influence of corneal biomechanical properties on intraocular pressure measurement: quantitative analysis. *J Cataract Refract Surg.* 2005;31(1):146–155.

Other Imaging Modalities

Confocal Microscopy

Confocal microscopy is a noninvasive technique for in vivo imaging of the cornea. The basic principle of confocal microscopy is that a tissue site can be illuminated by a point source of light or laser and simultaneously imaged by a camera in the same plane (ie, confocal). This technique involves scanning a small region of tissue with thousands of spots of light, producing a high-resolution image at a cellular level. Tandem scanning, scanning-slit, and laser scanning confocal microscopes are popular options for clinic use. Laser scanning confocal systems can traverse nontransparent tissues to generate a series of images from extremely thin sections. The depth of focus is 5 μm to 7 μm in laser scanning, 7 μm to 9 μm in tandem scanning, and 26 μm in scanning-slit microscopes. Successful imaging requires a skilled operator and a cooperative patient.

CLINICAL PEARL

Confocal microscopy is useful for identifying causative agents in cases of infectious keratitis (eg, *Acanthamoeba* keratitis, fungal keratitis, microsporidiosis, and herpetic eye disease), examining corneal nerve morphology in diabetic neurotrophic keratitis, and evaluating neuropathic pain in ocular surface disease and after refractive surgery (Fig 2-19).

Confocal microscopy also may be performed to visualize the corneal endothelial layer (as an alternative to specular microscopy) or to differentiate certain corneal dystrophies (see Chapter 8).

Alzubaidi R, Sharif MS, Qahwaji R, Ipson S, Brahma A. In vivo confocal microscopic corneal images in health and disease with an emphasis on extracting features and visual signatures for corneal diseases: a review study. *Br J Ophthalmol.* 2016;100(1):41–55.

Petroll WM, Cavanagh HD, Jester JV. Confocal microscopy. In: Mannis MJ, Holland EJ, eds. *Cornea.* Vol. 1. 4th ed. Elsevier; 2017:180–191.

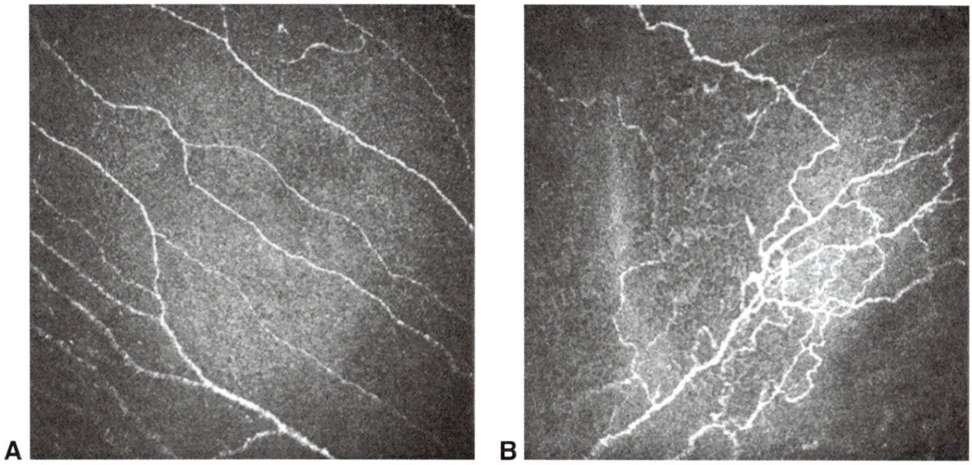

Figure 2-19 Confocal microscopy of corneal nerves. **A,** Normal nerve architecture. **B,** Tortuous branching patterns. *(Courtesy of Mina Massaro-Giordano, MD.)*

Anterior Segment Optical Coherence Tomography

Anterior segment optical coherence tomography is a noninvasive technology that produces 2-dimensional, high-resolution, high-definition cross-sectional images. AS-OCT images are similar to ultrasonographic images but are based on the emission and reflection of light (low-coherence interferometry). The achievable resolution (5–10 μm) allows for exquisite delineation of the layers of the cornea, the anterior chamber, and the iris. The primary types of AS-OCT are time-domain (TD-OCT) and frequency-domain (FD-OCT). A subtype of FD-OCT is spectral-domain OCT (SD-OCT). Swept-source OCT combines elements of TD-OCT and SD-OCT and has been applied in the office and as an attachment to the operating microscope for facilitating endothelial keratoplasty and epiretinal membrane peeling.

AS-OCT enables measurement of depth, width, and angle of the anterior chamber (Fig 2-20) as well as corneal thickness. The pachymetry feature is useful in the preoperative evaluation of patients with Fuchs endothelial corneal dystrophy. In postoperative follow-up of endothelial keratoplasty cases, the shape, thickness, and attachment of donor tissue can be visualized and quantified with AS-OCT. This tool also may be applied in LASIK cases to measure the thickness of the corneal flap and the residual stromal bed as indicators of enhancement/retreatment safety. Additional software is available for assessing corneal curvature and epithelial thickness in patients considering refractive surgery and in determining true corneal power for IOL power calculation after LASIK or photorefractive keratectomy.

Jancevski M, Foster CS. Anterior segment optical coherence tomography. *Semin Ophthalmol.* 2010;25(5–6):317–323.

Kaufman SC, Kelly A. Anterior segment imaging: Anterior segment OCT and confocal microscopy. *Focal Points: Clinical Practice Perspectives.* American Academy of Ophthalmology; 2017, Volume XXXV number 1.

Zhou SY, Wang CX, Cai XY, Huang D, Liu YZ. Optical coherence tomography and ultrasound biomicroscopy imaging of opaque corneas. *Cornea.* 2013;32(4):e25–e30.

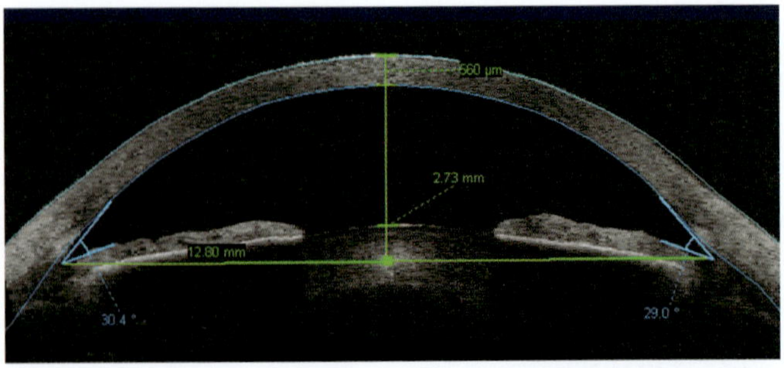

Figure 2-20 Anterior segment optical coherence tomography (AS-OCT) image of a phakic eye. The central anterior chamber depth is 2.73 mm; note the moderate narrowing of the anterior-chamber angle. *(Reproduced from Goins KM, Wagoner MD. Imaging the anterior segment.* Focal Points: Clinical Modules for Ophthalmologists. *American Academy of Ophthalmology; 2009, module 11.)*

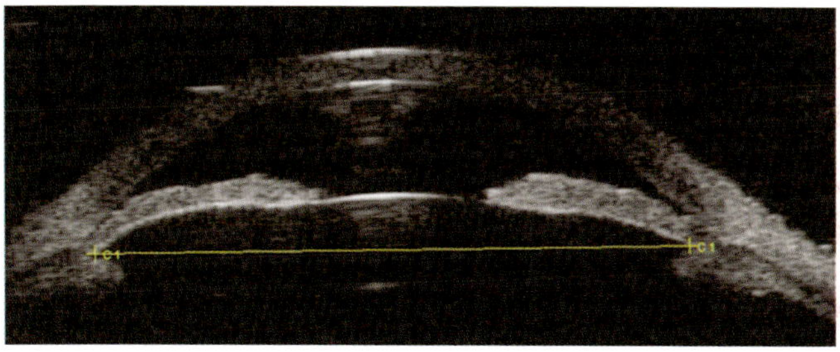

Figure 2-21 Ultrasound biomicroscopic visualization of the entire anterior segment, including structures behind the iris pigment epithelium, for precise sulcus-to-sulcus measurement prior to implantation of a phakic refractive intraocular lens. *(Reproduced from Goins KM, Wagoner MD. Imaging the anterior segment.* Focal Points: Clinical Modules for Ophthalmologists. *American Academy of Ophthalmology; 2009, module 11.)*

Ultrasound Biomicroscopy

High-frequency ultrasound biomicroscopy (UBM) provides high-resolution in vivo imaging of the anterior segment (Fig 2-21). UBM is applicable to many tissues, including the cornea, the anterior and posterior surface of the iris, the ciliary body, zonular fibers, angle structures, and the anterior lens capsule. UBM technology incorporates 50- to 100-MHz transducers into a B-mode clinical scanner, allowing for higher resolution of structures in the anterior segment with less penetration than a traditional B-scan. Unlike AS-OCT, UBM allows the examiner to view structures through an opaque cornea and total hyphema. The scleral spur, located where the trabecular meshwork meets an interface line between the sclera and ciliary body, is a valuable landmark for examining various angle configurations.

UBM is helpful in the following scenarios:

- assessing angle anomalies
  - angle recession
  - cyclodialysis cleft
  - foreign bodies
  - malignant glaucoma
  - narrow angles
  - pupillary block
  - plateau iris
- assessing ciliary body pathology
  - cysts
  - tumors
- confirming accurate placement of phakic IOLs
- determining IOL haptic positions and in the angle
- identifying pigment dispersion syndrome
- locating iridocorneal or iridolenticular adhesions in Peters anomaly

Goins KM, Wagoner MD. Imaging the anterior segment. *Focal Points: Clinical Modules for Ophthalmologists.* American Academy of Ophthalmology; 2009, module 11.

CHAPTER 3

Clinical Approach to Ocular Surface Disease

This chapter includes a related video. Go to www.aao.org/bcscvideo_section08 or scan the QR code in the text to access this content.

Indicates selected key points within the chapter.

Highlights

- It is helpful both diagnostically and therapeutically to divide dry eye disease into 2 categories: (1) aqueous tear deficiency (ATD) and (2) evaporative dry eye due to meibomian gland dysfunction (MGD).
- Discharge is common in patients with moderate to severe ATD (mucous) and in patients with infectious conjunctivitis (purulent); consequently, ATD is frequently misdiagnosed as infectious conjunctivitis.
- Patients with primary Sjögren syndrome are at increased risk for the development of lymphoma.
- MGD and blepharitis are commonly associated with dry eye; therefore, effective treatment of eyelid disease is an important adjunct to dry eye management.
- Basal cell, squamous cell, and sebaceous cell carcinoma can masquerade as chalazia or chronic blepharitis.

Common Clinical Findings in Ocular Surface Disease

This chapter will introduce and define the common clinical findings of the external eye and cornea (Table 3-1), such as dry eye and blepharitis, and explain how these findings aid in the diagnosis and management of ocular surface disease (OSD).

Conjunctival Signs of Inflammation

Table 3-2 lists conjunctival findings, with examples of commonly associated ocular and systemic conditions in the differential diagnosis of OSD.

Papillae Papillae are localized, elevated conjunctival lesions consisting of a central vascular core surrounded by connective tissue septa that anchor the palpebral conjunctiva to the tarsus (Fig 3-1).

Table 3-1 Common Clinical Findings of the External Eye, Sclera, and Cornea

Tissue	Finding	Description
Eyelid	Bulla	Large blister
	Eczema	Scaly crust on a red base
	Erosion	Excoriated epidermal defect
	Keratosis	Scaling from accumulated keratinized cells
	Macule	Flat lesion of skin color change
	Papule	Small, solid elevation of the skin
	Pustule	Pus-filled blister
	Ulcer	Epidermal erosion with dermal tissue loss
	Vesicle	Blister filled with serous fluid
Conjunctiva	Chalasis	Laxity of conjunctiva; tissue may roll up onto the eyelid margin or cover the lacrimal punctum
	Chemosis	Conjunctival edema caused by a transudate leaking through fenestrated conjunctival capillaries as a result of altered vascular integrity (eg, inflammation and vasomotor changes) or hemodynamic changes (eg, impaired venous drainage or intravascular hyposmolarity)
	Discharge	Exudate on the conjunctival surface, varying from proteinaceous (serous) to cellular (purulent)
	Epiphora	Excess tears from increased lacrimation or impaired lacrimal outflow
	Epithelial defect	Focal area of epithelial loss
	Follicle	Focal lymphoid nodule with accessory peripheral vascularization
	Granuloma	Nodule consisting of chronic inflammatory cells with fibrovascular proliferation
	Hyperemia	Focal or diffuse dilation of the subepithelial plexus of blood vessels; other changes include fusiform vascular dilations, saccular aneurysms, petechiae, and intraconjunctival hemorrhage
	Membrane	Inflammatory coagulum penetrating the conjunctival epithelium that bleeds when stripped; bleeding from a true membrane occurs when the conjunctival stromal vessels are ruptured when stripped
	Mucus excess	Increased amount of mucin relative to aqueous component of tears
	Papillae	Dilated, telangiectatic, conjunctival blood vessels surrounded by edema and a mixed inflammatory cell infiltrate
	Phlyctenule	Nodule consisting of chronic inflammatory cells, often at or near the limbus, and associated with neovascularization
	Pseudomembrane	Inflammatory coagulum on the conjunctival surface that has minimal bleeding during removal; bleeding from a pseudomembrane is more prevalent when there is significant hyperemia (see Video 11-1)
	Punctate epithelial erosion	Loss of individual epithelial cells in a stippled pattern
	Symblepharon	Subconjunctival scarring and fibrosis that often leads to shortening of the conjunctival fornices
Sclera	Episcleritis	Focal or diffuse dilation of radial superficial episcleral vessels
	Necrotizing scleritis	Area of avascular scleral erosion
	Nonnecrotizing scleritis	Dilated deep episcleral vessels with scleral edema

Table 3-1 *(continued)*

Tissue	Finding	Description
Cornea	Bulla	Fluid pocket within or under the epithelium
	Dendrite	Branching linear epithelial ridge with swollen cells, terminal bulbs, and possible central ulceration
	Epithelial defect	Focal area of epithelial loss, caused by trauma (abrasion) or other condition
	Epithelial edema	Swollen epithelial cells (intraepithelial edema) or intercellular vacuoles (microcystic edema)
	Filament	A single strand or clump (mucous plaque) of mucus and degenerating epithelial cells attached to an altered ocular surface
	Nonsuppurative stromal keratitis	Focal gray-white infiltrate of lymphocytes and other mononuclear cells; also called *interstitial keratitis,* especially when accompanied by stromal neovascularization
	Punctate epithelial erosion	Fine, slightly depressed stippling caused by altered or desquamated superficial epithelial cells that stain positively with fluorescein dye
	Punctate epithelial keratitis	Swollen, slightly raised epithelial cells that can be finely scattered, coarsely grouped, or arranged in an arborescent pattern that stain negatively with fluorescein dye
	Subepithelial infiltrate	Coin-shaped (nummular) inflammatory opacity in the anterior portion of Bowman layer
	Suppurative stromal keratitis	Focal yellow-white infiltrate of neutrophils
	Ulcer	Epithelial defect, stromal loss, stromal inflammation, or any combination of these changes

An acute, mild papillary reaction produces a smooth, velvety appearance (Fig 3-2A). Chronic changes result in enlarged vascular tufts that appear as elevated, polygonal, hyperemic mounds (Fig 3-2B). Each papilla has a central red dot that represents a dilated central capillary core viewed end-on.

Prolonged, recurrent, or severe conjunctival inflammation causes the anchoring fibers of the tarsal conjunctiva to stretch and weaken, leading to confluent papillary hypertrophy. *Giant papillae* are defined as those with a diameter greater than 0.3 mm (Fig 3-2C). Furrows between these enlarged fibrovascular structures collect mucus and purulent material. Following treatment, a fibrotic subepithelial scar may be seen at the apex of former giant papillae (Fig 3-2D).

Follicles Conjunctival lymphoid tissue is normally present within the substantia propria except in neonates, who do not have visible follicles. Conjunctival follicles are round or oval clusters of lymphocytes (Fig 3-3). Small follicles are often visible in the lower fornix. Clusters of enlarged, noninflamed follicles are occasionally seen in the forniceal or inferior palpebral conjunctiva of children and adolescents, a condition known as *benign lymphoid folliculosis* (Fig 3-4).

Follicular conjunctivitis is characterized by the following:

- conjunctival injection
- presence of new or enlarged follicles (Fig 3-5)

Table 3-2 Conjunctival Findings and Associated Differential Diagnoses

Finding	Typical Ocular or Systemic Conditions
Cicatrization	Chemical injury Chronic conjunctivitis Mucous membrane pemphigoid Prior epidemic keratoconjunctivitis Stevens-Johnson syndrome Trachoma
Erosion or ulceration	Factitious conjunctivitis Graft-vs-host disease Mechanical or chemical trauma Mucous membrane pemphigoid Stevens-Johnson syndrome
Follicular conjunctivitis	Adenovirus conjunctivitis Benign lymphoid folliculosis Chlamydial conjunctivitis Drug-induced conjunctivitis (eg, from brimonidine) Herpes simplex virus conjunctivitis Molluscum contagiosum blepharoconjunctivitis
Granuloma	Cat-scratch disease Foreign-body reaction Ligneous conjunctivitis Sarcoidosis
Papillary conjunctivitis	Allergic conjunctivitis Bacterial conjunctivitis Giant papillary conjunctivitis (contact lens–related)
Pseudomembrane or membrane	Chemical burn Severe viral or bacterial conjunctivitis Stevens-Johnson syndrome

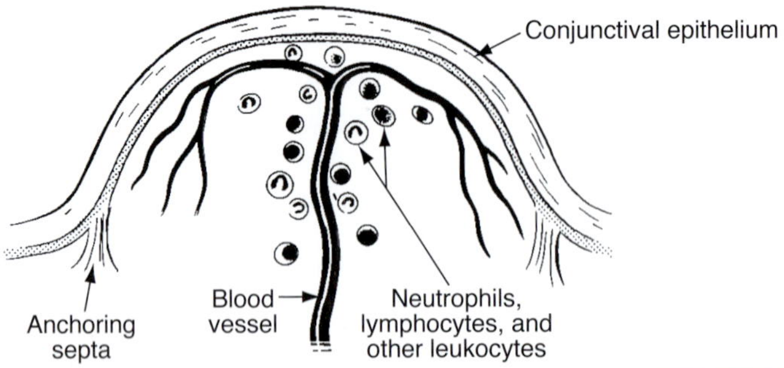

Figure 3-1 Cross-sectional diagram of a conjunctival papilla with a central vascular tuft surrounded by acute and chronic leukocytes.

- vessels that surround the raised surface of follicles but are not visible within the follicle
- follicles typically seen in the palpebral conjunctiva and, less often, on the bulbar or limbal conjunctiva

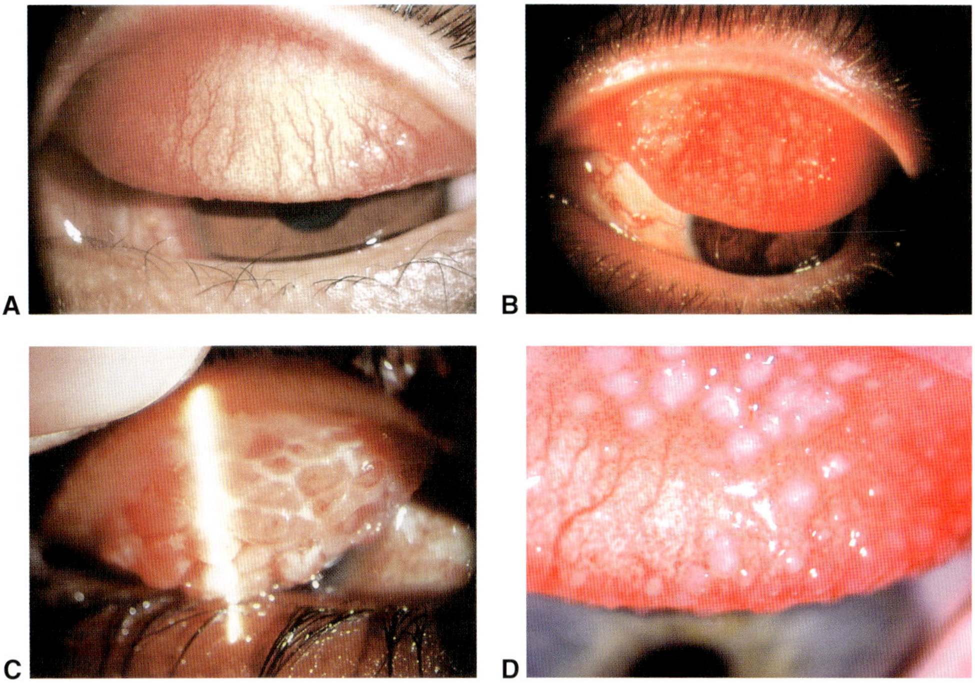

Figure 3-2 Papillary conjunctivitis. **A,** Mild papillae. **B,** Moderate papillae. **C,** Marked (giant) papillae. **D,** Fibrosis seen with moderate papillae. *(Part D courtesy of Joseph D. Iuorno, MD.)*

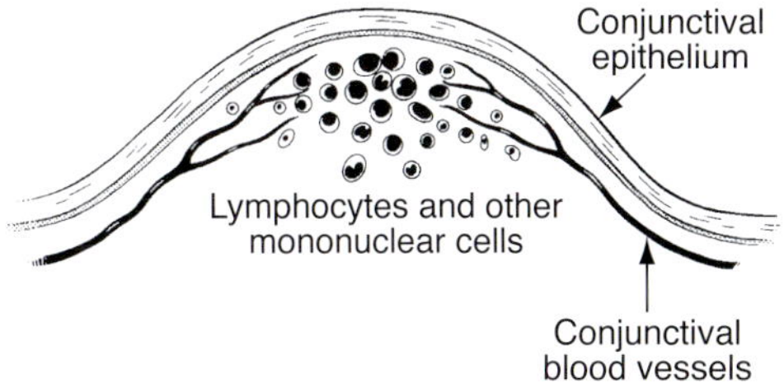

Figure 3-3 Cross-sectional diagram of a conjunctival follicle with mononuclear cells obscuring conjunctival blood vessels.

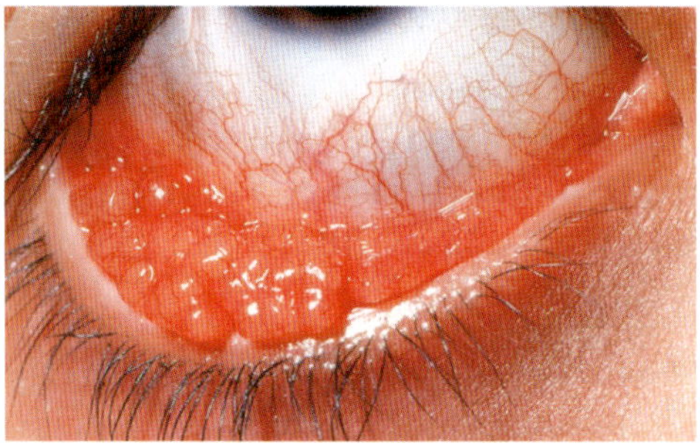

Figure 3-4 Benign lymphoid folliculosis. *(Courtesy of Kirk R. Wilhelmus, MD.)*

Follicular conjunctivitis must be differentiated from cysts produced by tubular epithelial infoldings associated with chronic inflammation and lymphangiectasis.

See also BCSC Section 4, *Ophthalmic Pathology and Intraocular Tumors.*

American Academy of Ophthalmology Cornea/External Disease Committee, Hoskins Center for Quality Eye Care. Preferred Practice Pattern Guidelines. *Conjunctivitis.* American Academy of Ophthalmology; 2018. www.aao.org/ppp

Stern G. Chronic conjunctivitis, Parts 1–2. *Focal Points: Clinical Modules for Ophthalmologists.* American Academy of Ophthalmology; 2012, modules 11–12.

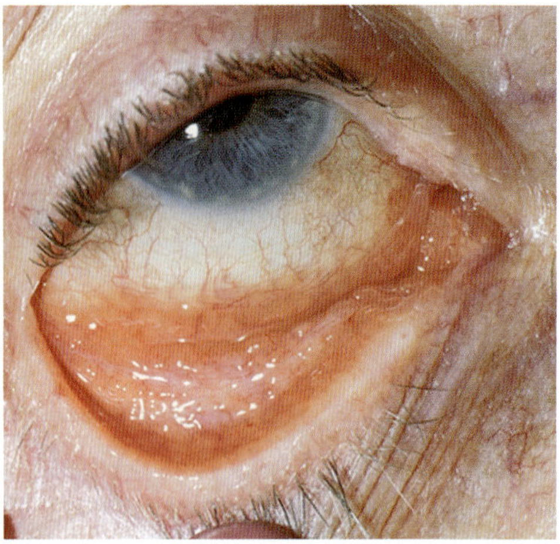

Figure 3-5 Follicular conjunctivitis of the inferior palpebral conjunctiva and fornix. *(Courtesy of John E. Sutphin, MD.)*

Corneal Signs of Inflammation

Table 3-3 lists corneal findings associated with inflammation, as well as common conditions to consider in the differential diagnosis.

The pattern of corneal inflammation, or *keratitis,* can be described by the following:

- *distribution:* diffuse, focal, or multifocal
- *depth:* epithelial, subepithelial, anterior stromal, deep stromal, or endothelial
- *location:* central, paracentral, or peripheral
- *shape:* dendritic, disciform, or geographic

Epithelial inflammation Punctate epithelial keratitis (PEK) is a nonspecific term that encompasses a spectrum of biomicroscopic changes, which include inflammatory changes; punctate epithelial erosions (Fig 3-6A) that stain positively with fluorescein; punctate epithelial granularity (Fig 3-6B), associated with negative fluorescein staining, as seen in Thygeson epithelial keratitis; and the "stuck on" appearance of the lesions seen in herpes zoster keratitis (Fig 3-6C).

Stromal inflammation Stromal inflammation occurs when inflammatory cells enter the cornea stroma from the tear film, through an epithelial defect and/or direct interlamellar infiltration at the limbus (eg, after laser in situ keratomileusis [LASIK]). In the presence of endothelial injury, inflammatory cells can also enter the stroma from the aqueous humor. In a vascularized cornea, inflammatory cells can enter the stroma directly from infiltrating blood and lymphatic vessels.

Stromal inflammation is characterized by the following:

- *degree of inflammation:* suppurative or nonsuppurative (Fig 3-7)
- *distribution:* focal or multifocal
- *location:* central, paracentral, or peripheral
- *depth:* subepithelial, anterior, or deep stromal

Stromal inflammation can lead to opacification. Altered stromal keratocytes make new collagen fibers that are disorganized, scatter light, and cause scarring that can incorporate

Table 3-3 Corneal Findings and Associated Differential Diagnoses

Finding	Typical Ocular Conditions
Endothelial keratitis	Keratoplasty immune rejection Herpes simplex virus endothelial keratitis Varicella-zoster virus endothelial keratitis
Peripheral keratitis	Blepharitis-associated marginal infiltrates Mooren ulcer Peripheral ulcerative keratitis associated with autoimmune disease
Punctate epithelial erosions	Atopic keratoconjunctivitis Dry eye Toxic reaction
Punctate epithelial keratitis	Adenovirus keratoconjunctivitis Herpes simplex virus epithelial keratitis Herpes zoster virus epithelial keratitis Thygeson superficial punctate keratitis
Stromal keratitis, nonsuppurative	Acanthamoeba keratitis Adenoviral keratoconjunctivitis Cogan syndrome Herpes simplex virus stromal keratitis Varicella-zoster virus stromal keratitis Lyme disease Leprosy (Hansen disease) Onchocerciasis Rheumatoid arthritis or other collagen vascular diseases Stromal graft rejection Syphilitic interstitial keratitis Tuberculosis
Stromal keratitis, suppurative	Bacterial keratitis Fungal keratitis Anesthetic abuse Retained foreign body

calcium complexes, lipids, and proteinaceous material. Dark pigmentation of a residual corneal opacity is often a result of incorporated melanin or iron salts. Stromal inflammation can also lead to neovascularization. Subepithelial fibrous within the peripheral cornea is called *pannus* or *vascularized pannus* (Fig 3-8). Neovascularization may invade the cornea at deeper levels, depending on the nature and location of the inflammatory stimulus.

Endothelial inflammation Endothelial inflammation results in dysfunction that can lead to reversible or irreversible endothelial decompensation, which can result in epithelial and stromal edema. Swollen endothelial cells called *inflammatory pseudoguttae* are visible on specular reflection as dark areas of the normal endothelial mosaic pattern. *Keratic precipitates (KPs)* are clumps of inflammatory cells that adhere to the back of the cornea and come from leakage of the iris vasculature during the course of keratitis or uveitis. The clinical appearance of typical KPs depends on their composition:

- Fibrin and proteins coagulate into small dots and strands.

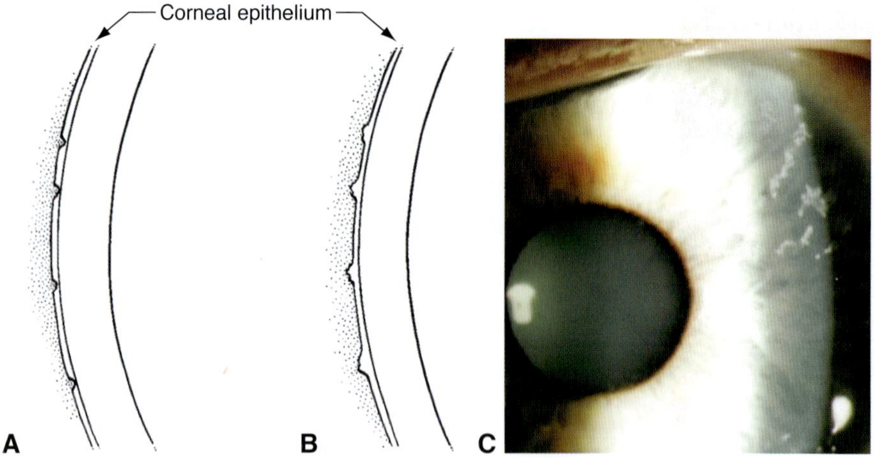

Figure 3-6 Punctate lesions of the corneal epithelium. **A,** Illustration of punctate epithelial erosions. **B,** Illustration of punctate epithelial keratitis. **C,** Clinical photo of the stuck-on lesions typical of epithelial keratitis in herpes zoster keratitis. *(Part C courtesy of Robert S. Feder, MD.)*

- Neutrophils and lymphocytes aggregate into punctate, round, or stellate opacities.
- Macrophages form larger "mutton-fat" clumps.

KPs and focal stromal edema are seen in both disciform keratitis associated with herpes zoster and simplex and in endothelial graft rejection. An inflammatory plaque of fibrin and debris on the endothelium can be seen in eyes with fungal keratitis and may indicate spread of infection through Descemet membrane.

Ciralsky J, Lai E, Waring GO III, Bouchard CS. A matrix of pathologic responses in the cornea. In: Mannis MJ, Holland EJ, eds. *Cornea.* Vol 1. 4th ed. Elsevier; 2017:46–71.

Clinical Approach to Dry Eye

Dry eye is defined as a multifactorial disease of the ocular surface characterized by a loss of homeostasis of the tear film that is accompanied by ocular discomfort and/or blurred vision. Tear film instability and hyperosmolarity, ocular surface inflammation and damage, and neurosensory abnormalities play etiological roles in this disease.

Dry eye results from disturbance of the lacrimal functional unit, an integrated system comprising the lacrimal glands, ocular surface (cornea, conjunctiva, and limbus), and eyelids, as well as the sensory and motor nerves connecting these components. See Chapter 1 for a discussion and illustration of the lacrimal functional unit.

Worldwide dry eye demographics include the following:

- increasing prevalence with age (10% of individuals aged 30–60 and 15% of adults older than 65 years)
- higher prevalence among women
- no racial or ethnic predisposition

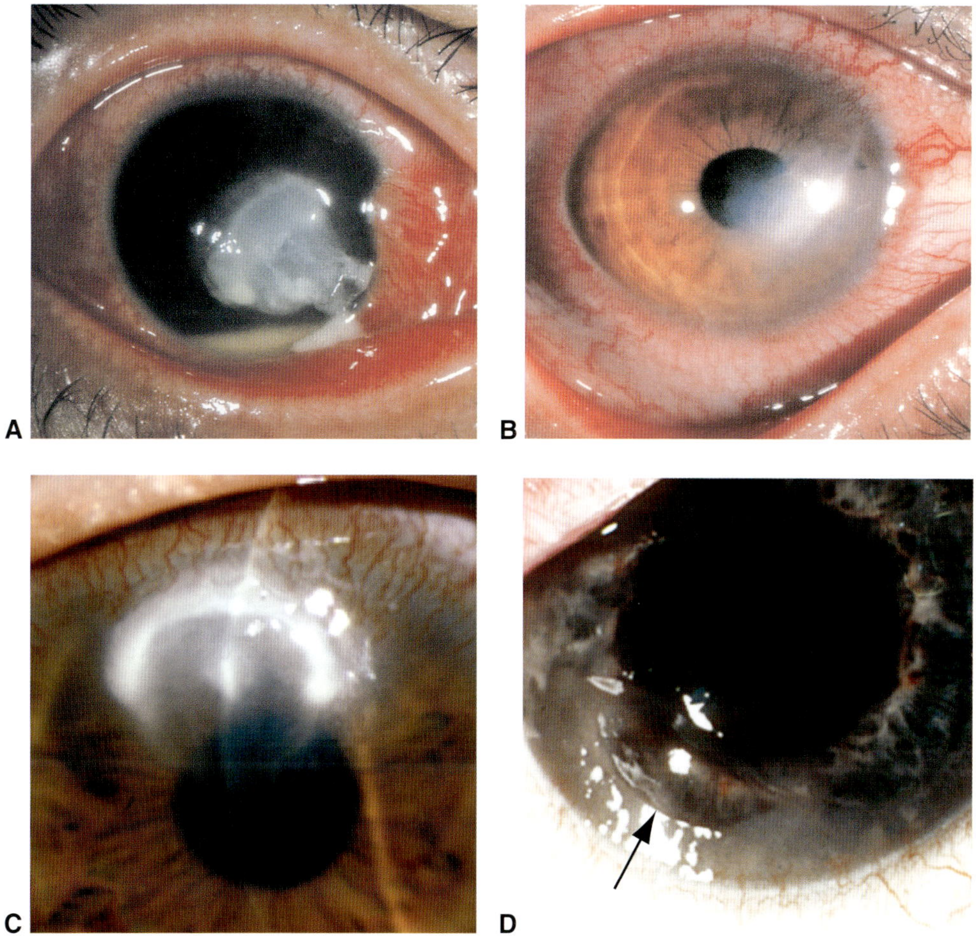

Figure 3-7 Inflammation of the corneal stroma. **A,** Suppurative keratitis. **B,** Nonsuppurative, nonnecrotizing (disciform) stromal keratitis. **C,** Immune ring. **D,** Peripheral ulcerative keratitis. An ovoid area of thinning *(arrow)* can be seen in the inferonasal quadrant. *(Parts C and D courtesy of Robert S. Feder, MD.)*

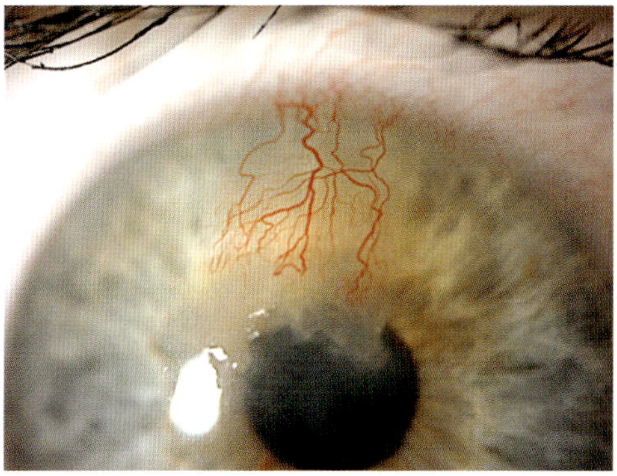

Figure 3-8 Corneal pannus. *(Courtesy of Danielle Trief, MD.)*

Table 3-4 Risk Factors for Dry Eye Disease

	Consistent [a]	Probable [b]	Inconclusive [c]
Nonmodifiable	Aging Female sex Asian race Meibomian gland dysfunction Connective tissue diseases Sjögren syndrome	Diabetes Rosacea Viral infection Thyroid disease Psychiatric conditions Pterygium	Hispanic ethnicity Menopause Acne Sarcoidosis
Modifiable	Androgen deficiency Computer use Contact lens wear Hormone replacement therapy Hematopoietic stem cell transplantation Environment: Pollution, low humidity, sick building syndrome Medications: Antihistamines, antidepressants, anxiolytics, isotretinoin	Low fatty acids intake Refractive surgery Allergic conjunctivitis Medications: Anticholinergic medications, β-blockers, diuretics	Smoking Alcohol Pregnancy Demodex infestation Botulinum toxin injection Medications: Multivitamins, oral contraceptives

[a] Consistent evidence implies the existence of at least 1 adequately powered and otherwise well-conducted study published in a peer-reviewed journal, along with the existence of a plausible biological rationale and corroborating basic research or clinical data.

[b] Suggestive evidence implies the existence of either inconclusive information from peer-reviewed publications or inconclusive or limited information to support the association, but either not published or published somewhere other than in a peer-reviewed journal.

[c] Inconclusive evidence implies either directly conflicting information in peer-reviewed publications, or inconclusive information but with some basis for a biological rationale.

Modified with permission from Stapleton F, Alves M, Bunya VY, et al. TFOS DEWS II Epidemiology Report. *Ocul Surf.* 2017;15(3):350.

Table 3-4 lists the risk factors associated with dry eye disease.

Dry eye is one of the most common reasons for ophthalmic office visits. Patients who develop psychological problems associated with this potentially highly symptomatic, chronic disease can require considerable support. Organizations such as the Sjögren's Foundation (www.sjogrens.org) can provide valuable resources for these patients. For certain patients, consultation with physicians who specialize in pain management and/or psychiatry can be very helpful.

CLINICAL PEARL

Results of quality-of-life studies have shown that the impact of moderate to severe dry eye is similar to that of moderate to severe angina.

Craig JP, Nichols KK, Akpek EK, et al. TFOS DEWS II Definition and Classification Report. *Ocul Surf.* 2017;15(3):276–283.

Schiffman RM, Walt JG, Jacobsen G, et al. Utility assessment among patients with dry eye disease. *Ophthalmology.* 2003;110(7):1412–1419.

Stapleton F, Alves M, Bunya VY, et al. TFOS DEWS II Epidemiology Report. *Ocul Surf.* 2017;15(3):334–365.

Mechanisms of Dry Eye

As mentioned, dry eye is a multifactorial disease. Tear hyperosmolarity stresses the surface epithelium, leading to the release of inflammatory mediators that disrupt the junctions between the superficial epithelial cells. T cells can infiltrate the epithelium and produce pro-inflammatory cytokines such as tumor necrosis factor-alpha (TNF-α) and interleukin 1 (IL-1). These cytokines promote accelerated detachment of the epithelial cells and apoptosis (programmed cell death), which results in further disruption of intercellular junctions and influx of inflammatory cells, creating a vicious cycle; this cycle is an important factor in the etiology of dry eye (Fig 3-9).

Dry eye can be divided into 2 major categories: aqueous tear deficiency (ATD) and evaporative dry eye (Fig 3-10). Patients may have elements of both conditions. In patients with ATD, T-cell–mediated inflammation of the lacrimal gland occurs, leading to diminished tear

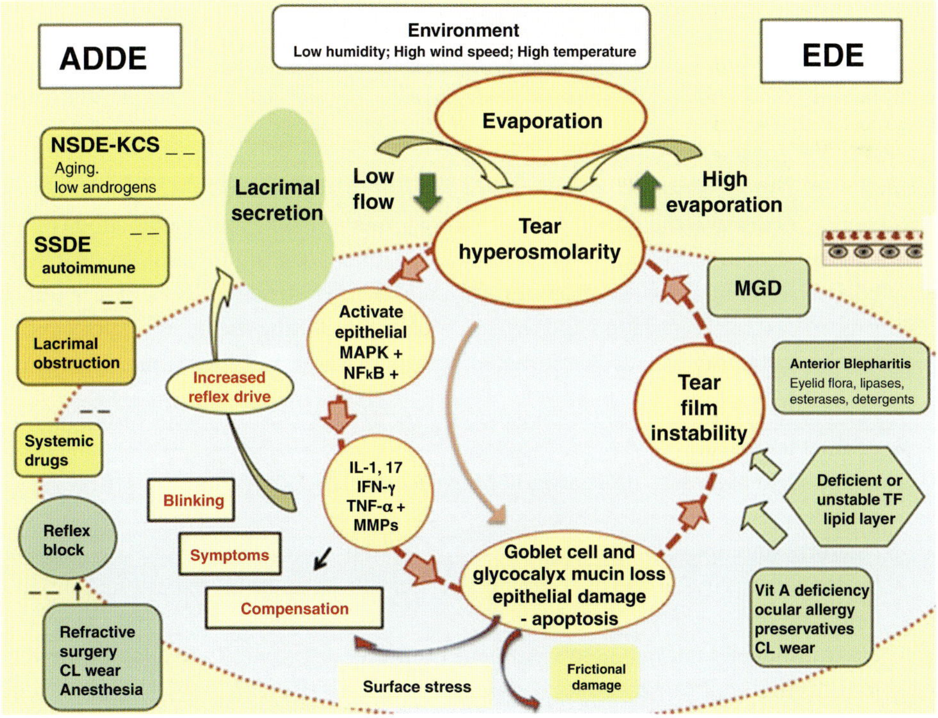

Figure 3-9 Inflammatory mediators in dry eye. ADDE = aqueous deficient dry eye; CL = contact lens; EDE = evaporative dry eye; IFN-γ = interferon gamma; IL-1, 17 = interleukins 1 and 17; KCS = keratoconjunctivitis sicca; MAPK = mitogen-activated protein kinase; MGD = meibomian gland dysfunction; MMPs = matrix metalloproteinases; NFκB = nuclear factor kappa-light-chain-enhancer of activated B cells; NSDE = Non-Sjögren dry eye; SSDE = Sjögren syndrome dry eye; TNF-α = tumor necrosis factor alpha; TF = tear film. *(Modified with permission from Craig JP, Nelson JD, Azar DT, et al. TFOS DEWS II Report executive summary.* Ocul Surf. *2017;15(4):802–812. With permission from Elsevier.)*

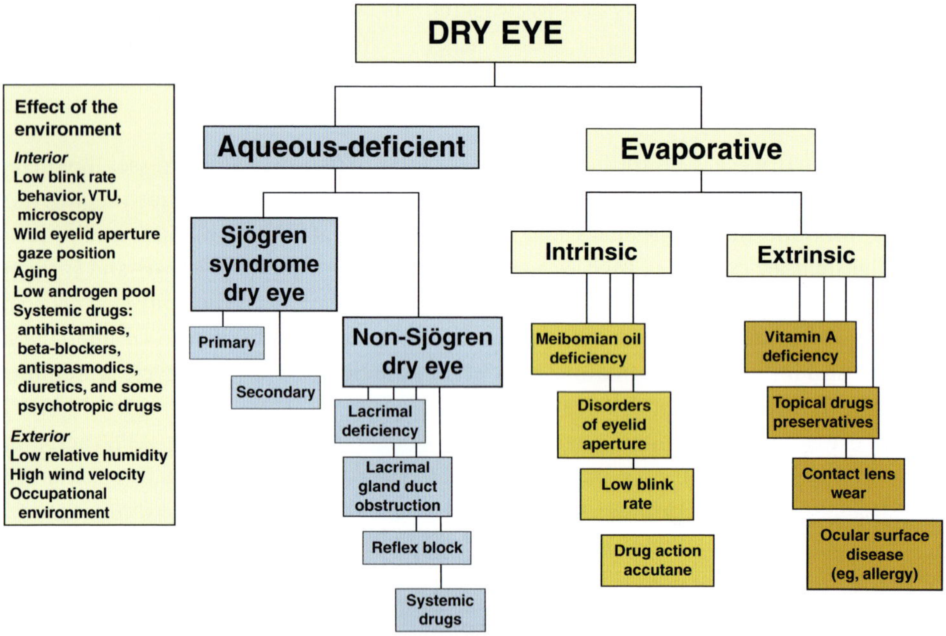

Figure 3-10 Diagnostic classification for dry eye disorders. *(Modified with permission from Craig JP, Nichols KK, Akpek EK, et al. TFOS DEWS II Definition and Classification Report.* Ocul Surf. *2017;15(3):276–283. With permission from Elsevier.)*

production and propagation of inflammatory mediators on the ocular surface. In patients with evaporative dry eye, the primary abnormality is meibomian gland dysfunction (MGD), in which altered lipid metabolism of the meibum causes a transition from unsaturated to saturated fats, resulting in obstruction of the glands. This obstruction leads to tear film instability as well as tear evaporation and hyperosmolarity, initiating the inflammatory cycle.

Tear film instability can also be initiated by other conditions, including

- ocular allergy
- contact lens wear
- a high ratio of dietary omega-6 to omega-3 essential fatty acids
- diabetes
- cigarette smoking
- prolonged driving or use of computers (especially in upgaze), cell phones, or handheld tablets
- environmental factors (eg, low ambient humidity or proximity to a fan or air vent)
- long-term use of preserved topical ocular medications
- xerophthalmia

Epithelial injury stimulates corneal nerve endings, resulting in symptoms such as ocular discomfort, increased blinking, and compensatory reflex lacrimal tear secretion. Loss of normal mucins on the ocular surface contributes to these symptoms by increasing frictional resistance between the eyelids and globe. During this period of abnormal corneal nerve stimulation, the high reflex input may cause neurogenic inflammation within the lacrimal gland.

Tear delivery may be obstructed by cicatricial conjunctival scarring or reduced by a reduction in the sensory reflex drive to the lacrimal gland (eg, following LASIK and photorefractive keratectomy), long-term contact lens wear, or chronic use of topical anesthetics.

American Academy of Ophthalmology Cornea/External Disease Committee, Hoskins Center for Quality Eye Care. Preferred Practice Pattern Guidelines. *Dry Eye Syndrome.* American Academy of Ophthalmology; 2018. www.aao.org/ppp

Bohm KJ, Djalilian AR, Pflugfelder SC, Starr CE. Dry eye. In: Mannis MJ, Holland EJ, eds. *Cornea.* Vol 1. 4th ed. Elsevier; 2017:377–396.

Bron AJ, de Paiva CS, Chauhan SK, et al. TFOS DEWS II pathophysiology report. *Ocul Surf.* 2017;15(3):438–510.

Nichols KK, Foulks GN, Bron AJ, et al. The International Workshop on Meibomian Gland Dysfunction: Executive Summary. *Invest Ophthalmol Vis Sci.* 2011;52(4):1922–1929.

Pflugfelder SC. Tear dysfunction and the cornea: LXVIII Edward Jackson Memorial Lecture. *Am J Ophthalmol.* 2011;152(6):900–909.

Stevenson W, Chauhan SK, Dana R. Dry eye disease: an immune-mediated ocular surface disorder. *Arch Ophthalmol.* 2012;130(1):90–100.

Aqueous Tear Deficiency

Symptoms and characteristics of ATD

- include burning, itching, dry sensation, or gritty or sandy irritation
- include sticky discharge
- include photophobia
- include blurred vision that may improve with blinking
- worsen as the day goes on
- worsen with sustained vision tasks
- worsen with environmental exposure to wind or low humidity

CLINICAL PEARL

Mucous discharge is common in patients with moderate to severe ATD and in those with infectious conjunctivitis; consequently, ATD can be misdiagnosed as infectious conjunctivitis. Similarly, symptoms of itching can lead to the misdiagnosis of allergic conjunctivitis.

The clinical presentation of ATD ranges from mild ocular irritation with minimal ocular surface disease to severe and disabling disease. Clinical signs of ATD include

- bulbar injection
- decreased tear meniscus
- an irregular corneal surface
- debris and/or mucus in the tear film
- punctate keratopathy
- filamentary keratitis

Diagnosis The volume of tear production can be evaluated by the Schirmer test, which can be conducted with or without topical anesthesia. Topical anesthesia decreases the amount of reflex tearing. A reading of greater than 10 mm of wetting is considered to be normal, whereas a reading of less than 5 mm is considered abnormal and consistent with ATD. The tear breakup time (TBUT) test helps to assess the quality and stability of the tear film. A rapid TBUT of less than 10 seconds is consistent with rapid image degradation.

SLIT-LAMP EXAMINATION Examination at the slit lamp may reveal a reduced inferior tear meniscus (which is normally 1.0 mm in height). Epithelial keratopathy, which can be fine and granular, coarse, or confluent, is best demonstrated following the instillation of fluorescein, rose bengal, or lissamine green dye. Rose bengal and lissamine green staining (Fig 3-11) can be more sensitive than fluorescein because these dyes stain devitalized epithelium rather than areas of absent epithelium. It is important to evaluate the entire surface, not simply the cornea. Lissamine green is particularly helpful for evaluating the conjunctiva; the staining may be seen at the nasal and temporal limbus, the inferior paracentral or midperipheral cornea *(exposure staining)*, and/or within the intrapalpebral conjunctiva (Fig 3-12).

Filaments (strands of degenerating epithelial cells attached to the corneal surface over a core of mucus), as well as mucous plaques, may be seen in patients with severe ATD. Filamentary keratopathy can be quite painful, because these strands are firmly attached to the richly innervated surface epithelium and move with blinking (Fig 3-13). Marginal or paracentral corneal thinning and even perforation can occur in cases of severe dry eye. Incomplete blinking is frequently noted. Advanced disease may also involve calcium deposition or band keratopathy (see Chapter 7), particularly in association with certain topical medications (especially glaucoma medications), and keratinization of the cornea and conjunctiva. Table 3-5 presents a grading scheme for dry eye severity. See Chapter 2 for

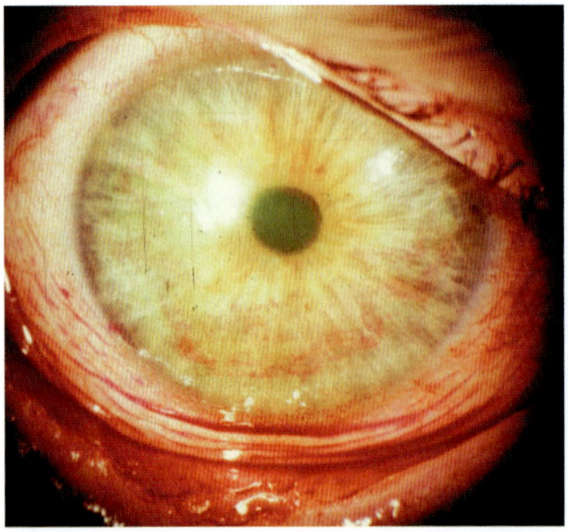

Figure 3-11 Rose bengal dye stains devitalized epithelial cells and is helpful in evaluating patients with dry eye. The dye can cause irritation; topical anesthetic should be considered. *(Courtesy of Robert S. Feder, MD.)*

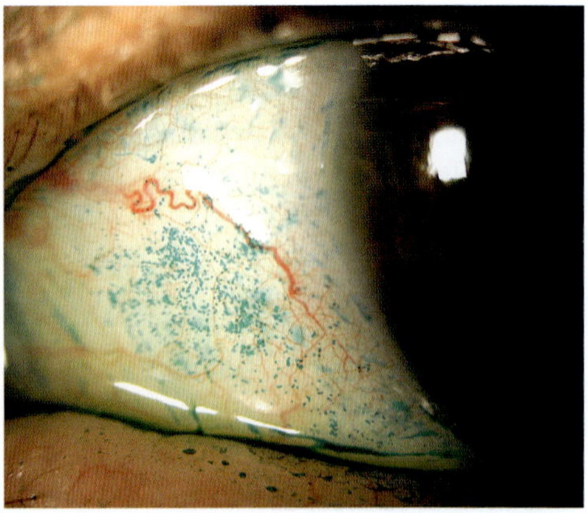

Figure 3-12 Photograph showing lissamine green staining of the nasal bulbar conjunctiva in the right eye of a patient with dry eye. This dye is particularly helpful in assessing the conjunctiva. *(Courtesy of Robert S. Feder, MD.)*

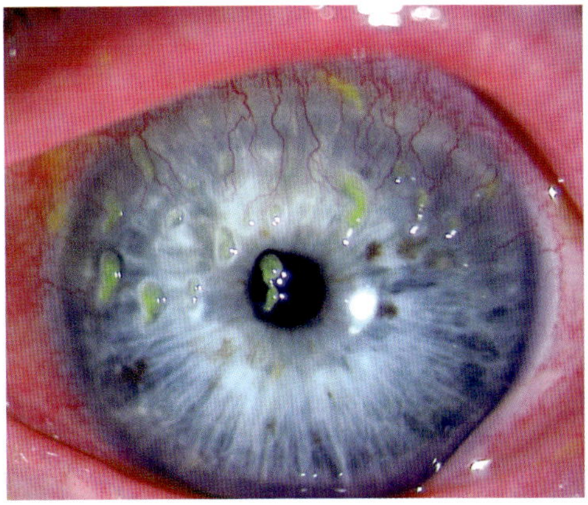

Figure 3-13 Filamentary keratitis in a vascularized cornea. *(Courtesy of Joseph D. Iuorno, MD.)*

Table 3-5 Dry Eye Severity Grading Scheme

Signs and Symptoms	Dry Eye Severity Level 1	2	3	4[a]
Discomfort, severity, and frequency	Mild and/or episodic; occurs under environmental stress	Moderate episodic or chronic, stress or no stress	Severe frequent or constant without stress	Severe and/or disabling and constant
Visual symptoms	None or episodic mild fatigue	Annoying and/ or activity-limiting, episodic	Annoying, chronic and/ or constant, limiting activity	Constant and/ or possibly disabling
Conjunctival injection	None to mild	None to mild	+/–	+/++
Conjunctival staining	None to mild	Variable	Moderate to marked	Marked
Corneal staining (severity/ location)	None to mild	Variable	Marked central	Severe punctate erosions
Corneal/tear signs	None to mild	Mild debris, ↓ tear meniscus	Filamentary keratitis, mucus clumping, ↑ tear debris	Filamentary keratitis, mucus clumping, ↑ tear debris, ulceration
Eyelid/ meibomian glands	MGD variably present	MGD variably present	MGD frequently present	Trichiasis, keratinization, symblepharon
TBUT (seconds)	Variable	≤10	≤5	Immediate
Schirmer score (mm wetting after 5 min)	Variable	≤10	≤5	≤2

MGD = meibomian gland dysfunction; TBUT = fluorescein tear break-up time; ↓ = reduced; ↑ = increased.
[a] Must have signs and symptoms.

Reprinted from The definition and classification of dry eye disease: report of the Definition and Classification Subcommittee of the International Dry Eye Workshop (2007). *Ocul Surf.* 2007;5(2):75–92. Copyright 2007. With permission from Elsevier.

a discussion on tear production evaluation and tear film quantitative tests. The American Academy of Ophthalmology's Preferred Practice Pattern guideline on dry eye syndrome referenced earlier in this chapter is a useful resource and has a complete list of diagnostic tests.

Sjögren syndrome

Patients with ATD are considered to have Sjögren syndrome if they have associated hypergammaglobulinemia, collagen vascular disease, or specific circulating autoantibodies (eg, SS-A, SS-B). It is estimated that Sjögren syndrome is present in 10% of patients with clinically significant ATD. The international classification criteria for Sjögren syndrome appear in Table 3-6. Although the precise causes of ATD in Sjögren syndrome are unknown, ATD is generally considered to be a T-cell–mediated inflammatory disease that

Table 3-6 Criteria for the Classification of Sjögren Syndrome

1. **Ocular symptoms**
   Definition: A positive response to at least 1 of the following 3 questions:
   a. Have you had daily, persistent, troublesome dry eyes for more than 3 months?
   b. Do you have a recurrent sensation of sand or gravel in the eyes?
   c. Do you use tear substitutes more than 3 times a day?
2. **Oral symptoms**
   Definition: A positive response to at least 1 of the following 3 questions:
   a. Have you had a daily feeling of dry mouth for more than 3 months?
   b. Have you had recurrent or persistently swollen salivary glands as an adult?
   c. Do you frequently drink liquids to aid in swallowing dry foods?
3. **Ocular signs**
   Definition: Objective evidence of ocular involvement, determined on the basis of a positive result on at least 1 of the following 2 tests:
   a. Schirmer I test (<5.5 mm after 5 minutes)
   b. Rose bengal score (>4 van Bijsterveld score)
4. **Histopathologic features**
   Definition: Focus score >1 on minor salivary gland biopsy (*focus* defined as a conglomeration of at least 50 mononuclear cells; *focus score* defined as the number of foci in 4 mm^2 of glandular tissue)
5. **Salivary gland involvement**
   Definition: Objective evidence of salivary gland involvement, determined on the basis of a positive result on at least 1 of the following 3 tests:
   a. Salivary scintigraphy: delayed uptake and/or secretion
   b. Parotid sialography: diffuse sialectasis without obstruction
   c. Unstimulated salivary flow (<1.5 mL in 15 minutes)
6. **Autoantibodies**
   Definition: Presence of at least 1 of the following serum autoantibodies:
   a. Antibodies to Ro/SS-A antigens
   b. Antibodies to La/SS-B antigens

Exclusion criteria: Preexisting lymphoma, acquired immunodeficiency syndrome, sarcoidosis, or chronic graft-vs-host disease; prior head and neck irradiation; hepatitis C; use of anticholinergic medications

Primary Sjögren syndrome: Presence of 4 of 6 items or presence of 3 of 4 objective criteria (items 3–6)

Secondary Sjögren syndrome: A combination of a positive response to item 1 or 2 plus a positive response to at least 2 items from among items 3, 4, and 5

Modified with permission from Vitali C, Bombardieri S, Jonnson R, et al; European Study Group on Classification Criteria for Sjögren's Syndrome. Classification criteria for Sjögren's syndrome: a revised version of the European criteria proposed by the American-European Consensus Group. *Ann Rheum Dis.* 2002;61(6):557. With permission from BMJ Publishing, Ltd.

leads to destruction of the lacrimal glands, in part by increasing the rate of apoptosis (programmed cell death). Involvement of the salivary glands is common in Sjögren syndrome, resulting in dry mouth and predisposing the patient to periodontal disease. Mucous membranes throughout the body (eg, vaginal, gastric, and respiratory mucosae) may also be affected, which can significantly impact quality of life.

Sjögren syndrome can be divided into 2 clinical subsets, primary and secondary. In primary Sjögren syndrome, patients either have ill-defined systemic immune dysfunction or lack any evidence of immune dysfunction or connective tissue disease. When compared with systemic lupus erythematosus and rheumatoid arthritis, primary Sjögren syndrome is associated with the highest risk of developing lymphoma.

CLINICAL PEARL

About 5% of patients with Sjögren syndrome develop some form of lymphoid malignancy; however, this risk appears to be cumulative with age.

In secondary Sjögren syndrome, patients have a well-defined, generalized connective tissue disease, most commonly rheumatoid arthritis; however, many other autoimmune and systemic diseases are associated with secondary Sjögren syndrome (Table 3-7).

Gomes JA, Azar DT, Baudouin C, et al. TFOS DEWS II iatrogenic report. *Ocul Surf.* 2017;15(3): 511–538.

Nishishinya MB, Pereda CA, Muñoz-Fernández S, et al. Identification of lymphoma predictors in patients with primary Sjögren's syndrome: a systematic literature review and meta-analysis. *Rheumatol Int.* 2015;35(1):17–26.

Voulgarelis M, Skopouli FN. Clinical, immunologic, and molecular factors predicting lymphoma development in Sjögren's syndrome patients. *Clin Rev Allergy Immunol.* 2007;32(3):265–274.

Zintzaras E, Voulgarelis M, Moutsopoulos HM. The risk of lymphoma development in autoimmune diseases: A meta-analysis. *Arch Intern Med.* 2005;165(20):2337–2344.

Evaporative Dry Eye

As mentioned, the primary abnormality associated with evaporative dry eye is meibomian gland dysfunction (MGD). According to the International Workshop on Meibomian Gland Dysfunction, MGD can be secondary to a hyposecretory state or obstructive disease. Obstructive MGD can be cicatricial (eg, trachoma, mucous membrane pemphigoid, or atopy) or noncicatricial (eg, seborrheic dermatitis, rosacea, or atopy). MGD is more common in people of Asian ethnicity than it is in White individuals.

Symptoms of evaporative dry eye, which are often worse in the morning, include

- burning
- foreign-body sensation
- redness of the eyelids
- conjunctival injection
- filmy vision

Table 3-7 Systemic Diseases and Other Conditions Associated With Dry Eye

Autoimmune disorders
- Primary Sjögren syndrome
- Secondary Sjögren syndrome associated with:
  - Rheumatoid arthritis
  - Systemic lupus erythematosus
  - Progressive systemic sclerosis (scleroderma)
  - Polymyositis and dermatomyositis
  - Primary biliary cirrhosis
- Graft-vs-host disease
- Immune reactions after radiation to head and neck

Infiltrative processes
- Amyloidosis
- Hemochromatosis
- Lymphoma
- Sarcoidosis

Infectious processes
- HIV-diffuse infiltrative lymphadenopathy syndrome
- Trachoma

Neuropathic dysfunction
- Alzheimer disease
- Cranial neuropathies (Bell palsy, vasculitis)
- Multiple sclerosis
- Parkinson disease

Endocrine dysfunction
- Androgen deficiency

Miscellaneous
- Adie syndrome
- Anhidrotic ectodermal dysplasia
- Congenital alacrima
- Familial dysautonomia (Riley-Day syndrome)
- Shy-Drager syndrome (idiopathic autonomic dysfunction with orthostatic hypotension and multiple system atrophy)

Clinical signs associated with this disease include

- seborrheic and eczematoid changes of the anterior eyelid margin and eyelid skin
- telangiectatic blood vessels and metaplasia of the eyelid margins
- pouting of the meibomian gland orifices
- foamy discharge of the posterior eyelid margin
- turbid, cheesy, or toothpaste-like meibomian secretions (Fig 3-14)
- posteriorly displaced meibomian gland orifices
- irregularity of the posterior eyelid margin

Occasionally, a patient is symptomatic but the meibomian glands appear normal. Compression of the lower eyelid reveals obstruction of the glands. More forceful expression produces a thin filamentous secretion, which is due to narrowing of the ducts, near the orifice. This condition has been described as nonobvious MGD (NOMGD) and is believed to be a precursor to clinically apparent disease. Gland expression can be performed using a cotton swab, a commercially available handheld device, or digital pressure with a finger (Video 3-1).

VIDEO 3-1 Meibomian gland expression following probing.
Courtesy of Frank W. Bowden III, MD.

Extensive atrophy of the meibomian gland acini may develop after years of inflammation from MGD, preventing expression of secretions with compression. Derangement of glandular architecture with shortening or tortuosity of the meibomian glands can be seen on transillumination of the everted eyelid using a muscle light or infrared photography (meibography) (see Chapter 2).

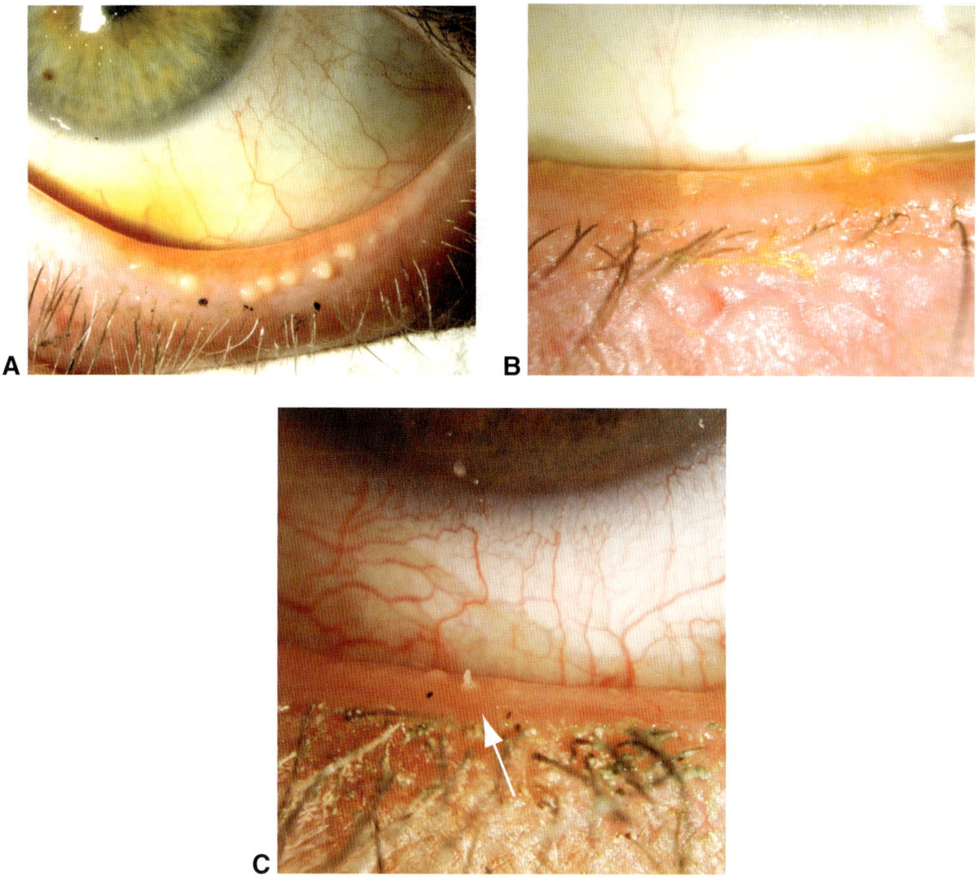

Figure 3-14 Meibomian gland dysfunction. **A,** Turbid, creamy expression of meibum after eyelid margin compression. **B,** Thickened, gelatinous, expression of meibum after eyelid margin compression. **C,** Toothpaste-like expression of meibum after eyelid margin compression. *(Part A courtesy of Arie L. Marcovich, MD, PhD; parts B and C courtesy of Gregg J. Berdy, MD.)*

In MGD, the stability of the tear film is disrupted, causing a rapid TBUT (ie, <10 seconds). See Chapter 2 for an explanation of the TBUT. In addition to the previously mentioned eyelid margin findings, which are found in evaporative dry eye and MGD, the following clinical signs are seen in MGD:

- papillary reaction on the inferior tarsus
- linear punctate fluorescein staining along the inferior cornea
- fine epithelial and subepithelial infiltrates in the midperipheral cornea
- corneal neovascularization or pannus
- corneal scarring or thinning

Patients with MGD frequently have acne rosacea, which is discussed later in this chapter. Corneal vascularization is more typical of MGD, while punctate staining is more typical of staphylococcal blepharitis.

American Academy of Ophthalmology Cornea/External Disease Committee. Preferred Practice Pattern Guidelines. *Blepharitis.* American Academy of Ophthalmology; 2018. www.aao.org/ppp

Bowden FW. Advances in the diagnoses and treatment of dry eye disease. *Focal Points: Clinical Practice Perspectives.* American Academy of Ophthalmology; 2020, module 8.

Foulks GN. Meibomian gland dysfunction. *Focal Points: Clinical Modules for Ophthalmologists.* American Academy of Ophthalmology; 2014, module 12.

Tomlinson A, Brom AJ, Korb DR, et al. The International Workshop on Meibomian Gland Dysfunction: Report of the Diagnosis Subcommittee. *Invest Ophthalmol Vis Sci.* 2011;52(4):2006–2049.

Treatment of Dry Eye

Before treatment of dry eye is initiated, it is important to carefully examine the eye to rule out structural and exogenous disorders that can cause symptoms similar to those of dry eye. Refer to the sidebar for examples of disorders that may cause dry eye–like symptoms. In addition, the clinician should inquire if the patient has any associated systemic conditions (see Table 3-7) or has used medications that can contribute to dry eye (Table 3-8). Medications with antihistaminic or anticholinergic properties increase dry eye symptoms. See the sidebar for disorders that can cause symptoms similar to dry eye.

Table 3-8 Medications That Decrease Tear Production

Anesthetics
Bisphosphonates
Enflurane
Halothane
Nitrous oxide

Antihypertensives
Clonidine
Diuretics, sometimes in combination with other antihypertensive drugs
Guanethidine, methyldopa
Prazosin
Propranolol
Reserpine

Antidepressants and psychotropic drugs
Amitriptyline, nortriptyline
Amoxapine, trimipramine
Clomipramine, desipramine, imipramine
Diazepam, nitrazepam
Doxepin
Phenelzine, tranylcypromine
Phenothiazines

Antihistamines

Antiulcer agents
Atropine-like agents
Metoclopramide, other drugs that decrease gastric motility

Cardiac antiarrhythmia drugs
Amiodarone
Disopyramide
Mexiletine

Decongestants (nonprescription cold remedies)
Ephedrine
Pseudoephedrine

Hormones
Androgen antagonists
Estrogen replacement

Muscle spasm medications
Cyclobenzaprine
Methocarbamol

Parkinson disease medications
Benztropine
Biperiden
Procyclidine
Trihexyphenidyl

DISORDERS THAT CAUSE SYMPTOMS SIMILAR TO DRY EYE

- Conjunctivochalasis
- Floppy eyelid syndrome
- Superior limbic keratoconjunctivitis
- Nighttime lagophthalmos
- Parkinson disease
- Mucous membrane pemphigoid

ATD and evaporative dry eye frequently coexist in ocular surface disease. The TFOS DEWS II (Tear Film and Ocular Surface Society Dry Eye Workshop II) diagnostic classification scheme presents a clinical decision algorithm that incorporates symptoms and signs of OSD that inform treatment protocols (Fig 3-15). Certain therapeutic interventions, such as artificial tear supplements, topical cyclosporine, topical lifitegrast, short pulses of topical corticosteroids, and omega-3 fatty acid supplements, can be helpful for both conditions. However, certain treatments for ATD may exacerbate evaporative dry eye. For example, punctal occlusion in the presence of active MGD increases the retention of the toxic meibum secretions. This therapy can be utilized once treatment of OSD inflammation is well under way.

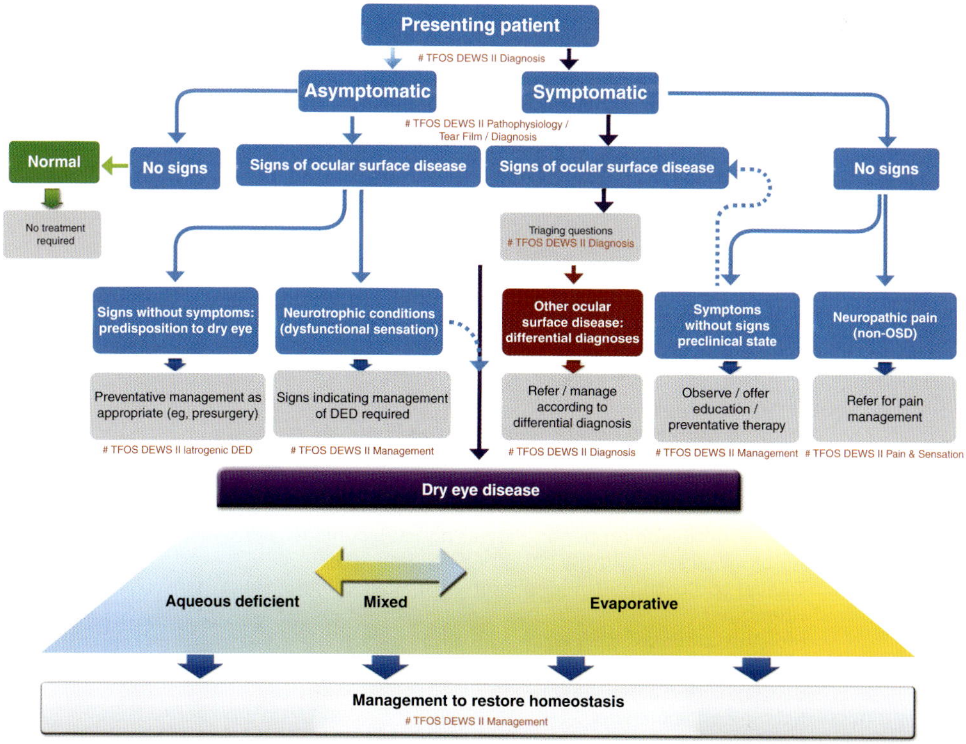

Figure 3-15 Classification scheme of dry eye disease, including symptoms and signs. DED = dry eye disease; OSD = ocular surface disease. *(Modified with permission from Craig JP, Nelson JD, Azar DT, et al. TFOS DEWS II Report executive summary.* Ocul Surf. *2017;15(4):802–812. With permission from Elsevier.)*

Medical management of aqueous tear deficiency

Selection of the treatment modalities for ATD depends on the severity of disease (Table 3-9). Because smoking is a risk factor for dry eye, advice should be given regarding cessation to patients who smoke. Also, it may be appropriate to modify the patient's environment to reduce evaporation of the tear film, for example, with a desktop humidifier or even moisture shields, which can be helpful in severe cases.

Changing or discontinuing topical or systemic medications that may contribute to ATD can be considered, although this is not always practical. Topical β-blockers have been associated with an increased incidence of dry eye, and many systemic medications (eg, diuretics, antihistamines, and anticholinergic and psychotropic drugs) decrease aqueous tear production and increase dry eye symptoms. These drugs should be avoided, if possible, in patients with symptoms of ATD (see Table 3-8).

Tear substitutes The mainstay of treatment for ATD is the use of tear substitutes (drops, gels, and ointments). Demulcents are polymers that can be added to artificial tear formulations to help improve lubricant properties; demulcent solutions have properties similar to mucomimetic agents, which can substitute for tear glycoproteins lost late in the disease process. However, demulcents alone cannot restore lost glycoproteins or conjunctival goblet cells, reduce corneal cell desquamation, or decrease tear film osmolarity. Liposomal sprays, applied to the closed eyelids by a sterile spray mechanism, may help support the tear film. Hydroxypropyl cellulose inserts are occasionally helpful for patients unable to instill artificial tears frequently.

Table 3-9 Therapeutic Options for Aqueous Tear Deficiency

Severity of ATD	Therapeutic Options
Mild	Tear substitutes with preservatives up to 4 times daily Lubricating ointment at bedtime Hot compresses and eyelid massage/compression
Moderate	Tear substitutes without preservatives 4 times daily to hourly Lubricating ointment at bedtime Topical anti-inflammatory treatment (cyclosporine A 0.05% or 0.09% twice daily or lifitegrast 5% twice daily) Omega-3 supplement [a] Reversible punctal occlusion (plugs), lower puncta Systemic immunosuppression if ATD is associated with inflammatory connective tissue disease
Severe	All of the above, plus 1 or more of the following: Punctal occlusion (upper and lower puncta); consider permanent occlusion Autologous serum drops (20–50%) 4–8 times daily Topical corticosteroids (nonpreserved if available) on a short-term basis Humidifier Moisture chamber glasses Tarsorrhaphy (lateral and/or medial) Bandage contact lenses (rarely) Scleral contact lenses Systemic cholinergic agonist (eg, pilocarpine; in rare cases)

ATD = aqueous tear deficiency.

[a] Benefits of omega-3 supplementation are controversial.

CLINICAL PEARL

Preservative-free tear substitutes are recommended for use in all patients to avoid the toxic effects of preservatives that can occur with dosing more than 4 times daily.

Topical anti-inflammatory agents In patients with ATD, topical anti-inflammatory agents offer significant benefit in controlling the associated inflammation in the ocular surface, and their use is typically initiated early in the course of disease. Topical cyclosporine A 0.05% and 0.09% address the inflammatory component of moderate to severe ATD. Therapy is often initiated in combination with a short course of topical corticosteroids to provide an initial reduction in surface inflammation. Patients should be advised that stinging upon instillation is possible, and further it may take several weeks to months of use before they obtain symptomatic relief.

Topical lifitegrast 5% may inhibit the migration and activation of T-cells and the subsequent release of inflammatory cytokines. Patients may see results within 2 to 6 weeks of beginning treatment. Lifitegrast can cause mild irritation, transient blurred vision, and altered taste perception.

Autologous serum, hyaluronic acid, and hormonal therapies Other treatments that have been successful in patients with severe ATD include dilute solutions of autologous serum and hyaluronic acid. Autologous serum drops require blood drawn from the patient. The tubes are spun to separate the serum and are sent to a compounding pharmacy, which prepares a 20% to 50% solution for use by the patient. There are companies in the United States that facilitate specimen collection and then prepare and ship serum tears. In advanced dry eye disease, hormonal therapies such as topical 0.03% testosterone eyedrops and topical progesterone cream have been effective in reducing signs and improving symptoms.

Treatment of filamentary keratopathy Treating the filamentary keratopathy associated with severe ATD can be challenging. Filaments are debrided with a cotton swab moistened with topical anesthetic or a jeweler's forceps. Treatment directed at improving the tear film function may reduce the severity of recurrence. In addition to tear supplementation and punctal occlusion, topical acetylcysteine 10%, a mucolytic agent formulated by a compounding pharmacy, can further reduce filament formation. Although therapeutic bandage soft contact lenses (BSCLs) may help impede the formation of filaments, they are not typically used to reduce symptoms in patients with ATD because of the associated increased risk of infectious keratitis. Close observation is warranted in patients with ATD who wear BSCLs. In contrast, scleral contact lenses have been found to be quite helpful in patients with advanced dry eye symptoms.

Moisture chamber glasses In cases of severe ATD, the use of moisture chamber glasses (glasses or sunglasses incorporating a moisture shield or seal, or goggles) can decrease tear evaporation. Unfortunately, many affected patients may find this therapy cosmetically objectionable.

Pharmacologic stimulation and neurostimulation of tear secretion In more severe cases of dry eye, pharmacologic stimulation of tear secretion has been attempted with varying degrees of success. The cholinergic agonists pilocarpine and cevimeline hydrochloride stimulate muscarinic receptors present in salivary and lacrimal glands, thereby increasing secretion. Although studies have shown these agents to be effective in treating both xerostomia and dry eye in patients with Sjögren syndrome, they are approved by the US Food and Drug Administration (FDA) only for the treatment of xerostomia. It is uncertain whether these agents provide long-term benefits, and they are associated with significant adverse effects.

Neurostimulation of tear secretion was previously accomplished with a device called TrueTear (Allergan), which used electrical current to intranasally stimulate the nasolacrimal nerve, a branch of cranial nerve V. This device was quite costly but could be performed by the patient at home. However, the device is currently no longer available.

Dietary supplementation Supplementation with omega-3 fatty acids has been shown to increase average tear production and tear volume. Certain fish (eg, salmon, tuna, cod, flounder) and crustaceans (eg, shrimp, crab), flaxseed oil, dark leafy greens, and walnuts are rich in omega-3 fatty acids, which block proinflammatory eicosanoids and cytokines. Commercial preparations of oral omega-3 fatty acids are also available. The Dry Eye Assessment and Management (DREAM) Study compared patients who were given 3000 mg of omega-3 fatty acid supplementation to patients who were given a placebo, 5000 mg of olive oil. The results demonstrated no statistical difference between the 2 groups; both groups showed improvement in predetermined endpoints. A potentially confounding element in the study design was that subjects were able to continue and/or change other treatment modalities for dry eye during the duration of the study.

Asbell PA, Maguire MG, Peskin E, et al. Dry Eye Assessment and Management (DREAM) Study: Study design and baseline characteristics. *Contemp Clin Trials.* 2018;71:70–79.

Epitropoulos AT, Donnenfeld ED, Shah ZA, et al. Effect of oral re-esterified omega-3 nutritional supplementation on dry eyes. *Cornea.* 2016;35(9):1185–1191.

Kojima T, Higuchi A, Goto E, Matsumoto Y, Dogru M, Tsubota K. Autologous serum eye drops for the treatment of dry eye diseases. *Cornea.* 2008;27(Suppl 1):S25–S30.

Shtein RM, Shen JF, Kuo AN, Hammersmith KM, Li JY, Weikert MP. Autologous serum-based eye drops for treatment of ocular surface disease: A report by the American Academy of Ophthalmology. *Ophthalmology.* 2020;127(1):128–133.

Wojtowicz JC, Butovich I, Uchiyama E, Aronowicz J, Agee S, McCulley JP. Pilot, prospective, randomized, double-masked, placebo-controlled clinical trial of an omega-3 supplement for dry eye. *Cornea.* 2011;30(3):308–314.

Surgical management of aqueous tear deficiency

Surgical treatment is generally reserved for patients in whom medical treatment is either inadequate or impractical. Patients with moderate to severe ATD may benefit from punctal occlusion, which can be temporary, semipermanent, or permanent.

Reversible punctal occlusion Reversible punctal occlusion, which has varying degrees of effectiveness, can be performed by applying topical anesthesia, dilating the punctum, and inserting either a collagen or silicone punctal plug (Fig 3-16). Collagen plugs usually dissolve within days and do not provide complete canalicular occlusion. Intracanalicular

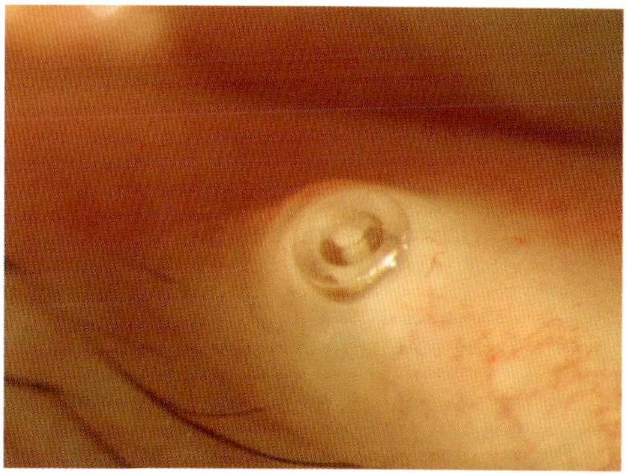

Figure 3-16 Silicone punctal plug. *(Courtesy of Robert S. Feder, MD.)*

plugs can be viewed by transillumination of the eyelid, enabling clinicians to monitor if they have dissolved, fallen out, or migrated. Both permanent and temporary intracanalicular plugs have been associated with infectious canaliculitis and sterile inflammation, which may require canaliculotomy and dacryocystorhinostomy.

Silicone plugs may remain in place for months or years unless they are undersized or are manually displaced. Some plugs have a small hole bored through the center to reduce the likelihood of epiphora. Most silicone plugs are continuously visible at the slit lamp, so it is readily apparent if they fall out or migrate into the canaliculus.

If inserted too forcefully, punctal plugs can be inadvertently inserted into the canaliculus and may require surgical removal. If a plug protrudes from the punctum, conjunctival irritation or abrasion may occur. If granuloma formation at the punctal opening occurs, removal of the plug and possible excision may be required.

Permanent punctal occlusion A disposable cautery, a hyfrecator, or a radiofrequency probe may be used to perform permanent punctal occlusion. Local anesthesia is typically required. Although the procedure is usually permanent, the canaliculus and puncta may subsequently reopen.

The value of punctal occlusion for patients with ocular surface disease other than tear deficiency is unproven. The procedure is recommended primarily for patients who have minimal basal tear secretion and punctate keratopathy but no significant ocular surface inflammation or infection.

Correction of eyelid malposition and tarsorrhaphy Another potentially beneficial treatment for patients with dry eye symptoms is correction of eyelid malposition (eg, entropion and ectropion). Reduction of the palpebral aperture by means of lateral and/or medial tarsorrhaphy can be performed in cases of severe keratoconjunctivitis sicca (KCS) when more conservative measures have failed. However, lateral tarsorrhaphy may limit the temporal visual field and produce an undesirable cosmetic deformity.

Marcet MM, Shtein RM, Bradley EA, et al. Safety and efficacy of lacrimal drainage system plugs for dry eye syndrome: A report by the American Academy of Ophthalmology. *Ophthalmology.* 2015;122(8):1681–1687.

Mazow ML, McCall T, Prager TC. Lodged intracanalicular plugs as a cause of lacrimal obstruction. *Ophthalmic Plast Reconstr Surg.* 2007;23(2):138–142.

Medical management of evaporative dry eye

Eyelid hygiene In the management of MGD, eyelid hygiene is an essential part at all stages of the disease; the goal is improving meibomian gland function and meibum quality (Tables 3-10 and 3-11). Application of warm compresses to the eyelids twice daily for 3–5 minutes liquefies thickened meibomian gland secretions and softens adherent crusts

Table 3-10 Clinical Summary of the MGD Staging Used to Guide Treatment

Stage	MGD Grade	Symptoms	Corneal Staining
1	+ (minimally altered expressibility and secretion quality)	None	None
2	++ (mildly altered expressibility and secretion quality)	Minimal to mild	None to limited
3	+++ (moderately altered expressibility and secretion quality)	Moderate	Mild to moderate; mainly peripheral
4	++++ (severely altered expressibility and secretion quality)	Marked	Marked; central in addition
"Plus" disease	Coexisting or accompanying disorders of the ocular surface and/or eyelids		

MGD = meibomian gland dysfunction.

Reproduced with permission from Nichols KK, Foulks GN, Bron AJ, et al. The International Workshop on Meibomian Gland Dysfunction: Executive Summary. *Invest Ophthalmol Vis Sci.* 2011;52(4):1922–1929.

Table 3-11 Treatment Algorithm for Meibomian Gland Dysfunction

Stage	Clinical Description	Treatment
1	No ***symptoms*** of ocular discomfort, itching, or photophobia ***Clinical signs*** of MGD based on gland expression: • Minimally altered secretions: grade ≥2 to 4 • Expressibility: 1 • No ocular surface ***staining***	*Inform* patient about MGD, the potential impact of diet, the effect of work/home environments on tear evaporation, and the possible drying effect of certain systemic medications *Consider* eyelid hygiene, including warming/expression as described below (±)
2	Minimal to mild ***symptoms*** of ocular discomfort, itching, or photophobia Minimal to mild MGD ***clinical signs:*** • Scattered eyelid margin features • Mildly altered secretions: grade ≥4 to <8 • Expressibility: 1 • None to limited ocular surface ***staining***: DEWS grade 0–7; Oxford grade 0–3 [a]	*Advise* patient on improving ambient humidity, optimizing workstations, and increasing dietary omega-3 fatty acid intake (±) *Institute* eyelid hygiene with eyelid warming (a minimum of 4 minutes, once or twice daily) followed by moderate to firm massage and expression of MG secretions (+) *All of the above, plus* (±) • Artificial lubricants (for frequent use, nonpreserved preferred) • Topical azithromycin • Topical emollient lubricant or liposomal spray • Consider oral tetracycline derivatives

Table 3-11 *(continued)*

Stage	Clinical Description	Treatment
3	Moderate ***symptoms*** of ocular discomfort, itching, or photophobia with limitation of activities Moderate MGD ***clinical signs:*** • ↑ Eyelid margin features: plugging, vascularity • Moderately altered secretions: grade ≥8 to <13 • Expressibility: 2 • Mild to moderate conjunctival and peripheral corneal ***staining,*** often inferior: DEWS grade 8–23; Oxford grade 4–10	*All of the above, plus* • Oral tetracycline derivatives (+) • Lubricant ointment at bedtime (±) • Anti-inflammatory therapy for dry eye as indicated (±)
4	Marked ***symptoms*** of ocular discomfort, itching, or photophobia with definite limitation of activities Severe MGD ***clinical signs:*** • ↑ Eyelid margin features: dropout, displacement • Severely altered secretions: grade ≥13 • Expressibility: 3 • Increased conjunctival and corneal ***staining,*** including central staining: DEWS grade 24–33; Oxford grade 11–15 • ↑ Signs of inflammation: ≥ moderate conjunctival hyperemia, phlyctenules	*All of the above, plus* • Anti-inflammatory therapy for dry eye (+)
"Plus" disease	Specific conditions occurring at any stage and requiring treatment. May be causal of or secondary to MGD, or may occur incidentally	
	1. Exacerbated inflammatory ocular surface disease 2. Mucosal keratinization 3. Phlyctenular keratitis 4. Trichiasis (eg, in cicatricial conjunctivitis, mucous membrane pemphigoid) 5. Chalazion 6. Anterior blepharitis 7. *Demodex*-related anterior blepharitis, with cylindrical dandruff	1. Pulsed soft steroid as indicated 2. Bandage contact lens/scleral contact lens 3. Steroid therapy 4. Epilation, electrolysis using radiofrequency 5. Intralesional steroid or excision 6. Topical antibiotic or antibiotic/steroid 7. Tea tree oil scrubs

DEWS = Dry Eye Workshop; MG = meibomian gland; MGD = meibomian gland dysfunction.

Meibum quality is assessed in each of eight glands of the central third of the lower eyelid on a scale of 0 to 3 for each gland: 0, clear; 1, cloudy; 2, cloudy with debris (granular); and 3, thick, like toothpaste (total score range, 0–24). *Expressibility* is assessed on a scale of 0 to 3 in five glands in the lower or upper eyelid, according to the number of glands expressible: 0, all glands; 1, three to four glands; 2, one to two glands; and 3, no glands. *Staining scores* are obtained by summing the scores of the exposed cornea and conjunctiva. Oxford staining score range, 1–15; DEWS staining score range, 0–33.

[a] Oxford grade: see Anthony.bron@eye.ex.ac.uk.

Modified with permission from Nichols KK, Foulks GN, Bron AJ, et al. The International Workshop on Meibomian Gland Dysfunction: Executive Summary. *Invest Ophthalmol Vis Sci.* 2011;52(4):1922–1929.

on the eyelid margins. The patient should be warned to avoid excessive or uneven heat if a microwave is used for the compress. The application of heat is followed by moderate-force, firm, and continuous (4-second hold) compression of the eyelid margin to express meibomian secretions. Compression can be followed by cleansing of the closed eyelid margin with a clean washcloth or a commercially available pad. A solution prepared by mixing a nonirritating shampoo and water, or commercially available solutions containing hypochlorous acid designed for this purpose may facilitate cleansing.

Topical antibiotic for eyelid disease Administered in short-term or pulsed, periodic use, topical antibiotics reduce the bacterial load on the eyelid margin. Topical azithromycin ophthalmic solution may be particularly efficacious, because it is a lipophilic antibiotic that reduces the production of bacterial lipases and improves the composition of meibomian lipids. The high viscosity of the drop prolongs the contact time and aids its penetration into the glands. Long-term use of topical antibiotics or subtherapeutic dosing can result in the development of resistant organisms; however, due to the high minimum inhibitory coefficient (MIC) value of azithromycin, this should not be expected.

Topical corticosteroids In cases with moderate to severe inflammation of the eyelids, topical corticosteroids may be required for short periods, particularly if corneal infiltrates and vascularization are present.

> **CLINICAL PEARL**
>
> Patients treated with topical corticosteroids should be warned about the potential complications associated with long-term use, including elevated intraocular pressure and cataract formation.

Dietary changes and omega-3 supplementation Patients with obstructive MGD may benefit from dietary changes and omega-3 supplementation. Several studies have found that omega-3 nutritional supplementation improved symptoms, tear film stability, and meibomian secretions. In one study, supplementation with fish oil showed no significant effect on meibum lipid composition or aqueous tear evaporation rate, but average tear production and tear volume increased. The DREAM study showed no benefit to the participants taking an omega-3 supplement over the control group.

Asbell PA, Maguire MG, Peskin E, et al. Dry Eye Assessment and Management (DREAM) Study: Study design and baseline characteristics. *Contemp Clin Trials.* 2018;71:70–79.

Epitropoulos AT, Donnenfeld ED, Shah ZA, et al. Effect of oral re-esterified omega-3 nutritional supplementation on dry eyes. *Cornea.* 2016;35(9):1185–1191.

Macsai MS. The role of omega-3 dietary supplementation in blepharitis and meibomian gland dysfunction. *Trans Am Ophthalmol Soc.* 2008;106:336–356.

Oral tetracycline Treatment with oral tetracyclines can be very effective; however, patients with MGD should be informed that therapy may only control their condition, not eliminate it. Because tetracycline should be taken on an empty stomach and requires more frequent dosing, doxycycline and minocycline are typically used. Doxycycline can be started at 50 mg twice daily and tapered to 50 mg daily. Larger doses are usually unnecessary, and lower doses are less likely to cause stomach upset. Minocycline is typically administered as 100 mg daily. Lower doses of both drugs may also be effective. A typical course is 4 to 6 weeks, but can be repeated, or continued for several months, to achieve long-term control. An alternative long-term approach is to use the medication for 3 weeks followed by 1 week off the medication, repeated monthly. Erythromycin can be used as alternative therapy in children or in patients with known hypersensitivity to tetracycline.

Adverse effects of oral tetracyclines include

- photosensitization, which can result in severe sunburn
- gastrointestinal upset
- azotemia in rare instances
- oral or vaginal candidiasis in susceptible patients
- potentiated effect of certain anticoagulants (eg, warfarin)
- reduced efficacy of oral contraceptives
- purple discoloration of skin and cartilage due to deposition of minocycline in the tissues; looks like bruising
- permanent discoloration of teeth and bones in children younger than 14 years

CLINICAL PEARL

The use of tetracyclines is contraindicated during pregnancy, in women who are breastfeeding, and in patients with a known hypersensitivity to these agents. These agents should be used with caution in women of childbearing age, women with a family history of breast cancer, and patients with a history of liver disease.

Oral azithromycin is an alternative treatment, but there are conflicting reports about the potential risk of cardiac arrhythmia with its use.

Ohara H, Nakamura Y, Watanabe Y, et al. Azithromycin can prolong QT interval and suppress ventricular contraction, but will not induce torsade de pointes. *Cardiovasc Toxicol.* 2015:15(3);232–240.

Ray WA, Murray KT, Hall K, Arbogast PG, Stein CM. Azithromycin and the risk of cardiovascular death. *N Engl J Med.* 2012;366(20):1881–1890.

Svanström H, Pasternak B, Hviid A. Use of azithromycin and death from cardiovascular causes. *N Engl J Med.* 2013;368(18):1704–1712.

New treatment modalities Mechanical meibomian gland probing can be performed using special instruments (Maskin Meibomian Gland Intraductal Probe; Katena Products Inc) to lyse a fibrovascular membrane covering the ductule openings, which can facilitate gland function and permit normal secretion of meibum. The LipiFlow Thermal Pulsation System (Johnson & Johnson) combines pulsatile pressure and thermal energy to increase blood flow to the eyelid and open obstructed meibomian gland ductules; it may be an appropriate alternative when conventional treatment has failed. Variable improvement in dry eye symptoms has been reported; however, it is not currently covered by insurance plans. LipiFlow should not be used in the presence of active infection, postoperatively, or in the presence of functional abnormalities of the eyelid. The Systane iLUX MGD Thermal

Pulsation System (Alcon) is a handheld device that utilizes light-based heat followed by compression of the eyelid under direct visualization. Intense Pulsed Light (IPL) technology (Lumenis), a concentrated heat treatment, may also be used to treat MGD.

The efficacy of IPL therapy has not been proven in well-designed, prospective, randomized, controlled studies; however, improvement in symptoms and meibomian gland function has been reported.

American Academy of Ophthalmology Cornea/External Disease Committee. Preferred Practice Pattern Guidelines. *Blepharitis.* American Academy of Ophthalmology; 2018. www.aao.org/ppp

Foulks GN, Lemp MA. Meibomian gland dysfunction and seborrhea. In: Mannis MJ, Holland EJ, eds. *Cornea.* Vol 1. 4th ed. Elsevier; 2017:357–365.

Geerling G, Tauber J, Baudouin C, et al. The International Workshop on Meibomian Gland Dysfunction: Report of the Subcommittee on Management and Treatment of Meibomian Gland Dysfunction. *Invest Ophthalmol Vis Sci.* 2011;52(4):2050–2064.

Eyelid Conditions Associated With Ocular Surface Disease

Rosacea

Rosacea (sometimes called *acne rosacea*) is a chronic dermatological disease that can affect the skin of both the face and the eyelids. Women are typically affected more often than men. People of all races are affected, and the onset is typically in middle age; however, rosacea can be seen in children and young adults and is often underdiagnosed. The findings tend to be more subtle in young patients, but recurrent chalazia may be an early sign.

CLINICAL PRESENTATION The clinical presentation of rosacea includes facial and eyelid findings as well as associated ocular conditions.

Facial findings (Fig 3-17) associated with rosacea include

- midfacial erythema (can also affect the forehead and chin)
- episodic facial flushing
- recurrent pustules and papules
- telangiectasias
- rhinophyma (thickening of the skin and connective tissue of the nose)

Eyelid findings associated with rosacea include

- excessive sebum secretion
- chronic blepharitis and MGD
- eyelid margin telangiectasia with hyperemia and induration
- recurrent chalazia

Ocular conditions associated with rosacea include

- chronic conjunctivitis
- stromal keratitis (Fig 3-18)
- marginal keratitis (Fig 3-19A)

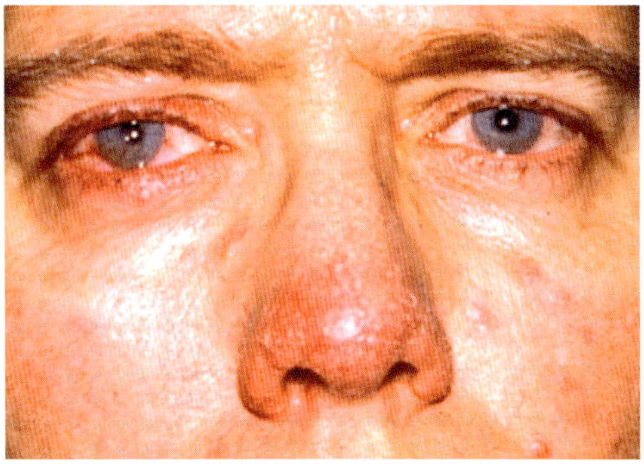

Figure 3-17 Facial characteristics of moderate acne rosacea, including facial erythema, papules, and rhinophyma. *(Courtesy of Robert S. Feder, MD.)*

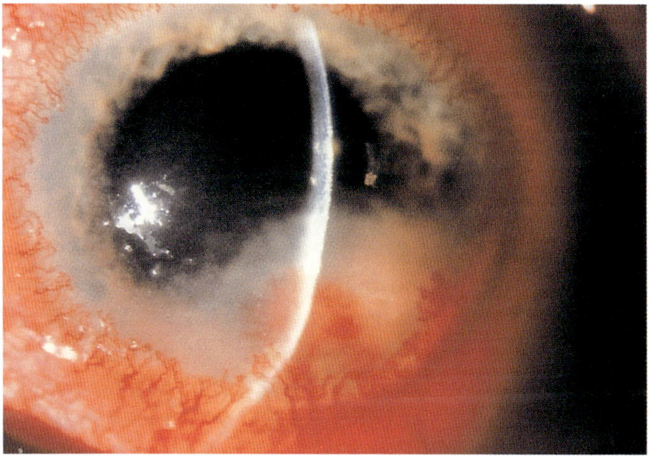

Figure 3-18 Stromal keratitis associated with rosacea.

A

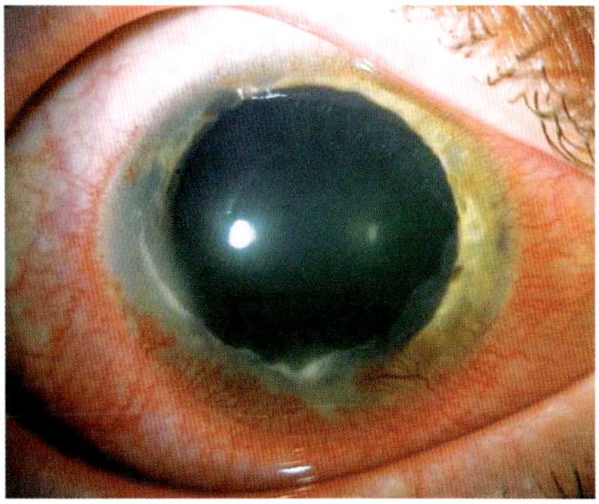

B

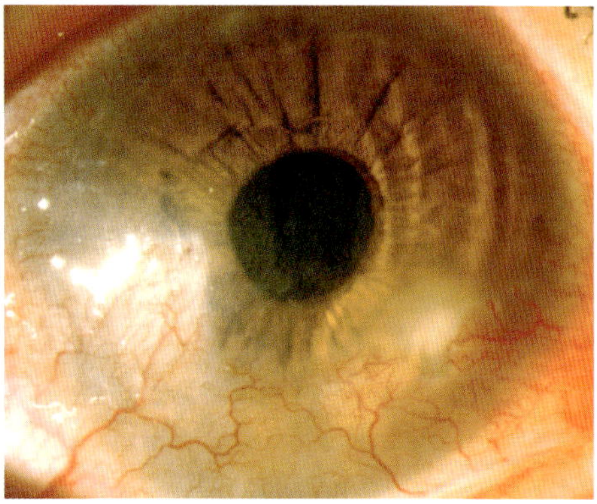

Figure 3-19 Ocular conditions associated with rosacea. **A,** Rosacea-associated marginal keratitis with possible episcleritis. **B,** Corneal neovascularization and scarring associated with rosacea. *(Courtesy of Mark Mannis, MD.)*

- sterile ulceration
- episcleritis (see Fig 3-19A)
- iridocyclitis

PATHOGENESIS Rosacea has no proven cause; staphylococcal bacteria and *Demodex* mites have been implicated. Rosacea is associated with cutaneous sebaceous gland dysfunction of the face, neck, and shoulders. Although rosacea has generally been thought to be more common in fair-skinned individuals, it may simply be more difficult to diagnose in patients with dark skin. Alcohol consumption can contribute to a worsening of facial redness because of its effect on vasomotor stability with dilatation of vessels; however, most patients with rosacea do not have a history of excessive alcohol intake. In some patients, exacerbation can be triggered by emotional stress, ingestion of hot or spicy foods, or a hot or cold environment. Repeated bouts of ocular surface inflammation can cause corneal neovascularization and scarring (Fig 3-19B).

MANAGEMENT If properly treated, the corneal involvement can be controlled with few sequelae. Oral tetracyclines are the mainstay of therapy for both the ocular and dermatologic disease. Tetracyclines have anti-inflammatory properties that include suppression of leukocyte migration, reduced production of nitric oxide and reactive oxygen species, inhibition of matrix metalloproteinases, and inhibition of phospholipase A2. In addition, tetracyclines may reduce irritative free fatty acids and diglycerides by suppressing bacterial lipases. Erythromycin or azithromycin may be used when tetracyclines are not appropriate.

With time, oral therapy with doxycycline or minocycline can be tapered. In addition to oral therapy, topical therapy with metronidazole gel 0.75%, metronidazole cream 1%, or azelaic acid gel 15% applied to the affected facial areas can significantly reduce facial erythema. Azelaic acid 15% is thought to suppress rosacea through anti-inflammatory and antimicrobial mechanisms.

Ulcerative keratitis associated with rosacea can result from an infectious or a sterile inflammatory process. If it is determined that the ulcer is noninfectious, topical corticosteroids, used judiciously, can play a significant role in reducing inflammation and promoting reepithelialization of the cornea. In advanced cases with scarring and neovascularization, conservative therapy is generally recommended. Penetrating keratoplasty is a high-risk procedure in patients with rosacea due to corneal vascularization, corneal thinning, and a compromised ocular surface. Deep anterior lamellar keratoplasty (DALK) could be considered in patients who need a corneal transplant.

National Rosacea Society website. www.rosacea.org

Schittek B, Paulmann M, Senyürek I, Steffen H. The role of antimicrobial peptides in human skin and in skin infectious diseases. *Infect Disord Drug Targets.* 2008;8(3):135–143.

Seborrheic Blepharitis

CLINICAL PRESENTATION Seborrheic blepharitis may occur alone or in combination with staphylococcal blepharitis, MGD, or seborrheic dermatitis. Inflammation occurs primarily at the anterior eyelid margin.

Clinical symptoms of seborrheic blepharitis include

- chronic eyelid redness
- burning
- foreign-body sensation

Clinical signs include

- eyelid scaling or scurf (Fig 3-20), typically oily or greasy consistency
- scaling of the eyelashes, eyebrows, scalp, and facial skin folds
- increased meibomian gland secretions that appear turbid
- inferior punctate erosions
- keratitis or conjunctivitis (in 15% of affected patients)
- evaporative dry eye (in 33% of affected patients)

See Table 3-12 for additional information on seborrheic and other types of blepharitis.

MANAGEMENT Eyelid hygiene (discussed earlier in this chapter) is the primary treatment for seborrheic blepharitis as well as the associated MGD or staphylococcal blepharitis. Concurrent treatment of the scalp disease with selenium sulfide shampoos is recommended.

Demodicosis should be considered in patients who do not improve with traditional blepharitis treatments. Eyelash sleeves or cylindrical dandruff is typically seen in these patients (Fig 3-21A; also see Fig 3-20). A small case series found that symptoms and signs improved among participants when weekly 50% tea tree oil eyelid scrubs and daily tea tree oil shampoo scrubs were used for a minimum of 6 weeks in a group of patients who had not previously improved with eyelid hygiene and concurrent scalp treatment. Eyelid treatments with hypochlorous acid have been shown to be clinically effective; laboratory studies have demonstrated that it effectively kills the nymph form of the Demodex mites. Oral ivermectin has also been reported to be of benefit in some cases of recalcitrant *Demodex* blepharitis.

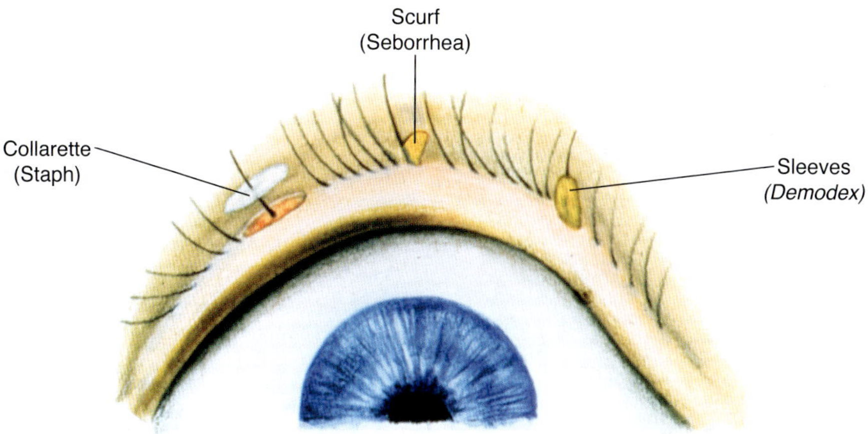

Figure 3-20 Illustration showing the clinical signs of blepharitis.

Table 3-12 Types of Blepharitis

	Staphylococcal	Meibomian Gland	Seborrheic
Location	Anterior eyelid margin	Posterior eyelid margin	Anterior eyelid margin
Eyelash loss and whitening	Varying degrees	(–)	Rare
Eyelid crusting	Hard, fibrinous scales; hard, matted crusts (often accompany ulcerative form)	+/–	Oily or greasy
Eyelid ulceration	Occasional	(–)	(–)
Conjunctivitis	Papillary (occasionally with mucopurulent discharge)	Mild to moderate injection, papillary tarsal reaction	Mild injection, follicular or papillary tarsal reaction
Keratitis	Inferior PEE, marginal infiltrates, vascularization, phlyctenulosis	Inferior PEE, marginal infiltrates, vascular pannus	Inferior PEE
Rosacea	(–)	Common	Less common

PEE = punctate epithelial erosion.

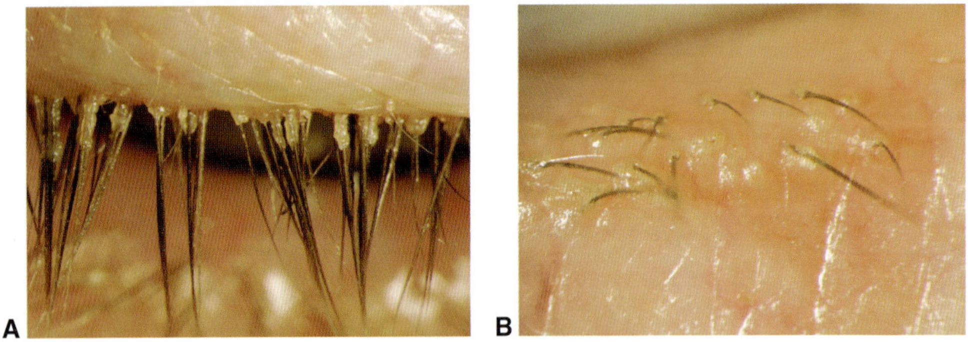

Figure 3-21 Photographs showing the clinical signs of blepharitis. **A,** Eyelash sleeves, referred to as cylindrical dandruff, typical of demodicosis. **B,** Staphylococcal blepharitis. *(Part A courtesy of Robert S. Feder, MD; part B courtesy of Robert W. Weisenthal, MD.)*

Staphylococcal Blepharitis

In general, the term *staphylococcal blepharitis* (caused typically by *Staphylococcus aureus* but occasionally by other species) refers to cases in which bacterial infection of the eyelids (and frequently the conjunctiva) is predominant. In contrast, MGD and seborrheic blepharitis are primarily inflammatory noninfectious conditions. Clinical features that may help in the differential diagnosis of these conditions are summarized in Table 3-12.

CLINICAL PRESENTATION Staphylococcal blepharitis is seen more commonly in younger individuals with symptoms that are worse in the morning and improve as the day progresses.

Clinical symptoms of staphylococcal blepharitis include

- burning
- itching
- foreign-body sensation
- crusting, particularly upon awakening

Clinical signs include

- fibrinous scales and matted, flattened crusts surrounding individual cilia (collarettes) (Fig 3-21B)
- small ulcers of the anterior eyelid margin, visible when the crusts are removed (see Fig 3-20)
- injection and telangiectasis of the anterior and posterior eyelid margins
- white lashes (poliosis), loss of lashes (madarosis), and trichiasis in varying degrees, worsening with increased severity and duration

MANAGEMENT Effective treatment addresses both the infection and the associated inflammation. Eyelid hygiene, with either commercially available eyelid scrubs, warm water mixed with baby shampoo, or hypochlorous acid sprays may help reduce bacterial colonization and the accumulation of sebaceous secretions. These treatments should focus on the base of the lashes, where colonization and seborrhea are the greatest. Aggressive scrubbing should be discouraged. Topical antibiotics such as bacitracin, erythromycin, azithromycin, or tobramycin may be applied to the eyelid margin to reduce both the bacterial load and associated inflammation. As stated, ATD and/or lipid-induced tear film instability may occur concomitantly; these should be treated to improve patient comfort.

Topical corticosteroids can be helpful in selected cases. Patients with routine staphylococcal blepharitis or blepharoconjunctivitis obtain rapid symptomatic relief with a short course of topical corticosteroids. If epithelial defects are noted over the corneal infiltrates, diagnostic cultures should be considered before corticosteroid treatment is begun. Long-term or indiscriminate use of corticosteroids is not recommended.

Staphylococcal Blepharoconjunctivitis

CLINICAL PRESENTATION Staphylococcal blepharoconjunctivitis may present as a chronic (>4-week duration) unilateral or bilateral conjunctivitis.

CHRONIC UNILATERAL CONJUNCTIVAL INFLAMMATION

If unilateral signs or symptoms persist, the clinician should consider an obstruction of the nasolacrimal system and perform a dye disappearance test or perhaps irrigation of the nasolacrimal system. Giant fornix syndrome and mucus fishing syndrome could be included in the differential diagnosis of chronic unilateral mucopurulent conjunctivitis, as could *Chlamydial* conjunctivitis. Tumors (eg, sebaceous cell carcinoma) can masquerade as unilateral conjunctivitis. Finally, molluscum contagiosum can cause unilateral follicular conjunctivitis, but is typically not mucopurulent in nature.

Clinical symptoms of staphylococcal blepharoconjunctivitis include

- burning
- itching
- discharge
- crusting

Clinical signs include

- matted, honey-colored crusts and ulcers on the anterior eyelid margin
- papillary reaction of the tarsal conjunctiva, particularly near the eyelid margin
- mild injection of the bulbar and tarsal conjunctiva
- scant mucopurulent discharge
- concomitant ATD and/or lipid-induced tear film instability

Clinical findings can at times provide a clue to the causative organism. *S aureus* is often associated with honey-colored crusting, marginal keratitis, and, in rare cases, conjunctival or corneal phlyctenules. *Moraxella lacunata* may cause a chronic angular blepharoconjunctivitis, with crusting and ulceration of the skin in the lateral canthal angle and a papillary or follicular reaction on the tarsal conjunctiva, sometimes with adjacent keratitis. *Moraxella* angular blepharoconjunctivitis is frequently associated with concomitant *S aureus* blepharoconjunctivitis.

LABORATORY EVALUATION Eyelid and conjunctival cultures can be performed in suspected cases of staphylococcal blepharoconjunctivitis when the initial diagnosis is in doubt, the treatment response is poor, or the infection is worsening. An antibiotic washout period of at least 3 days should be employed prior to culture.

CLINICAL PEARL

In chronic unilateral conjunctivitis refractory to therapy, canaliculitis, conjunctival malignancy (eg, sebaceous cell carcinoma), and factitious illness should be considered.

The characteristic laboratory finding in staphylococcal blepharoconjunctivitis is a heavy, confluent growth of *S aureus.* Nevertheless, the finding of a light to moderate growth of bacteria and/or the isolation of staphylococcal species other than *S aureus* does not exclude the diagnosis, particularly if a predominant manifestation of the disease is punctate epithelial keratopathy, marginal infiltrates, or phlyctenulosis. Susceptibility testing may be useful in guiding treatment in cases that have been refractory to empiric antibiotic therapy.

MANAGEMENT See the “Management” subsection under Staphylococcal Blepharitis.

Marginal Keratitis

CLINICAL PRESENTATION Several forms of keratitis may develop in association with staphylococcal blepharoconjunctivitis. Punctate epithelial keratopathy manifests as erosions

A B

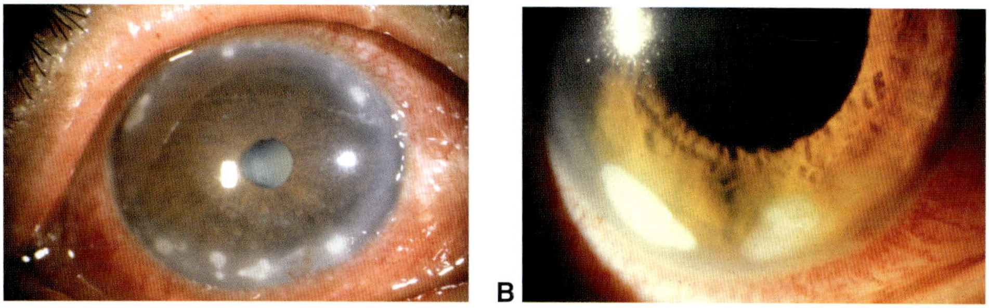

Figure 3-22 Marginal keratitis in association with staphylococcal blepharoconjunctivitis. **A**, Staphylococcal marginal corneal infiltrates are typically oval, white opacities. **B,** These infiltrates typically demonstrate a clear zone between the lesions and the limbus. *(Part A courtesy of David Rootman, MD; part B courtesy of Arie L. Marcovich, MD, PhD.)*

distributed across the inferior cornea that stain with fluorescein. A diffuse pattern may also be observed, and asymmetric or unilateral keratopathy is not uncommon.

CLINICAL PEARL

Marginal keratitis can occur even when eyelid inflammation is minimal, a circumstance that may lead to diagnostic confusion. Marginal corneal infiltrates have a distinctive clinical appearance, with creamy white elliptical opacities typically separated from the limbus by a relatively lucent zone. They most often occur near the point of intersection of the eyelid margin and the limbus, that is, at 10, 2, 4, and 8 o'clock (Fig 3-22).

There may or may not be an associated epithelial defect. Although the above findings are typical, the marginal lesions can occur at other locations and without a clear zone.

MANAGEMENT See the "Management" subsection under Staphylococcal Blepharitis. In addition, staphylococcal marginal keratitis readily responds to judicious use of topical steroids used in concert with antibiotic therapy and eyelid hygiene. If the condition does not improve or worsens with topical steroid treatment, consideration of an infectious etiology is advised.

Phlyctenular Keratoconjunctivitis (Phlyctenulosis)

CLINICAL PRESENTATION Phlyctenules are hyperemic, focal nodules consisting of chronic inflammatory cells. They often present unilaterally at or near the limbus, on the bulbar conjunctiva or cornea, as small, round, elevated, gray or yellow nodules accompanied by a zone of engorged hyperemic vessels (Fig 3-23A). Phlyctenules typically become necrotic and ulcerate centrally; they then spontaneously involute over a period of 2–3 weeks. Conjunctival phlyctenules do not lead to scarring, but residual wedge-shaped fibrovascular corneal scars form along the limbus. When such scars are bilateral and inferior, they may suggest previous phlyctenulosis. Corneal involvement can be recurrent, and migration of successive inflammatory lesions with a leash of neovascularization may occur, affecting vision if untreated (Fig 3-23B). Occasionally, such inflammation leads to corneal thinning and, in rare cases, perforation.

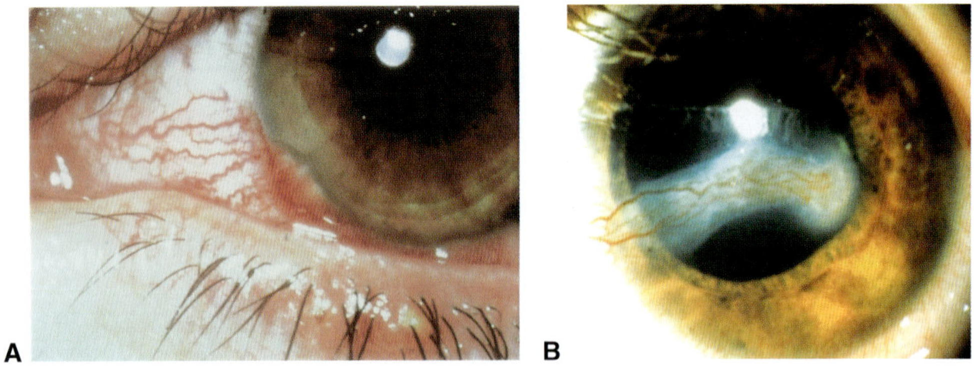

Figure 3-23 Phlyctenule. **A,** Confluent phlyctenules secondary to staphylococcal blepharitis. **B,** Recurrent phlyctenular involvement may result in fibrovascular scarring that progresses across the cornea and into the visual axis. *(Part B courtesy of Robert S. Feder, MD.)*

PATHOGENESIS Phlyctenulosis is believed to represent a T cell–mediated, or delayed, hypersensitivity (type IV) response induced by microbial antigens such as the cell wall components of staphylococcus. In this disease, 2 specific requirements are necessary to develop a delayed hypersensitivity reaction: (1) sensitization of the cornea and conjunctiva to an antigen; and (2) repeated exposure to this antigen. Phlyctenulosis is most frequently associated with *S aureus* but can also be associated with *Mycobacterium tuberculosis* infection affecting malnourished individuals in tuberculosis-endemic areas of the world. It is therefore important to question the patient or family members regarding contacts with individuals with chronic cough.

MANAGEMENT See the "Management" subsection under Staphylococcal Blepharitis. In addition, as with staphylococcal marginal keratitis, phlyctenulosis readily responds to judicious use of topical steroids used in concert with antibiotic therapy and eyelid hygiene. Serologic or skin testing is advised if associated tuberculosis is a possibility based on family history or review of systems.

Hordeola and Chalazia

CLINICAL PRESENTATION Hordeola present as painful, tender, red nodular masses near the eyelid margin (Fig 3-24). Those occurring on the anterior eyelid in the glands of Zeis or lash follicles are called *external hordeola,* or *styes.* Hordeola occurring on the posterior eyelid from meibomian gland inspissation are termed *internal hordeola.* Both types are associated with a localized purulent abscess, usually caused by *S aureus,* and may rupture, producing a purulent drainage. Hordeola are generally self-limited, improving spontaneously over the course of 1–2 weeks.

Internal hordeola occasionally evolve into chalazia, which are chronic lipogranulomatous nodules involving the meibomian glands. The lesion resolves in weeks to months. A small amount of scar tissue or calcium inclusions may remain. Occasionally, patients with a chalazion experience blurred vision secondary to astigmatism induced by its pressure on the globe.

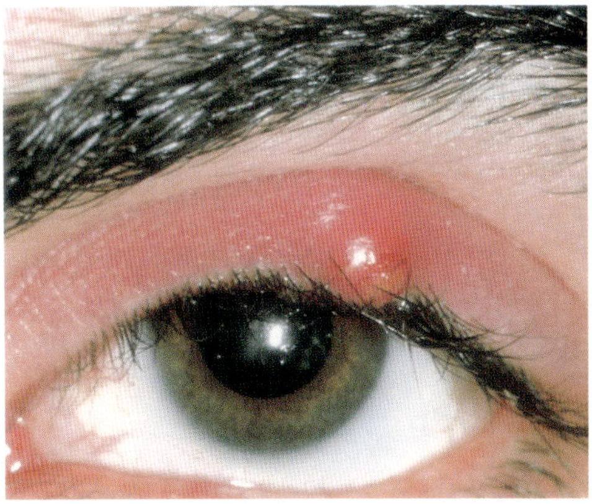

Figure 3-24 Hordeolum. *(Courtesy of Vincent P. deLuise, MD.)*

CLINICAL PEARL

Basal cell, squamous cell, and sebaceous cell carcinoma can masquerade as chalazia or chronic blepharitis. The histopathological examination of persistent, recurrent, or atypical chalazia is therefore important. Lash loss occurring over a chronic lesion is suggestive of malignancy.

MANAGEMENT Cultures are not indicated for isolated, uncomplicated cases of hordeolum or chalazion. Warm compresses can facilitate spontaneous drainage. Topically applied antibiotics are generally not effective and, therefore, are not indicated unless an accompanying infectious blepharoconjunctivitis is present. Systemic antibiotics are generally indicated only in cases of secondary eyelid cellulitis. If the patient has accompanying MGD or recurrent chalazia, oral doxycycline can be helpful.

If an internal hordeolum evolves into a chalazion that fails to respond to warm compresses and eyelid hygiene, intralesional injection of a corticosteroid (eg, 0.1–0.2 mL of triamcinolone 40 mg/mL), incision and curettage, or both may be necessary. In general, intralesional corticosteroid injection works best with small chalazia, chalazia on the eyelid margin, and multiple chalazia. Intralesional corticosteroid injection in patients with dark skin may lead to eyelid skin depigmentation and thus should be used with caution.

Large chalazia are best treated with surgical drainage and curettage. Internal chalazia require vertical incisions through the tarsal conjunctiva along the meibomian gland to facilitate drainage and avoid horizontal scarring of the tarsal plates. Surgical drainage usually requires perilesional, local anesthesia. A biopsy for pathological evaluation should be performed for recurrent chalazia to rule out meibomian gland carcinoma.

Oral doxycycline has been shown to be of proven benefit in reducing the incidence of recurrent chalazion. See also BCSC Section 7, *Oculofacial Plastic and Orbital Surgery,* for further discussion of chalazion.

CHAPTER 4

Eyelid, Conjunctival, and Corneal Conditions Associated With Ocular Surface Disorders

Indicates selected key points within the chapter.

Highlights

- Patients with floppy eyelids should be evaluated for obstructive sleep apnea and keratoconus.
- Exposure keratopathy is common in patients with Parkinson syndrome, who exhibit poor blinking, and in patients after blepharoplasty, who often demonstrate incomplete blinking.
- Exposure of the ocular surface in the presence of a neurotrophic cornea or corneal anesthesia is an ophthalmic emergency because of the risk of a stromal melt.
- Recurrent corneal erosion can result from corneal dystrophies or trauma and can usually be successfully treated with topical hypertonic sodium chloride drops or ointment, a bandage contact lens, anterior stromal puncture, epithelial debridement, or an excimer laser.
- Patching followed by topical lubrication and recognition with possible correction of the underlying cause are important in the management of dellen.

Introduction

The stability and refractive function of the ocular surface are maintained by a close relationship among the eyelids, conjunctiva, and cornea epithelium. When any part of this triad is disturbed, the ocular surface is compromised, resulting in significant ocular comorbidities. Each element of this triad will be considered along with the pertinent associated conditions.

Eyelid Disease

Floppy Eyelid Syndrome

CLINICAL PRESENTATION Floppy eyelid syndrome (FES) is an ophthalmic disorder consisting of chronic ocular inflammation and characterized by a lax upper tarsus that everts with minimal force applied to the eyelid. Clinical findings include small to large papillae on the upper palpebral conjunctiva, mucous discharge, and corneal involvement ranging from mild punctate epitheliopathy to superficial vascularization (Fig 4-1). Common symptoms include redness, foreign-body sensation (FBS), and mucous discharge most prominent upon waking.

PATHOGENESIS FES may result in spontaneous eversion of the upper eyelid during face-down sleeping, which allows the eye to come into contact with the pillow or other bed linens. Contact with the ocular surface can result in trauma to the corneal epithelium or upper tarsal conjunctiva, inducing inflammation and chronic irritation. The condition is usually bilateral but can be asymmetric or unilateral if the patient has a strong preference for the side on which they sleep. The syndrome is most frequently observed in obese individuals, who often also have obstructive sleep apnea. Keratoconus has also been reported in patients with FES. See Chapter 9 for more information on keratoconus. The differential diagnosis for FES includes vernal conjunctivitis, giant papillary conjunctivitis, atopic keratoconjunctivitis, bacterial conjunctivitis, and toxic keratopathy.

MANAGEMENT Treatment consists of applying ointment to the eye at night and either protecting the affected eye with a shield or taping the eyelids closed at night to prevent eyelid eversion. If symptoms persist, a surgical procedure can be performed to tighten the upper eyelid to manage the condition See BCSC Section 7, *Oculofacial Plastic and Orbital Surgery*.

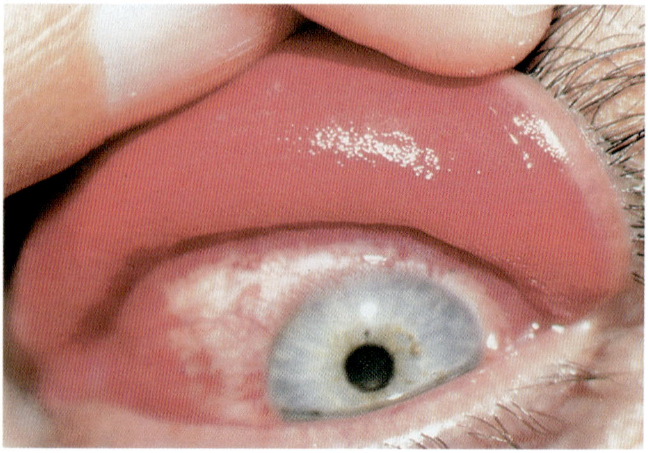

Figure 4-1 Floppy eyelid syndrome with a papillary response on the superior tarsus. *(Courtesy of Vincent P. deLuise, MD.)*

Pham TT, Perry JD. Floppy eyelid syndrome. *Curr Opin Ophthalmol.* 2007;18(5):430–433.
Stern GA. Chronic conjunctivitis, parts 1–2. *Focal Points: Clinical Modules for Ophthalmologists.* American Academy of Ophthalmology; 2012, modules 11–12.

Distichiasis and Trichiasis

Distichiasis is a congenital (often autosomal dominant) or acquired condition in which an extra row of eyelashes emerges from the orifices of the meibomian glands. These eyelashes may be fine and well tolerated or coarse and a threat to corneal surface integrity (Fig 4-2A).

Trichiasis is an acquired condition in which eyelashes emerging from their normal anterior origin curve inward toward the cornea. It can be idiopathic or secondary to serious chronic inflammatory conditions such as mucous membrane pemphigoid (MMP; also known as ocular cicatricial pemphigoid [OCP]), Stevens-Johnson syndrome, or chronic ocular graft-vs-host disease. It may also occur following chemical or thermal injury or even blepharitis. Many cases are probably the result of subtle cicatricial entropion of the eyelid margin (Fig 4-2B). This should be distinguished from an inturned eyelid (ie, entropion).

Just as poor eyelid position and movement should be corrected, so should aberrant eyelashes. Aberrant eyelashes may be removed by mechanical epilation, electrolysis with a radiofrequency probe (also known as hyfrecation), ablation with an argon laser, or cryotherapy. Mechanical epilation provides only temporary relief because the eyelashes normally grow back in as little as 3 weeks. Electrolysis works well for removing only a few eyelashes; however, it may be preferable in younger patients for cosmetic reasons. Cryotherapy is still a common treatment for aberrant eyelashes, but freezing can result in eyelid margin thinning, loss of skin pigmentation, loss of adjacent normal eyelashes, and persistent lanugo (fine hairs), which may continue to abrade the cornea. It is important to limit treatment at −20°C to minimize complications. The preferred surgical technique for aberrant eyelashes due to marginal cicatricial entropion is tarsotomy with eyelid margin rotation. See BCSC Section 7, *Oculofacial Plastic and Orbital Surgery,* for additional discussion of trichiasis and cicatricial entropion.

A 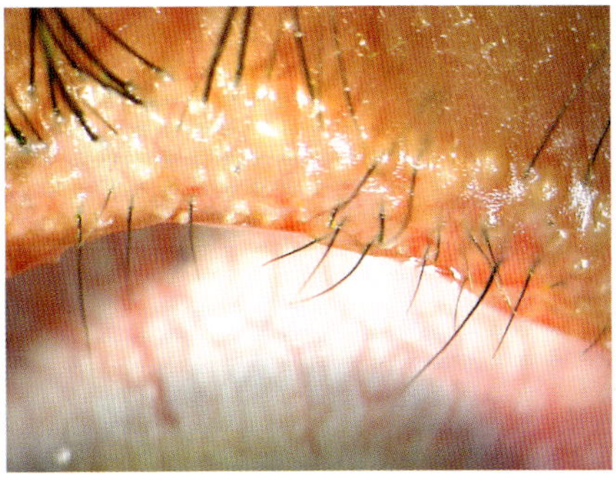 B 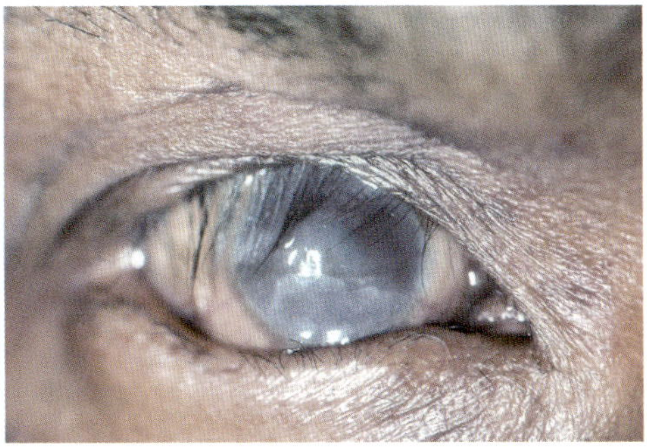

Figure 4-2 Eyelash disorders. **A,** Distichiasis is a congenital or acquired condition in which an aberrant extra row of eyelashes emerges from the orifices of the meibomian glands. **B,** Trichiasis is diagnosed when eyelashes emerge from their normal anterior origin and curve inward toward the cornea. *(Part A courtesy of Joseph D. Iuorno, MD; part B courtesy of Robert S. Feder, MD.)*

In older adults, MMP can present with trichiasis. Hallmarks of the disease are fibrosis of the tarsal conjunctiva, foreshortening of the cul-de-sac, and symblepharon. Treating this underlying cause of trichiasis can preserve vision and reduce associated morbidity.

Woreta F, Muñoz B, Gower E, Alemayehu W, West SK. Three-year outcomes of the Surgery for Trichiasis, Antibiotics to Prevent Recurrence trial. *Arch Ophthalmol.* 2012;130(4): 427–431.

Conjunctival Disease

Superior Limbic Keratoconjunctivitis

Superior limbic keratoconjunctivitis (SLK) is a chronic, recurrent inflammatory condition involving the superior tarsal and bulbar conjunctiva, as well as the superior limbus and cornea.

CLINICAL PRESENTATION Symptoms of SLK can include irritation, light sensitivity, and FBS. Vision is not usually affected. SLK is often bilateral but can be asymmetric. The condition can be associated with aqueous tear deficiency (ATD) or blepharospasm. Ocular findings may include the following:

- injection and thickening of the superior bulbar conjunctiva
- hypertrophy of the superior limbus
- fine punctate fluorescein, lissamine green, or rose bengal staining of the superior bulbar conjunctiva extending above the limbus with involvement of the superior cornea adjacent to the limbus (Fig 4-3A)
- a fine "velvety" papillary reaction on the superior tarsal conjunctiva (Fig 4-3B)
- superior filamentary keratitis

SLK is most frequently observed in women and may recur over a period of 1–10 years. SLK is associated with thyroid disease. In 1 study, 90% of SLK patients had some type of

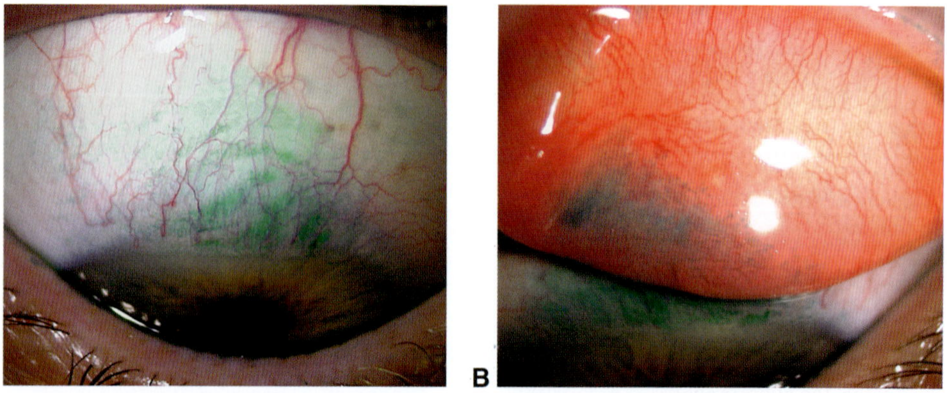

A B

Figure 4-3 Superior limbic keratoconjunctivitis. **A,** Note the superior conjunctival injection and staining with lissamine green. **B,** The staining pattern extends to the superior palpebral conjunctiva, which has a fine, "velvety" papillary reaction as well. *(Courtesy of Joseph D. Iuorno, MD.)*

thyroid-related ophthalmopathy; 49% required orbital decompression. Therefore, SLK is a prognostic indicator for thyroid eye disease.

> **CLINICAL PEARL**
>
> Whereas the percentage of patients with thyroid disorders who develop SLK is low, the prevalence of thyroid dysfunction in patients with SLK ranges from 20% to 65%.

PATHOGENESIS The pathogenesis of SLK has not been established, but the condition is thought to result from mechanical trauma transmitted from the upper eyelid to the superior bulbar and tarsal conjunctiva. In addition, SLK has been associated with graft-vs-host disease and has been observed following blepharoplasty. It can also be associated with lax conjunctiva, known as conjunctival chalasis. It is important to differentiate this condition from contact lens–induced keratoconjunctivitis (CLK), which is in effect a focal limbal stem cell deficiency. Unlike in SLK, vision in CLK may be impaired by punctate keratopathy, which extends through the visual axis. Also, in cases of CLK, filamentary keratitis does not typically occur, and contact lens wear is a cause, not a treatment.

LABORATORY EVALUATION Hyperproliferation, acanthosis, loss of goblet cells, and keratinization are observed in histologic sections of the superior bulbar conjunctiva. SLK can often be diagnosed clinically. However, scrapings or impression cytology of the superior bulbar conjunctiva showing characteristic features of nuclear pyknosis with "snake nuclei," an increased epithelial cytoplasm–nucleus ratio, goblet cell loss, or keratinization may be helpful in the diagnosis of mild or confusing cases. It is recommended that patients with SLK undergo thyroid function tests, including free thyroxine (T_4), thyroid-stimulating hormone (TSH), and thyroid antibodies.

MANAGEMENT A variety of therapies have been reported to provide temporary or permanent relief of symptoms, but in general, medical treatment of SLK is less effective than surgical treatment. The goal of medical treatment is to reduce inflammation and friction between the upper tarsal and bulbar conjunctiva. Table 4-1 lists medical and surgical treatment options for SLK.

Table 4-1 Treatment of Superior Limbic Keratoconjunctivitis

Medical Treatment[a]	Surgical Treatment
Nonpreserved artificial tears	Punctal occlusion
Topical anti-inflammatory agents	Thermocauterization of the superior bulbar conjunctiva
Topical cyclosporine	Resection of the affected superior limbal and bulbar conjunctiva
Topical mucolytic agent (10% *N*-acetyl cysteine)	Amniotic membrane transplantation
Autologous serum drops	Conjunctival fixation sutures
Large-diameter bandage soft contact lenses (protect the superior bulbar conjunctiva from the mechanical action of the upper eyelid)	

[a] Can be used in combination.

Sheu MC, Schoenfield L, Jeng BH. Development of superior limbic keratoconjunctivitis after upper eyelid blepharoplasty surgery: support for the mechanical theory of its pathogenesis. *Cornea.* 2007;26(4):490–492.

Stern GA. Chronic conjunctivitis, parts 1–2. *Focal Points: Clinical Modules for Ophthalmologists.* American Academy of Ophthalmology; 2012, modules 11–12.

Theodore FH, Ferry AP. Superior limbic keratoconjunctivitis. Clinical and pathological correlations. *Arch Ophthalmol.* 1970;84(4):481–484.

Udell IJ, Kenyon KR, Sawa M, Dohlman CH. Treatment of superior limbic keratoconjunctivitis by thermocauterization of the superior bulbar conjunctiva. *Ophthalmology.* 1986;93(2):162–166.

Yamada M, Hatou S, Mochizuki H. Conjunctival fixation sutures for refractory superior limbic keratoconjunctivitis. *Br J Ophthalmol.* 2009;93(12):1570–1571.

Conjunctivochalasis

Conjunctivochalasis is a term used to describe laxity or redundancy of the otherwise normal conjunctiva.

CLINICAL PRESENTATION Patients present with symptoms similar to dry eye disease (chronic redness, FBS, and chronic epiphora); however, these symptoms do not typically respond to treatment with a topical lubricant or topical corticosteroid. In addition to the conjunctival folds on the eyelid margin, punctate staining may be observed. This surface disruption is presumably caused by conjunctival tissue chafing against itself with movement of the eye. These patients may be predisposed to recurrent subconjunctival hemorrhages. Severity of conjunctival chalasis can range from mild to marked (Fig 4-4). This tissue may roll on or over the eyelid margin or cover the lacrimal punctum, obstructing tear outflow. In 1998, Meller and Tseng proposed a grading system that may help characterize the findings in this underrecognized condition.

Meller D, Tseng SCG. Conjunctivochalasis: literature review and possible pathophysiology. *Surv Ophthalmol.* 1998;43(3):225–232.

PATHOGENESIS The pathogenesis has not been established but may be similar to that of SLK (see the previous section Superior Limbic Keratoconjunctivitis). Histologic studies have revealed elastosis and chronic nongranulomatous inflammation. In addition, collagenolysis may explain the conjunctival laxity.

MANAGEMENT It is reasonable to try topical lubricants, topical antihistamines, a short course of topical corticosteroids, or nocturnal patching. Cauterization of the redundant folds is sometimes effective. Alternatively, the clinician may consider excision of excess conjunctival tissue with primary closure using fibrin adhesive to relieve the chronic ocular irritation and the obstruction of the lacrimal punctum, thereby restoring tear drainage (see Fig 4-4). Amniotic tissue grafting and conjunctival fixation are alternative surgical procedures. See Chapter 5 for further discussion of surgical management.

Yamamoto Y, Yokoi N, Ogata M, et al. Correlation between recurrent subconjunctival hemorrhages and conjunctivochalasis by clinical profile and successful surgical outcome. *Eye Contact Lens.* 2015;41(6):367–372.

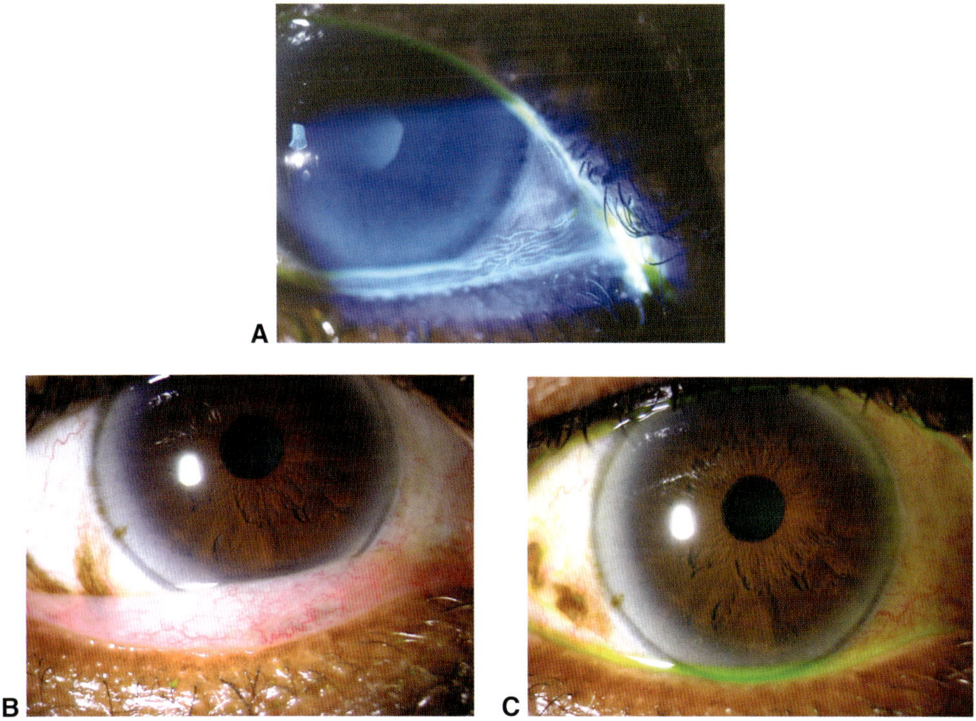

Figure 4-4 Conjunctivochalasis. **A,** Mild chalasis seen with fluorescein highlighting the redundant conjunctival folds temporally. **B,** Demonstration of redundant conjunctival tissue overlapping the lower eyelid margin. **C,** Restoration of inferior eyelid margin and tear drainage after excision of redundant conjunctival tissue. *(Part A courtesy of Cornea Service, Paulista School of Medicine, Federal University of São Paulo; parts B and C courtesy of Joseph D. Iuorno, MD.)*

Surface Disorders of the Cornea

Exposure Keratopathy

CLINICAL PRESENTATION When corneal sensation is normal, the symptoms of exposure keratopathy are similar to those of evaporative dry eye, including FBS and photophobia. Exposure keratopathy is characterized by punctate epithelial erosions that usually involve the inferior one-third of the cornea; however, in severe cases the entire corneal surface may be involved. Large, coalescent epithelial defects may result, which may in turn lead to infectious or sterile ulceration and occasionally perforation. Exposure in the presence of a neurotrophic cornea or corneal anesthesia is an ophthalmic emergency because of the risk of a stromal melt (see the section Neurotrophic Keratopathy, later in this chapter).

PATHOGENESIS Exposure keratopathy can develop as a result of proptosis or any disease associated with poor blinking or limitation of eyelid closure. Lagophthalmos is defined as the inability to completely close the eyelids. Exposure keratopathy can result from lagophthalmos associated with

- neurogenic disease such as cranial nerve (CN) VII palsy
- degenerative neurologic conditions such as Parkinson disease
- cicatricial or restrictive eyelid diseases such as ectropion
- drug abuse
- following eyelid surgery (blepharoplasty), scarring, or trauma
- dermatological disorders (eg, Stevens-Johnson syndrome, dermatomyositis, and xeroderma pigmentosum)
- proptosis (eg, due to thyroid eye disease or other inflammatory or infiltrative orbital disease)
- prolonged lack of eyelid closure, as observed in the obtunded patient
- incomplete blink with poor Bell phenomenon or associated lower lid lag (eg, nocturnal exposure)

MANAGEMENT Therapy is similar to that for severe evaporative dry eye. In the earliest stages, as seen in patients with an incomplete blink and poor Bell phenomenon, nonpreserved artificial tears instilled during the day and/or punctal occlusion and ointment applied at bedtime may suffice. Taping the eyelid shut at bedtime can help if the exposure occurs mainly while sleeping. Caution is warranted when using bandage contact lenses in patients with exposure keratopathy because of the risk of desiccation and infection. For cases in which the problem is likely to be temporary or self-limited, temporary tarsorrhaphy using tissue adhesive or sutures may be helpful. However, if the problem is likely to be long-standing, a more permanent surgical approach is advised.

Most commonly, surgical management consists of permanent lateral and/or medial tarsorrhaphy (see Chapter 5). Insertion of gold or platinum weights into the upper eyelid is also an effective, more cosmetically pleasing approach to facilitate eyelid closure. Reported complications of gold weight implants include infection, implant malposition, extrusion, induced astigmatism, unacceptable ptosis, and noninfectious inflammatory response to the gold. The weights remain stable during magnetic resonance imaging. In addition, correction of any associated eyelid abnormalities, such as ectropion, entropion, and/or trichiasis, is indicated. For example, in cases of paralytic ectropion of the lower eyelid, a horizontal tightening procedure may also be beneficial.

See BCSC Section 7, *Oculofacial Plastic and Orbital Surgery,* for further discussion of thyroid eye disease, lagophthalmos, and proptosis.

Neurotrophic Keratopathy

CLINICAL PRESENTATION Persistent corneal epithelial defects on neurotrophic corneas typically occur in the central or paracentral cornea and tend to be located inferiorly or inferonasally because of the protective effect of the Bell phenomenon on the superior cornea. The round or oval erosions frequently have elevated gray-white edges of "heaped-up" epithelium, which are associated with underlying stromal inflammation (Fig 4-5). Left untreated, persistent corneal epithelial defects can progress to vascularization and corneal

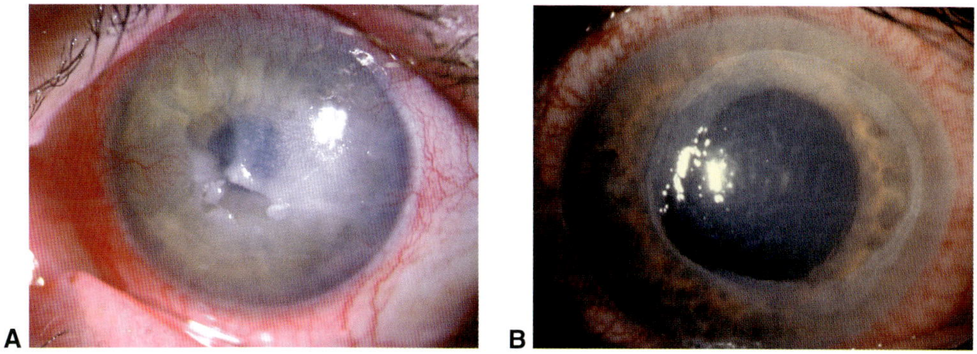

Figure 4-5 Neurotrophic keratopathy. **A,** Neurotrophic cornea ulcer secondary to chronic herpetic keratitis. Note the "heaped-up" epithelial edges. Peripheral vascularization indicates chronicity. **B,** Large ovoid corneal neurotrophic ulceration with typical heaped-up gray-white epithelial edges. *(Part A courtesy of Joseph D. Iuorno, MD; part B courtesy of Stephen E. Orlin, MD.)*

opacification or corneal thinning and possible perforation. Secondary bacterial keratitis may also occur in these patients.

PATHOGENESIS Neurotrophic keratopathy is typically caused by damage to CN V or to the branches of CN V that innervate the cornea, resulting in corneal hypoesthesia or anesthesia (Table 4-2). Healthy innervation of the cornea provides a trophic effect that is necessary for an optimal corneal surface. The most common cause of neurotrophic keratopathy is probably herpetic keratitis, which can be associated with persistent or recurrent corneal epithelial defects or chronic punctate keratopathy in the absence of replicating virus or active inflammation. A neurotrophic cornea can also occur in the early postoperative period following keratoplasty, laser in situ keratomileusis (LASIK) surgery, or surgery near CN V (eg, gamma knife radiotherapy treatment for temporomandibular joint pain). Diabetic neuropathy is a potential cause of neurotrophic keratopathy and nonhealing epithelial defects.

Table 4-2 Causes of Neurotrophic Keratopathy

Postsurgical
- Limbal relaxing incisions
- Penetrating keratoplasty
- Laser in situ keratomileusis (LASIK)
- Corneal implants/inlays
- Gamma knife radiotherapy

Compressive
- Aneurysm
- Tumors (acoustic neuroma, angioma, neurofibroma)

Vascular
- Cerebrovascular accident
- Diabetes (types 1 and 2)

Genetic
- Familial dysautonomia (Riley-Day syndrome)

Inflammatory
- Multiple sclerosis

Infectious
- Herpes simplex virus
- Herpes varicella zoster virus
- Acanthamoeba
- Leprosy (Hanson disease)

Toxic
- Topical medications (eg, anesthetics, β-blockers, carbonic anhydrase inhibitors, nonsteroidal anti-inflammatory drugs)

> **CLINICAL PEARL**
>
> Persistent epithelial defects often occur in patients with long-standing diabetes who require epithelial debridement in the course of vitreoretinal surgery.

MANAGEMENT Management of neurotrophic keratopathy with or without persistent epithelial defects begins with eliminating or limiting the use of potentially aggravating topical medications. Frequent lubrication with nonpreserved drops, gels, or ointments is suggested. Autologous serum drops (20%–50%), which contain growth factors and fibronectin, may be useful. In cases involving significant dry eye, temporary or permanent punctal occlusion may be effective in improving the volume and stability of the tear film and restoring the ocular surface.

For years, pressure patching or eyelid taping in conjunction with ophthalmic ointments has been the mainstay of treatment of persistent epithelial defects. Recently, low-water-content bandage contact lenses (soft, thin, highly oxygen-permeable lenses) or scleral contact lenses with a fluid-filled reservoir have shown efficacy in facilitating reepithelialization or improving keratopathy in the short term for patients who are not surgical candidates.

In cases associated with stromal melting, a medication with specific activity against matrix metalloproteinases, such as a tetracycline administered orally, may help prevent or arrest keratolysis. Most recently, the use of a topical recombinant human nerve growth factor, cenegermin 20 µmcg/mL (Oxervate) administered 6 times daily for 8 weeks, has been shown to be beneficial in the treatment of neurotrophic keratitis. Some patients experience eye pain in the course of this treatment. Amniotic membrane transplantation has been reported to encourage healing of persistent epithelial erosions. Lateral and/or medial tarsorrhaphy may be required to prevent ocular surface desiccation. Tarsorrhaphy, which can be performed in a temporary or permanent manner, decreases the ocular surface exposure area and reduces tear film evaporation. Partial or total Gundersen conjunctival flap surgery can prevent keratolysis, or corneal melting; however, due to the permanent nature of this procedure, it is typically used as a last-resort option. Cornea neurotization, or transposition of intact nerve branches to the subconjunctival space near the limbus in the affected eye, is a recent surgical technique designed to reestablish cornea sensation in neurotrophic patients. See Chapter 5 for further discussion of surgical management of ocular surface disorders.

Jeng BH. Persistent epithelial defects. *Focal Points: Clinical Practice Perspectives.* American Academy of Ophthalmology; 2016, module 9.

Jeng BH. Use of autologous serum in the treatment of ocular surface disorders. *Arch Ophthalmol.* 2011;129(12):1610–1612.

Koaik M, Baig K. Corneal neurotization. *Curr Opin Ophthalmol.* 2019;30(4):292–298.

Pflugfelder SC, Massaro-Giordano M, Perez VL, et al. Topical recombinant human nerve growth factor (cenegermin) for neurotrophic keratopathy: a multicenter randomized vehicle-controlled pivotal trial. *Ophthalmology.* 2020;127(1):14–26.

Sacchetti M, Lambiase A. Diagnosis and management of neurotrophic keratitis. *Clin Ophthalmol.* 2014;8:571–579.

Recurrent Corneal Erosion

CLINICAL PRESENTATION Recurrent erosion syndrome (RES) classically refers to a recurrent condition that results from a traumatic corneal injury (eg, from a fingernail, paper cut, or tree branch). Patients present with a sudden onset of eye pain, typically during sleep or upon first awakening, accompanied by FBS, redness, photophobia, and tearing.

> **CLINICAL PEARL**
>
> In patients with RES, the initial epithelial abrasion and occasionally subsequent erosions may heal rapidly, at times leaving no clinical evidence of damage by the time of the office examination.

After an interval from the initial erosion ranging from days to years, symptoms suddenly recur without any obvious precipitating event. Episodes usually last from 30 minutes to several hours. More severe episodes may last for several days and are often associated with greater pain, extreme photophobia, eyelid edema, or decreased vision and may have associated stromal keratitis or anterior uveitis. Many patients seem to experience ocular discomfort that is out of proportion to the degree of observable pathology. Slit-lamp examination using a broad oblique beam with direct, indirect, or retroillumination, or with fluorescein showing negative staining (see Fig 8-4) can enhance the typical corneal abnormalities (eg, epithelial cysts or fingerprint lines) (see Fig 8-1).

During an acute attack, the epithelium in the involved area often appears heaped up, edematous, and sloughed (Fig 4-6).

PATHOGENESIS Recurrent erosions are caused by disruption of the epithelial basement membrane complex, resulting in a lack of epithelial adherence and an increased likelihood of occurrence of an epithelial defect. The precise nature of these abnormalities has yet to be fully determined. The corneal epithelium is loosely attached to the underlying

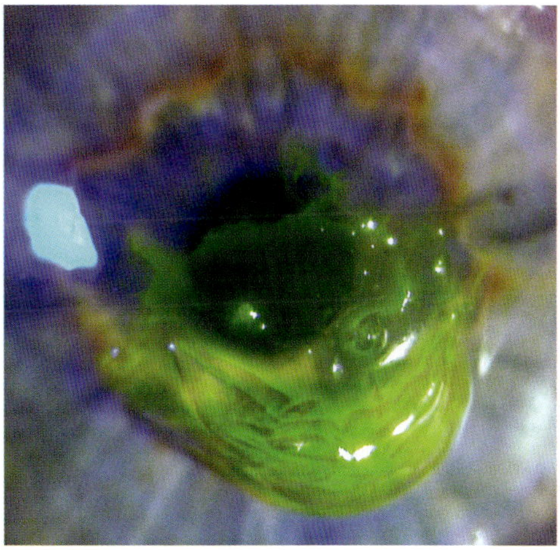

Figure 4-6 Corneal abrasion in a patient with recurrent erosion syndrome demonstrates heaping of sloughed epithelium inferior to the abrasion. *(Courtesy of Joseph D. Iuorno, MD.)*

basement membrane and Bowman layer, both at the time of a recurrent attack and between attacks, when the cornea appears to be entirely healed. Typically, epithelial basement membrane dystrophy (see Chapter 8) is associated with recurrent corneal erosions that produce FBS throughout the day.

In order to distinguish between posttraumatic erosion syndrome and corneal erosion caused by other corneal pathology (eg, epithelial basement membrane dystrophy), obtaining a thorough patient history, including onset of recurrent symptoms, is helpful. A careful examination of the contralateral eye following maximal pupillary dilation to enhance retroillumination is also of benefit.

The presence of dystrophic changes in the epithelium of the unaffected eye suggests a primary basement membrane abnormality as the root cause, whereas the absence of such findings in combination with a corroborating history may indicate a posttraumatic etiology (Fig 4-7).

Occasionally, subtle areas of loosely adherent corneal epithelium can be identified by applying gentle pressure with a surgical sponge following instillation of topical anesthetic. In anterior stromal dystrophies, subepithelial deposits can disrupt the epithelial

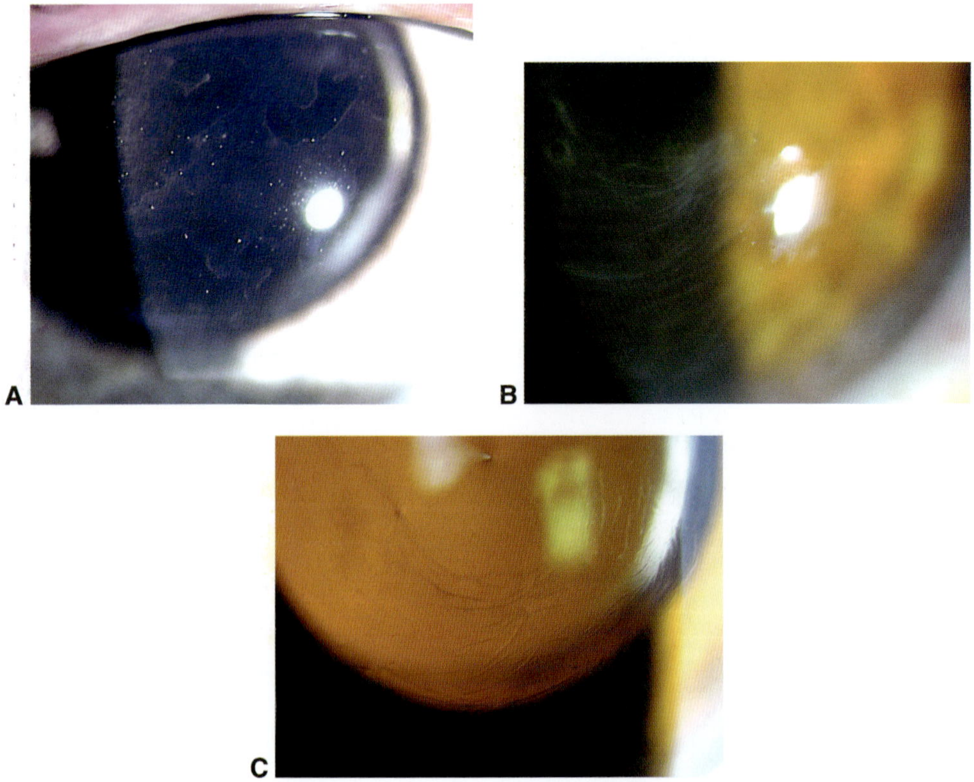

Figure 4-7 Epithelial basement membrane dystrophy (EBMD), also known as map-dot-fingerprint dystrophy. **A,** A broad oblique slit beam is useful to illustrate maps seen in EBMD (tiny dots represent artifact). **B,** Indirect illumination highlights fingerprint findings. **C,** Fingerprints are also well visualized on retroillumination. *(Courtesy of Joseph D. Iuorno, MD.)*

basement membrane complex, resulting in poor adherence of the epithelium. In patients with endothelial dystrophies, stromal edema develops, which places stress on the epithelial basement membrane and can predispose to recurrent corneal erosions (see Chapter 8). Corneal edema due to endothelial disruption can also cause microcystic edema or bullous keratopathy, which may result in recurrent corneal erosions and FBS that are typically worse in the morning, when the cornea is most edematous.

MANAGEMENT Traditional therapy for the acute phase of RES consists of patching with topical antibiotic ointments and cycloplegia, followed by use of nonpreserved lubricants or hypertonic saline solution or ointment (5% sodium chloride) during the day and sodium chloride ointment at bedtime for at least 6 weeks to provide protection during epithelial attachment. Hypertonic agents provide lubrication and may transiently produce an osmotic gradient, drawing fluid from the epithelium and theoretically promoting the adherence of epithelial cells to the underlying tissue. Some patients find hypertonic medications unacceptably irritating, whereas many patients do quite well with this therapy indefinitely. The use of low-dose oral doxycycline and short-term use of topical corticosteroids to inhibit of matrix metalloproteinases have been effective in treating some patients with recurrent erosions.

A bandage soft contact lens may be used as an alternative to patching in the short term but is a less desirable option for long-term management. Proper patient education regarding the risks associated with contact lens wear and judicious monitoring during use are crucial to a successful outcome. The ideal bandage lens fits without excessive movement and has high oxygen transmissibility (Dk). New-generation soft contact lenses with lens-surface treatments that decrease bacterial adherence may offer a better safety profile than older lens designs. Concomitant use of a topical broad-spectrum antibiotic 2–4 times daily may reduce the possibility of secondary infection but may also increase the risk of toxicity and bacterial resistance over the long term. Some cornea specialists prefer not to prescribe topical antibiotics for a patient using a bandage contact lens. Alternatively, large-diameter scleral contact lenses can provide a precorneal fluid reservoir effective in treating patients with chronic RES. Patients with intractable recurrent corneal erosions despite the above treatment modalities may benefit from protecting the affected eye with a rigid shield during sleep.

When consistent conservative management fails to control symptoms, surgical therapy may be indicated. Surgical management of recurrent corneal erosion includes epithelial debridement and anterior stromal puncture (ASP) (see Chapter 5). Some clinicians prefer to use debridement for central erosions or erosions related to corneal dystrophy and stromal puncture in patients with posttraumatic recurrent erosions. Diamond burr superficial keratectomy has been used to treat recurrent erosions, but it can result in irregular astigmatism if the treatment is too aggressive. Because diamond burr and ASP are occasionally associated with visually significant anterior stromal scarring, some clinicians prefer laser ablation for areas of recurrent erosion within the central visual axis. Excimer laser ablation can be performed with either phototherapeutic keratectomy (PTK) or photorefractive keratectomy (PRK). It is important to caution patients undergoing PTK about the possibility of induced refractive error. See Chapter 5 in this volume and BCSC Section 13, *Refractive Surgery,* for further discussion.

Lin SR, Aldave AJ, Chodosh J. Recurrent corneal erosion syndrome. *Br J Ophthalmol.* 2019;103(9):1204–1208.

Dellen

Dellen are saucerlike depressions in the corneal surface caused by focal stromal dehydration. Desiccation of the corneal epithelium and subepithelial tissues occurs at or near the limbus, adjacent to conjunctival surface elevations such as those associated with pterygium, recess-resect procedures, or in the presence of large filtration blebs. Normal blinking does not wet the involved area properly because the tear film is interrupted by these surface elevations. After an active blink, a transient bubble that temporarily displaces the tear film may be observed overlying the dellen. This can cause a dysesthesia that enhances the development of dellen. Nonpreserved artificial tear therapy alone is effective only in rare cases. The use of viscous lubricants and ointments or a bandage contact lens may help restore the focal desiccation of the cornea. Patching followed by frequent topical lubrication is most effective in rapidly restoring stromal hydration, although resolution of the conjunctival surface elevation may be necessary for permanent resolution of dellen.

Limbal Stem Cell Deficiency

The ocular surface comprises populations of epithelial cells, which are regularly replaced by proliferation from a distinct subpopulation of cells known as *stem cells.* Corneal stem cells are located in the basal cell layer of the limbus, whereas conjunctival stem cells may be uniformly distributed throughout the bulbar surface or the fornices (see Chapter 1).

CLINICAL PRESENTATION Stem cell deficiency of the cornea can be found in several ocular surface disorders. A whorl-like irregularity of the ocular surface emanating from the limbus is typical and is easily observed after the instillation of topical fluorescein (Fig 4-8). Neovascularization is invariably present in the involved cornea. Another sign of limbal stem cell deficiency (LSCD) is loss of architecture of the palisades of Vogt (see Chapter 1). Recurrent ulceration and decreased vision may develop in some patients as a result of the irregular corneal surface.

PATHOGENESIS To ensure normal ocular resurfacing, approximately 25%–33% of the limbus must remain intact. The normal limbus acts as a barrier to prevent neovascularization extending from the conjunctiva and invasion of conjunctival cells from the bulbar surface. When the limbal stem cells are congenitally absent, injured, or destroyed, conjunctival cells migrate onto the ocular surface, often accompanied by surface irregularity and superficial neovascularization (Fig 4-9). The absence of limbal stem cells reduces the effectiveness of epithelial wound healing, as evidenced by compromised ocular surface integrity with an irregular ocular surface and recurrent epithelial breakdown.

Stem cell deficiency can result from both primary and secondary causes. An example of a primary cause is aniridia or sclerocornea (*PAX6* gene mutation). Secondary causes include chemical burns, thermal burns, radiation, contact lens wear, and immune-based

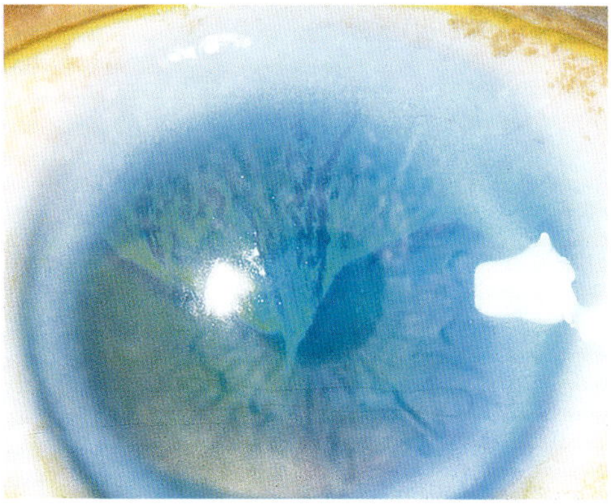

Figure 4-8 Mild stem cell deficiency secondary to contact lens wear. A whorl-like irregularity of the ocular surface is seen following instillation of topical fluorescein. *(Courtesy of James J. Reidy, MD.)*

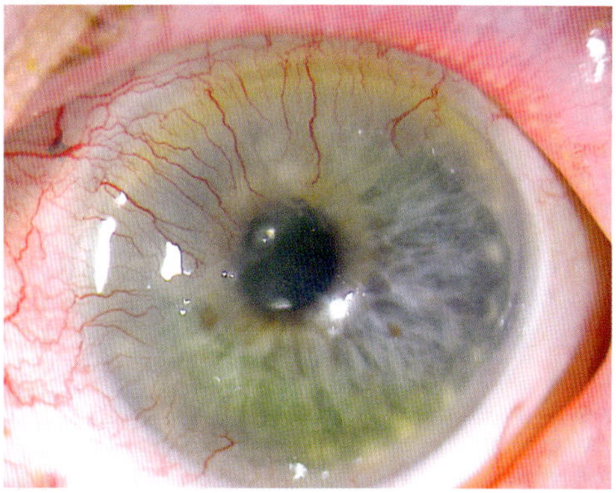

Figure 4-9 Limbal stem cell deficiency secondary to chemical injury. Neovascularization is evidence of long-standing stem cell damage. *(Courtesy of Joseph D. Iuorno, MD.)*

mucous membrane conjunctivitis (eg, MMP, Stevens-Johnson syndrome, ocular graft-vs-host disease). Other causes are listed in Table 4-3.

MANAGEMENT In mild or focal cases associated with local factors such as contact lens use or topical medications, the inciting cause should be discontinued. In addition to topical lubrication and/or punctal occlusion, medical interventions include topical corticosteroids, topical cyclosporine, topical vitamin A, and oral doxycycline. In some cases, a scleral contact lens may be helpful.

If the stem cell deficiency is focal or sectoral, the abnormal epithelium can be debrided in the hope of resurfacing of the denuded area from healthy adjacent stem cells.

If the above treatments are not effective, replacement of stem cells by limbal transplantation is an alternative. When the limbus is focally affected in 1 eye (eg, pterygium), a limbal or conjunctival autograft can be harvested from the same eye. For unilateral, moderate, or severe chemical injuries, a limbal autograft can be obtained from the healthy fellow eye. Simple limbal epithelial transplantation (SLET) is an autologous limbal stem cell transplant from a healthy fellow eye to the affected eye with LSCD (see Chapter 5 and Video 5-3). For bilateral limbal deficiency, such as in Stevens-Johnson syndrome or bilateral chemical burns, a limbal allograft from a human leukocyte antigen (HLA)–matched living related

Table 4-3 Etiologic Classification of Limbal Stem Cell Deficiency

Ocular diseases
- Anterior segment ischemic syndrome
- Atopic keratoconjunctivitis
- Infections (eg, herpes, trachoma)
- Neoplasia (eg, CIN, OSSN)
- Degenerations (pterygium, Salzmann nodular degeneration)
- Neurotrophic keratitis
- Peripheral corneal ulcers (eg, Fuchs marginal keratitis)

Congenital aniridia (*PAX6* mutation) and hereditary conditions
- Ectodactyly-ectodermal dysplasia; clefting syndrome
- Erythrokeratodermia
- KID syndrome
- LADD syndrome (Levy-Hollister syndrome)
- MEN type II
- Sclerocornea
- Xeroderma pigmentosa

Traumatic
- Chemical exposure
- Thermal burn

Iatrogenic
- *Topical*
  - Contact lens medications (eg, mitomycin C, anesthetics, preservatives)
  - Severe infection
  - Radiation exposure
  - Following ocular surgery (cryotherapy, excessive conjunctival resection, multiple ocular surface operations)
- *Systemic*
  - Graft-vs-host disease
- *Medication*
  - Hydroxyurea

Autoimmune diseases
- Mucous membrane pemphigoid
- Stevens-Johnson syndrome
- Linear IgA deficiency
- Drug-induced pemphigoid disease

Idiopathic

CIN = corneal/conjunctival intraepithelial neoplasia; IgA = immunoglobulin A; KID = keratitis-ichthyosis-deafness; LADD = lacrimo-auriculo-dento-digital; MEN = multiple endocrine neoplasia; OSSN = ocular surface squamous neoplasia.

donor or an eye bank donor can be considered; however, systemic immunosuppression is required following limbal allograft transplantation (see Chapter 5). Another alternative in cases of severe limbal cell deficiency is a keratoprosthesis (see Chapters 15 and 16).

Kim BY, Riaz KM, Bakhtiari P, et al. Medically reversible limbal stem cell disease: clinical features and management strategies. *Ophthalmology.* 2014; 121(10):2053–2058.

Sangwan VS, Sharp JAH. Simple limbal epithelial transplantation. *Curr Opin Ophthalmol.* 2017,28(4):382–386.

Zhao Y, Ma L. Systematic review and meta-analysis on transplantation of ex vivo cultivated limbal epithelial stem cell on amniotic membrane in limbal stem cell deficiency. *Cornea.* 2015;34(5):592–600.

Toxic Corneal Epithelial Cell Reactions to Topical Ophthalmic Medications

CLINICAL PRESENTATION Punctate staining of the corneal or conjunctival epithelium, erosive changes, and subepithelial corneal infiltrates are all indicative of direct toxicity. Mucopurulent discharge and conjunctival injection with a follicular response are signs of acute toxicity. Mild to severe papillary reaction may indicate chronicity. Occasionally, the discharge may be copious and mimic bacterial conjunctivitis. Infrequently, a monocular reaction occurs despite the medication being applied to both eyes.

More severe cases of toxic keratitis can present with a diffuse punctate epitheliopathy, occasionally in a whorl pattern called *vortex* or *hurricane keratopathy*. The most severe cases may present with a central or inferior corneal epithelial defect, stromal opacification, and neovascularization, which may be compounded by extensive damage to the limbal stem cells. This can result from prolonged use of preserved topical medications or agents that block fibrin formation (eg, mitomycin C).

PATHOGENESIS Toxic ocular surface disease can occur as a complication of exposure to various substances (Table 4-4). Epithelial keratopathy secondary to use of topical ophthalmic medications can result in a dose-dependent cytotoxic effect on the ocular surface. One of the most common toxic ingredients in these preparations is the preservative benzalkonium chloride (BAK). Corneal and conjunctival epithelial cells absorb and retain preservatives; residual amounts of preservative are detectable in the corneal epithelium days after a single application of a topical preserved medication. This condition is sometimes referred to as *toxic ulcerative keratopathy*.

In some cases, pericentral pseudodendritiform lesions and pseudogeographic defects may occur. These clinical findings are often misinterpreted as a worsening of the underlying disease and thus may lead to more frequent dosing of the offending medication. Other topical medications most frequently implicated in toxic ocular surface disease include

- anesthetics
- nonsteroidal anti-inflammatory drugs (NSAIDs)
- corticosteroids
- trifluridine
- glaucoma drops (eg, β-blockers and carbonic anhydrase inhibitors)
- eyedrops containing a preservative such as BAK

Mitomycin C, even when used with care, has been associated with prolonged, irreversible stem cell damage with a resultant chronic keratopathy. Localized application of

Table 4-4 Toxic Reactions to Topical Ophthalmic Medications

Keratoconjunctivitis	Follicular Conjunctivitis
Aminoglycosides	Glaucoma medications
Gentamicin sulfate	*Miotics*
Neomycin	Carbachol
Tobramycin sulfate	Pilocarpine
Antiviral agent	*α-adrenergic agonists*
Trifluridine (trifluorothymidine)	Apraclonidine hydrochloride
Antineoplastic agent	Brimonidine tartrate
Mitomycin C	Dipivefrin
Topical anesthetics	Epinephrine
Proparacaine	Cycloplegics
Tetracaine	Atropine sulfate
Preservatives	Homatropine hydrobromide
Benzalkonium chloride	
Thimerosal	

mitomycin C in a low concentration (≤0.4 mg/mL) applied only to the surgical site using a cellulose surgical sponge, as in trabeculectomy or pterygium excision, followed by copious irrigation is believed to reduce the risk of limbal stem cell damage.

Toxic keratitis that manifests as peripheral corneal infiltrates in the epithelium and anterior stroma, with a clear zone between the lesions and the limbus, is typically associated with aminoglycoside antibiotics, antiviral agents, or medications preserved with BAK or thimerosal.

Chronic follicular conjunctivitis generally involves both the upper and the lower palpebral conjunctiva but is usually most prominent inferiorly. Bulbar follicles are uncommon but, when present, are highly suggestive of a toxic etiology (Fig 4-10). The medications most commonly associated with toxic follicular conjunctivitis are presented in Table 4-4. Inferior punctate epithelial erosions may occasionally accompany toxic follicular conjunctivitis.

Contact lens solutions can also cause severe epithelial damage and pain when contact lenses soaked in cleaning or preservative-laden solutions are inadvertently placed in the eye without rinsing. The alkaline cleaning material or preservative (often thimerosal) can cause chemical injury of the cornea.

Asymptomatic subconjunctival fibrosis is sometimes associated with the long-term use of topical ophthalmic drugs (eg, miotics, β-blockers); however, in a small minority of affected patients, a more severe type of progressive subconjunctival scarring develops, which can lead to contraction of the conjunctival fornix, symblepharon formation, punctal stenosis, and corneal pannus formation.

Due to the rapid turnover of epithelial cells, drugs that inhibit DNA synthesis may be toxic to the epithelium when used systemically in high doses. Cytarabine, for example, can cause punctate keratopathy and refractile epithelial microcysts, which are associated with pain, photophobia, FBS, and reduced vision.

MANAGEMENT Treatment of ocular toxicity requires that the offending topical medications be discontinued. Severe cases may take months to resolve completely; thus, failure of symptoms and signs to resolve within a period of days to a few weeks is not inconsistent with a toxic etiology. Patients who are experiencing significant ocular irritation may find

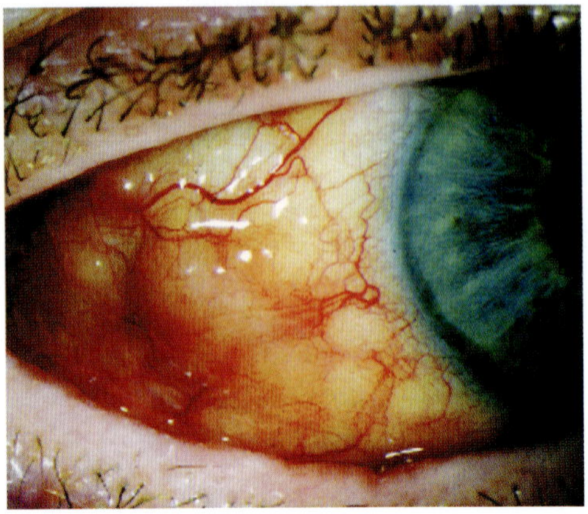

Figure 4-10 Bulbar follicles seen in drug-induced chronic follicular conjunctivitis. *(Courtesy of James J. Reidy, MD.)*

relief with nonpreserved topical lubricant drops or ointment. It is important to emphasize that toxic reactions to ocular medications can lead to irreversible changes, for example, conjunctival scarring and/or shrinkage.

A conjunctival biopsy showing the characteristic diffuse, nonlinear immunofluorescent staining that confirms antibody deposition would typically indicate the diagnosis of the autoimmune disease MMP, rather than drug-induced scarring (ie, pseudopemphigoid). However, even in patients with MMP, a conjunctival biopsy can be negative in up to 50% of cases. Withdrawal of the medication is generally followed by a lag of weeks before progressive scarring can be stabilized (see Chapter 13); MMP would be expected to progress.

Huang LC, Wong JR, Alonso-Llamazares J, et al. Pseudopemphigoid as caused by topical drugs and pemphigus disease. *World J Ophthalmol.* 2015;5(1):1–15.

Self-Induced Ocular Surface Disorders

Ocular surface disorders related to corneal injuries include a spectrum of self-induced disorders with associated symptoms or physical findings. Eyes with these disorders usually show evidence of mechanical injury to the inferior and nasal quadrants of the cornea and conjunctiva. The areas of involvement show sharply delineated borders. The conjunctival tissues usually show no evidence of inflammation on pathologic examination.

Mucus-fishing syndrome

Mucus-fishing syndrome is characterized by a well-circumscribed pattern of rose bengal or lissamine green staining on the nasal and inferior bulbar conjunctiva. All patients have a history of increased mucus production as a nonspecific response to ocular surface damage. The inciting event is typically keratoconjunctivitis sicca. Patients usually demonstrate vigorous eye rubbing and compulsive removal of strands of mucus from the fornix (mucus fishing). The resultant epithelial injury heightens the ocular surface irritation, which in turn stimulates additional mucus production, resulting in a vicious cycle.

Topical anesthetic abuse

Clinical application of topical anesthetics is an integral part of the modern practice of ophthalmology. However, indiscriminate use of topical anesthetics can cause serious ocular surface toxicity and complications. Health care workers and other individuals with access to topical anesthetics may be more likely to abuse these agents. Local anesthetics are known to inhibit epithelial cell migration and division. Loss of microvilli, reduction of desmosomes and other intercellular connections, and swelling of mitochondria and lysosomes have been reported in ultrastructural studies. The characteristic clinical feature of anesthetic abuse is failure of the presenting condition, for example, corneal abrasion or keratitis, to respond to appropriate therapy.

Initially, a punctate keratopathy is observed. As the abuse continues, the eye becomes more injected, and epithelial defects develop heaped up or rolled edges suggestive of neurotrophic keratopathy (see Fig 4-5). As the process continues, keratic precipitates and hypopyon develop, thus mimicking an infectious etiology. Common presenting signs at an advanced stage include diffuse stromal edema, dense stromal infiltrates, and a large ring opacity (Fig 4-11). Stromal vascularization may occur with chronic abuse, and infection

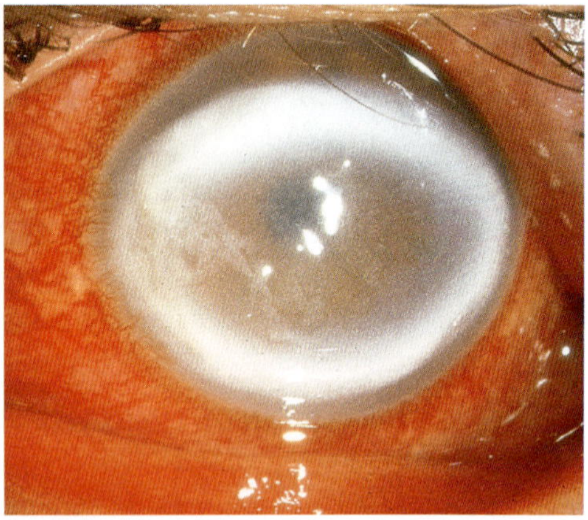

Figure 4-11 Topical anesthetic overuse with persistent corneal epithelial defect and necrotic ring opacity. *(Courtesy of Kirk R. Wilhelmus, MD.)*

or even perforation may ensue. Because of the presence of corneal infiltrates and anterior segment inflammation, it is important to consider the possibility of infectious keratitis and to evaluate the eye with corneal scraping, culture, or biopsy as needed.

The differential diagnosis includes bacterial, fungal, herpetic, and amebic keratitis. Suspicion of anesthetic abuse is warranted in any patient with negative culture results who does not respond to appropriate therapy. In suspected cases, a trial of patching, with the patch appropriately labeled to detect removal, may be therapeutic as well as diagnostic. Often, the condition is diagnosed only when the patient is discovered concealing the anesthetic drops. Once the diagnosis is made and the offending anesthetics are removed, corneal healing usually ensues. Psychiatric counseling may be helpful.

CHAPTER 5

Therapeutic Interventions for Ocular Surface Disorders

This chapter includes related videos. Go to www.aao.org/bcscvideo_section08 or scan the QR code in the text to access this content.

Indicates selected key points within the chapter.

Highlights

- Leaving sclera bare after pterygium excision is associated with higher morbidity and recurrence rates than covering the defect with tissue.
- Tissue glue can be used effectively to secure a conjunctival graft.
- The recurrence rate after pterygium surgery may be lower with use of a conjunctival graft than with amniotic membrane.
- Mitomycin C should be used with caution in pterygium surgery because its potential toxicity can result in significant complications.
- Tarsorrhaphy is an underutilized procedure for treatment of corneal surface disorders.

Introduction

This chapter covers common surgical procedures and other therapeutic interventions used in the management of ocular surface disorders (Table 5-1). More detailed descriptions of these procedures and discussion of alternative surgical techniques can be found in surgical textbooks and other resources (see the references in this chapter).

Conjunctival Interventions for Ocular Surface Disorders

Pterygium Excision

A pterygium is a wing-shaped degenerative fibrovascular growth that extends from the conjunctiva to the superficial cornea (see Chapter 7). Indications for pterygium excision include ocular discomfort, conjunctival inflammation, decreased vision secondary to induced astigmatism, progression of the pterygium toward the visual axis (Fig 5-1), restricted ocular motility, and cosmesis. The goal of pterygium surgery is to achieve a

Table 5-1 Indications for Ocular Surface Reconstruction

Conjunctival Autograft	Limbal Autograft[a]	Limbal Allograft[b]	Amniotic[c] or Mucous Membrane Transplantation
Cicatricial strabismus Fornix reconstruction (unilateral) Postexcision of conjunctival tumor Pterygium surgery Symblepharon repair	Chemical injury Chronic medication toxicity Contact lens keratopathy Limbal depletion after multiple surgeries Persistent epithelial defect (various etiologies) Thermal burn	Aniridia Atopy Mucous membrane pemphigoid Stevens-Johnson syndrome	Chemical injury[d] Conjunctival tumor removal Fornix reconstruction (bilateral) Immune keratolysis Mucous membrane pemphigoid Pterygium surgery Stevens-Johnson syndrome

[a] A limbal autograft from the contralateral eye is preferable only in unilateral cases.
[b] A limbal allograft from donor tissue is preferable for bilateral disease.
[c] May be used in conjunction with a limbal autograft or allograft.
[d] May need fornix reconstruction after cicatrization.

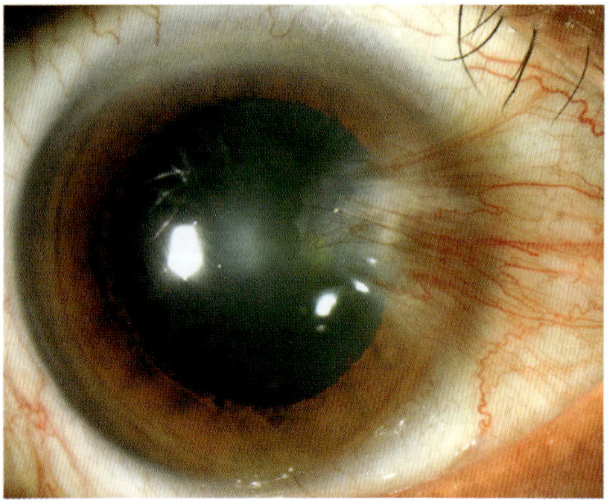

Figure 5-1 Clinical photograph of a nasal pterygium inducing 3.00 diopters (D) of with-the-rule astigmatism. *(Courtesy of Arie L. Marcovich, MD, PhD.)*

relatively clear and topographically regular ocular surface. After excision, the most commonly used technique for coverage of exposed sclera is an autologous free graft from the same or fellow eye. Surgical excision is performed on an outpatient basis. The choice of anesthesia varies according to the degree of involvement and surgeon preference. Options include topical, subconjunctival, and peribulbar or retrobulbar anesthesia (the latter providing postoperative pain relief). Peribulbar or retrobulbar options are particularly useful in cases such as recurrent pterygium complicated by excessive Tenon-layer proliferation.

Surgical technique

The surgical technique for pterygium excision can be summarized as follows:

1. A corneal traction suture (eg, 8-0 silk or polyglactin) on a spatulated needle is placed at the superior limbus. A traction suture can also be placed at the temporal or nasal limbus opposite the pterygium. The traction sutures provide maximal exposure of both the pterygium and the superior bulbar conjunctival donor site.

2. The pterygium margins are marked with a surgical pen to delineate conjunctival resection margins.
3. The epithelium anterior to the pterygium head is scraped using a flat crescent or other rounded-tip blade to create a smooth tissue plane toward the limbus between the pterygium and underlying corneal tissue (ideally leaving Bowman layer intact).
4. Dissection down to bare sclera is performed at the limbus using scissors. Caution is necessary when dissecting Tenon tissue posteriorly because of the risk of significant bleeding and inadvertent trauma to the underlying rectus muscle.
5. The pterygium base and underlying Tenon layer are excised at the conjunctival marks using scissors.
6. After the excision, pressure using a pledget is applied to the sclera for hemostasis. Extensive cautery is preferably avoided. A relatively smooth surface at the site of dissection is a desirable endpoint (Video 5-1).

VIDEO 5-1 Pterygium excision with conjunctival graft using fibrin glue.
Courtesy of Arie L. Marcovich, MD, PhD.

Leaving the sclera bare following excision is associated with a higher recurrence rate (32%–88%) than if the sclera were covered (Table 5-2). It also increases the likelihood of postoperative pain, pyogenic granuloma, and scleral melt, as well as corneal complications such as dellen and vascularization.

CLINICAL PEARL

Covering the entire pterygium excision site decreases postoperative inflammation and speeds reepithelialization of the ocular surface.

Table 5-2 Recurrence Rates of Pterygium With Different Surgical Treatment Options

Surgical Option		Recurrence Rate, %
Bare sclera excision	Isolated	32–88
	With postoperative topical MMC[a]	0–38
	With intraoperative MMC[a]	3–38
Amniotic membrane transplantation	Isolated	7–41
	With intraoperative MMC[a]	16
Conjunctival autograft[b]	Isolated	1–17
	With postoperative MMC[a] eyedrops	4–21
	With intraoperative MMC[a]	0–16
	With fibrin glue	0–9
	With suture	9–16
Conjunctival–limbal autograft	Isolated	0–7
	With MMC[a]	0–5

MMC = mitomycin C.
[a] Various concentrations of and regimens for MMC.
[b] Conjunctival autograft refers to a free graft or a rotational or sliding flap.

Techniques for coverage of bare sclera using fibrin glue or sutures for fixation include the following:

- free conjunctival graft from the same or fellow eye
- conjunctival–limbal autograft
- amniotic membrane graft
- conjunctival flap from contiguous tissue
- simple limbal epithelial transplantation (SLET)

Conjunctival autografts and other techniques for coverage of bare sclera

Covering small to moderate bare areas Following pterygium excision, many surgeons cover small bare areas using a sliding flap technique. This procedure is performed by undermining contiguous conjunctival tissue and rotating it in place without tension. If there is a larger defect, coverage with conjunctival autograft transplantation using tissue from the superior bulbar conjunctiva is optimal. With a surgical pen, the area to be harvested is marked 0.5–1.0 mm larger than the size of the defect to account for retraction of the graft. It is essential to procure thin donor conjunctival tissue with only minimal or no Tenon tissue. The donor material is oriented in the host bed so that the limbal side of the graft is adjacent to the cornea in the excision site. A gap of 0.5–1.0 mm is left between the graft and the limbus. The superior bulbar donor site under the eyelid can be left bare. At the conclusion of surgery, some surgeons apply a bandage contact lens for 1–4 weeks, which may reduce pain and facilitate healing (Fig 5-2; see Video 5-1). Figure 5-3 shows various types of surgical wound closures after pterygium excision.

When either a sliding flap or free graft is used, the conjunctival tissue is secured to adjacent conjunctiva with either 10-0 polyglactin (absorbable) sutures or 10-0 nylon (nonabsorbable) sutures, with or without incorporating episcleral tissue. Alternatively, commercially available fibrin glue can be used, which eliminates the need for sutures, reduces surgical time, and decreases postoperative pain and inflammation.

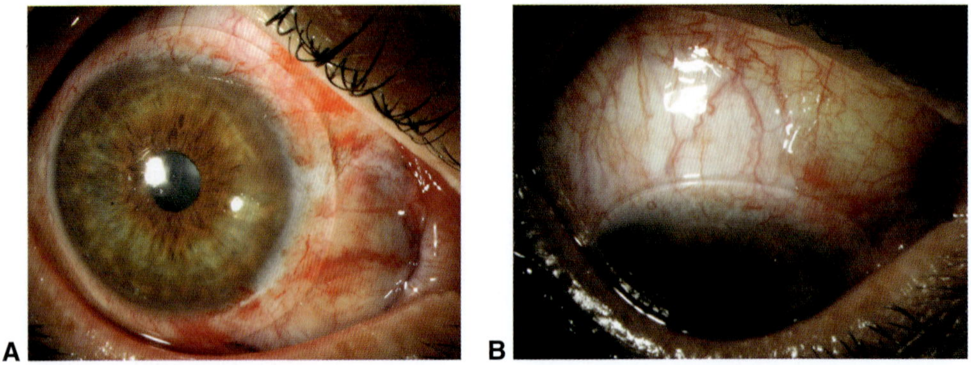

Figure 5-2 Postoperative appearance of a pterygium excision with conjunctival autograft. **A,** Nasal conjunctival graft was secured with fibrin glue. A bandage contact lens promotes healing and provides comfort. **B,** The superior excision site of the harvested donor conjunctiva. *(Courtesy of Arie L. Marcovich, MD, PhD.)*

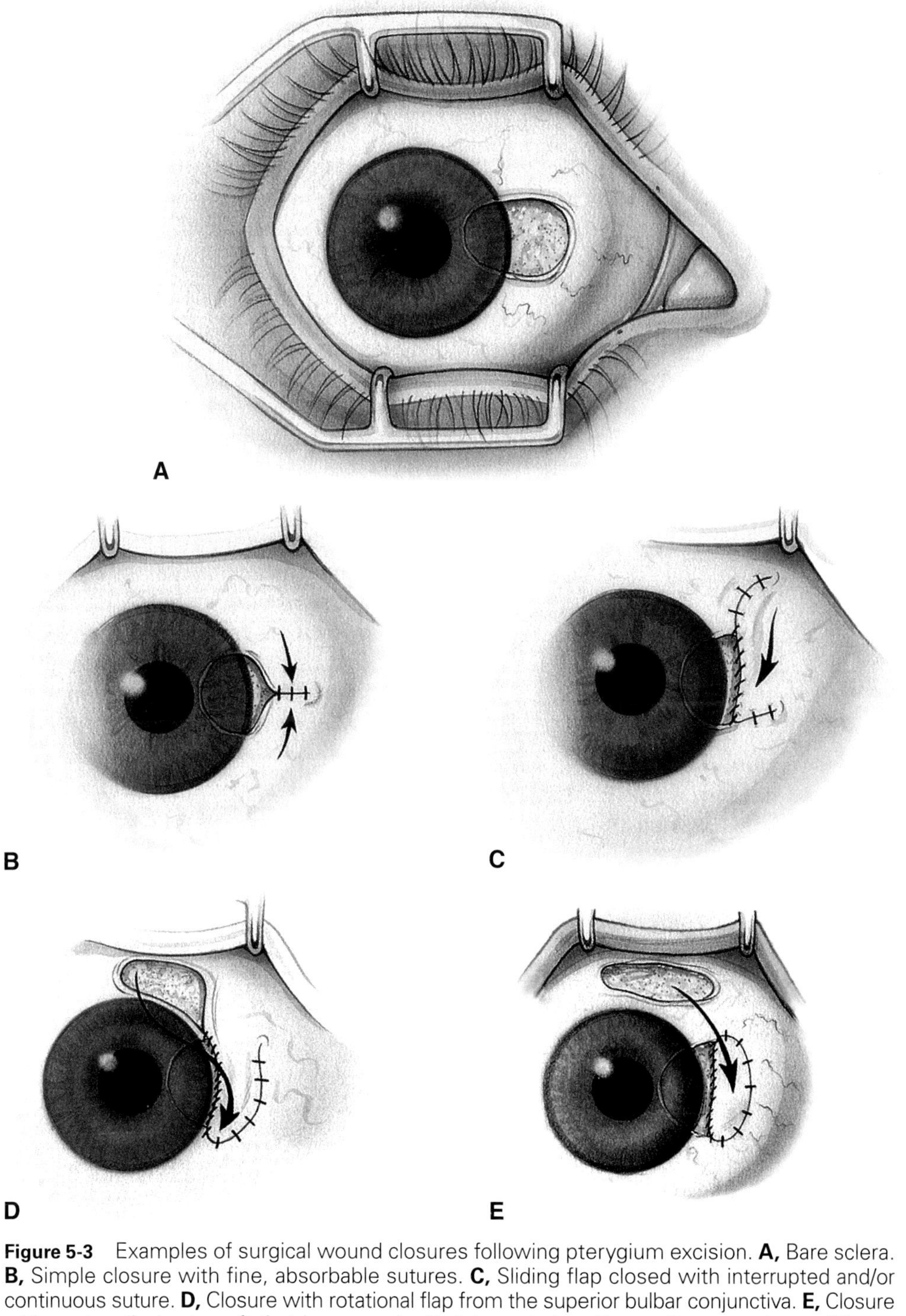

Figure 5-3 Examples of surgical wound closures following pterygium excision. **A,** Bare sclera. **B,** Simple closure with fine, absorbable sutures. **C,** Sliding flap closed with interrupted and/or continuous suture. **D,** Closure with rotational flap from the superior bulbar conjunctiva. **E,** Closure with conjunctival autograft that is secured with interrupted and/or continuous sutures. Alternatively, wounds can be secured with fibrin glue. *(Reproduced from Gans LA. Surgical treatment of pterygium.* Focal Points: Clinical Modules for Ophthalmologists. *American Academy of Ophthalmology; 1996, module 12. Illustration by Christine Gralapp.)*

Use of fibrin glue Fibrin glue mimics natural fibrin formation. Several fibrin sealants are approved by the US Food and Drug Administration (FDA) and commercially available. Sealants contain pooled human plasma components, usually without bovine ingredients. Fibrin glue prepared from the patient's own serum is seldom used due to the preparation time. Currently, use of these products in pterygium surgery is considered off-label. Also, because pooled human plasma is used to obtain some components of these sealants, clinicians should be aware of the small potential risk for disease transmission with their use.

Covering large bare areas Bare areas considerably larger than what can be covered with an autologous conjunctival graft present a challenge that can be remedied with an amniotic membrane graft. However, comparative studies showed that use of conjunctival autograft was superior to amniotic membrane for reducing recurrence. In cases of recurrent pterygium, use of a conjunctival–limbal graft lowers recurrence rates. In this procedure, a piece of superior corneal limbus is transferred with adjacent bulbar conjunctiva from the same eye or from the fellow eye (Video 5-2). The procedure is more demanding and may be associated with pseudopterygium at the donor site. SLET is another surgical technique that optimizes the use of limbal tissue from the healthy fellow eye by combining it with amniotic membrane (Video 5-3); see the section Limbal Stem Cell Transplantation, later in the chapter, for a more detailed description.

VIDEO 5-2 Pterygium excision with conjunctival–limbal graft using fibrin glue.
Courtesy of Arie L. Marcovich, MD, PhD.

VIDEO 5-3 Simple limbal epithelial transplantation technique and outcomes.
Courtesy of Cristos Ifantides, MD; Shobha Mocherla, PhD; and Virender S. Sangwan, MS.

Use of mitomycin C Mitomycin C (MMC) used in association with conjunctival graft has been shown to reduce the pterygium recurrence rate after surgical excision. However, further studies are necessary to determine the dose and optimal route of administration, as well as the duration of treatment with MMC and its long-term effects. In various reports, MMC is applied intraoperatively at a concentration of 0.2 mg/mL (0.02%) for up to 2 minutes or injected subconjunctivally before surgery. Use of topical postoperative MMC application for several days has declined because of possible serious adverse effects. Reported recurrence rates with conjunctival–limbal or conjunctival autograft with or without MMC are similar. Topical MMC is used with caution because it can potentially be toxic and may cause visually significant complications, such as aseptic scleral necrosis and infectious sclerokeratitis. These complications may occur months or even years after use of the drug. If use of MMC is being considered, it is safer to apply this agent intraoperatively rather than topically during the postoperative period.

Al Fayez MF. Limbal–conjunctival vs conjunctival autograft transplant for recurrent pterygia: a prospective randomized controlled trial. *JAMA Ophthalmol.* 2013;131:11–16.

Clearfield E, Muthappan V, Wang X, et al. Conjunctival autograft for pterygium. *Cochrane Database Syst Rev.* 2016;2:CD011349.

Ganelis IB. Conjunctival surgery: pterygium excision with transplantation surgery. In: *Basic Techniques of Ophthalmic Surgery.* 3rd ed. American Academy of Ophthalmology; 2019:73–80.

Hernández-Bogantes E, Amescua G, Navas A, et al. Minor ipsilateral simple limbal epithelial transplantation (mini-SLET) for pterygium treatment. *Br J Ophthalmol.* 2015;99(12):1598–1600.

Kheirkhah A, Hashemi H, Adelpour M, Nikdel M, Rajabi MB, Behrouz MJ. Randomized trial of pterygium surgery with mitomycin C application using conjunctival autograft versus conjunctival-limbal autograft. *Ophthalmology.* 2012;119(2):227–232.

Romano V, Cruciani M, Conti L, Fontana L. Fibrin glue versus sutures for conjunctival autografting in primary pterygium surgery. *Cochrane Database Syst Rev.* 2016;12(12):CD011308.

Young AL, Ho M, Jhanji V, Cheng LL. Ten-year results of a randomized controlled trial comparing 0.02% mitomycin C and limbal conjunctival autograft in pterygium surgery. *Ophthalmology.* 2013;120(12):2390–2395.

Postoperative care

After pterygium surgery, topical antibiotic drops are typically used until reepithelialization occurs and while a bandage contact lens is left in place. Topical steroid drops are applied for approximately 4–12 weeks or as needed until inflammation has subsided. The intraocular pressure is monitored regularly. Most recurrences occur in the first few months, and almost all in the first year. The use of bevacizumab in primary pterygium excision has not been reported to reduce the recurrence rate of this condition.

Complications

Complications of pterygium excision include conjunctival graft edema, corneoscleral dellen, epithelial cysts, and, if MMC is used, scleral melting with possible infection. Pyogenic granuloma due to exposed Tenon fibrovascular tissue may also occur, as may chronic nonhealing wounds if exposed sclera remains uncovered by autologous conjunctiva. Persistent corneal epithelial defect may lead to thinning and perforation (Fig 5-4). Nonhealing corneoscleral wounds should be treated promptly, using either a bandage contact lens or

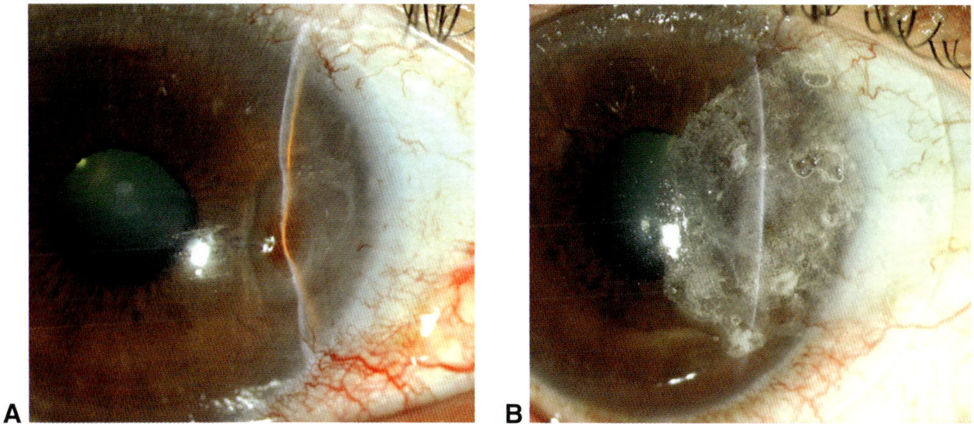

Figure 5-4 Slit-lamp photographs of corneal melting and perforation 2 weeks after nasal pterygium excision with conjunctival graft secured with tissue glue. **A,** The iris is attached to the perforation site with pupil distortion. **B,** Sealing of the perforation was performed with cyanoacrylate adhesive. A bandage contact lens was applied. *(Courtesy of Arie L. Marcovich, MD, PhD.)*

preferably temporary tarsorrhaphy (see the section on tarsorrhaphy later in this chapter). Diplopia may result from severe scarring around the medial rectus muscle. Postoperative infections are rare, but cases reported in the literature reveal a poor visual outcome; thus, attention to postoperative care is essential.

Kaufman SC, Jacobs DS, Lee WB, Deng SX, Rosenblatt MI, Shtein RM. Options and adjuvants in surgery for pterygium: a report by the American Academy of Ophthalmology. *Ophthalmology.* 2013;120(1):201–208.

Masters JS, Harris DJ Jr. Low recurrence rate of pterygium after excision with conjunctival limbal autograft: a retrospective study with long-term follow-up. *Cornea.* 2015;34(12): 1569–1572.

Autologous Conjunctival Transplantation

Autologous conjunctival transplantation is useful when conjunctival loss is not associated with extensive damage to the limbal epithelial stem cells. Although it is most commonly used in association with pterygium excision, autologous conjunctival transplantation has also been used to treat fornix foreshortening resulting from retinal detachment surgery with a scleral buckle, strabismus surgery, or excision of ocular surface tumors or nevi. Systemic conditions associated with fornix obliteration (eg, mucous membrane pemphigoid and Stevens-Johnson syndrome) usually affect both eyes, so there is no ready source of uninvolved conjunctiva. Another indication for conjunctival transplantation is clinically significant pinguecula causing chronic ocular redness and irritation.

Conjunctival Flap for Corneal Disease

Indications

A conjunctival flap can be used to cover an unstable or painful corneal surface when there is little chance of resolution by normal corneal wound healing or other means. A conjunctival flap provides a vascularized tissue cover for the cornea and, although helpful for healing, is not optically clear. Conjunctival flap surgery is performed less frequently than in the past because of the availability of bandage and scleral contact lenses, commercial availability of amniotic membrane, use of tarsorrhaphy, and broadened indications for keratoplasty (see Chapter 16). Nevertheless, use of the conjunctival flap remains an effective method for managing inflammatory and structural corneal disorders when restoration of vision is not the primary concern. The use of a conjunctival flap is controversial in patients with either active microbial keratitis or corneal perforation because residual infectious organisms may proliferate in the avascular corneal stroma beneath the flap, and corneal perforation may continue to leak under a flap.

The principal indications for use of a conjunctival flap are as follows:

- chronic, sterile, nonhealing epithelial defects (eg, stromal herpes simplex or herpes zoster keratitis, chemical and thermal burns, keratoconjunctivitis sicca, postinfectious ulcers, neurotrophic keratopathy)
- closed but unstable corneal wounds
- painful bullous keratopathy in a patient who is not a candidate for keratoplasty
- a phthisical eye being prepared for a prosthetic shell

Some disadvantages of conjunctival flap surgery include a reduced view of the anterior chamber and the creation of a potential barrier to drug penetration through the cornea into the anterior chamber. However, a successful conjunctival graft, free of buttonholes, will thin out over time and, if blood vessels regress, may eventually enable some usable vision.

Massop DJ, Johnson DA. Conjunctival surgery: Gundersen flap. In: *Basic Techniques of Ophthalmic Surgery.* 3rd ed. American Academy of Ophthalmology; 2019:99–104.

Surgical technique

Placement of a complete (Gundersen) flap (Figs 5-5, 5-6) can be highly successful if the surgeon pays close attention to several fundamental principles for covering the corneal surface with vascularized tissue and keeping this tissue in place (Video 5-4):

- use of retrobulbar, peribulbar, or general anesthesia
- complete removal of the corneal epithelium and debridement of necrotic tissue from the cornea
- reinforcement of thin areas with corneal or scleral tissue
- inferior displacement of the eye with a traction suture (8-0 silk or polyglactin) placed at the superior limbus
- subconjunctival injection of lidocaine 1%–2% with or without epinephrine, taking care not to pierce the flap area
- dissection of a mobile, thin conjunctival flap without buttonholes, starting from the limbus or superior fornix and followed by 360° peritomy with relaxing incisions
- undermining of the flap to allow coverage of the entire cornea without tension on the margins, to avoid flap retraction
- positioning of the flap over the cornea and suturing it to the sclera with 8-0 or 10-0 polyglactin or 10-0 nylon sutures so that the flap is placed just posterior to the limbus superiorly and inferiorly

VIDEO 5-4 Gundersen flap.
Courtesy of D. Brian Kim, MD.

Occasionally it may be necessary to invert the eyelid and remove the palpebral conjunctiva or conjunctiva and tarsus to obtain sufficient tissue for a Gundersen flap.

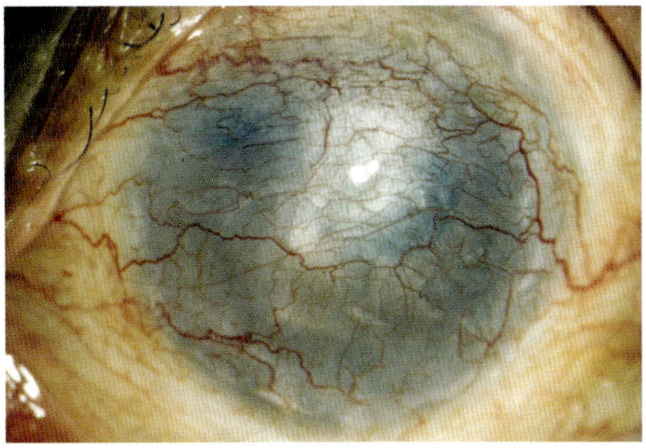

Figure 5-5 Clinical photograph of a Gundersen conjunctival flap. *(Courtesy of David Rootman, MD.)*

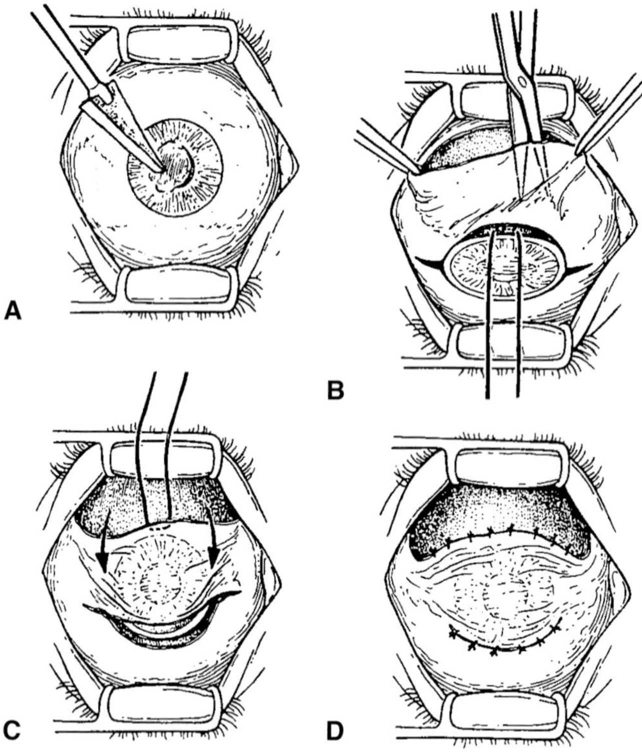

Figure 5-6 Surgical steps for placement of a Gundersen conjunctival flap. **A,** Removal of the corneal epithelium using cellulose sponges. **B,** A 360° peritomy with relaxing incisions, placement of a superior limbal traction suture, a superior forniceal incision, and dissection of a thin flap. **C,** Positioning of the flap. **D,** Suturing of the flap into position with multiple interrupted sutures. *(Reproduced with permission from Mannis MJ. Conjunctival flaps.* Int Ophthalmol Clin. *1988;28(2):165–168.)*

Alternatives to the Gundersen flap include smaller or temporary conjunctival flaps (Fig 5-7) such as

- bipedicle flap
- advancement flap
- single pedicle flap

These flaps may be used for temporary coverage of small peripheral corneal wounds or areas of ulceration. The advantage is that only small or partial areas of the cornea are covered; thus, details of the anterior chamber can be visualized, and the patient may regain functional vision. Because retraction is a common feature of these temporary flaps, the surgeon should take care to minimize tension on any conjunctival flap when it is placed.

Complications

Retraction is the most common complication of conjunctival flaps and occurs in approximately 10% of cases. Other complications include hemorrhage beneath the flap and epithelial cysts. In some cases, inclusion cysts enlarge to the point of requiring excision or marsupialization. Ptosis, usually due to levator dehiscence in elderly patients, may also occur postoperatively and may or may not be related to the flap itself. Unsatisfactory

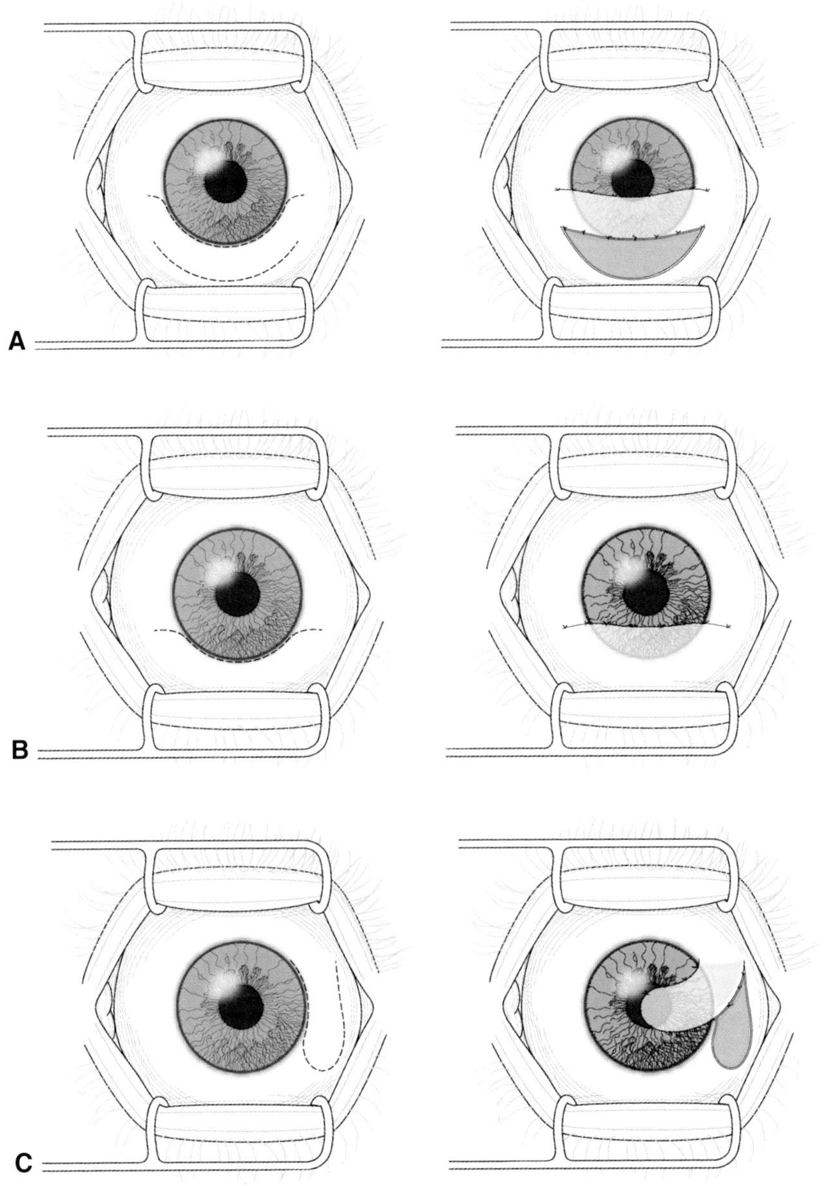

Figure 5-7 Alternatives to the Gundersen flap. **A,** Bipedicle flap. **B,** Advancement flap. **C,** Single pedicle flap. *(Illustration by Mark Miller.)*

cosmetic appearance can be improved with a cosmetic contact lens. Progressive corneal disease under any type of conjunctival flap is a concern in patients with infectious or autoimmune conditions.

Considerations in removal of a flap

If PK or lamellar keratoplasty is to be performed in an eye with a conjunctival flap, the flap may be removed either as a separate procedure or at the time of keratoplasty. Removal of the flap (without keratoplasty) usually does not succeed in restoring vision, as the underlying cornea is almost always opaque from subepithelial scarring and/or thinning. Because the conjunctival flap procedure tends to destroy or displace most limbal stem cells, a limbal autograft or allograft after removal of the flap may be necessary to provide a permanent source of normal corneal epithelial cells before an optical keratoplasty is attempted.

Zemba M, Stamate AC, Tataru CP, Branisteanu DC, Balta F. Conjunctival flap surgery in the management of ocular surface disease (review). *Exp Ther Med.* 2020;20(4): 3412–3416.

Conjunctival Biopsy

Indications

A conjunctival biopsy can be helpful in evaluating chronic conjunctivitis and unusual ocular surface diseases, including

- squamous lesions of the conjunctiva (eg, ocular surface squamous neoplasia [OSSN])
- pigmented conjunctival lesions (eg, primary acquired melanosis [PAM])
- cicatrizing conjunctivitis (eg, mucous membrane pemphigoid [MMP]; also referred to as ocular cicatricial pemphigoid [OCP])
- conjunctival lymphoid tumors
- lichen planus
- pemphigus vulgaris
- graft-vs-host disease

Surgical technique

Topical anesthetic eyedrops, as well as a pledget soaked with lidocaine 1% or 2%, are applied to the lesion or biopsy site for approximately 30 seconds. Subconjunctival anesthesia (lidocaine 1% or 2% with or without epinephrine) may also be used. The advantages of the lidocaine injection are improved analgesia, blanching of the conjunctival vessels, and reduced bleeding. Forceps and scissors are used to snip a conjunctival specimen sufficient for histologic examination. For cases of MMP, it is helpful to also submit some normal-appearing tissue near the lesion. For a subepithelial lesion, a wedge- or block-shaped specimen is excised. Grasping only the edge of the specimen minimizes crushing and preserves tissue integrity. Gentle cauterization can facilitate hemostasis after the specimen has been removed.

Leung TG, Thorne JE. Conjunctival surgery: conjunctival biopsy. In: *Basic Techniques of Ophthalmic Surgery.* 3rd ed. American Academy of Ophthalmology; 2019:95–98.

Tissue processing

Typically, the sample is placed in the proper anatomical orientation on a carrier (eg, filter paper) and inserted into the appropriate fixative, such as 10% neutral-buffered formalin (for histology), 3% glutaraldehyde (for electron microscopy), or Michel or Zeus transport medium (for immunofluorescence microscopy). Tissue wrapped in a gauze pad soaked with balance salt solution may be submitted to the surgical pathologist for immediate processing if prearranged. Consulting with the pathologist prior to surgery is advised to ensure proper handling and staining of specimens. See BCSC Section 4, *Ophthalmic Pathology and Intraocular Tumors,* for further discussion of tissue processing.

Treatment of Conjunctivochalasis

Conjunctivochalasis is characterized by the presence of redundant conjunctival folds positioned between the globe and the lower eyelid margin (see Chapter 4 and Fig 4-4). Surgical procedures used to treat these redundant folds include superficial cauterization, conjunctival fixation, resection, and amniotic membrane grafting.

Superficial cauterization

A topical anesthetic (eg, proparacaine hydrochloride 0.5%) is administered. The patient is instructed to look upward and remains in this position throughout the procedure. After either topical anesthetic or subconjunctival injection of 0.2 mL of lidocaine 1% is given, the surgeon grasps the redundant conjunctiva 4 mm from the limbus and cauterizes it, starting with low-voltage (power level 0.6) bipolar cauterization and gradually increasing the voltage until the conjunctiva coagulates. Coagulation is considered adequate when the conjunctiva turns white. Coagulation is performed at 5–10 sites in an arc on the inferior bulbar conjunctiva. The slack conjunctiva shrinks and tightens immediately after coagulation. This procedure can also be done at the slit lamp using topical anesthetic and low-temperature cautery.

Nakasato S, Uemoto R, Mizuki N. Thermocautery for inferior conjunctivochalasis. *Cornea.* 2012;31(5):514–519.

Conjunctival fixation (plication)

The lower bulbar conjunctiva is pulled inferiorly, stretched to flatten, and sutured to the inferior sclera with 3 interrupted 6-0 absorbable sutures or 10-0 nylon on a CU-5 needle using episcleral bites inserted 8–10 mm posterior to the limbus. The resulting fold of bulbar conjunctiva must be well below the eyelid margin to prevent the patient from experiencing a foreign-body sensation after the procedure.

Resection

The surgical technique used for resection of the conjunctiva involves making a crescent excision of the inferior bulbar conjunctiva 5 mm from the limbus, followed by excision of redundant tissue and suture closure. A modified sutureless technique involves making 2 small radial incisions on either side of the area of redundant tissue several millimeters posterior to the limbus. Fibrin glue can be introduced into the subconjunctival space in this area. An angled forceps is applied to the surface of the globe incorporating the redundant tissue. The excess tissue is excised, and the edges of the wound pinched together. Excess fibrin can be trimmed (Video 5-5).

VIDEO 5-5 Paste-pinch-cut conjunctivoplasty using fibrin glue for conjunctivochalasis.
Courtesy of Yakov Goldich, MD, and Biana Dubinsky-Pertzov, MD.

Amniotic membrane grafts

After excision of the redundant crescent of conjunctiva, an amniotic membrane is fitted to cover the entire defect and placed with the basement membrane surface up to cover the conjunctival wound. The membrane is secured to the surrounding conjunctival edge with interrupted fine, absorbable, or nylon sutures with episcleral bites. The surgeon must take care to flatten the membrane tightly onto the scleral surface as well as at or beneath the epithelial edge.

Doss LR, Doss EL, Doss RP. Paste-pinch-cut conjunctivoplasty: subconjunctival fibrin sealant injection in the repair of conjunctivochalasis. *Cornea.* 2012;31(8):959–962.

Marmalidou A, Palioura S, Dana R, Kheirkhah A. Medical and surgical management of conjunctivochalasis. *Ocul Surf.* 2019;17(3):393–399.

Limbal Stem Cell Transplantation

The peripheral corneal epithelium is derived from stem cells residing in the basal layer of the corneal limbus. However, when the limbal stem cells are not functioning properly, the conjunctival epithelium proliferates over the surface of the cornea. Conjunctival cells do not have the pluripotency of limbal stem cells and cannot differentiate into the corneal phenotype. Replacement of the corneal epithelium by conjunctival epithelium is characterized by surface irregularity and opacity, vascularization, absence of the limbal palisades of Vogt, and poor epithelial adhesion. Impression cytology studies may show goblet cells. This process is called *corneal conjunctivalization.*

Minor disturbances to the corneal limbal stem cell function or surface may be reversible with medical therapy using frequent topical lubrication, topical corticosteroid drops, topical cyclosporine, oral doxycycline, punctal occlusion, or a combination of these modalities.

The current surgical procedures for the treatment of corneal stem cell deficiency are listed in Table 5-3.

Table 5-3 Surgical Procedures for Limbal Stem Cell Transplantation

Type[a]	Surgical Procedure	Success, %
Conjunctival–limbal autograft (CLAU)	Transplantation of 2 grafts of limbal epithelium with conjunctiva from fellow eye; 2 clock-hours each	33–100
Conjunctival–limbal allograft (CLAL) from living related donor	Transplantation of 2 grafts of limbal epithelium with conjunctiva from living related donor; 2 clock-hours each	72–87
Keratolimbal allograft (KLAL) from cadaver (sometimes combined with CLAL)	Transplantation of circumlimbal tissue from a fresh cadaver donor cornea	33–83
Simple limbal epithelial transplantation (SLET)	8–10 pieces of limbal epithelium are cut from a 2 × 2-mm strip taken from fellow eye; pieces are secured with fibrin adhesive onto amniotic membrane previously glued with fibrin adhesive onto recipient cornea	70–84
Cultivated autologous limbal epithelial transplantation (auto-CLET)	Transplantation of cultured limbal epithelial cells from a 1 × 1-mm limbal explant from fellow eye onto amniotic membrane	37–72
Cultivated allogeneic limbal epithelial transplantation (allo-CLET)	Transplantation of cultured limbal epithelial cells from several limbal segments from fresh cadaver donor cornea onto amniotic membrane	0–70

[a] Other abbreviations for the same procedures are used in the literature.

Unilateral total loss of limbal stem cells The unilateral total loss of limbal stem cells can be treated with an autograft of limbal epithelium from the fellow eye; this treatment allows for normal corneal epithelium to repopulate the diseased cornea (Fig 5-8). In this procedure, the unhealthy corneal epithelium, conjunctiva, and pannus are removed from within 2–4 mm of the limbus of the recipient eye, and 2 thin limbal autografts from the fellow eye are attached to the limbus to facilitate the regeneration and proliferation of corneal epithelial cells (Video 5-6; Fig 5-9).

VIDEO 5-6 Superficial keratectomy with limbal autograft from the fellow eye.
Courtesy of Arie L. Marcovich, MD, PhD.

Simple limbal epithelial transplantation SLET is a promising technique for unilateral stem cell injury that obviates the need for intensive systemic immunosuppression, which conventional allograft transplantation requires (see also the section Pterygium Excision, earlier in the chapter). After a superficial keratectomy to remove pannus, the cornea is covered with amniotic membrane. A small 2×2-mm strip of donor limbal tissue from the healthy fellow eye is divided into 8–10 pieces; these pieces are placed evenly over the cornea with fibrin adhesive and then covered with a bandage contact lens (see Video 5-3).

Cell culture of corneal stem cells (*cultivated limbal epithelial transplantation [CLET]*) has been shown to be an effective source of corneal surface repopulation; however, the long-term survival of these grafts remains uncertain. The procedure is expensive and requires regulatory approval and a sophisticated laboratory for cell preparation. Epithelial cells present in the oral mucosa and the human umbilical cord are emerging as important sources of cultured stem cells. At present, these approaches remain experimental and are available in few centers worldwide.

Basu S, Sureka SP, Shanbhag SS, Kethiri AR, Singh V, Sangwan VS. Simple limbal epithelial transplantation: long-term clinical outcomes in 125 cases of unilateral chronic ocular surface burns. *Ophthalmology.* 2016;123(5):1000–1010.

Borderie VM, Ghoubay D, Georgeon C, et al. Long-term results of cultured limbal stem cell versus limbal tissue transplantation in stage III limbal deficiency. *Stem Cells Transl Med.* 2019;8(12):1230–1241.

Kim BY, Riaz KM, Bakhtiari P, et al. Medically reversible limbal stem cell disease: clinical features and management strategies. *Ophthalmology.* 2014;121(10):2053–2058.

Movahedan A, Cheung AY, Eslani M, Mogilishetty G, Govil A, Holland EJ. Long-term outcomes of ocular surface stem cell allograft transplantation. *Am J Ophthalmol.* 2017;184:97–107.

Shanbhag SS, Nikpoor N, Donthineni RP, Singh V, Chodosh J, Basu S. Autologous limbal stem cell transplantation: a systematic review of clinical outcomes with different surgical techniques. *Br J Ophthalmol.* 2020;104(2):247–253.

Shanbhag SS, Saeed HN, Paschalis EI, Chodosh J. Keratolimbal allograft for limbal stem cell deficiency after severe corneal chemical injury: a systematic review. *Br J Ophthalmol.* 2018;102(8):1114–1121.

Suh LH, Chuck RS. Conjunctival surgery: limbal stem cell transplantation. In: *Basic Techniques of Ophthalmic Surgery.* 3rd ed. American Academy of Ophthalmology; 2019:89–94.

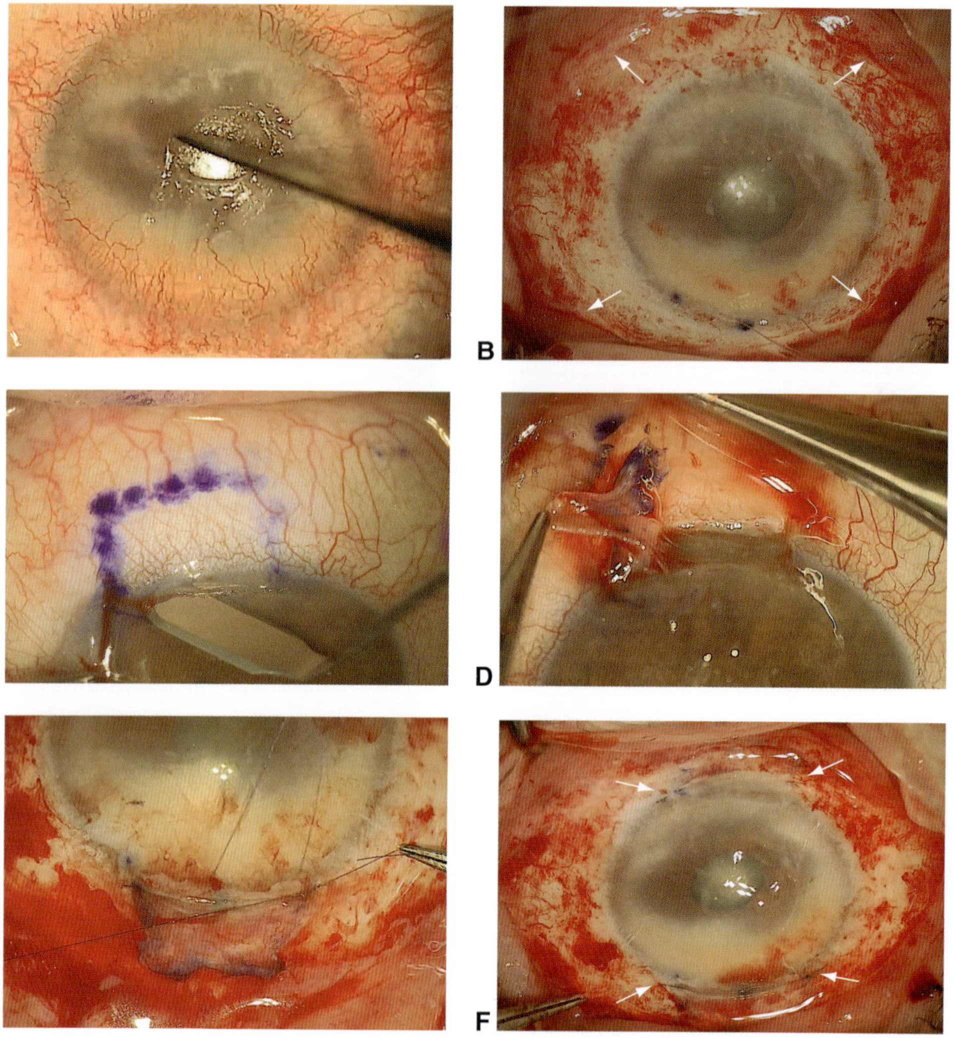

Figure 5-8 Conjunctival–limbal autograft procedure. **A,** Abnormal corneal epithelium and fibrovascular pannus are stripped by blunt dissection using a metal spatula or rounded blade and tissue forceps. **B,** The conjunctiva is undermined with blunt scissors, recessed 2–3 mm posterior to the limbus *(arrows),* and attached to the sclera with 10-0 polyglactin sutures or fibrin glue. A superior corneal traction suture is placed to facilitate exposure. **C,** Superior and inferior conjunctival–limbal grafts are delineated in the donor eye with a marking pen. A superficial incision is made within clear cornea with a crescent blade. **D,** The bulbar conjunctival part of the graft is undermined and thinly dissected from its limbal attachment. **E,** The limbal grafts are transferred to their corresponding sites in the recipient eye and secured with 10-0 nylon sutures at the corneal edge and 10-0 polyglactin sutures or fibrin glue at the conjunctival margin. **F,** Superior and inferior limbal grafts *(arrows)* at the conclusion of surgery. *(Courtesy of Arie L. Marcovich, MD, PhD.)*

Bilateral total loss of limbal stem cells Bilateral total loss of limbal stem cells can be treated with stem cells from a living, related donor (ie, a limbal stem cell allograft) or from an eye bank donor cornea (ie, a keratolimbal allograft). Use of a limbal stem cell allograft

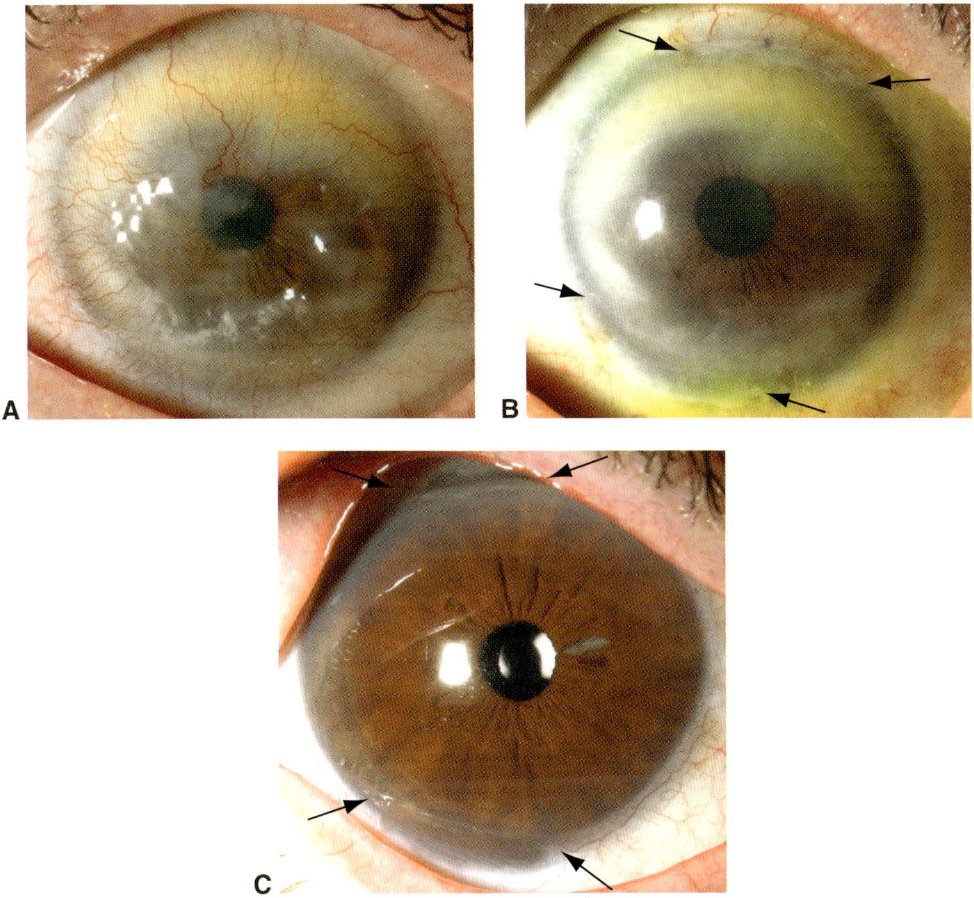

Figure 5-9 Clinical photographs of a patient treated for a unilateral alkali burn with an autograft of limbal epithelium. **A,** Conjunctivalized cornea of the left eye after unilateral alkali burn. **B,** Photograph taken 3 months after superior and inferior limbal transplantation from the right fellow eye. *Arrows* outline the edges of the transplanted limbal segments. **C,** Right eye, showing superior and inferior sites of limbal harvesting *(arrows)*. *(Courtesy of Arie L. Marcovich, MD, PhD.)*

may decrease the risk of rejection but still requires systemic immunosuppression; it also enables more conjunctiva to be harvested and transplanted than does a keratolimbal allograft. Although host cells may eventually reject or replace such tissue, good long-term results have been reported with both techniques. Poor epithelial viability and complications from systemic immunosuppression are considerable concerns, but dramatic success has been observed in some cases.

Mucous Membrane Grafts

In the absence of healthy conjunctiva (eg, in bilateral cicatricial conjunctival disease), extraocular mucous membrane may be used to restore the conjunctival surface to a more functional state.

The goals of the mucous membrane graft are to

- create a more normal fornix
- reduce ocular surface inflammation
- minimize corneal damage from the abnormal eyelid–globe relationships (eg, entropion, trichiasis)
- avoid chronic exposure (eg, lagophthalmos)
- avoid direct corneal trauma from palpebral conjunctival keratinization, common in bilateral cicatricial disorders (see Table 5-1)
- increase ocular surface wetting

Mucous membrane grafts increase ocular surface wetting by improving eyelid movement and distribution of the tear film over the cornea, thereby reducing exposure and evaporation. These grafts also provide suitable extracellular matrix substrate for epithelial cell migration and adhesion, but they are not effective in replacing normal stem cells.

Mucous membrane grafting can be performed in patients with inactive cicatricial disorders such as late-stage, nonprogressive Stevens-Johnson syndrome and quiescent mucous membrane pemphigoid (MMP). However, mucosa in the mouth is thicker than in the conjunctiva, and any surgical procedure in patients with these disorders can incite severe inflammation. A combination of limbal allograft, amniotic membrane transplantation, and tarsorrhaphy, followed by the use of serum-derived tears and systemic immunosuppression, helps make reconstruction of the ocular surface possible. Patients with advanced, progressive stage III or IV MMP require advanced immunosuppressive treatment to reduce active inflammation prior to any graft procedure (see the discussion of MMP in Chapter 13). Keratoprosthesis is another treatment option for patients with late-stage cicatricial disease (see Chapter 16), although it is less successful in severely dry eyes.

Multiple surgical techniques for mucosal grafts are available. The reader is encouraged to consult a surgical textbook or video for discussion and illustration of these techniques (see the reference list that follows). Potential complications, regardless of the technique, include buttonhole development, graft retraction, trichiasis, surface keratinization of the graft, ptosis, blepharophimosis, depressed eyelid blink, lagophthalmos, submucosal abscess formation, and persistent nonhealing epithelial defects of the cornea.

Black EH, Nesi FA, Gladstone G, Levine MR, Calvano CJ, eds. *Smith and Nesi's Ophthalmic Plastic and Reconstructive Surgery.* 3rd ed. Springer-Verlag; 2012.

Chun YS, Park IK, Kim JC. Technique for autologous nasal mucosa transplantation in severe ocular surface disease. *Eur J Ophthalmol.* 2011;21(5):545–551.

Fu Y, Liu J, Tseng SC. Oral mucosal graft to correct lid margin pathologic features in cicatricial ocular surface diseases. *Am J Ophthalmol.* 2011;152(4):600–608.e1.

Liu J, Sheha H, Fu Y, Giegengack M, Tseng SC. Oral mucosal graft with amniotic membrane transplantation for total limbal stem cell deficiency. *Am J Ophthalmol.* 2011;152(5):739–747.

Sant'Anna AE, Hazarbassanov RM, de Freitas D, Gomes JA. Minor salivary glands and labial mucous membrane graft in the treatment of severe symblepharon and dry eye in patients with Stevens-Johnson syndrome. *Br J Ophthalmol.* 2012;96(2):234–239.

Takeda K, Nakamura T, Inatomi T, Sotozono C, Watanabe A, Kinoshita S. Ocular surface reconstruction using the combination of autologous cultivated oral mucosal epithelial transplantation and eyelid surgery for severe ocular surface disease. *Am J Ophthalmol.* 2011;152(2):195–201.

Corneal Interventions for Ocular Surface Disorders

Superficial Keratectomy and Corneal Biopsy

Indications

In superficial keratectomy, the surgeon excises the superficial layers of cornea (epithelium, Bowman layer, or superficial stroma) without replacing the tissue. Frequently, scraping the surface with a rounded blade alone without excision is sufficient.

The primary indications for superficial keratectomy are

- removal of hyperplastic or necrotic tissue (eg, corneal dermoid, pterygium, Salzmann nodular degeneration, epithelial basement membrane dystrophy with scarring, degenerative calcification)
- excision of retained foreign material in the cornea
- obtaining tissue for diagnostic studies (histologic or microbiologic)
- excision of scar tissue or superficial corneal dystrophic tissue

If corneal biopsy is performed for histopathologic studies, preservation of tissue integrity and anatomical orientation is important. A small specimen can be placed on filter paper or a thin card to maintain the tissue orientation before fixation or cryosection. For microbiologic workup, the biopsy specimens can be minced or homogenized before inoculation of the culture media or prepared for histochemical staining.

Surgical techniques

Mechanical keratectomy If the corneal lesion is superficial, it may be possible to scrape or peel it away without sharp dissection. Often, the surgeon can obtain a smooth anatomical tissue plane anterior to Bowman layer by using sweeping strokes taken parallel to the tissue while keeping the metal spatula or blade perpendicular to the cornea. Alternatively, a cellulose sponge can be used. In some cases, such as in Salzmann nodular degeneration, the abnormal tissue can be peeled off gently by using a 0.12 forceps (see Chapter 7, Video 7-2). When deeper dissection is required, the surgeon can either mark the area freehand with an adjustable-depth blade or use a trephine. A 2- to 3-mm disposable dermatologic skin punch trephine blade can be used to create a partial-thickness incision, and forceps and scissors are then used to excise a lamellar flap of cornea. The specimen is generally split into 2 pieces, or separate biopsies are taken, so that tissue can be sent for both histologic and microbiologic examination.

Alió JL, Agdeppa MC, Uceda-Montanes A. Femtosecond laser–assisted superficial lamellar keratectomy for the treatment of superficial corneal leukomas. *Cornea.* 2011;30(3):301–307.

Mian SI. Corneal surgery: corneal biopsy. In: *Basic Techniques of Ophthalmic Surgery.* 3rd ed. American Academy of Ophthalmology; 2019:113–118.

Phototherapeutic keratectomy Excimer laser can be used to remove superficial stromal tissue. However, corneal scars or calcium or other deposits may ablate at rates that differ from those of healthy tissue. An uneven surface can result even if the original surface was smooth. Manual techniques are more likely to respect Bowman layer and maintain a smooth ocular surface, unlike the laser, which does not respect anatomical planes. Frequent application of viscous liquid to the corneal surface (as a masking agent) during laser ablation can fill gaps in the surface and help achieve a smooth surface after ablation. Most patients experience a hyperopic shift after phototherapeutic keratectomy (PTK) from the corneal-flattening effect of the procedure. Nevertheless, when manual techniques are not feasible, PTK is an excellent option in patients with superficial (<100-μm deep) stromal scarring or dystrophies. Treatment with PTK may result in postponing or eliminating the need for corneal transplantation. Topical MMC applied to the corneal ablation zone for a brief period following PTK has been shown to decrease postoperative scar formation. Usually MMC 0.2 mg/mL is applied for 20–30 seconds. Oral vitamin C has been used prophylactically to reduce haze formation following PTK (see Chapter 4 for additional information on recurrent corneal erosions).

Hindman HB, MacRae SM. Phototherapeutic keratectomy. In: *Basic Techniques of Ophthalmic Surgery.* 3rd ed. American Academy of Ophthalmology; 2019:173–180.

Nagpal R, Maharana PK, Roop P, et al. Phototherapeutic keratectomy. *Surv Ophthalmol.* 2020;65(1):79–108.

Surgical Management of Recurrent Corneal Erosion

Recurrent corneal erosion results from poor adhesion of the corneal epithelium to the underlying basement membrane and Bowman layer. This can occur after trauma, such as an injury caused by a fingernail, or in association with a corneal dystrophy, such as epithelial basement membrane dystrophy or a dystrophy that results in deposition at the level of the epithelial basement membrane complex (see Chapters 4 and 8). When treatment with hypertonic sodium chloride ointment and drops or bandage contact lens fail to control the erosion symptoms, a surgical approach is warranted.

Epithelial debridement

Removal of the loose epithelium or an area that contains microcysts, maps, or fingerprints can allow healthy surrounding epithelium to fill this defect. The procedure is easily done at the slit lamp after instillation of topical anesthetic and 5% povidone-iodine. After insertion of a self-retaining speculum, a blunt spatula or rounded blade can be used to remove the abnormal area. The surrounding epithelium can be quite loose; it is important to avoid removing more tissue than necessary. Treatment with topical antibiotic, cycloplegic, and corticosteroid, along with a bandage soft contact lens, reduces risk of infection and inflammation and promotes healing. Once the epithelium has healed, continued treatment with hypertonic 5% sodium chloride is recommended.

Anterior stromal puncture

Anterior stromal puncture is best performed at the slit lamp for the treatment of recurrent corneal erosions failing to respond to medical treatment. Some clinicians prefer anterior stromal puncture for the treatment of traumatic recurrent erosions and favor epithelial debridement for dystrophic recurrent erosions. After application of topical anesthesia and 5% povidone-iodine drops, an eyelid speculum is placed. Puncture of the anterior corneal stroma through the epithelium in the area of loose epithelium is performed using an 18-gauge needle or 25-gauge bent needle. After the procedure, a bandage contact lens can be applied for several weeks with topical antibiotic and corticosteroid treatment. In the absence of a contact lens, topical hypertonic sodium chloride 5% ointment may be continued at bedtime (Fig 5-10). Anterior stromal puncture can be tried if epithelial debridement is unsuccessful or vice-versa.

Zauberman NA, Artornsombudh P, Elbaz U, Goldich Y, Rootman DS, Chan CC. Anterior stromal puncture for the treatment of recurrent corneal erosion syndrome: patient clinical features and outcomes. *Am J Ophthalmol.* 2014;157(2):273–279.

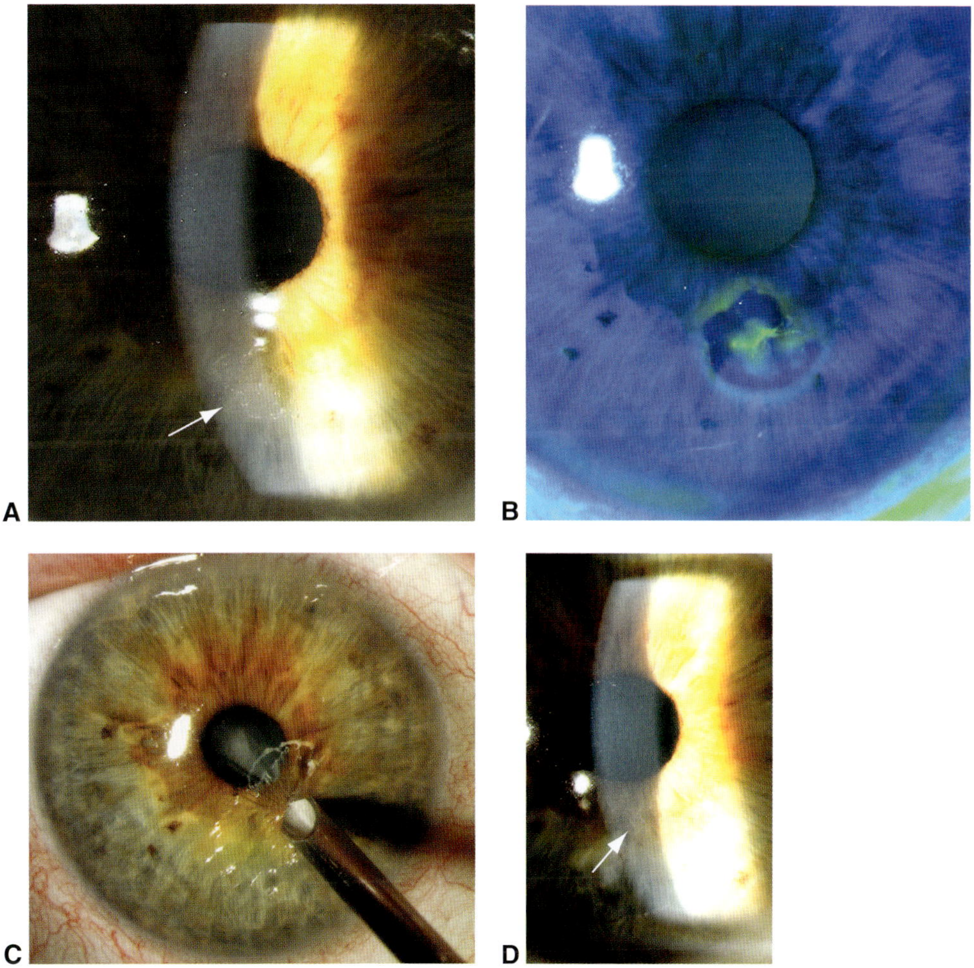

Figure 5-10 Clinical photographs of a patient with recurrent corneal erosions. **A,** Slit-lamp photograph of loose corneal epithelium *(arrow)*. **B,** Fluorescein-negative staining of the irregular epithelium with a small linear epithelial defect. **C,** Anterior stromal puncture using 18-gauge needle distributed over the area of loose epithelium. **D,** Slit-lamp photograph of the same eye taken 2 months after treatment, with resolution of the erosions. There are faint stromal scars at the puncture area *(arrow)*. *(Courtesy of Arie L. Marcovich, MD, PhD.)*

Excimer laser

The excimer laser can be used to induce adherence of the corneal epithelium. However, this may not be the most cost-effective approach. Depending on the refractive error, hyperopic photorefractive keratectomy (PRK) or myopic PRK can be considered. PRK is appropriate for a patient hoping to correct both recurrent erosion and refractive error, provided the area of erosion is within the proposed ablation zone. PTK can be used as well and has the advantage of a smooth tissue ablation; however, a hyperopic shift may occur, which might be problematic for the patient. Postoperatively, the patient is treated as described in the preceding sections.

Management of Persistent Corneal Epithelial Defects, Thinning, and Perforation

Although persistent epithelial defects are often associated with neurotrophic cornea, they also occur after chemical injury or moderate to severe infectious keratitis. Reepithelialization of the cornea tends to be slow in the presence of stromal inflammation (see Chapter 4 for further discussion).

> **CLINICAL PEARL**
>
> Factors that may complicate healing of epithelial defects include surface disease related to dry eye, conjunctival cicatrization, or limbal stem cell deficiency; chronic exposure due to poor blinking, lagophthalmos, or abnormal eyelid position; and trichiasis, eyelid inflammation, or corneal edema.

Correcting these underlying factors, if possible, can be quite helpful. A long-standing epithelial defect can contribute to the chronic inflammation that can lead to stromal thinning and even perforation.

Patching

Persistent epithelial defects can be managed by patching on a short-term basis. Trauma from eyelids during normal blinking may retard reepithelialization. Some patients may require part-time patching with slow tapering to maintain epithelial stability. Proper placement of the patch ensures that it will not rub on the cornea. It is difficult to sustain patching long-term because the patch interferes with the administration of medication, compromises corneal oxygenation, and impairs vision. If progress toward reepithelialization stops, an alternative measure is recommended.

Use of bandage contact lenses

Application of a thin, oxygen-permeable, continuous-wear soft contact lens as a therapeutic bandage can protect loosely adherent remaining or regenerating epithelium from the rubbing action of the eyelids. Use of bandage contact lenses has significantly enhanced the management of persistent epithelial defects. These lenses help reduce stromal leukocyte infiltration and promote regeneration of basement membrane and restoration of tight epithelial–stromal adhesion without compromising corneal oxygenation, patient comfort, or vision. For comfortable wear, a contact lens with an appropriate base curve is fitted (see BCSC Section 3, *Clinical Optics and Vision Rehabilitation,* for more information on contact lens fitting).

Careful consideration is needed in the choice of a soft contact lens for patients with severe dry eye syndrome. In general, patients with dry eye have a higher risk of infection with contact lens use. Punctal occlusion can be performed in these patients to improve comfort and reduce this risk. Contact lenses with high oxygen transmissibility are theoretically the most appropriate choice in these patients. Lenses should be replaced periodically. Frequent lubrication, antibiotic administration, and close follow-up are important, especially in patients with decreased corneal sensitivity or dry eyes. The use of prophylactic antibiotics after the defect has healed is recommended by many clinicians but remains controversial. If a conventional soft lens is not tolerated, an acrylic scleral lens may be a better choice.

Continuous wear of a soft lens can relieve the symptoms of painful bullous or filamentary keratopathy. However, long-term use of a bandage contact lens can also lead to hypoxia, limbal stem cell damage, and vascularization, all of which can compromise the success of future keratoplasty for vision rehabilitation.

A lateral or medial tarsorrhaphy, either temporary or permanent, may be considered for patients who have not responded to patching or application of bandage contact lenses. The tarsorrhaphy procedure is described later in this chapter.

Treatment of corneal thinning/descemetocele

The presence of dellen, resulting from focal stromal dehydration, is a potential cause of corneal thinning that can occur when tear film is uneven. Dellen typically appear at the limbus next to an area of elevated or edematous conjunctiva. An epithelial defect may be present (Fig 5-11). Short-term patching or a bandage contact lens is helpful. Addressing the underlying cause is necessary for recurrent dellen.

A descemetocele is defined as corneal thinning down to the level of Descemet membrane (Fig 5-12). Its presence is typically due to stromal infection or sterile inflammation and signals that the patient is at risk for corneal perforation. Deep radial folds are commonly observed toward the area of extreme thinning. The goals of therapy are to treat the infection and inflammation while facilitating reepithelialization, in an effort to prevent perforation.

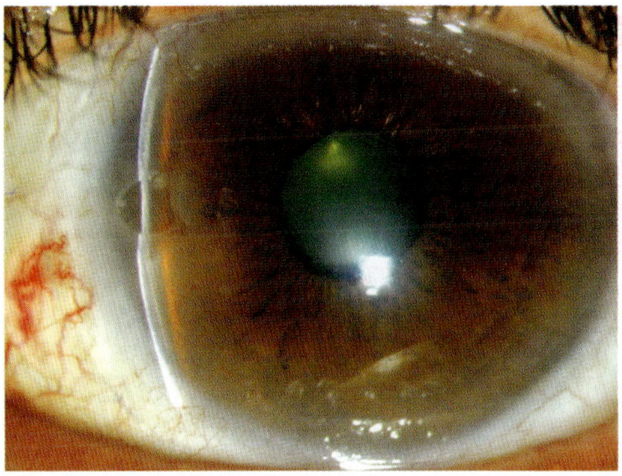

Figure 5-11 Clinical photograph of corneal dellen after nasal pterygium excision with conjunctival graft secured using tissue glue. The slit beam demonstrates thinning of the cornea. An epithelial defect was present. Dellen resolved with return to normal stromal thickness using a bandage contact lens and topical antibiotic and steroid drops. *(Courtesy of Arie L. Marcovich, MD, PhD.)*

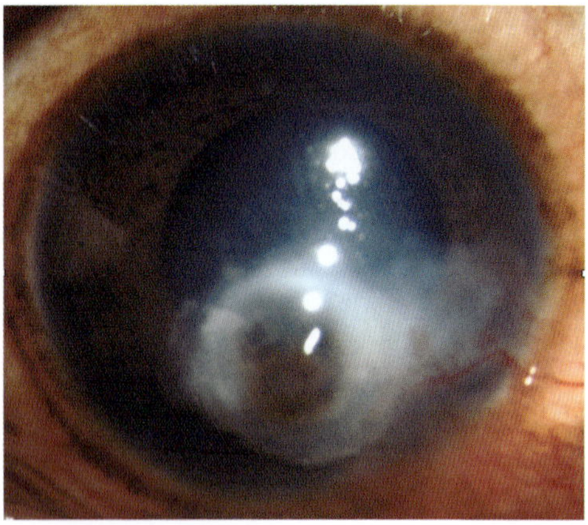

Figure 5-12 Clinical photograph of a large descemetocele, including typical findings of a clear zone in the center of the stromal haze, with smooth contour and increased anterior curvature. *(Courtesy of Robert S. Feder, MD.)*

The first order of therapy is to use appropriate antibiotics and anti-inflammatory medications. Topical steroids may reduce inflammation but also may potentiate collagen breakdown. A bandage lens or even tarsorrhaphy may facilitate reepithelialization. In patients with underlying autoimmune conditions and sterile peripheral ulcerative keratitis, adequately treating the systemic disease is essential. Oral doxycycline is used by some clinicians as a protease inhibitor. Conjunctival resection in the area of a peripheral melt may arrest keratolysis and promote epithelialization. Application of cyanoacrylate glue is helpful in treating impending perforation. The key is to use the glue sparingly. A bandage contact lens is typically applied.

Use of an amniotic membrane graft is an alternative treatment for a sterile melt. The graft is cut to the shape of the defect and placed as a patch over the descemetocele. The patch may be held in place with a larger amniotic membrane graft that is sutured or held in place with fibrin glue. With time, scar tissue will reinforce the deficient area and may reduce the need for keratoplasty.

Liu T, Lindquist TP, Lee WB. Conjunctival surgery: amniotic membrane transplantation. In: *Basic Techniques of Ophthalmic Surgery.* 3rd ed. American Academy of Ophthalmology; 2019:81–88.

Treatment of perforation

Some corneal perforations are small and seal spontaneously before ophthalmic examination, with no intraocular damage, iris prolapse, or adherence. In such cases only systemic and/or topical antibiotic therapy, along with close observation, may be needed. If a corneal wound is leaking but the anterior chamber remains formed, the leakage may be sealed through a combination of pharmacologic suppression of aqueous production (using a topical ocular hypotensive medication or systemic carbonic anhydrase inhibitor), patching, and/or a bandage contact lens. The wound can be sealed with cyanoacrylate glue (see Fig 5-4). Perforations larger than 1 mm are usually not amenable to tissue adhesive and require use of a tissue patch graft (Fig 5-13).

Use of cyanoacrylate glue Although cyanoacrylate glues are not FDA approved for ophthalmic use, they are used widely and have a long track record for safety and efficacy in

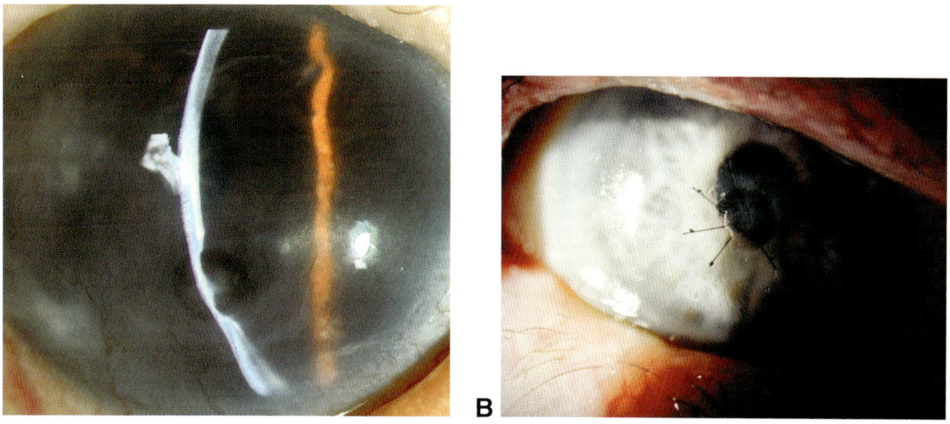

Figure 5-13 Management of a small descemetocele. **A,** Slit-beam view of a smaller descemetocele. **B,** Clinical photograph showing a corneal patch graft for a small central perforation unresponsive to gluing. *(Part A courtesy of Arie L. Marcovich, MD, PhD; part B courtesy of Woodford S. Van Meter, MD.)*

sealing impending or small (<1 mm) perforations. Cyanoacrylate glue applied to thinned or ulcerated cornea may prevent further thinning and can prevent leakage during the healing process. After the lesion is sealed, corneal vascularization and scar formation will help ensure the integrity of the area by providing nutrients and antiproteases.

SURGICAL TECHNIQUE Cyanoacrylate glue can usually be applied on an outpatient basis using topical anesthetic. However, if adherent or prolapsed uvea in the leakage site or a flat chamber is encountered, the procedure may be performed best in the operating room using balanced salt solution and/or viscoelastic to re-form the anterior chamber. An eyelid speculum is necessary to keep the eyelids open and immobilized, and the area is dried with a cellulose sponge. The glue will not adhere well to necrotic tissue or loose epithelium.

An operating microscope is used. A small drop of the fluid adhesive is applied to the corneal wound with the tip of a 30-gauge needle or anterior chamber cannula. Because the glue does not polymerize on plastic, an alternative way to apply the adhesive is to spread a small amount on a section of sterile plastic wrapping taken from any medical product and cut into a 3- to 4-mm disk shape using a skin trephine. The plastic disk is attached with ointment to the wooden tip of a cotton swab (Video 5-7). The glue polymerizes completely within 20–60 seconds and usually adheres well to the deepithelialized surface (see Fig 5-4B).

VIDEO 5-7 Sealing a perforation with cyanoacrylate glue.
Courtesy of Arie L. Marcovich, MD, PhD.

The adhesive plug has a rough surface and can be irritating, so a bandage contact lens is necessary to protect the upper tarsal conjunctiva and to prevent the plug from being dislodged by the eyelid during blinking. The glue usually detaches after several weeks but can remain in place for months.

Anchouche S, Harissi-Dagher M, Segal L, Racine L, Darvish-Zargar M, Robert M-C. Cyanoacrylate tissue adhesive for the treatment of corneal thinning and perforations: a multicenter study. *Cornea.* 2020;39(11):1371–1376.

Suh LH, Akpek EK. Corneal surgery: corneal gluing. In: *Basic Techniques of Ophthalmic Surgery.* 3rd ed. American Academy of Ophthalmology; 2019:119–122.

Tarsorrhaphy

Tarsorrhaphy—the surgical fusion of the upper and lower eyelid margins—is performed to reduce the exposed surface area of the cornea. It is among the safest, most effective, and most underutilized procedures for healing difficult-to-treat corneal lesions. Tarsorrhaphy is performed most often to protect the cornea from exposure caused by inadequate eyelid coverage, as may occur in neurotrophic cornea, thyroid eye disease, or facial nerve dysfunction such as Bell palsy. It can also be used to aid in the healing of indolent corneal ulceration, as sometimes occurs with tear film deficiency, herpes simplex or herpes zoster infection, or stem cell dysfunction.

Tarsorrhaphies are classified as lateral (Fig 5-14), medial, or central and as temporary or permanent according to the position of the adhesion of the eyelids and the desired duration of the adhesion. Because the cosmetic effect of a tarsorrhaphy is significant, patients may be reluctant to undergo this procedure and should be counseled on its therapeutic benefits. Eyelid anatomy and surgical technique for tarsorrhaphy are discussed in detail in BCSC Section 7, *Oculofacial Plastic and Orbital Surgery.*

The Frost suture is a temporary lid closure involving use of a transtarsal plate suture to keep the eyelids closed without intramarginal adhesion; it can be employed to partially occlude the eyelids for up to 2–3 weeks (Video 5-8). Eye inspection can be performed through the nasal or temporal opening. A releasable knot may be placed to allow for periodic examination (Fig 5-15). If closure for longer than 3 weeks is desired, or the length of time needed is uncertain, permanent but reversible adhesion is induced by denuding the eyelid margin (Video 5-9). Plastic bolsters can be used to protect the eyelids from tight

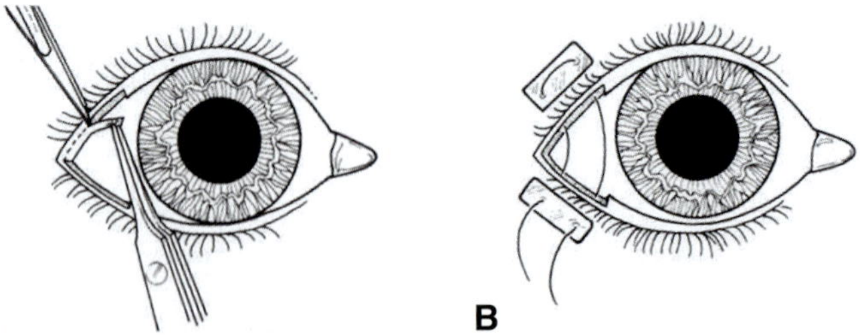

Figure 5-14 Lateral tarsorrhaphy technique. **A,** A strip of eyelid margin is shaved over the gray line. **B,** One or two mattress sutures are passed through the upper and lower eyelids to secure the tarsorrhaphy. Sutures are threaded through bolsters (#40 silicone band or sterile rubber band) and tied. Each suture end is placed through the skin of the upper eyelid approximately 5 mm above the lash line, traverses the upper tarsal plate, exits through the denuded wound surface of the upper eyelid margin, enters through the denuded wound surface of the lower eyelid margin, traverses the lower tarsal plate, and exits through the skin of the lower eyelid approximately 5 mm from the lash line. *(Reproduced with permission from Hersh PS, Zagelbaum BM, Cremers SL.* Ophthalmic Surgical Procedures. *2nd ed. Thieme Medical Publishers; 2009:253.)*

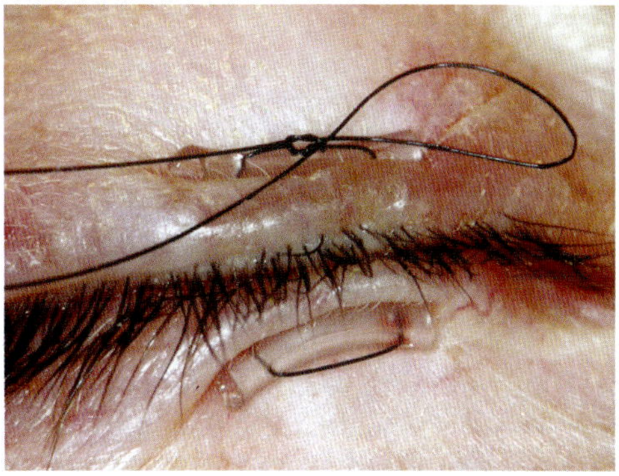

Figure 5-15 Central temporary tarsorrhaphy. A transtarsal plate suture passed through bolsters (tubing) occludes the eyelids. Examination and drop installation can be performed through the nasal or temporal opening. *(Courtesy of Arie L. Marcovich, MD, PhD.)*

sutures (see Fig 5-15). Alternatively, small incisions in the eyelid skin can be performed for absorbable suture burial to reduce patient discomfort due to the sutures. Finally, a vertical mattress suture of 6-0 nylon can be placed in the tarsus of the upper and lower eyelid through the lid margin and tied temporally or nasally. The suture can remain in place for 2 weeks.

VIDEO 5-8 Temporary tarsorrhaphy.
Courtesy of Arie L. Marcovich, MD, PhD.

VIDEO 5-9 Temporal permanent tarsorrhaphy.
Courtesy of Asher Milstein, MD.

A tarsorrhaphy can be opened using local anesthesia in the office. After infiltration of local anesthetic, a muscle hook is placed under the tissue, and a hemostat is placed (for 5 seconds) across the adhesion to be released. A blade or scissors are used to incise the adhesion parallel to the upper and lower eyelid margins. If the status of the corneal exposure is uncertain, the tarsorrhaphy can be opened in stages, a few millimeters at a time. If the tarsorrhaphy has been performed properly, eyelid margin deformity is minimal.

Alternatives to tarsorrhaphy

Injection of botulinum toxin A into the levator palpebrae superioris muscle to paralyze its function can cause pharmacologic ptosis and, mimicking surgical tarsorrhaphy, can impart a protective effect that can last several months. Application of cyanoacrylate adhesive (discussed earlier in this chapter) to the eyelid margins may also result in temporary closure of the eyelids. It is important to avoid inadvertent application of glue to the cornea. In both procedures, the surgeon cannot control how long the effect will last.

Tape may also be used to close the eyelids temporarily, but tape rarely adheres for longer than 24 hours and irritates the skin. Use of moisture-retaining eyewear (also called moisture chamber glasses) is another temporary measure that may be used to minimize desiccation and help protect the ocular surface. These devices are available commercially or may be constructed with plastic wrap and taped over the eyelids.

Sadiq SA, Dharmasena A. Superior rectus underaction following botulinum toxin injection to induce protective upper eye lid ptosis—a comparative study of two techniques. *Strabismus.* 2014;22(3):111–114.

Trivedi D, McCalla M, Squires Z, Parulekar M. Use of cyanoacrylate glue for temporary tarsorrhaphy in children. *Ophthal Plast Reconstr Surg.* 2014;30(1):60–63.

Corneal Tattooing

Corneal tattooing has been used for centuries to improve the cosmetic appearance of a blind eye with an unsightly leukoma (Fig 5-16). It has also been used occasionally in seeing eyes to reduce the glare from scars and to eliminate monocular diplopia in patients with large iridectomies, traumatic loss of iris, and congenital iris colobomas (Fig 5-17). For small iris defects, applying a marking pen to the cornea over the affected area can simulate the effect of tattooing. Although the effect is temporary, this practice allows patients to experience the effect of the procedure.

Different techniques may be used to create a tattoo. One involves applying a platinum-ion solution to the cornea. When this solution reacts with a second agent, a black precipitate is formed in the cornea, producing a dark deposit that can simulate a pupil. Another technique involves adapting standard methods used in skin tattooing to the corneal setting: applying a paste of colored pigment (either India ink or a metal oxide) to the

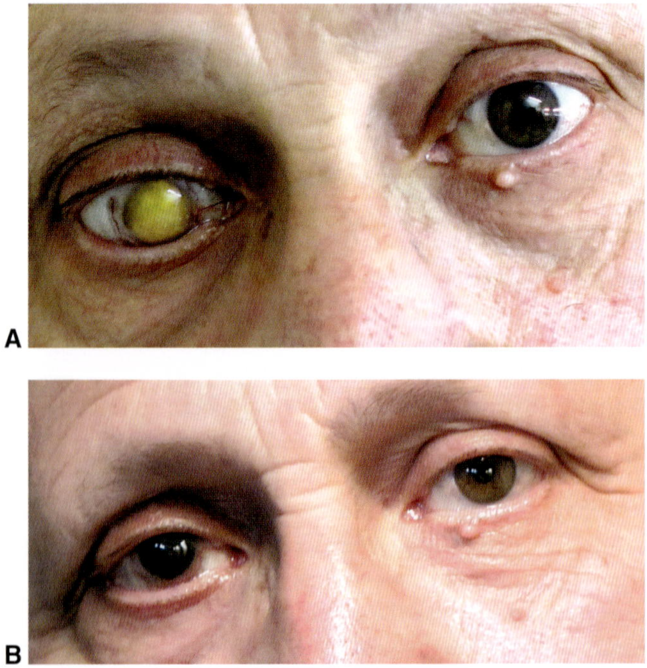

Figure 5-16 Cosmetic use of corneal tattooing. **A,** Photograph of a patient with a corneal leukoma in a blind right eye. **B,** Marked cosmetic improvement after microkeratome-assisted anterior lamellar keratoplasty with tattooing under the graft (see Video 5-10). *(Courtesy of Aaron Grinbaum , MD.)*

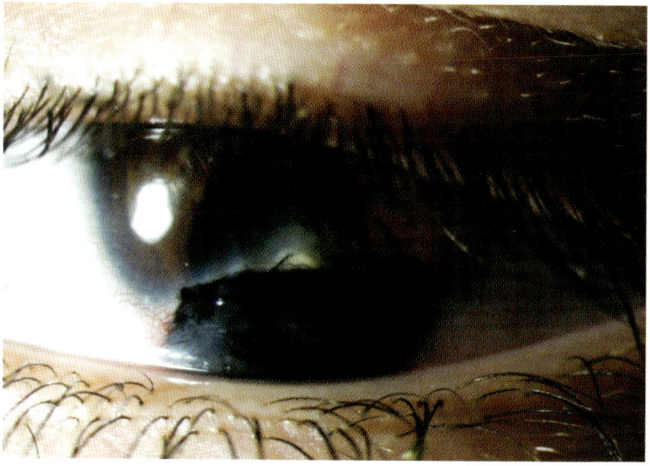

Figure 5-17 Clinical photograph showing a corneal tattoo for a cosmetically displeasing inferior scar in a young woman. *(Courtesy of Robert W. Weisenthal, MD.)*

cornea and then using a hypodermic needle or angled blade to drive the pigment into the corneal stroma in the area that needs coverage. Multiple superficial punctures are made until enough pigment has been applied; additional pigment colors can be used to give a more natural appearance. However, the method is time-consuming and often needs to be repeated if pigment uptake is inadequate, or the pigment migrates. Pigment application under a corneal lamellar flap created by a microkeratome or femtosecond laser can be performed with or without lamellar keratoplasty (Video 5-10).

VIDEO 5-10 Corneal tattooing with microkeratome-assisted anterior lamellar keratoplasty.
Courtesy of Aaron Grinbaum, MD.

Alio JL, Al-Shymali O, Amesty, MA, Rodriguez AE. Keratopigmentation with micronised mineral pigments: complications and outcomes in a series of 234 eyes. *Br J Ophthalmol.* 2018;102(6):742–747.

Hasani H, Es'haghi A, Rafatnia S, Alilou S, Abolmaali M. Keratopigmentation: a comprehensive review. *Eye (Lond).* 2020;34(6):1039–1046.

CHAPTER 6

Congenital Anomalies of the Cornea and Sclera

This chapter includes related videos. Go to www.aao.org/bcscvideo_section08 or scan the QR codes in the text to access this content.

Indicates selected key points within the chapter.

Highlights

- Anterior segment dysgenesis arises from the disruption of anterior segment embryogenesis early in gestation.
- Imaging, such as high-frequency ultrasound, can be helpful in evaluating an infant with congenital corneal opacity to uncover underlying anatomic abnormalities.
- Anterior segment dysgenesis disorders are undergoing reclassification based on underlying genetic factors and the recognition that widely variable phenotypes may share common genotypes.
- Infants with congenital corneal opacities should be managed by a multidisciplinary team, with collaboration from various ophthalmologic subspecialties where appropriate, as well as the pediatrician.
- Patients with congenital glaucoma can present with enlarged corneas, which may be misdiagnosed as megalocornea.

Developmental Anomalies of the Anterior Segment

Table 6-1 summarizes the developmental anomalies of the anterior segment. Congenital anomalies are also discussed in depth in BCSC Section 6, *Pediatric Ophthalmology and Strabismus.* See also BCSC Section 2, *Fundamentals and Principles of Ophthalmology.*

Anomalies of Size and Shape of the Cornea

The cornea of a neonate measures approximately 10 mm; it grows to approximately 12 mm by 2 years of age. Table 6-2 summarizes key measurements in the normal and anomalous cornea.

Table 6-1 Developmental Anomalies of the Anterior Segment

Anomaly	Unilateral/ Bilateral	Clinical Findings	Associated Ocular Anomalies	Associated Systemic Anomalies	Inheritance	Gene Loci
Microcornea	Unilateral or bilateral	Corneal diam. <10 mm (<9 mm in infant); flat corneas with shallow anterior chamber; hyperopia	Persistent fetal vasculature, congenital cataracts, anterior segment dysgenesis, optic nerve hypoplasia, cornea plana	Myotonic dystrophy, fetal alcohol syndrome, Ehlers-Danlos syndrome, achondroplasia	Autosomal dominant (more common) or recessive	11p13: *PAX6*
Megalocornea	Bilateral	Corneal diam. ≥13 mm (>12 mm in an infant); typically seen in males	Iris hypoplasia or translucency, pigment dispersion, miosis, goniodysgenesis, glaucoma, cataract, ectopia lentis, iridodonesis, arcus juvenilis, central cloudy dystrophy	Craniosynostosis, frontal bossing, hypertelorism, facial anomalies, facial hemiatrophy, hypotonia, dwarfism, intellectual disability, Down syndrome, Marfan syndrome, Alport syndrome, osteogenesis imperfecta, mucolipidosis II	X-linked recessive Autosomal dominant and recessive (rare)	Xq23: *CHRDL1*
Cornea plana	Bilateral	Corneal curvature <43 D, typically 30–35 D; peripheral corneal haze; high hyperopia is typical	Cataracts, anterior and posterior colobomas, narrow angle, angle closure, microcornea or sclerocornea	Ehlers-Danlos syndrome	Autosomal dominant and recessive; Finnish ancestry	12q22: *KERA*

Anomaly	Unilateral/ Bilateral	Clinical Findings	Associated Ocular Anomalies	Associated Systemic Anomalies	Inheritance	Gene Loci
Sclerocornea	90% bilateral; often asymmetric	Nonprogressive, noninflammatory scleralization of cornea; may be partial or complete; ill-defined limbus; vascularization	Cornea plana, angle anomalies	Multiple systemic anomalies reported	Usually sporadic; autosomal dominant and recessive inheritance patterns reported	22q11 2p25
Posterior embryotoxon	Usually bilateral	Thickened, anteriorly displaced Schwalbe line; seen in 8%–30% of normal eyes	Usually none	Arteriohepatic dysplasia (alagille syndrome), X-linked ichthyosis, familial aniridia, Axenfeld-Rieger syndrome	Usually autosomal dominant	—
Axenfeld-Rieger syndrome	Bilateral	Anteriorly displaced Schwalbe line (posterior embryotoxon) with attached iris strands	Iris hypoplasia, corectopia, pseudopolycoria, glaucoma	Skeletal, craniofacial, dental, umbilical anomalies, hypospadias	Usually autosomal dominant, may be sporadic	6p25: *FOXC1* 4q25: *PITX2* 13q14: *FOX01A* 11p13: *PAX6*
Peters anomaly	80% bilateral	Central corneal opacity present at birth; variable degrees of iridocorneal adhesion (type 1); cataractous lens or corneolenticular adhesions (type 2)	Congenital glaucoma, microcornea, aniridia, persistent fetal vasculature, cataract, retinal detachment	Intellectual disability, heart defects, external ear anomalies, hearing loss, CNS deficits, GI and GU anomalies, facial clefts, skeletal anomalies, spinal defects, short stature	Most cases sporadic; autosomal dominant and recessive inheritance patterns reported	11p13: *PAX6* 4q25–26: *PITX2* 2p22–21: *CYP1B1* 6p25: *FOXC1* 1p32: *FOXE3* 13q12.3: *B3GALTL* (Peters plus) Trisomy 13–15

(Continued)

Table 6-1 *(continued)*

Anomaly	Unilateral/ Bilateral	Clinical Findings	Associated Ocular Anomalies	Associated Systemic Anomalies	Inheritance	Gene Loci
Posterior keratoconus	Typically unilateral	Localized central or paracentral indentation of posterior cornea with normal anterior topography; overlying stromal haze; focal pigment deposits and guttae often present at margins of the opacity	Astigmatism and amblyopia may occur	Usually none	Sporadic	—
Keratoglobus	Bilateral	Diffuse protrusion and thinning, particularly in the periphery	Blue sclerae	Ehlers-Danlos syndrome type VI	Usually sporadic	—
Congenital anterior staphyloma	Typically unilateral	Large, ectatic cornea protruding between the eyelids at birth; lined by uveal tissue	Anterior segment anomalies, glaucoma, cataract	None	Sporadic	—
Keratectasia	Typically unilateral	Large, ectatic cornea protruding between the eyelids at birth, not lined by uveal tissue	Anterior segment anomalies, glaucoma, cataract	None	Sporadic	—

CNS = central nervous system; D = diopters; GI = gastrointestinal; GU = genitourinary.

Table 6-2 Dimensions of the Cornea

	Horizontal Diameter at Birth	Horizontal Diameter After 2 Years Old	Keratometry of Central Cornea
Normal	9.5–10.5 mm	10.5–12.5 mm	43 D
Microcornea	<9 mm	<10 mm	Usually flat
Megalocornea	>12 mm	>13 mm	Usually steep
Cornea plana	Variable	Variable	Flat, often 30–35 D

D = diopters.

Microcornea

Microcornea refers to a clear cornea of normal thickness with a diameter of less than 10 mm (or <9 mm in an infant) (Fig 6-1). It is important to distinguish microcornea from microphthalmos (a small globe with anatomical malformations) and nanophthalmos (a small but normal globe). Ultrasound imaging and axial length measurements can be helpful in differentiating these conditions. The etiology of microcornea is unknown, but it may be related to fetal arrest of corneal growth in the fifth month of gestation. Alternatively, it may be related to overgrowth of the anterior tips of the optic cup, which leaves less space for the cornea to develop. Microcornea is inherited as an autosomal dominant (most commonly) or recessive trait. There is no sex predilection. Because the cornea is relatively flat in microcornea, these eyes are usually hyperopic, and it is associated with an increased incidence of angle-closure glaucoma. Open-angle glaucoma develops later in life in 20% of patients in whom angle-closure glaucoma does not occur.

Important ocular anomalies often associated with microcornea include

- persistent fetal vasculature (PFV)
- congenital cataracts
- anterior segment dysgenesis
- optic nerve hypoplasia

Significant systemic associations include

- myotonic dystrophy
- fetal alcohol syndrome
- Ehlers-Danlos syndrome
- achondroplasia

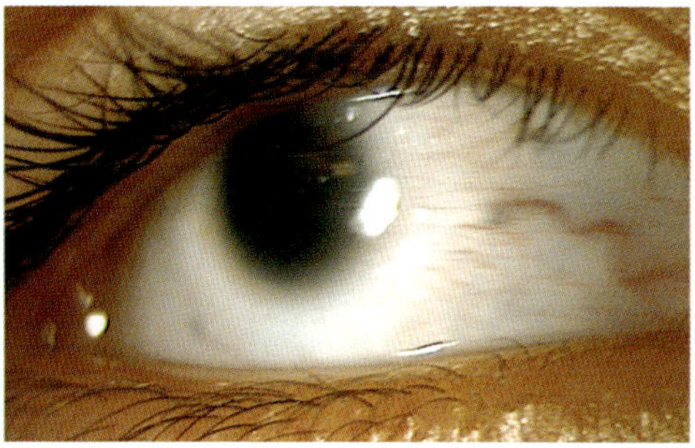

Figure 6-1 Microcornea. *(Courtesy of Danielle Trief, MD.)*

When microcornea occurs as an isolated finding, the visual prognosis is excellent if spectacles are used to treat the hyperopia resulting from the flat cornea. Concurrent ocular pathologic conditions such as refractive amblyopia, cataract, PFV, and glaucoma may require additional medical or surgical treatment.

Robert MC, Colby K. Congenital anomalies. In: Colby K, ed. *Corneal Diseases in Children.* Springer International Publishing; 2017:69–85.

Wang P, Sun W, Li S, Xiao X, Guo X, Zhang Q. *PAX6* mutations identified in 4 of 35 families with microcornea. *Invest Ophthalmol Vis Sci.* 2012;53(10):6338–6342.

Megalocornea

Megalocornea is a bilateral, nonprogressive enlargement of the cornea. On histologic examination, the cornea is normal but measures greater than or equal to 13 mm in diameter (or >12 mm in an infant) (Fig 6-2). The etiology may be related to failure of the optic cup to grow and of its anterior tips to close, leaving a larger space for the cornea to fill. Alternatively, megalocornea may represent arrested buphthalmos (enlargement of the entire globe) and exaggerated growth of the cornea in relation to the rest of the eye. An abnormality in collagen production is suggested by the association of megalocornea with systemic disorders of collagen synthesis (eg, Marfan syndrome). Males are affected more often than females, because it is often inherited as an X-linked recessive condition, but the corneal diameter may also be slightly increased in heterozygous females.

Associated anomalies Ocular anomalies associated with megalocornea include iris translucency (diaphany), pigment dispersion, miosis, goniodysgenesis, cataract, ectopia lentis, arcus juvenilis, and glaucoma (but not congenital glaucoma). Nonocular and systemic associations may include craniosynostosis, frontal bossing, hypertelorism, facial anomalies, facial hemiatrophy, dwarfism, intellectual disability, hypotonia, Down syndrome, Marfan syndrome, Alport syndrome, osteogenesis imperfecta, mucolipidosis II, or occasionally other genetic syndromes.

Differential diagnosis The differential diagnosis for megalocornea typically consists primarily of congenital glaucoma (discussed later in the chapter), which can be ruled out by intraocular pressure measurement and careful biomicroscopy. The presence of pigmentary dispersion, iris transillumination defects, and/or a Krukenberg spindle and the

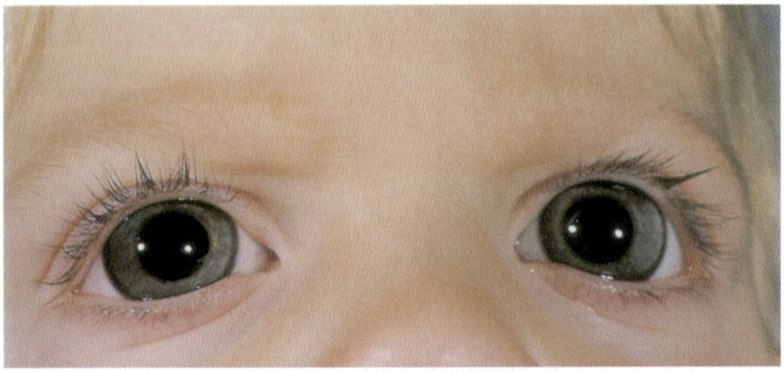

Figure 6-2 Megalocornea.

absence of Haab striae and previous breaks in Descemet membrane can also help distinguish megalocornea from congenital glaucoma. Ultrasonography may be of value in demonstrating the short vitreous length, deep lens and iris position, and normal axial length that distinguish megalocornea from buphthalmos caused by congenital glaucoma. Myopia and with-the-rule astigmatism, which are common in megalocornea, are managed in typical fashion.

CLINICAL PEARL

Lens instability and subluxation, iridodonesis, and poor zonular fiber integrity are associated with megalocornea and present additional risks and challenges in the management of cataracts, particularly in terms of the selection and placement of an intraocular lens (IOL) after cataract surgery (Video 6-1).

VIDEO 6-1 Phacoemulsification with intraocular lens implantation for megalocornea.
Courtesy of Robert W. Weisenthal, MD.

Smith JEH, Traboulsi EI. Malformations of the anterior segment of the eye. In: Traboulsi EI, ed. *Genetic Diseases of the Eye.* 2nd ed. Oxford University Press; 2012:92–108.

Webb TR, Matarin M, Gardner JC, et al. X-linked megalocornea caused by mutations in *CHRDL1* identifies an essential role for ventroptin in anterior segment development. *Am J Hum Genet.* 2012;90(2):247–259.

Welder J, Oetting TA. Megalocornea. EyeRounds.org. September 17, 2010. Accessed November 13, 2021. www.EyeRounds.org/cases/121-megalocornea.htm

Cornea plana

Cornea plana is a rare condition in which the corneal curvature is quite flat, with typical keratometry readings of 30.00–35.00 diopters (D) (see Table 6-2). Additional hallmarks of cornea plana include high hyperopia (usually >10.00 D) and peripheral corneal haze or arcus. Corneal curvature that is the same as the curvature of the adjacent sclera is pathognomonic of this condition. Flat corneas are also a feature of sclerocornea (see Fig 6-3), but sclerocornea can be distinguished by the loss of corneal transparency and limbal architecture. Most isolated cases of cornea plana appear in patients of Finnish ancestry.

Both autosomal recessive and autosomal dominant forms of cornea plana have been associated with mutations of the *KERA* gene, which codes for keratan sulfate proteoglycans (keratocan, lumican, and mimecan). These proteins are thought to play an important role in the regular spacing of corneal collagen fibrils. Investigators have speculated that mutations in the *KERA* gene cause an alteration of the tertiary structure of the keratan sulfate proteoglycans that leads to the cornea plana phenotype.

Associated abnormalities The ocular abnormalities associated with cornea plana include central corneal clouding, cataracts, and anterior and posterior colobomas. Because of the morphologically shallow anterior chamber, angle-closure glaucoma occurs; open-angle glaucoma may develop because of angle abnormalities. Cornea plana is often seen in association with sclerocornea (discussed in the following section) or microcornea. Ehlers-Danlos syndrome can also be associated with cornea plana.

Medical or surgical treatment of this condition consists of correction of refractive errors and control of glaucoma. Loss of central corneal clarity may require deep anterior lamellar keratoplasty (DALK) or penetrating keratoplasty (PK).

Dudakova L, Vercruyssen JHJ, Balikova I, et al. Analysis of KERA in four families with cornea plana identifies two novel mutations. *Acta Ophthalmol.* 2018;96(1):87–91.
Khan AO. Cornea plana. In: Traboulsi EI, ed. *Genetic Diseases of the Eye.* 2nd ed. Oxford University Press; 2012:85–91.

Sclerocornea

Sclerocornea is a nonprogressive, noninflammatory scleralization of the cornea. The scleralization may be limited to the corneal periphery, or the entire cornea may be involved. The limbus is usually ill defined, and superficial vessels that are extensions of normal scleral, episcleral, and conjunctival vessels cross the corneal limbus (Fig 6-3). Sclerocornea is usually sporadic, but both autosomal dominant and autosomal recessive patterns of inheritance have been reported. No sex predilection is evident, and 90% of cases are bilateral.

The most common associated ocular finding is cornea plana, which occurs in 80% of cases. Angle structures are also commonly malformed. Multiple systemic anomalies have been reported in association with sclerocornea.

Ali M, Buentello-Volante B, McKibbin M, et al. Homozygous *FOXE3* mutations cause nonsyndromic, bilateral, total sclerocornea, aphakia, microphthalmia, and optic disc coloboma. *Mol Vis.* 2010;16:1162–1168.

Keratoglobus

Keratoglobus is a congenital ectasia of the cornea, characterized by bilateral steepening and thinning. It manifests as a globular corneal shape and is associated with Ehlers-Danlos

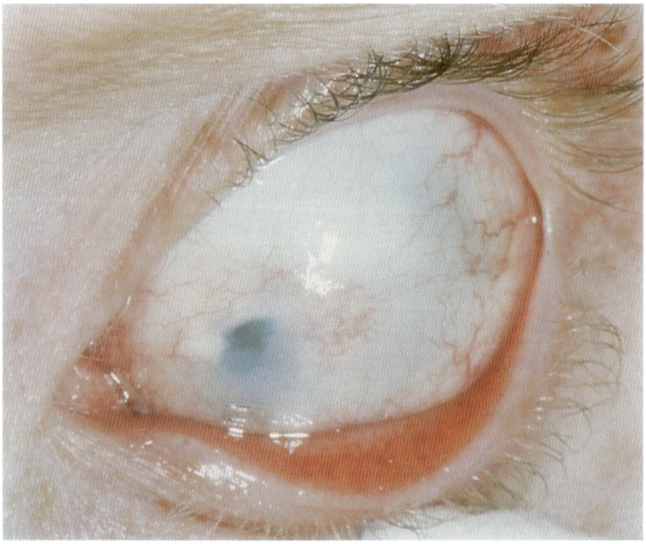

Figure 6-3 Sclerocornea.

syndrome type VI. It is present at birth, unlike keratoconus and pellucid marginal degeneration. Keratoglobus is discussed in further detail in Chapter 9.

Corneal Dystrophies

See Chapter 8 for discussion of congenital stromal corneal dystrophy and congenital hereditary endothelial dystrophy.

Developmental Anomalies of the Cornea and Associated Anterior Segment Structures

Beginning around the sixth week of gestation, anterior ocular structures are formed by 3 waves of neural crest migration that differentiate into corneal endothelium, corneal stroma, and iris stroma. Disruption at any point in this process can hinder subsequent development and differentiation of anterior segment structures (Video 6-2). The term *anterior segment dysgenesis* describes a spectrum of congenital anomalies that arise from miscues during anterior segment embryogenesis and affect any or all of the anterior segment structures, including the cornea, anterior chamber angle, iris, and lens. High-frequency ultrasound can be very helpful in determining underlying anatomical abnormalities in these conditions.

VIDEO 6-2 Development of the cornea.
Developed by Danielle Trief, MD.

Historically, this mixed group of anomalies was categorized by phenotypic, clinical, and anatomical presentation. Updated reclassification of anterior segment dysgenesis disorders is based on underlying genetic factors and the recognition that widely variable phenotypes may share common genotypes. Many of these conditions also have associated systemic anomalies as well as other ocular anomalies; where appropriate, a multidisciplinary approach with physicians from other specialties, as well as the child's pediatrician, is recommended. For further discussion, see the chapter on ocular development in BCSC Section 2, *Fundamentals and Principles of Ophthalmology.*

Mihelec M, St Heaps L, Flaherty M, et al. Chromosomal rearrangements and novel genes in disorders of eye development, cataract, and glaucoma. *Twin Res Hum Genet.* 2008;11(4):412–421.

Nischal KK. Genetics of congenital corneal opacification—impact on diagnosis and treatment. *Cornea.* 2015;34(Suppl 10):S24–S34.

Reis LM, Semina EV. Genetics of anterior segment dysgenesis disorders. *Curr Opin Ophthalmol.* 2011;22(5):314–324.

Posterior embryotoxon

The Schwalbe line, which represents the junction of the trabecular meshwork and the termination of Descemet membrane, is visible in 8%–30% of normal eyes as an irregular, opaque ridge 0.5–2.0 mm central to the limbus. The term *posterior embryotoxon* is used when the Schwalbe line is visible on external examination. In eyes with posterior embryotoxon, the Schwalbe line is thickened and anteriorly displaced (Fig 6-4). Posterior embryotoxon is usually bilateral and inherited as a dominant trait. It may occur as an isolated

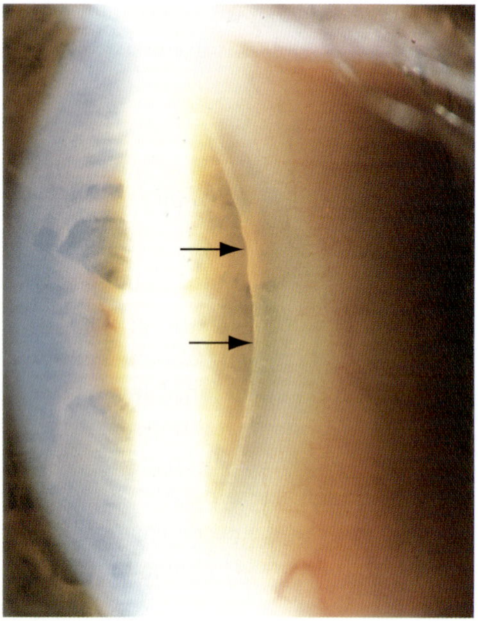

Figure 6-4 Posterior embryotoxon displaying a prominent and anteriorly displaced Schwalbe line *(arrows).*

finding or with other anterior segment anomalies that are part of ocular or systemic syndromes, such as Axenfeld-Rieger syndrome, arteriohepatic dysplasia (Alagille syndrome), X-linked ichthyosis, or familial aniridia.

Axenfeld-Rieger syndrome

The conditions previously referred to as *Axenfeld anomaly* or *syndrome* and *Rieger anomaly* or *syndrome* overlap genotypically and phenotypically and are now considered a single entity, *Axenfeld-Rieger syndrome.* This syndrome comprises a spectrum of disorders characterized by posterior embryotoxon with attached iris strands, iris hypoplasia, corectopia, pseudopolycoria, and glaucoma (in 50% of the cases occurring in late childhood or in adulthood). Associated craniofacial, dental, skeletal, and umbilical abnormalities are often present (Fig 6-5).

Autosomal dominant inheritance is most common (75% of cases), but transmission can be sporadic. The differential diagnosis of Axenfeld-Rieger syndrome includes iridocorneal endothelial (ICE) syndrome; irregular iris architecture is present in both conditions, and glaucoma is associated with both conditions. However, ICE, unlike Axenfeld-Rieger, is unilateral and sporadic, and the corneal endothelium is usually irregular (see Chapter 7, as well as BCSC Section 10, *Glaucoma*).

Seifi M, Walter MA. Axenfeld-Rieger syndrome. *Clin Genet.* 2018;93(6):1123–1130.

Peters anomaly (kerato-irido-lenticular dysgenesis)

Peters anomaly is characterized by the presence, at birth, of a central or paracentral corneal opacity (leukoma), which is due to the localized absence of the corneal endothelium and Descemet membrane beneath the area of opacity. Eighty percent of cases are bilateral. Most cases occur sporadically, but autosomal recessive and autosomal dominant modes of inheritance have been reported.

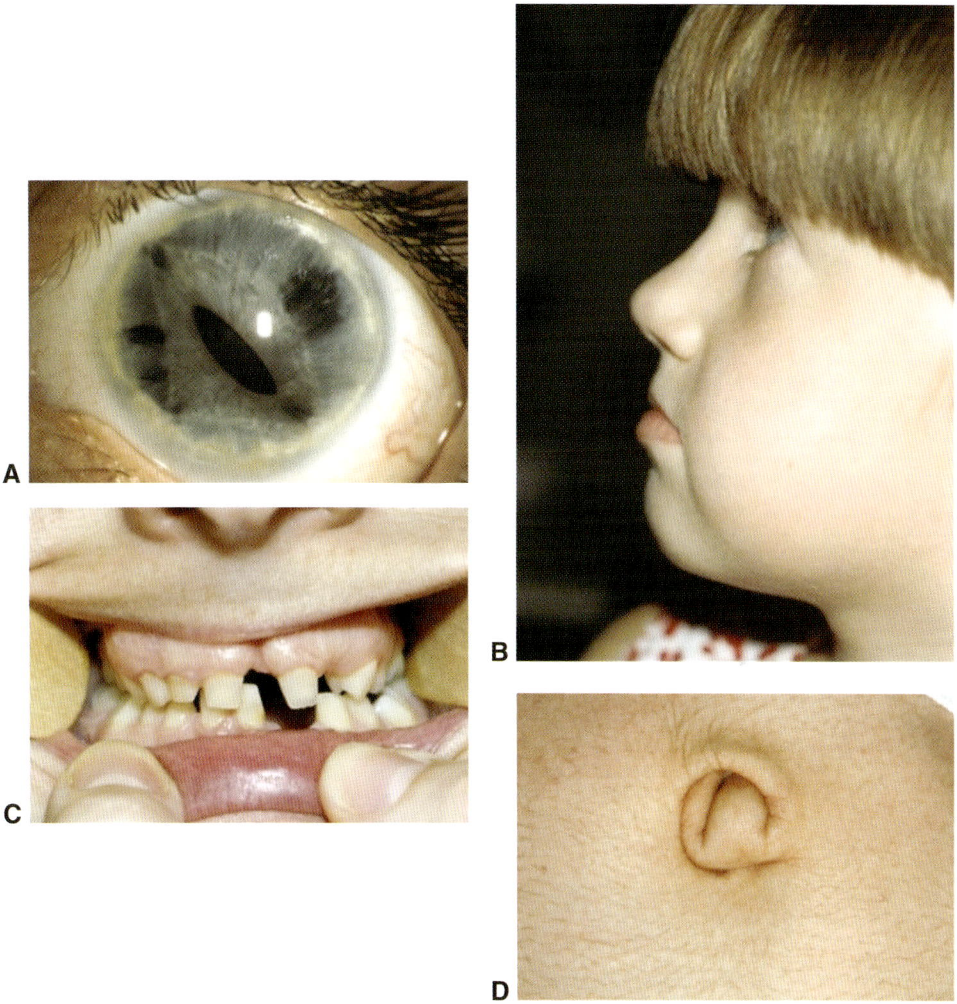

Figure 6-5 Ocular and systemic findings in Axenfeld-Rieger syndrome. **A,** Iris atrophy, corectopia, and pseudopolycoria. **B,** Maxillary hypoplasia with flat nasal bridge. **C,** Dental hypoplasia. **D,** Redundant umbilical skin. *(Courtesy of Irene Maumenee, MD.)*

Peters anomaly is classified into 2 types. Peters anomaly type 1 is characterized by iridocorneal adhesions. The corneal opacity is avascular and may be central, eccentric, or less commonly total. Peters anomaly type 2 is characterized by corneolenticular adhesions and/or cataract, along with a central or total corneal opacity that is usually vascularized (Fig 6-6). Peters anomaly type 2 is presumed to be due to a developmental failure in separation of the invaginating lens vesicle from the overlying surface ectoderm. The same genetic mutation can cause Peters type 1 to occur in 1 eye and type 2 in the contralateral eye. High-frequency ultrasonography can be very useful in differentiating Peters anomaly types 1 and 2.

Glaucoma is present in 50% of Peters anomaly cases. Additional associated ocular abnormalities include microcornea, aniridia, retinal detachment, and PFV. The prognosis for

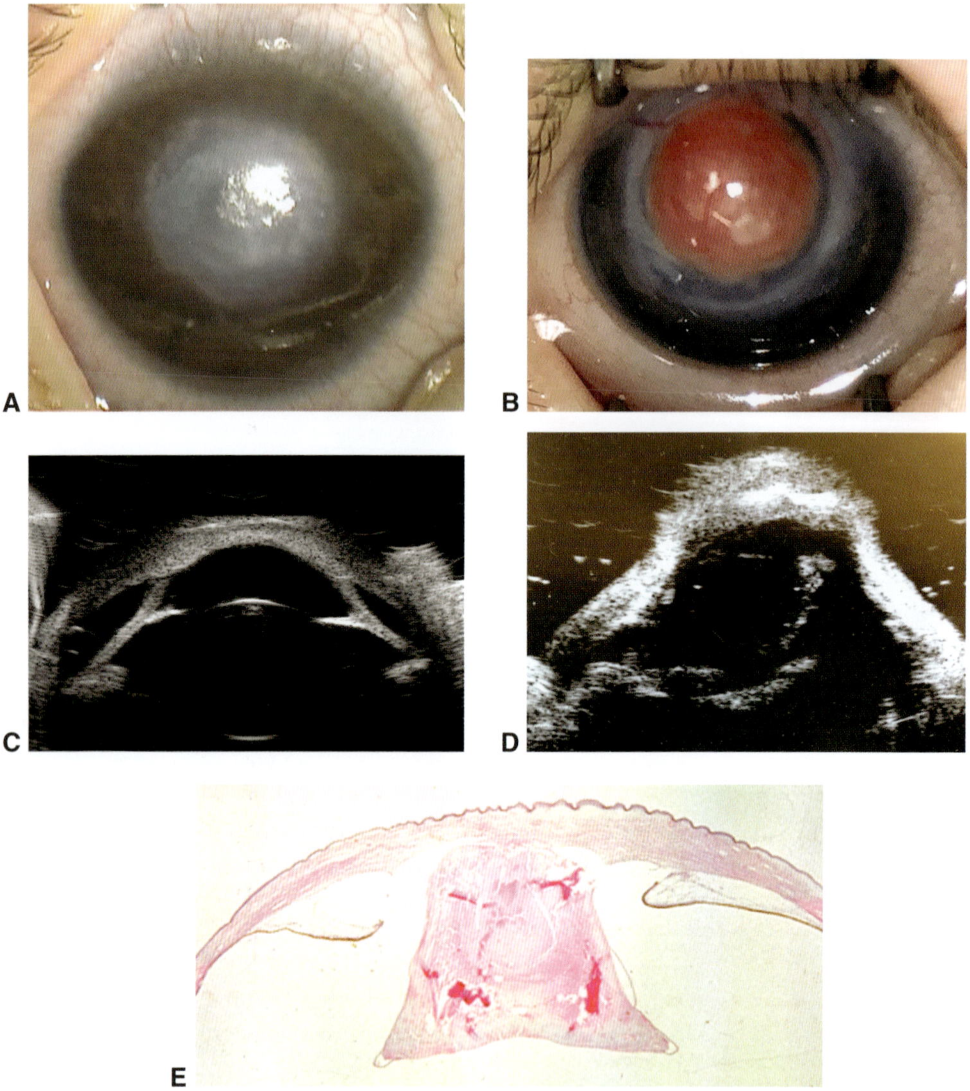

Figure 6-6 Peters anomaly types 1 and 2. **A,** Central corneal opacity. **B,** Vascularized central opacity. **C,** High-resolution ultrasound biomicroscopy image of the same patient as in **(A)** shows iridocorneal adhesions (Peters anomaly type 1). **D,** Anterior segment optical coherence tomography imaging of the same patient shown in **(C)** reveals corneolenticular adhesions (Peters type 2). **E,** Pathology specimen of Peters anomaly type 2 shows lens adherent to cornea. *(Parts A–D courtesy of Gerald Zaidman, MD; part E courtesy of Robert S. Feder, MD.)*

vision rehabilitation with corneal transplantation is better for patients with Peters anomaly type 1 than for those with type 2 (see Chapter 16). Peters anomaly is a major indication for pediatric keratoplasty. If the central opacity is small, a less invasive surgical procedure, such as an iridectomy, could also be considered.

Peters-plus syndrome Peters anomaly that is associated with systemic abnormalities is called *Peters-plus syndrome.* Systemic involvement is variable and may include

- cleft lip/palate
- short stature
- external ear abnormalities and hearing loss
- intellectual disability
- heart defects
- central nervous system deficits
- gastrointestinal and genitourinary defects
- skeletal defects

See also BCSC Section 4, *Ophthalmic Pathology and Intraocular Tumors;* Section 6, *Pediatric Ophthalmology and Strabismus;* and Section 10, *Glaucoma.*

Bhandari R, Ferri S, Whittaker B, Liu M, Lazzaro DR. Peters anomaly: review of the literature. *Cornea.* 2011;30(8):939–944.

Lesnik Oberstein SAJ, Ruivenkamp CAL, Hennekam RC. Peters plus syndrome. In: Adam MP, Ardinger HH, Pagon RA, Wallace SE, eds. *GeneReviews* [Internet]. University of Washington, Seattle; 1993–2021. Accessed November 13, 2021. www.ncbi.nlm.nih.gov/books/NBK1464

Posterior keratoconus

Posterior keratoconus is characterized by a usually localized central or paracentral indentation of the posterior cornea without protrusion of the anterior corneal surface, as is seen in typical keratoconus. Posterior excavation can occur in multiple areas; there is also a generalized form of this disease that can involve much of the cornea. Classification of posterior keratoconus as a congenital anomaly is supported by its association with an abnormal anterior banded layer of Descemet membrane and its presence at birth.

Posterior keratoconus may be a variant of Peters anomaly but can be distinguished by the presence of Descemet membrane (absent in Peters anomaly). Loss of stromal substance can lead to corneal thinning that approaches one-third of normal (Fig 6-7). Focal deposits of pigment and guttae are often present at the involved margins. Subtle anterior corneal irregularities overlying the area of posterior involvement can contribute to irregular astigmatism and amblyopia, which should be sought and treated appropriately. Corneal tomography can confirm the corneal thinning and posterior elevation. Most cases of posterior keratoconus are unilateral and sporadic. Although astigmatism can occur, the anterior curvature is usually not very irregular, like that seen in keratoconus. Acquired posterior keratoconus can also occur, usually following trauma.

Charles N, Charles M, Croxatto JO, Charles DE, Wertheimer D. Surface and Orbscan II slit-scanning elevation topography in circumscribed posterior keratoconus. *J Cataract Refract Surg.* 2005;31(3):636–639.

Krachmer JH, Rodrigues MM. Posterior keratoconus. *Arch Ophthalmol.* 1976;96:1867–1873.

Silas MR, Hilkert SM, Reidy JJ, Farooq AV. Posterior keratoconus. *Br J Ophthalmol.* 2018:102(7):863–867.

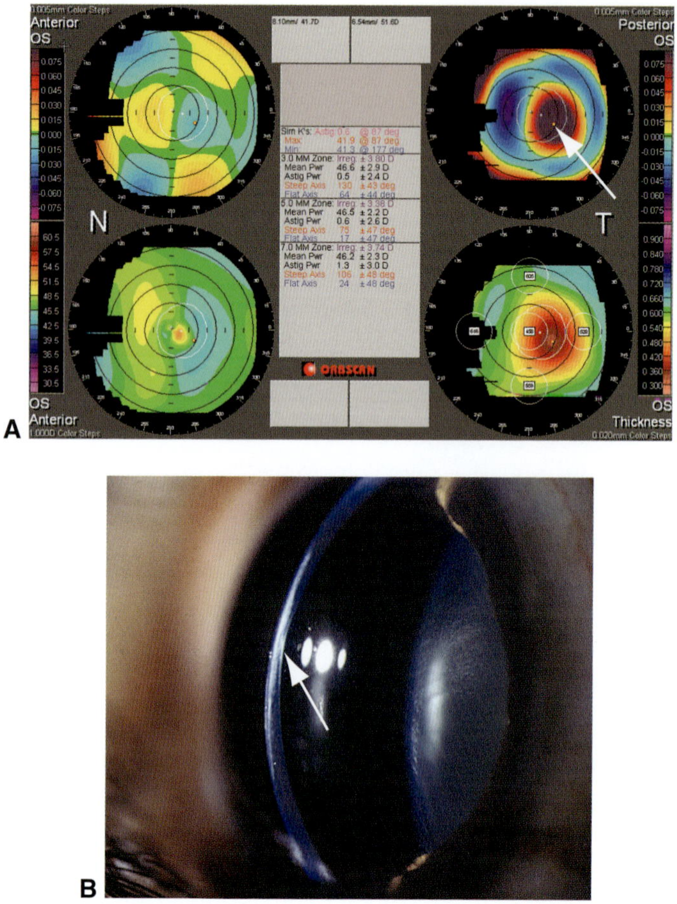

Figure 6-7 Posterior keratoconus. **A,** Scanning-slit corneal topography shows temporal paracentral posterior corneal vaulting *(arrow; top right)*. The anterior elevation map shows elevation nasally *(top left)* and the power map shows a nasally displaced corneal apex *(bottom left)*. The elevation seen in the posterior map is more pronounced compared to the anterior maps. The pachymetry map shows corresponding stromal thinning *(bottom right)*. **B,** Slit-lamp photograph shows loss of stromal thickness, stromal haze, and a craterlike depression in the posterior cornea *(arrow)*. *(Courtesy of Kenneth M. Goins, MD.)*

Congenital anterior staphyloma and keratectasia

Congenital anterior staphyloma is a rare developmental anomaly characterized by an opaque cornea protruding between the eyelids and partial or complete absence of Descemet membrane and endothelium (Fig 6-8A). A thin layer of uveal tissue lines the posterior cornea. The anterior segment is usually markedly abnormal, often with iridocorneal adhesions, iris hypoplasia, and lens opacity. Exposure may promote corneal scarring and keratinization. Inflammation is markedly absent. Unlike Peters anomaly, congenital anterior staphyloma is usually unilateral, but the contralateral eye frequently has some form of anterior segment abnormality. Typically, cases are sporadic, with no familial or systemic association.

On histologic examination, keratectasia differs from congenital anterior staphyloma only by the absence of a thin layer of uveal tissue lining the posterior cornea, which is

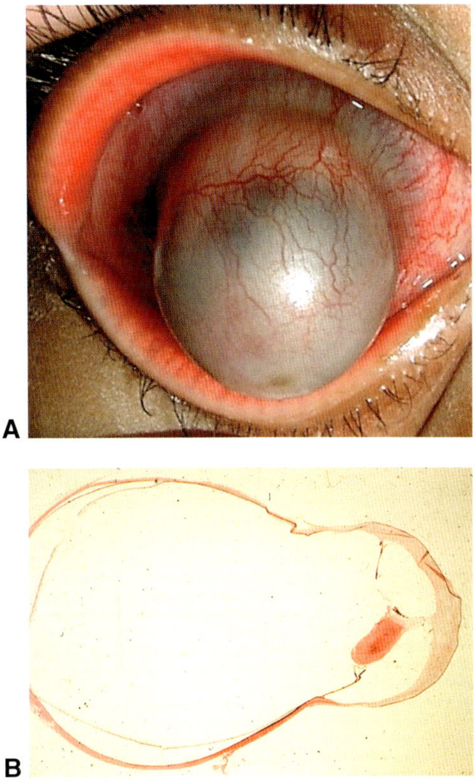

Figure 6-8 Congenital anterior staphyloma and keratectasia. **A,** Clinical photo of congenital anterior staphyloma. **B,** Pathology specimen demonstrates keratectasia; note the lack of uveal tissue lining the cornea that would be present in an eye with congenital anterior staphyloma. *(Part A courtesy of Gerald Zaidman, MD; part B courtesy of Robert S. Feder, MD.)*

present in congenital anterior staphyloma (Fig 6-8B). Keratectasia is possibly the result of intrauterine keratitis or vitamin deficiency and subsequent corneal perforation.

Except in very mild cases, the visual prognosis for both congenital anterior staphyloma and keratectasia is poor because of associated severe damage to the anterior segment. PK and sclerokeratoplasty may be useful to preserve the globe and improve cosmesis; however, enucleation may be required for a painful, blind glaucomatous eye.

Secondary Abnormalities Affecting the Infant Cornea

Intrauterine Keratitis: Bacterial and Syphilitic

Infections acquired in utero or during delivery can cause ocular damage in several ways:

- through direct involvement of the infectious agent, which damages tissue
- through a teratogenic effect that results in malformation
- through a delayed reactivation of the infectious agent after birth, with inflammation that damages fully developed tissue

Congenital syphilis is acquired in utero and caused by infection with the spirochete *Treponema pallidum.* It can lead to fetal death or premature delivery. A variety of systemic manifestations have been widely described. In children with untreated congenital syphilis, onset of interstitial keratitis is typically between 6 and 12 years of age. The keratitis presents as rapidly progressive corneal edema, followed by abnormal vascularization in the deep stroma adjacent to Descemet membrane. The cornea may assume a salmon-pink color because of intense vascularization, giving rise to the term *salmon patch.* Over several weeks to months, blood flow through these vessels gradually ceases, leaving empty "ghost" vessels in the corneal stroma.

CLINICAL PEARL

The presence of bilateral interstitial keratitis in an adult or child is highly likely to be secondary to congenital syphilis.

See Chapter 13 for a more complete discussion of interstitial keratitis and BCSC Section 6, *Pediatric Ophthalmology and Strabismus,* for additional discussion of congenital syphilis.

Congenital Corneal Keloid

A corneal keloid is reactive fibrous tissue proliferation that appears as a white raised mass. It is a relatively rare lesion, most commonly occurring following corneal perforation, trauma, or surgery. Congenital corneal keloids, which are often bilateral, have been described in Lowe (oculocerebrorenal) syndrome (an X-linked recessive disorder characterized by cataracts, renal failure, intellectual disability, and seizures), Rubinstein-Taybi syndrome, and ACL (*a*cromegaly, *c*utis verticis gyrata, corneal *l*eukoma) syndrome. Corneal keloids are not associated with cutaneous keloids except in Rubenstein-Taybi syndrome. Autosomal dominant inheritance has been observed in the ACL syndrome. Corneal keloids can occur in association with cataracts, aniridia, and glaucoma and may represent a developmental anomaly with failure of normal differentiation of corneal tissue. Histologic examination reveals thick collagen bundles haphazardly arranged, with focal areas of myofibroblastic proliferation.

Limbal Dermoid

Limbal dermoids (also called epibulbar dermoids) are benign congenital tumors that arise most frequently in the inferotemporal corneoscleral junction. They are choristomas, or mass lesions containing normal tissue in an atypical location. The lesions are typically raised and fleshy appearing and may contain hair, sebaceous glands, sweat glands, muscle, bone, or teeth (Fig 6-9). Limbal dermoids are usually unilateral and can vary greatly in size, often inducing astigmatism with secondary anisometropic amblyopia. They occasionally extend to the central cornea, can be full thickness, and can even involve the entire anterior segment. Limbal dermoids are associated with Goldenhar-Gorlin syndrome, trisomy 8 mosaicism syndrome, and linear nevus sebaceous syndrome (see Chapter 10 for further discussion).

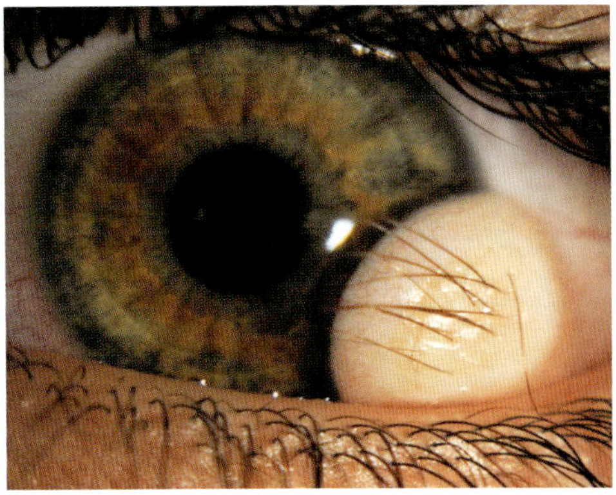

Figure 6-9 Limbal dermoid. These benign tumors are choristomas: tissue derived from germ layers that are foreign to that body site. This dermoid contains hair, adipose tissue, and squamous epithelium. *(Courtesy of Danielle Trief, MD.)*

Congenital Corneal Anesthesia

Congenital corneal anesthesia is a rare, usually bilateral, condition that is often misdiagnosed as herpes simplex virus keratitis, recurrent corneal erosion, or dry eye. Most patients present with painless corneal opacities and sterile epithelial ulcerations during infancy or childhood. The disorder can be subdivided into 3 distinct groups:

- *Group I.* Associated with isolated trigeminal anesthesia, which is probably due to primary hypoplasia of the hindbrain.
- *Group II.* Associated with mesenchymal anomalies, which include Goldenhar syndrome, Möbius syndrome, and familial dysautonomia (FD; also known as *Riley-Day syndrome*). FD is autosomal recessive.
- *Group III.* Associated with focal brainstem signs without evidence of mesenchymal dysplasia.

A thorough systemic examination, including neuroradiologic studies, is performed to rule out associated systemic conditions. CIPA (congenital insensitivity to pain with anhidrosis), another rare autosomal recessive condition associated with congenital corneal anesthesia, is linked to mutations in the *NTRK1* gene.

Treatment options for congenital corneal anesthesia include

- frequent topical lubrication
- punctal occlusion
- nighttime eyelid splinting
- permanent lateral tarsorrhaphy
- amniotic membrane transplantation
- scleral contact lenses
- conjunctival flap

Ramappa M, Chaurasia S, Chakrabarti S, Kaur I. Congenital cornea anesthesia. *J AAPOS.* 2014;18(5):427–432.

Verpoorten N, De Jonghe P, Timmerman V. Disease mechanisms in hereditary sensory and autonomic neuropathies. *Neurobiol Dis.* 2006;21(2):247–255.

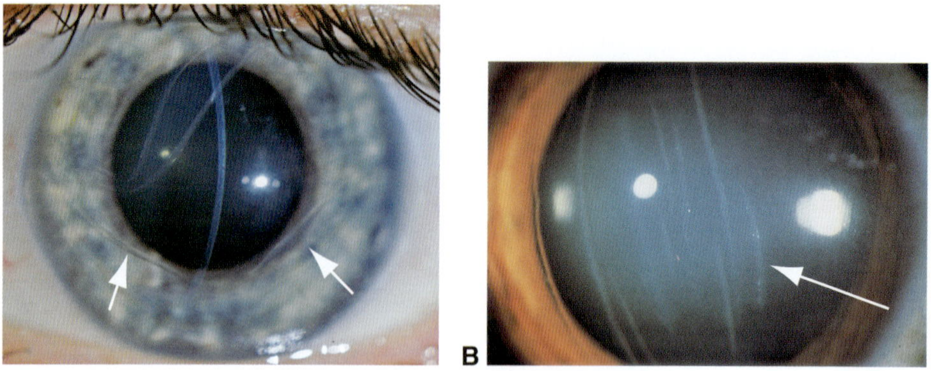

Figure 6-10 Haab striae. **A,** Horizonal or circumferential striae *(arrows)* are typical of primary congenital glaucoma. **B,** Vertical striae *(arrow)* in Descemet membrane are more typical of birth trauma. *(Part A courtesy of Danielle Trief, MD; part B courtesy of Vincent P. deLuise, MD.)*

Congenital Glaucoma

Primary congenital glaucoma (PCG) is evident either at birth or within the first 3 years of life. It is believed to be caused by dysplasia of the anterior chamber angle (dysgenesis and compression of the trabecular meshwork as well as an anterior insertion of the iris root) without other ocular or systemic abnormalities. PCG may be inherited as an autosomal recessive trait. Characteristic findings in newborns with PCG include the triad of epiphora, photophobia, and blepharospasm. External eye examination may reveal buphthalmos, with the cornea enlarging to more than 12 mm in diameter during the first year of life. Corneal edema due to increased intraocular pressure is present in 25% of affected infants at birth and in more than 60% by the sixth month of life; it may range from mild haze to dense stromal opacification. Tears in Descemet membrane resulting in *Haab striae* may occur acutely as a result of corneal stretching and are typically oriented horizontally or concentric to the limbus (Fig 6-10). This contrasts with birth trauma, in which the striae are usually vertical or oblique. For additional discussion, see BCSC Section 6, *Pediatric Ophthalmology and Strabismus,* and Section 10, *Glaucoma.*

Wiggs JL, Langgurth AM, Allen KF. Carrier frequency of *CYP1B1* mutations in the United States (an American Ophthalmological Society thesis). *Trans Am Ophthalmol Soc.* 2014;112:94–102.

Birth Trauma

Progressive corneal edema that develops during the first few postnatal days, accompanied by vertical or oblique posterior striae, may be caused by birth trauma (Fig 6-11). Ruptures occur in Descemet membrane and the corneal endothelium. These ruptures usually heal but leave a hypertrophic ridge of Descemet membrane. The left eye is affected more than the right because neonates assume a left occiput anterior position. The edema may or may not clear; if it does clear, the cornea can become edematous again at any time later in life. High astigmatism and amblyopia may be associated findings.

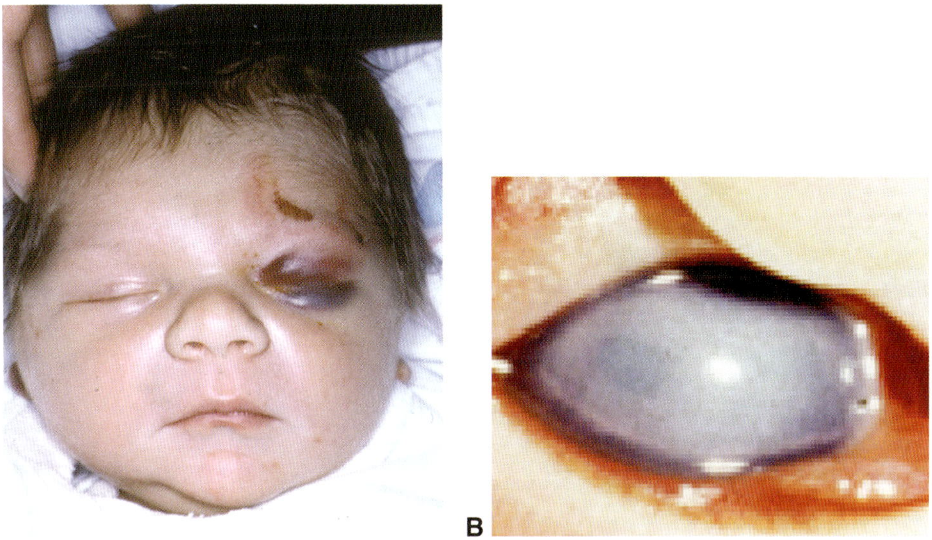

A B

Figure 6-11 Birth trauma. **A,** Birth trauma typically occurs on the left side. **B,** Marked corneal edema due to breaks in Descemet membrane is common. *(Courtesy of Robert S. Feder, MD.)*

Congenital glaucoma can present with similar findings and should be considered in the differential diagnosis.

Metabolic Disorders

The *mucopolysaccharidoses* and the *mucolipidoses* are disorders caused by abnormal carbohydrate metabolism. Affected patients present with corneal clouding. These conditions are discussed further in Chapter 10 of this volume and in BCSC Section 6, *Pediatric Ophthalmology and Strabismus.*

CHAPTER 7

Clinical Approach to Degenerations and Depositions of the Conjunctiva, Cornea, and Sclera

This chapter includes related videos. Go to www.aao.org/bcscvideo_section08 or scan the QR codes in the text to access this content.

Indicates selected key points within the chapter.

Highlights

- Pterygium is a fibrovascular degeneration of the conjunctiva with a characteristic appearance. The presence of atypical pigmentation, elevation, or vascularization warrants evaluation for neoplastic disease.
- Band keratopathy can affect both vision and comfort but may also be a manifestation of a systemic disease. An appropriate investigation as to the cause is recommended.
- Iridocorneal endothelial (ICE) syndrome has 3 clinical variants. An easy way to remember them is to consider ICE as an acronym: *I*ris nevus syndrome, *C*handler syndrome, and *E*ssential (progressive) iris atrophy.

Degenerations and Depositions of the Conjunctiva

Age-Related Changes

As a result of aging, the conjunctiva loses transparency and becomes thinner. The *substantia propria* (stroma) becomes less elastic, causing conjunctival laxity. In older individuals, the conjunctival vessels may become more prominent. Saccular telangiectasias, fusiform dilatory changes, or tortuosities may appear in the vessels. These changes are not necessarily uniform; they tend to be more pronounced in the region of the interpalpebral fissure, corresponding to the area most commonly exposed to the environment.

Pinguecula

A pinguecula is a common conjunctival condition that occurs typically on the nasal side of the bulbar conjunctiva, adjacent to the limbus in the interpalpebral zone. It is usually bilateral; appears as a yellow-white, elevated mass (Fig 7-1); and occurs as a result of the effects of aging, ultraviolet (UV) light exposure, and environmental insults such as dust and wind. Pingueculae are caused by an elastotic degeneration (the material stains for elastin but is not broken down by elastase) of subepithelial collagen with hyalinized connective tissue. The mass may enlarge gradually over long periods of time. Patients may develop recurrent inflammatory episodes known as pingueculitis. Topical lubrication to alleviate ocular irritation associated with pingueculitis is the mainstay of treatment. Judicious use of topical corticosteroids may be considered for patients with associated inflammation, but long-term corticosteroid therapy for pingueculae is strongly discouraged due to the adverse effects. Excision is indicated when pingueculae become chronically inflamed, are refractory to topical therapy, or interfere with contact lens wear. Excision is not typically performed for cosmesis.

Pterygium

A pterygium is a wing-shaped fibrovascular growth of conjunctiva involving the superficial cornea (Fig 7-2). The pathogenesis of pterygia is strongly correlated with UV light exposure, although environmental factors such as chronic exposure to dust, wind, or other irritants may contribute as well. There may also be a genetic predisposition to the development of pterygia. Nasal pterygia are more common than those with temporal involvement, presumably because the light exposure to the nasal limbus through the cornea is unobstructed, whereas the nose reduces light exposure to the temporal limbus. The prevalence

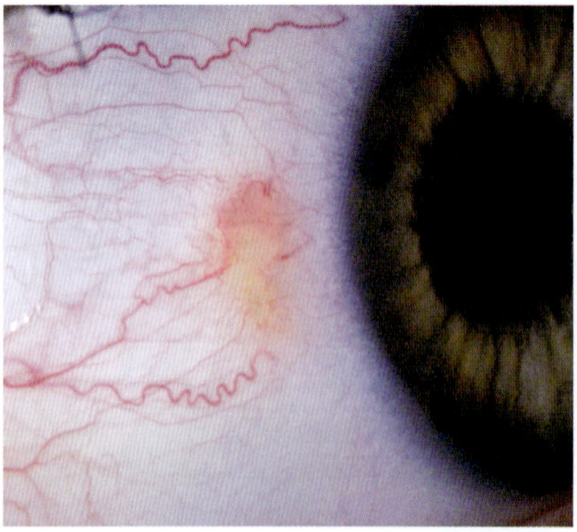

Figure 7-1 A pinguecula, shown in its typical location within the interpalpebral fissure, commonly a yellow, low-lying degeneration of the bulbar conjunctiva. *(Courtesy of Joseph D. Iuorno, MD.)*

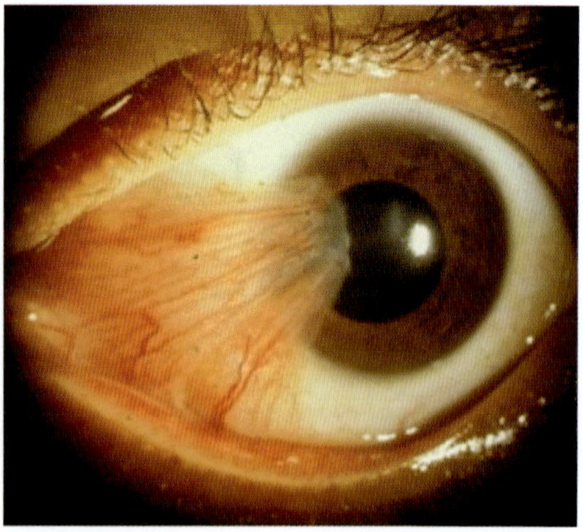

Figure 7-2 Pterygium, a triangular fibrovascular conjunctival lesion extending onto the superficial cornea. Note that the base is wider than the head (corneal portion) and extends posteriorly toward the caruncle. *(Courtesy of Robert S. Feder, MD.)*

of pterygia increases with geographic proximity to the equator, and the condition is more common in men than women and in people who work outdoors. The onset of the condition is typically between the ages of 20 and 30 years. The histopathology of pterygia is similar to that of pingueculae (basophilic degeneration of elastotic fibers), except that a pterygium invades the superficial cornea. Calcifications, leukoplakia, atypical elevation, irregular feeder vessels, and rapid growth are not typical of pterygia and may alert the clinician to the possibility of a masquerading malignancy. High-resolution optical coherence tomography (OCT) can help the clinician differentiate a pterygium from ocular surface squamous neoplasia (OSSN). Marked thickening of the epithelium, which is typical of OSSN, is not typical of pterygia (Fig 7-3). See BCSC Section 4, *Ophthalmic Pathology and Intraocular Tumors.*

As the pterygium progresses toward the visual axis, it will induce more visually significant regular and irregular astigmatism and scarring. A pigmented iron line *(Stocker line)* may be seen in the corneal epithelium, just central to the edge of the pterygium (Fig 7-4). A pterygium must be distinguished from a pseudopterygium, which may occur after trauma or chemical burns or secondary to inflammatory corneal disease.

Prophylactic treatment for pingueculae and pterygia includes UV-blocking sunglasses and a broad-brimmed hat, especially for patients chronically exposed to the sun, particularly tropical sun. Medical treatment with artificial tears can alleviate associated ocular irritation, but long-term use of topical corticosteroids for pterygia is not advisable. Excision is indicated if the pterygium causes persistent irritation, exhibits progressive growth that threatens the visual axis, or restricts motility. Patients in certain occupations (eg, modeling or television performance) may desire removal for aesthetic reasons; however, given the risk of recurrence and scarring, cosmesis is not a routine indication for surgery. To

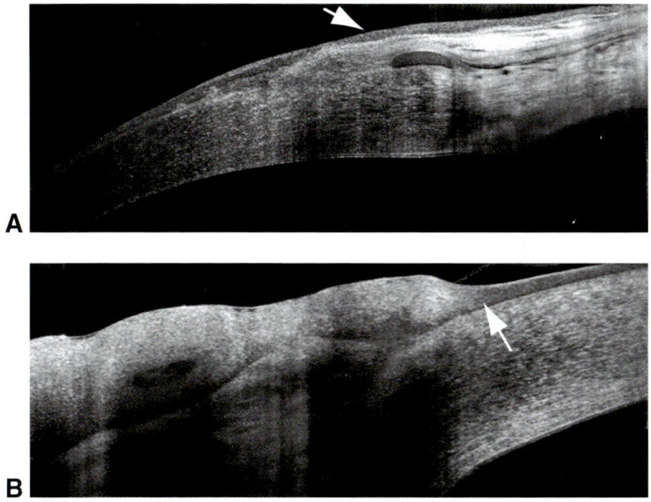

Figure 7-3 High-resolution anterior segment optical coherence tomography (OCT) can illustrate epithelial thickness, which can help differentiate pterygium from ocular surface squamous neoplasia (OSSN). **A,** Epithelium of normal thickness overlying subepithelial fibrosis seen in pterygium *(arrow).* **B,** Transition between normal epithelium and grossly thickened epithelium in OSSN *(arrow). (Courtesy of Carol L. Karp, MD.)*

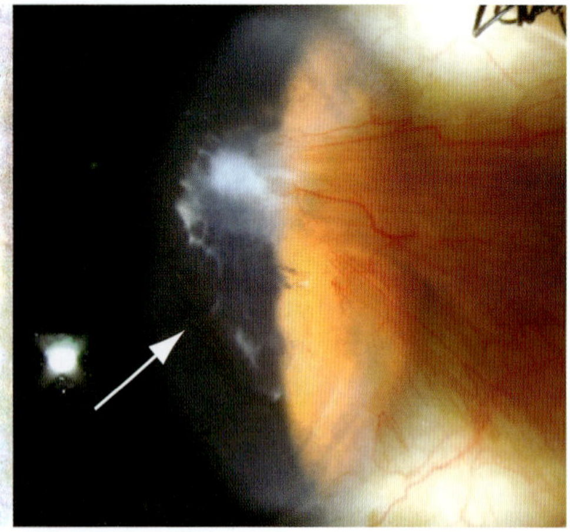

Figure 7-4 The Stocker line is iron deposition at the head of the pterygium *(arrow)*. *(Courtesy of Arie L. Marcovich, MD, PhD.)*

reduce the recurrence rate, most clinicians prefer to cover the bare sclera with tissue (eg, conjunctival autograft) at the time of surgery. See Chapter 5.

CLINICAL PEARL

In patients with visually significant cataract and pterygium, a staged surgical approach is indicated. After the pterygium is excised and the corneal contour has stabilized, cataract surgery can be planned; this approach can lead to improved long-term refractive results (Fig 7-5).

Conjunctival Concretions

Concretions appear as small cystic lesions, which are filled with epithelial and keratin debris, glycosaminoglycans (GAGs; previously called mucopolysaccharides), and mucin. They are visible as small, yellow-white dots in the palpebral conjunctiva (Fig 7-6) of older patients or patients who have had chronic conjunctivitis or meibomian gland dysfunction. Concretions are almost always asymptomatic, but they may erode through the overlying epithelium, causing foreign-body sensation. If symptomatic, concretions can be easily removed at the slit lamp with topical anesthesia and a 25-gauge needle.

Conjunctival Epithelial Inclusion Cysts

Conjunctival epithelial inclusion cysts are clear or transilluminating lesions that appear in either the bulbar conjunctiva or the conjunctival fornix and are typically incidental findings on examination. Because these cysts are usually asymptomatic, they generally do not require treatment. If large or elevated, a cyst can cause irritation (Fig 7-7). If the cyst is symptomatic, incision and drainage with a needle at the slit lamp may be sufficient. Piercing the cyst in multiple locations may prevent recurrence (Video 7-1). If the cyst recurs, complete excision may be necessary.

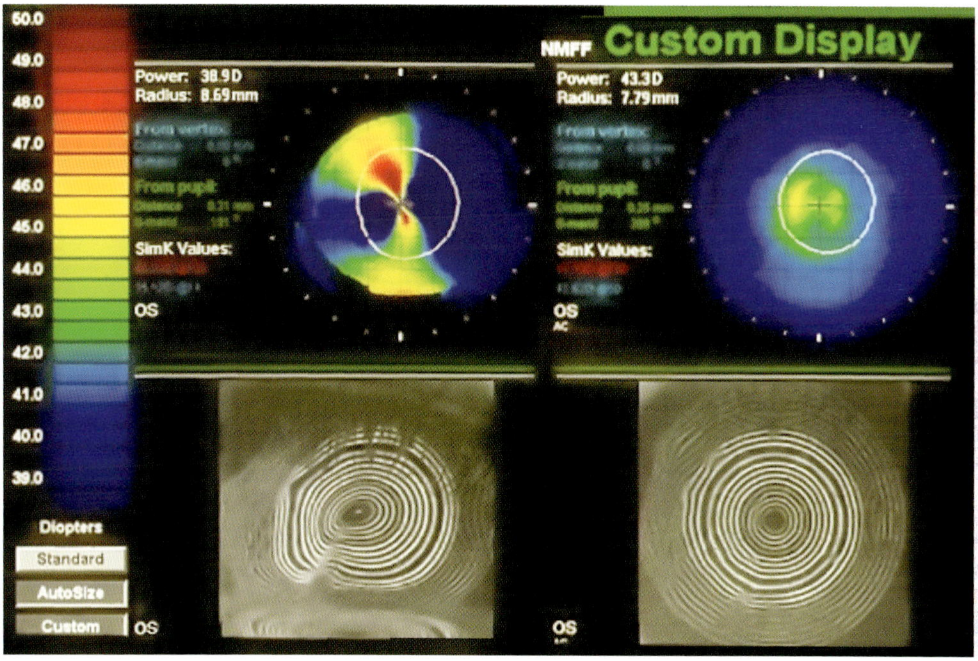

Figure 7-5 Change in astigmatism before and after pterygium excision. *Left:* Power map *(top)* demonstrates marked induced astigmatism due to nasal pterygium. Keratoscopic image *(bottom)* reveals irregular mires over the pterygium head. *Right:* Power map *(top)* 3 months after pterygium excision shows marked reduction in astigmatism. Keratoscopic image *(bottom)* shows more regular mires postoperatively. *(Courtesy of Robert S. Feder, MD.)*

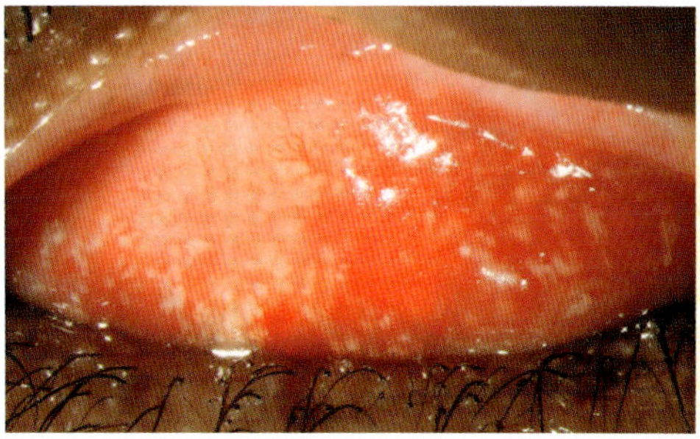

Figure 7-6 Conjunctival concretions. *(Courtesy of Arie L. Marcovich, MD, PhD.)*

VIDEO 7-1 Lancing of a conjunctival cyst.
Courtesy of Joseph D. Iuorno, MD.

Conjunctival inclusion cysts can be congenital or acquired. Most acquired cysts of the conjunctiva are derived from an inclusion of conjunctival epithelium within the substantia propria. The implanted cells proliferate to form a central fluid-filled cavity that is lined with nonkeratinized conjunctival epithelium. Conjunctival cysts may also form from ductal epithelium of the accessory lacrimal glands; these cysts are lined with a double layer of

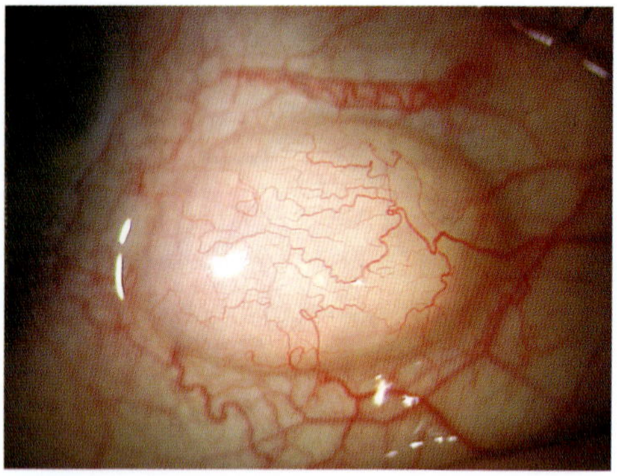

Figure 7-7 Large solitary conjunctival epithelial inclusion cyst. *(Courtesy of Joseph D. Iuorno, MD.)*

epithelium. Cysts can also result from chronic inflammation, trauma, and surgery. Dilated lymphatic channels may mimic a chain of inclusion cysts of the bulbar conjunctiva.

Conjunctivochalasis

Poor adherence of the bulbar conjunctiva that leads to redundancy is referred to as conjunctivochalasis. This condition is described in Chapter 4, and its treatment is discussed in Chapter 5.

Conjunctival Vascular Tortuosity and Hyperemia

There are many causes of conjunctival vascular tortuosity and hyperemia. A differential diagnosis is presented in Table 7-1.

Degenerations and Depositions of the Cornea

For a proper diagnosis, it is important to distinguish corneal degenerations from inherited corneal dystrophies (Table 7-2).

Age-Related Changes

As a result of aging, the cornea gradually becomes flatter in the vertical meridian, thinner, more rigid, and slightly less transparent. Its refractive index increases, and Descemet membrane becomes thicker, increasing from 3 μm at birth to 13 μm in adults. With increasing age, occasional peripheral endothelial guttae, sometimes known as *Hassall-Henle bodies,* may form (discussed later in this chapter). Age-related attrition of corneal endothelial cells results in a reduction in cell density from approximately 4000 cells/mm^2 at birth to 2500–3000 cells/mm^2 in older adults.

Epithelial and Subepithelial Degenerations and Depositions

Coats white ring

Coats white ring (Fig 7-8) refers to a small (1 mm or less in diameter) circular or oval area of discrete gray-white dots seen in the superficial corneal stroma. The ring consists of iron-containing fibrotic remnants of a metallic foreign body. Once these lesions mature and are free of any associated inflammation, they do not change. Therapy with corticosteroids or

Table 7-1 Causes of Conjunctival Vascular Conditions

Diffuse Vascular Tortuosity	Segmented Vascular Tortuosity	Subconjunctival Hemorrhage	Telangiectasia
Blood hyperviscosity disorders	Choriostoma	Ocular associations	Ataxia telangiectasia (Louis-Barr syndrome)
Carcinoid tumor	Epithelial cysts	Allergy	Telangiectasia of the conjunctiva and skin
Carotid-cavernous sinus fistula (trauma) and dural shunts	Ocular tumor	Conjunctival amyloidosis	Galactosialidosis (Goldenberg syndrome)
Diabetes	Pinguecula	Conjunctivitis (viral)	Hereditary hemorrhagic telangiectasia
Fabry disease	Pterygia	Conjunctivochalasis	Local conditions that dilate the conjunctiva
Hypertension		Orbital lymphangioma	Rendu-Osler-Weber syndrome
Mucolipidosis I		Related to ocular surgery	
Polycythemia vera		Systemic associations	
Sickle cell anemia		Bleeding disorders	
		Anticoagulants	
		Trauma/Valsalva maneuver	
		Hypertension	
		Head-down positioning	

Table 7-2 Differences Between Corneal Degenerations and Corneal Dystrophies

Degeneration	Dystrophy
Opacity often involves periphery	Opacity often centrally located with limbal sparing
May be bilateral but asymmetric	Typically bilateral and symmetric
Presents later in life	Presents early in life
Usually no inheritance	Typically inherited
May be associated with a systemic disease (eg, band keratopathy, sarcoidosis)	Usually not associated with systemic disease
Progression can vary from slow to rapid	Progression is usually slow

other anti-inflammatory agents is not beneficial. These lesions should be distinguished from corneal facets, which are small, gray-white, epithelium-filled defects in the anterior stroma.

Spheroidal degeneration

Spheroidal degeneration is characterized by the appearance of translucent, golden-brown, spheroidal deposits in the superficial stroma, at Bowman layer, and/or in the anterior stroma (Fig 7-9A). The conjunctiva can also be involved. Despite its appearance, the brown deposit is not lipid but rather proteinaceous material (Fig 7-9B).

Alternative names for spheroidal degeneration include

- actinic keratopathy
- climatic droplet keratopathy
- Bietti nodular dystrophy
- Labrador keratopathy

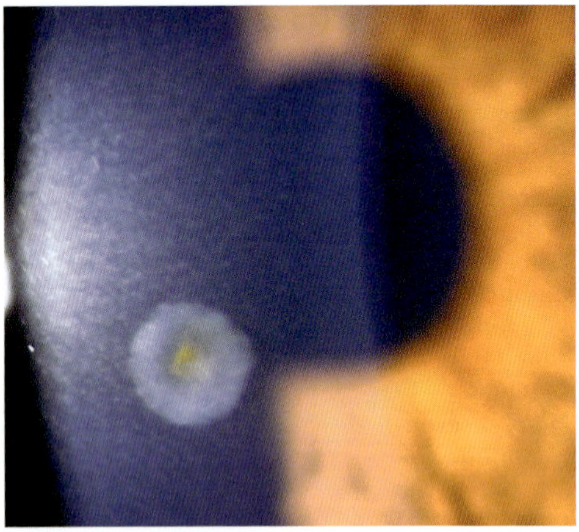

Figure 7-8 Coats white ring surrounding a metallic foreign body embedded in the cornea. *(Courtesy of Joseph D. Iuorno, MD.)*

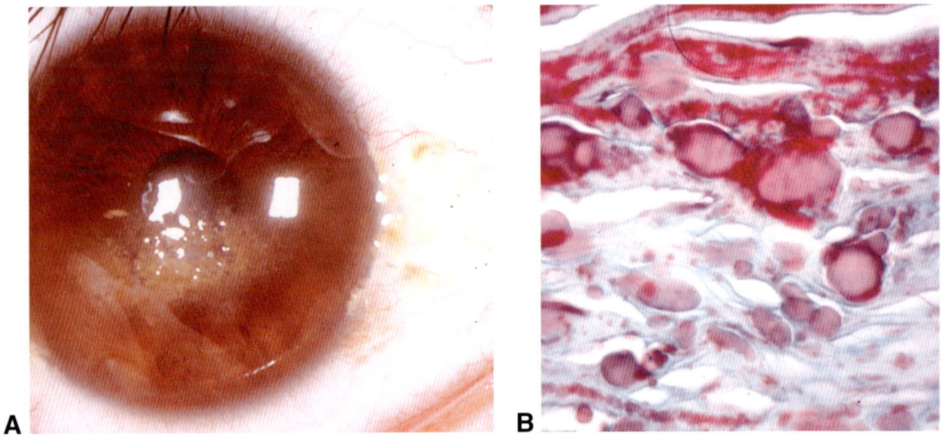

Figure 7-9 Spheroidal degeneration and histopathology. **A,** Spheroidal degeneration involving cornea and conjunctiva. **B,** Masson trichrome stain demonstrates deposition of protein rather than lipid. *(Courtesy of Robert S. Feder, MD.)*

Primary spheroidal degeneration In primary spheroidal degeneration, the deposits are bilateral and initially located in the nasal and temporal cornea. With age, they can extend onto the conjunctiva in the interpalpebral zone. The primary degeneration is unrelated to the coexistence of other ocular disease. In rare cases, generally in childhood, the spheroidal deposits extend across the interpalpebral cornea, producing a noncalcific band-shaped keratopathy. The etiology is controversial, but the deposits may develop from UV radiation–induced alteration of preexisting structural connective tissue components or from the synthesis of abnormal extracellular material in limbal conjunctiva.

Secondary spheroidal degeneration Secondary spheroidal degeneration is associated with ocular injury or inflammation. The deposits aggregate near the area of corneal scarring or vascularization. All cases show extracellular, proteinaceous, hyaline deposits with characteristics of elastotic degeneration. These deposits are thought to be secondary to the combined effects of genetic predisposition, actinic exposure associated with temperature extremes, age, and perhaps various kinds of environmental trauma, such as dust and wind.

Medical therapy is of little value, but ocular lubrication may help address uneven layering of the tear film over affected areas. In cases of central corneal involvement, superficial keratectomy, phototherapeutic keratectomy (PTK) using an excimer laser, or lamellar keratoplasty may be indicated.

Iron deposition

Iron lines are generally related to pooling of tears near areas of ocular surface irregularity (Fig 7-10; also see Fig 7-4). The iron is deposited at the level of the basal epithelium. An iron line surrounding a corneal lesion indicates that the lesion has been present for some time. Visualization of an iron line at the slit lamp is enhanced by use of diffuse illumination with a cobalt-blue filter prior to instilling fluorescein. A *Fleischer ring,* or iron deposition at the base of a cone in eyes with keratoconus, becomes narrower and more prominent as the disease progresses (see Chapter 9, Fig 9-4). It should not be confused with the Kayser-Fleischer ring (see Chapter 10). The Fleischer ring is an important diagnostic sign in keratoconus and can also aid in complete cone removal during keratoplasty. The *Hudson-Stähli line* is a horizontal opacity generally located at the junction of the upper two-thirds and lower one-third of the cornea; it is likely related to pooling of tears on the lower eyelid. Iron lines are also associated with keratorefractive surgery, particularly radial keratotomy. Various corneal iron lines are summarized in Table 7-3. In general, iron lines do not require treatment, although they can alert the clinician to an underlying pathology that may require intervention.

Calcific band keratopathy

Calcific band keratopathy is a degeneration of the superficial cornea that involves mainly Bowman layer. The degeneration begins as fine, dustlike, basophilic deposits at the level of Bowman layer. These changes are usually first seen peripherally at 3 and 9 o'clock. Eventually, the deposits may coalesce to form a dense horizontal band of plaques across the interpalpebral zone of the cornea (Fig 7-11). There is often a clear zone between the lesion and the limbus. In later stages, small cracks can occur in the band as a result of fractures in the

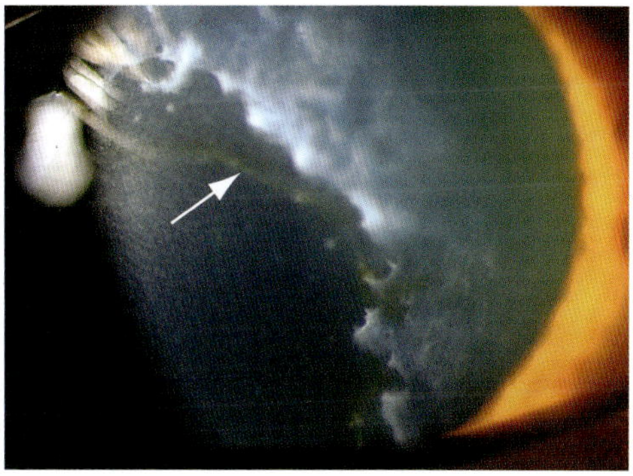

Figure 7-10 Iron deposition (iron line) *(arrow)* due to irregularity of the tear film, which results from subepithelial fibrosis. *(Courtesy of Robert W. Weisenthal, MD.)*

Table 7-3 Corneal Deposits

Location in Cornea	Pigment	Clinical Findings	Characteristics
Epithelium	Iron	Ferry line	Anterior to filtering bleb
		Fleischer ring	Surrounding base of the cone in keratoconus Can also be seen in iatrogenic keratectasia after refractive surgery
		Hudson-Stähli line	Horizontal line at junction of upper two-thirds and lower one-third of the cornea
		Stocker line	Anterior to head of pterygium
		LASIK line	Line, ring, or patch at margin of ablation zone or in flatter central cornea. Pseudo–Fleischer ring after hyperopic ablation. Paracentral star pattern seen after RK.
Epithelium and superficial stroma	Melanin-like pigment (alkapton)	Ochronosis	Peripherally; occurs in the metabolic disease alkaptonuria
Between basement membrane and Bowman layer; occurs in the conjunctiva as well	Melanin-like pigment (oxidized epinephrine)	Adrenochrome deposition	Occurs with topical epinephrine compounds for glaucoma or oral tetracycline or minocycline therapy
Stroma	Iron	Blood staining	Chiefly stroma; epithelium in some cases; can occur with hyphema related to duration and/or elevated IOP
	Iron (foreign body)	Siderosis	Chiefly stroma; epithelium in some cases
	Carbon	Corneal tattoo	In keratocytes or between collagen fibrils
	Gold	Chrysiasis	More often in the periphery
Deep stroma and Descemet membrane	Silver	Argyriasis	Slate-gray or silver discoloration
Descemet membrane	Copper	Kayser-Fleischer ring	Peripherally; in patients with hepatolenticular degeneration (Wilson disease) Biliary cirrhosis Chronic active hepatitis Copper deposition in cornea associated with multiple myeloma
		Chalcosis	Usually occurs with copper-containing foreign body
Endothelium	Melanin	Krukenberg spindle	In a vertical ellipse; sometimes associated with pigmentary glaucoma; most often bilateral

IOP = intraocular pressure; LASIK = laser in situ keratomileusis; RK = radial keratotomy.

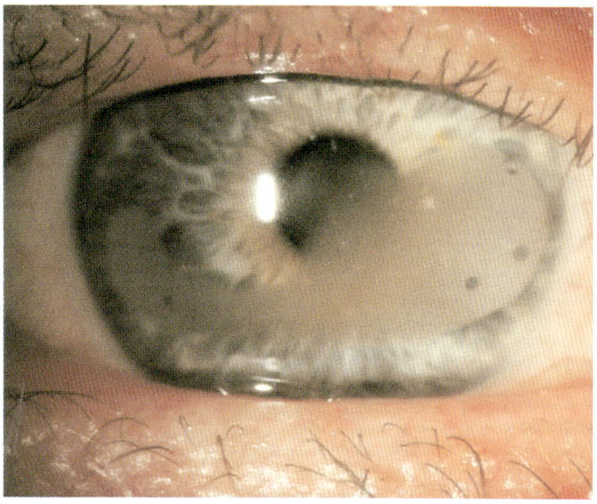

Figure 7-11 Band keratopathy. Note the clear zone between the limbus and the lesion and the Swiss cheese holes through which corneal nerves pierce through Bowman layer.

calcium deposits. In addition, small, lucent holes can be observed throughout the opacity, resembling the appearance of Swiss cheese and resulting from the penetration of corneal nerves through Bowman layer.

Common causes of band keratopathy are listed in Table 7-4. Typical band keratopathy can be idiopathic, confined to the eye as a consequence of ocular disease, or a manifestation of a systemic disease. Band keratopathy may also result from the corneal deposition of urates. The urates appear brown, unlike the gray-white calcific deposits observed in band keratopathy, and they may be associated with gout or hyperuricemia.

To rule out associated metabolic or renal disease, the clinician may conduct a basic workup consisting of

- serum calcium/phosphorus/uric acid
- blood urea nitrogen (BUN)/creatinine
- parathyroid hormone level
- urinalysis (checking for crystals, pH)
- angiotensin-converting enzyme (ACE) and serum lysozyme levels (particularly if sarcoidosis is suspected)
- chest x-ray (if sarcoidosis is suspected)

In order to reduce or slow the deposition of calcium, it is important to treat or control any underlying conditions, such as keratoconjunctivitis sicca or renal failure, to the extent possible; this may reduce the recurrence of band keratopathy after treatment. A combination of mechanical and chemical chelation with a neutral solution of disodium, ethylenediaminetetraacetic acid (EDTA), can be used to remove the calcium. The usual concentration of EDTA (0.05 mol/L), 3%–4%, can be obtained through a compounding pharmacy. The epithelium overlying the calcium is removed before the chelating solution is applied. One option for applying EDTA is to use any cylindrical tube that approximates the diameter of the area to be treated (eg, corneal trephine) to act as a reservoir to confine the chelating solution; alternatively, an EDTA-soaked cellulose sponge can be used to gently rub the affected area. A bandage contact lens is left in place until the epithelium

Table 7-4 Causes of Band Keratopathy

Systemic Conditions	Investigation/Serum Marker	
Hyperparathyroidism	Parathyroid hormone	Serum calcium
Vitamin D toxicity	Vitamin D	Serum calcium
Milk-alkali syndrome	Metabolic alkalosis	Serum calcium
Sarcoidosis	CXR/ACE	Serum calcium
Chronic renal failure	BUN/creatinine	
Mercury exposure	Mercury level	
Gout	Uric acid/urinalysis	
Juvenile idiopathic arthritis	Rheumatoid factor, antinuclear antibody	

Ocular Conditions	
Uveitis (especially in children)	Phthsis bulbi
Interstitial keratitis	Topical preservatives (phenylmercuric nitrate or acetate)
Severe superficial keratitis	

ACE = angiotensin-converting enzyme; BUN = blood urea nitrogen; CXR = chest x-ray.

has healed. The patient is treated with topical antibiotic and steroid until the surface has healed. Topical cycloplegia can help control postoperative discomfort.

Occasionally, calcium plaques can form on the cornea, which can cause irritation. These plaques can be removed at the slit lamp with forceps. Corneal epithelium will not grow over a calcium plaque. A fibrous pannus may accompany extensive calcific band keratopathy, especially if intracameral silicone oil is the underlying cause. PTK using an excimer laser is not advised as primary treatment, because calcium ablates at a different rate than stroma and may result in a severely irregular surface. If there is residual opacification after the initial EDTA chelation, PTK may be considered. Recurrence of band keratopathy can occur if the underlying ocular or systemic condition persists. EDTA chelation can be repeated. Continued follow-up of these patients is advised.

White limbal girdle of Vogt

Two forms of the white limbal girdle of Vogt have been described:

- *Type I* is a narrow, concentric, whitish superficial band running along the limbus within the palpebral fissure and is generally thought to represent early calcific band keratopathy. A lucid interval appears between the limbus and the girdle. This girdle is a degenerative change at the level of Bowman layer with chalklike opacities and small clear areas as seen in band keratopathy.
- *Type II* consists of small, white, needlelike flecks that are often seen at the nasal and temporal limbus in older patients. No clear interval separates these lesions from the limbus (Fig 7-12). Histologic examination reveals elastotic degeneration of collagen, similar to the changes seen in pingueculae.

Neither type I nor type II lesions are sight threatening, and no treatment is required.

Jhanji V, Rapuano CJ, Vajpayee RB. Corneal calcific band keratopathy. *Curr Opin Ophthalmol.* 2011;22(4):283–289.

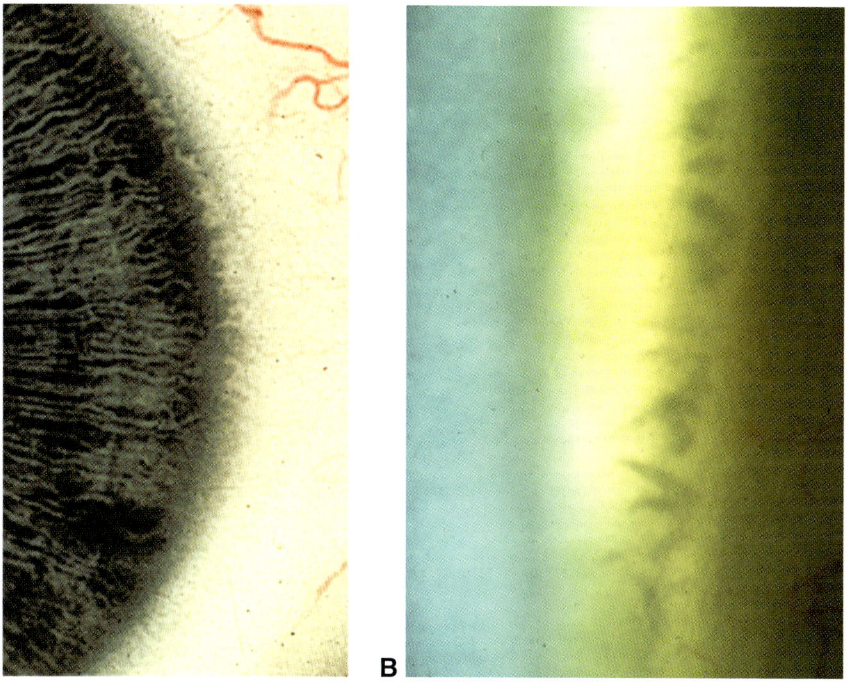

A B

Figure 7-12 White limbal girdle of Vogt, type II. **A,** Small, white, needlelike deposits are visible at the temporal limbus. **B,** Higher-magnification deposits are visible by indirect illumination. *(Courtesy of Robert S. Feder, MD.)*

Salzmann nodular degeneration

Salzmann nodular degeneration is an idiopathic noninflammatory corneal condition that can be bilateral and is typically seen in middle-aged and older women. The subepithelial elevated nodules are gray-white or blue-white (Fig 7-13) and often present in a roughly circular configuration involving the central or paracentral cornea. A variant of this condition occurs in association with dry eye, exposure, or long-standing keratitis (eg, phlyctenulosis, trachoma, or interstitial keratitis). It is observed at the ends of vessels associated with a pannus. The degeneration may not appear until years after the active keratitis has subsided. Subepithelial fibrosis can also occur at 3 and 9 o'clock in patients who wear hard contact lenses.

Histologic examination reveals localized replacement of Bowman layer with hyaline and fibrillar material, probably representing basement membrane and material similar to that found in spheroidal degeneration (discussed earlier in this chapter). Confocal microscopy reveals elongated basal epithelial cells and activated keratocytes in the anterior stroma, near the nodules; occasionally, subbasal nerves and tortuous stromal nerve bundles are also observed.

Treatment for mild cases consists of topical lubrication. Manual superficial keratectomy may be indicated in more severe cases associated with decreased vision due to

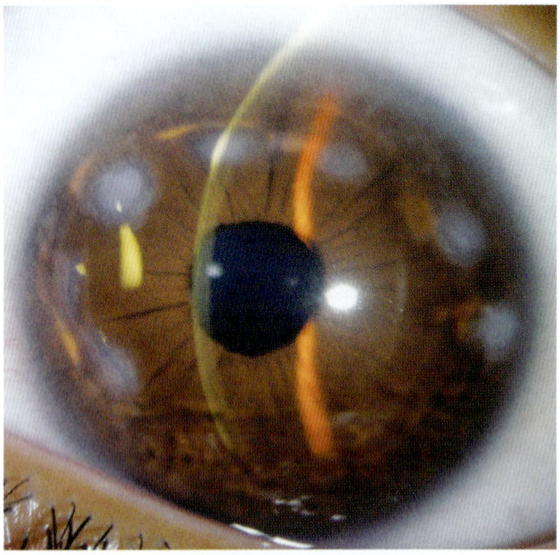

Figure 7-13 Slit-lamp biomicroscopy image shows elevated gray-white Salzmann nodules in a roughly circular configuration in the mid-peripheral cornea. *(Courtesy of Cornea Service, Paulista School of Medicine, Federal University of São Paulo.)*

irregular astigmatism, photophobia, and/or irritation. The simplicity of the surgical procedure used depends on the ability to find the correct corneal tissue plane. Once discovered by gently scraping with a rounded microsurgical blade, the nodule can be peeled off with jeweler's forceps (Video 7-2). This degeneration may recur after removal of the nodules. PTK has also been used to treat this condition but may result in an irregular contour or an undesirable refractive condition.

VIDEO 7-2 Superficial keratectomy of Salzmann nodule.
Courtesy of Joseph D. Iuorno, MD.

A variant of Salzmann nodular degeneration, called *peripheral hypertrophic subepithelial corneal degeneration,* has been described (Fig 7-14). It is most common in women and is typically bilateral, peripheral, and symmetrical. Adjacent superficial limbal vascularization with occasional pseudopterygium has been noted. Underlying chronic ocular surface inflammation is absent, and minimal relief of ocular irritation is achieved with topical corticosteroids.

Gore DM, Iovieno A, Connell BJ, Alexander R, Meligonis G, Dart JK. Peripheral hypertrophic subepithelial corneal degeneration: nomenclature, phenotypes, and long-term outcomes. *Ophthalmology.* 2013;120(5):892–898.

Roszkowska AM, Aragona P, Spinella R, Pisani A, Puzzolo D, Micali A. Morphologic and confocal investigation on Salzmann nodular degeneration of the cornea. *Invest Ophthalmol Vis Sci.* 2011;52(8):5910–5919.

Mid- and Deep Stromal Degenerations and Depositions

Corneal arcus

Corneal arcus is usually an involutional change that is modified by genetic factors and caused by the deposition of lipid in the peripheral corneal stroma The lipid is concentrated

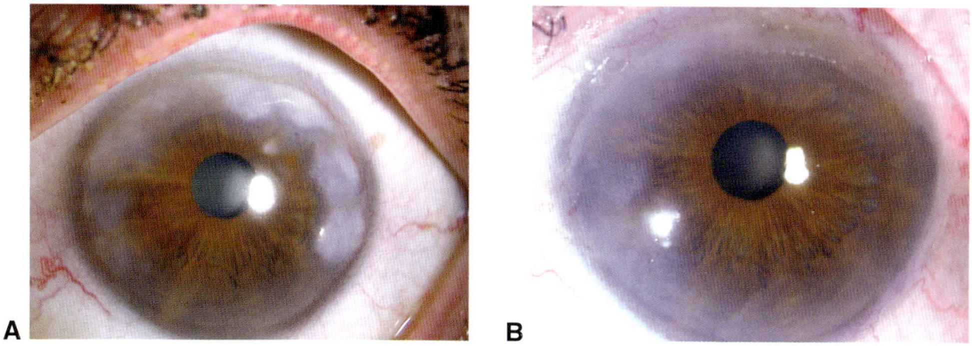

Figure 7-14 Peripheral hypertrophic subepithelial corneal degeneration, with elevated circumferential corneal opacities. **A,** Left eye with temporal and superior corneal degeneration. **B,** Same eye following superficial keratectomy surgery, resulting in a residual faint stromal scar and a significant reduction in symptoms. *(Courtesy of Joseph D. Iuorno, MD.)*

at 2 levels: (1) adjacent to Bowman layer and (2) near Descemet membrane. A relatively lucid interval is present between the peripheral edge of the arcus and the limbus because Bowman layer stops short of the insertion of Descemet membrane, which is at Schwalbe line. The arcus has a hazy white appearance, a sharp outer border, and an indistinct central border; it is denser superiorly and inferiorly (Fig 7-15). The arcus starts at the inferior and superior aspects of the cornea and ultimately involves the entire circumference.

The prevalence of corneal arcus is higher in African American individuals and in males; it also increases with age. Most patients older than 80 years have corneal arcus. Corneal arcus may also occur as a congenital anomaly *(arcus juvenilis).* In patients younger than 40 years, the presence of arcus may be indicative of a hyperlipoproteinemia with elevated serum cholesterol. An appropriate workup or referral is advised.

Unilateral corneal arcus is a rare condition associated with contralateral carotid artery disease or ocular hypotony. Corneal arcus is also seen in Schnyder corneal dystrophy (Chapter 8).

Crocodile shagreen

Crocodile shagreen, or *mosaic degeneration,* is a bilateral corneal opacity with a characteristic mosaic pattern reminiscent of a crocodile's back. It consists of centrally located,

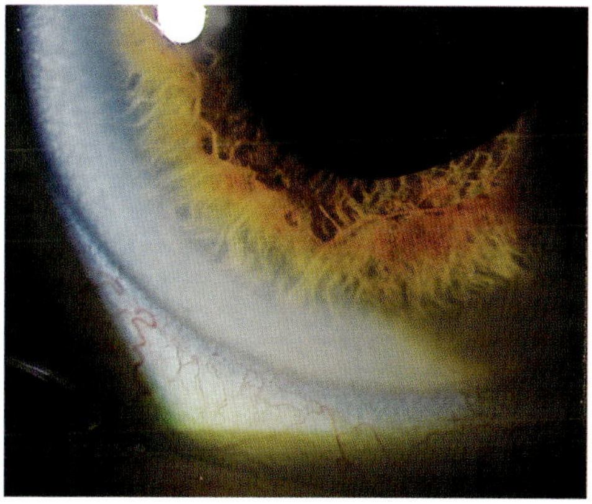

Figure 7-15 Corneal arcus. *(Courtesy of Robert W. Weisenthal, MD.)*

polygonal, gray opacities at the level of Bowman layer that are separated by clear zones. On histologic examination, Bowman layer is indented, forming ridges, and it may be calcified. Similar changes can occur in the deep stroma, near Descemet membrane, or in the corneal periphery. The condition is usually not visually significant.

Polymorphic amyloid degeneration

Polymorphic amyloid degeneration (PAD) is a bilateral, symmetric, primarily central, and slowly progressive corneal degeneration that appears later in life and is characterized by amyloid deposition. The crystalline deposits in PAD can resemble early lattice corneal dystrophy but are found primarily in the mid- to deep stroma and may appear to indent Descemet membrane. The opacities can appear gray-white and somewhat refractile and appear crystalline in retroillumination (Fig 7-16). The intervening stroma appears clear, and unless the condition is advanced, vision is usually minimally affected. Recurrent erosions do not occur, and cataract surgery can be performed without added risk. Refer to Chapters 8 and 10 for more information on amyloid in the cornea.

Furrow degeneration

Furrow degeneration is observed in older patients and is characterized by corneal arcus associated with peripheral thinning within the lucid interval. The corneal epithelium remains intact and there is no associated inflammation, vascularization, or potential for perforation. Vision is rarely affected, and no treatment is required. Although the thinning is generally slight, it can appear more prominent. Circumlimbal involvement may eventually occur; therefore, the cataract surgeon may consider using a scleral rather than clear corneal approach.

Terrien marginal degeneration

Terrien marginal degeneration (TMD) is a noninflammatory, slowly progressive thinning disorder of the peripheral cornea. It is usually bilateral but can be asymmetric. Although individuals of any age can be affected, this degeneration appears primarily in those older

A 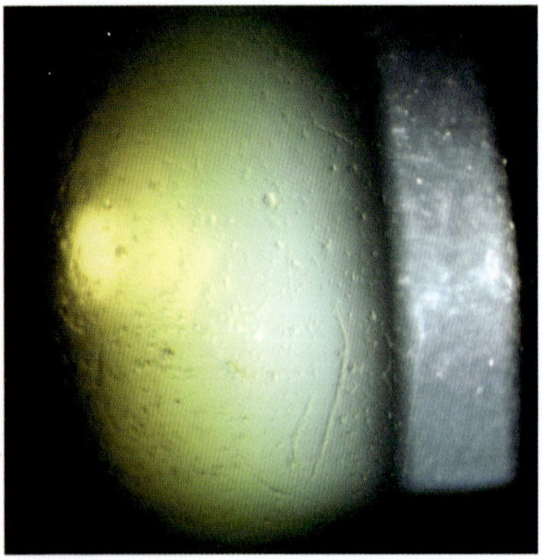 B 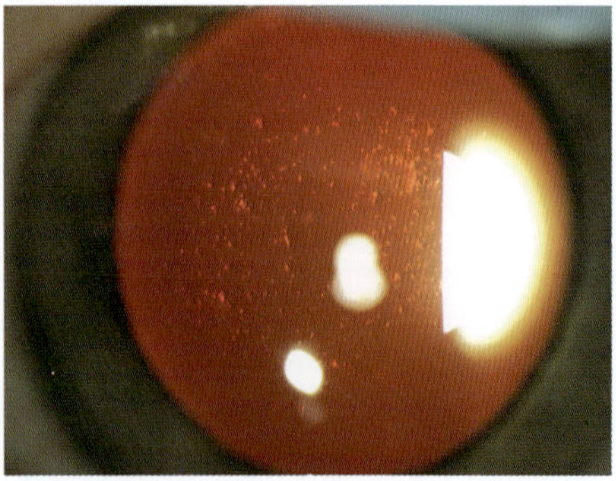

Figure 7-16 Polymorphic amyloid degeneration. **A,** Central mid- and deep stromal crystals observed with indirect illumination. **B,** Crystals observed with retroillumination. *(Part A courtesy of Robert W. Weisenthal, MD; part B courtesy of Robert S. Feder, MD.)*

than 40 years. Males are affected more frequently than females. The cause of this condition is unknown. The thinning typically presents superiorly but may spread circumferentially. It usually does not progress toward the central cornea but may involve the inferior limbus. Affected patients often are asymptomatic until bothered induced astigmatism.

The corneal epithelium remains intact, and a fine pannus typically traverses the area of peripheral stromal thinning. Lipid typically deposits at the central edge of the vascular pannus (Fig 7-17). Spontaneous perforation is rare, although it can occur with minor trauma. Acute corneal hydrops can result from a rupture in Descemet membrane.

An inflammatory condition known as *Fuchs superficial marginal keratitis* that occurs in children and young adults may resemble TMD. This condition may be part of the clinical spectrum of TMD.

CLINICAL PEARL

TMD may be confused with peripheral ulcerative keratitis (PUK); however, in the latter, the epithelium typically is not intact and there is no lipid deposition (see Chapter 9, Table 9-2). This distinction is important because PUK is often associated with an underlying systemic disease, and TMD is not.

Surgical intervention is indicated when progressive thinning results in marked astigmatism that significantly affects vision or threatens perforation. Crescent-shaped lamellar or full-thickness corneoscleral patch grafts may be used. Annular lamellar keratoplasty grafts may be considered in severe cases of 360° marginal degeneration.

Chan AT, Ulate R, Goldich Y, Rootman DS, Chan CC. Terrien marginal degeneration: clinical characteristics and outcomes. *Am J Ophthalmol.* 2015;160(5):867–872.e1.

Keenan JD, Mandel MR, Margolis TP. Peripheral ulcerative keratitis associated with vasculitis manifesting asymmetrically as Fuchs superficial marginal keratitis and Terrien marginal degeneration. *Cornea.* 2011;30(7):825–827.

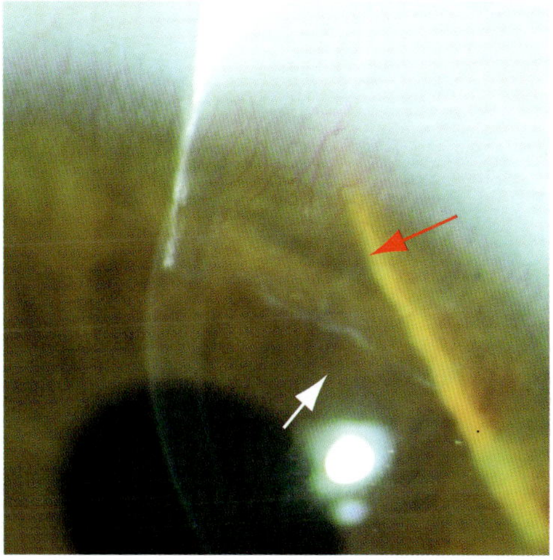

Figure 7-17 Terrien marginal degeneration. Note the leading edge of lipid *(white arrow)*, which serves as a border of the fine vessels that bridge the area of thinning *(red arrow)*. *(Courtesy of Joseph D. Iuorno, MD.)*

Corneal keloid

Corneal keloids are superficial, sometimes protuberant, glistening, white corneal masses that can involve the entire corneal surface. They are thought to be secondary to a vigorous fibrotic response to corneal injury or chronic ocular surface inflammation. Keloids can be congenital or primary, and they have been reported in association with many congenital conditions, such as Lowe disease (oculocerebrorenal syndrome). They have sometimes been confused with neurotrophic scars, Salzmann degeneration, or dermoids. Treatment of symptomatic patients may include superficial keratectomy or penetrating or lamellar keratoplasty (see Chapter 6).

Bakhtiari P, Agarwal DR, Fernandez AA, et al. Corneal keloid: report of natural history and outcome of surgical management in two cases. *Cornea.* 2013;32(12):1621–1624.

Lipid keratopathy

Lipid keratopathy has 2 forms. In *secondary lipid keratopathy* (Fig 7-18), yellow or cream-colored lipids containing cholesterol, neutral fats, and glycoproteins are deposited in the superficial or deep stroma, following corneal inflammation with vascularization (eg, chemical injury or interstitial keratitis related to herpes keratitis or syphilis). In rare instances, lipid keratopathy has been reported with no evidence of an antecedent infection, inflammatory process, or corneal damage; such cases are described as *primary lipid keratopathy.* Occasionally lipid keratopathy can be associated with focal stromal necrosis in the absence of significant inflammation. Treatment is indicated in cases of decreased vision or compromised cosmetic appearance. Controlling the neovascularization with topical corticosteroids may reduce or even stop progression of the keratopathy. Green laser treatment in the presence of few isolated vessels, photodynamic therapy with verteporfin, and subconjunctival and topical bevacizumab have been reported to reduce corneal neovascularization and lipid deposition.

Chang JH, Garg NK, Lunde E, Han KY, Jain S, Azar DT. Corneal neovascularization: an anti-VEGF therapy review. *Surv Ophthalmol.* 2012;57(5):415–429.
Goh YW, McGhee CN, Patel DV, Barnes R, Misra S. Treatment of herpes zoster–related corneal neovascularization and lipid keratopathy by photodynamic therapy. *Clin Exp Optom.* 2014;97(3):274–277.

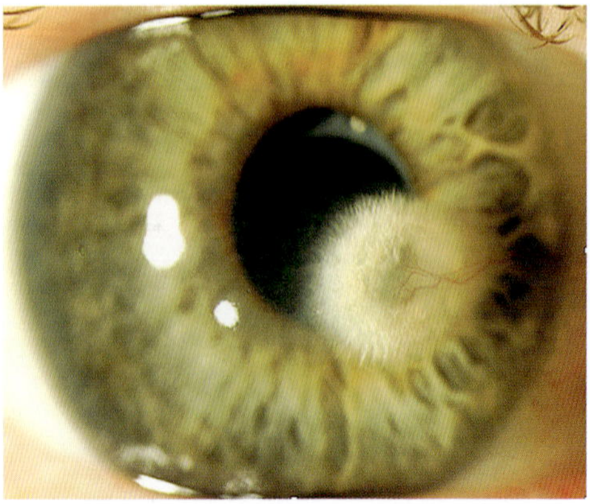

Figure 7-18 Lipid keratopathy occurred in this patient following the development of stromal vascularization. *(Courtesy of Robert S. Feder, MD.)*

Endothelium

Iridocorneal endothelial syndrome

Iridocorneal endothelial (ICE) syndrome is a spectrum of disorders characterized by varying degrees of iris changes, pupillary anomalies, structural and proliferative abnormalities of the corneal endothelium, and peripheral anterior synechiae. Three clinical variants of ICE syndrome have been identified. Coincidentally, I, C, and E are the first letters of each of the variants, which creates a convenient mnemonic (Table 7-5). The first variant, iris nevus syndrome *(Cogan-Reese syndrome),* is characterized by the presence of multiple pigmented iris nodules, which are also produced by the contracting endothelial membrane (Fig 7-19). When the disease is confined to the posterior corneal surface *(Chandler syndrome),* corneal edema may occur. When the abnormal corneal endothelium spreads onto the surface of the iris, the resulting contractile membrane may produce iris atrophy, corectopia, and polycoria—hallmarks of *essential (progressive) iris atrophy* (Fig 7-20). The syndrome occurs most commonly in middle-aged women and is almost always unilateral. Gonioscopy demonstrates broadened synechiae caused by proliferation and migration of abnormal endothelium over the anterior chamber angle, which result in outflow obstruction and secondary glaucoma.

The pathogenesis of ICE syndrome is unknown but appears to involve abnormal proliferation of endothelial cells that take on the ultrastructural characteristics of epithelial cells (ICE cells). It is not clear when the abnormal cloning occurs; however, herpesvirus has been implicated, because viral DNA has been identified in some specimens following keratoplasty and in the aqueous of some patients with ICE. ICE cells seen with specular microscopy (Fig 7-21) are typically abnormal, large, rounded, and pleomorphic. They show a characteristic reversal of the normal "light–dark" pattern; thus, the surface appears dark with an occasional central light spot, and the intercellular borders appear light. In vivo confocal microscopy shows ICE cells to be pleomorphic, epithelial-like endothelial cells with hyperreflective nuclei and cell borders that appear brighter than cell surfaces. Ultrasound biomicroscopy (UBM) is useful for detecting changes in angle structures in ICE syndrome, especially when corneal edema does not allow visualization with gonioscopy.

When diagnosing ICE syndrome as a cause of unilateral corneal edema, the clinician is advised to consider other possible differential diagnoses (Table 7-6).

Endothelial keratoplasty is the preferred treatment of the corneal component of this syndrome unless there is significant corneal scarring, in which case penetrating keratoplasty might be more appropriate. Long-term graft clarity depends on the successful control

Table 7-5 Iridocorneal Endothelial (ICE) Syndrome

I	Iris nevus (Cogan-Reese) syndrome	Abnormal endothelium spreads to and contracts iris, producing multiple clumps of pigmented nodules
C	Chandler syndrome	Abnormal endothelium is confined to the corneal surface, resulting in subnormal endothelial pump function (corneal edema)
E	Essential (progressive) iris atrophy	Abnormal endothelium spreads to iris, causing atrophy, corectopia, and polycoria

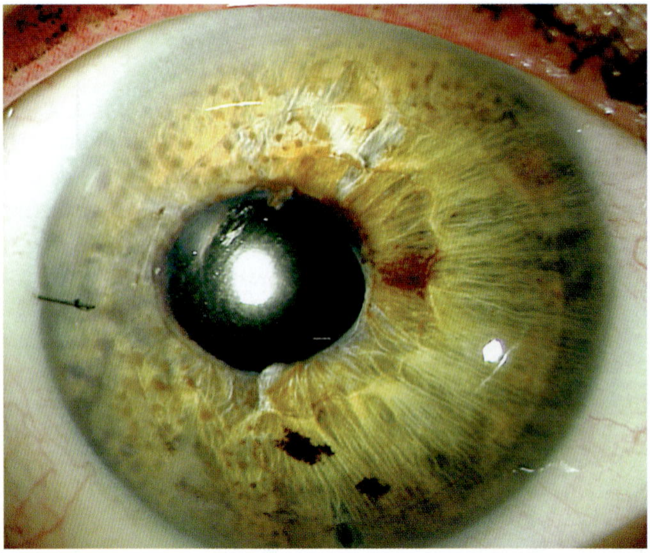

Figure 7-19 Iridocorneal endothelial syndrome, Cogan-Reese syndrome (iris nevus syndrome) variant. Note the multiple pigmented iris nodules, or nevi, produced by a contracting membrane. This patient had endothelial keratoplasty for corneal edema. *(Courtesy of Joseph D. Iuorno, MD.)*

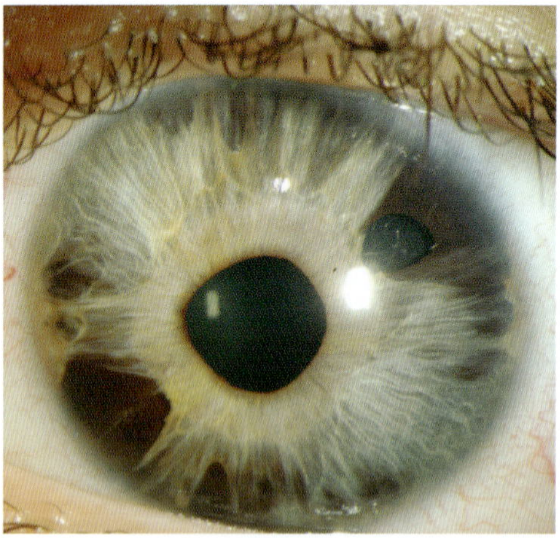

Figure 7-20 Iridocorneal endothelial syndrome, essential iris atrophy variant, with corectopia. *(Courtesy of Stephen E. Orlin, MD.)*

of intraocular pressure, which can be difficult (see BCSC Section 10, *Glaucoma*). Medical treatment of the glaucoma can be challenging. If filtering surgery is performed, the progressive growth of the abnormal endothelial membrane can block the filtration site. Tube shunt surgery may be more successful. Keratoprosthesis may be an alternative to repeated keratoplasty.

Carpel EF. Iridocorneal endothelial syndrome. In: Mannis MJ, Holland EJ, eds. *Cornea.* Vol 1. 4th ed. Elsevier; 2017:844–855.

Phillips DL, Goins KM, Greiner MA, Alward WL, Kwon YH, Wagoner MD. Boston type 1 keratoprosthesis for iridocorneal endothelial syndromes. *Cornea.* 2015;34(11):1383–1386.

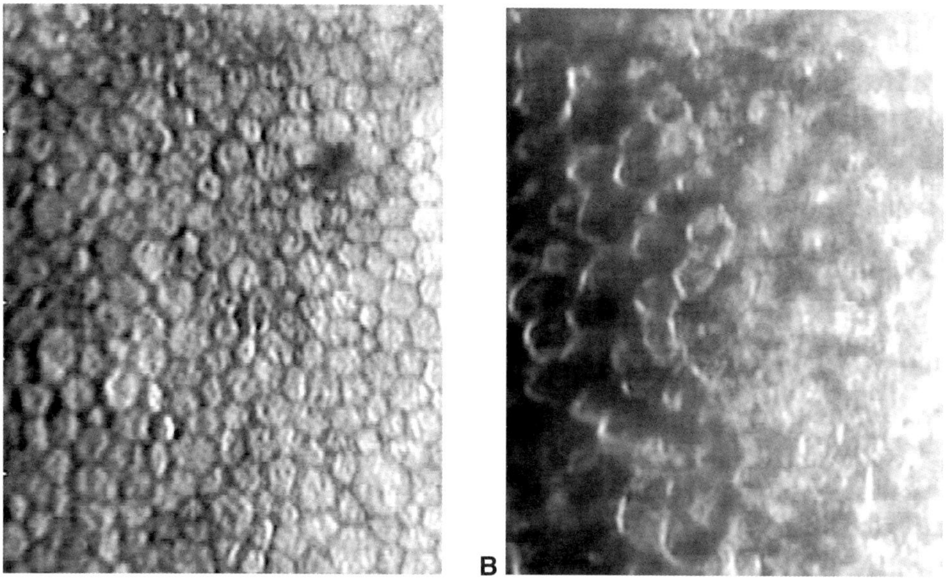

A B

Figure 7-21 Specular microscopy images of a normal eye and an eye from a patient with iridocorneal endothelial syndrome (ICE). **A,** Image of the normal cornea shows hexagon-shaped endothelial cells with white bodies and dark borders. **B,** Image of the cornea from a patient with ICE shows the reverse pattern: dark cell bodies and white borders. *(Courtesy of Arie L. Marcovich, MD, PhD.)*

Table 7-6 Differential Diagnosis of Unilateral Corneal Edema

Congenital	Acquired	
Glaucoma	Endothelial dysfunction	Acute angle-closure glaucoma
CHED	Aphakic	Posner-Schlossman syndrome
PPMD	Postoperative	Acute corneal hydrops
Birth trauma (forceps)	Pseudophakic	HSV/HZO trabeculitis or endotheliitis
	Contact lens overwear	ICE (Chandler syndrome)
	Tight lens syndrome	Cornea transplant
		Acute rejection
		Graft failure

CHED = congenital hereditary endothelial dystrophy; HSV = herpes simplex virus; HZO = herpes zoster ophthalmicus; ICE = iridocorneal endothelial; PPMD = posterior polymorphous corneal dystrophy.

Quek DTL, Wong CW, Wong TT, et al. Graft failure and intraocular pressure control after keratoplasty in iridocorneal endothelial syndrome. *Am J Ophthalmol.* 2015;160(3):422–429.e1.

Sacchetti M, Mantelli F, Marenco M, Macchi I, Ambrosio O, Rama P. Diagnosis and management of iridocorneal endothelial syndrome. *Biomed Res Int.* 2015;2015:763093.

Peripheral cornea guttae

Peripheral cornea guttae (Hassall-Henle bodies), which occur with aging, are small, wartlike excrescences that appear in the peripheral portion of Descemet membrane. They result from thickening of Descemet membrane, which takes place throughout life, and are seen on the

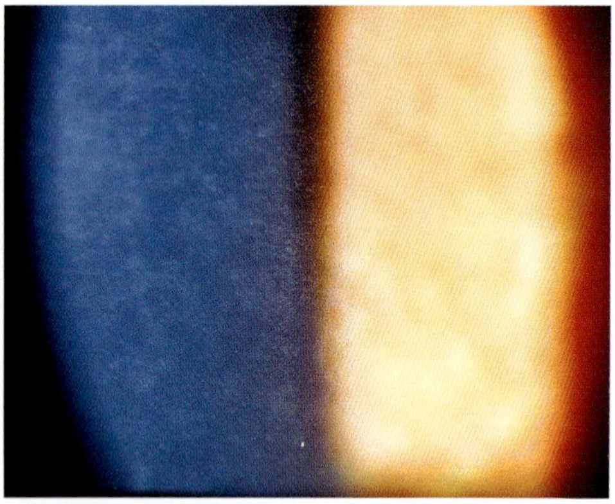

Figure 7-22 Cornea farinata, demonstrated with direct illumination. *(Courtesy of Robert W. Weisenthal, MD.)*

posterior corneal surface, protruding toward the anterior chamber. At the slit lamp, Hassall-Henle bodies appear as small, dark dimples within the endothelial mosaic. These are best seen with specular reflection. Hassall-Henle bodies are observed in patients younger than 20 years only in rare instances; they increase steadily in number with age. When they appear in the central cornea, they are pathologic. Central cornea guttae associated with progressive stromal and epithelial edema are key findings in Fuchs endothelial corneal dystrophy (see Chapter 8).

Cornea farinata

Cornea farinata is an involutional change that may be dominantly transmitted. The deep corneal stroma shows many delicate dotlike and comma-shaped opacities (Fig 7-22). *Farinata* means flourlike, which describes the appearance of the dusting that occurs just anterior to Descemet membrane. The location is similar to that of pre-Descemet corneal dystrophy, but the lesions in the latter are larger and more varied (see Chapter 8). These opacities are often best seen in indirect illumination. Confocal microscopy reveals highly reflective particles in the cytoplasm of keratocytes in the deep stroma, adjacent to the corneal endothelial layer. No abnormalities are detected in other layers of the cornea. The deposits may consist of lipofuscin, a degenerative pigment that appears in some aging cells. The condition does not affect vision and has no clinical significance, except that it is sometimes mistaken for a progressive dystrophy.

Pigment deposition

Deposits of melanin on the corneal endothelium can be seen in patients with glaucoma associated with pigment dispersion syndrome. The cluster of vertically oriented spindle-shaped pigment deposits is usually referred to as *Krukenberg spindle* (see Table 7-3). Transillumination defects in the midperipheral iris may also be observed. (See BCSC Section 10, *Glaucoma,* for a more detailed discussion of pigment dispersion.)

Degenerations and Depositions in the Sclera

The sclera becomes less elastic with age, and there is a relative decrease in scleral hydration and the amount of GAG. These changes are accompanied by subconjunctival deposition of fat, which gives the sclera a yellowish appearance. Calcium may also be deposited

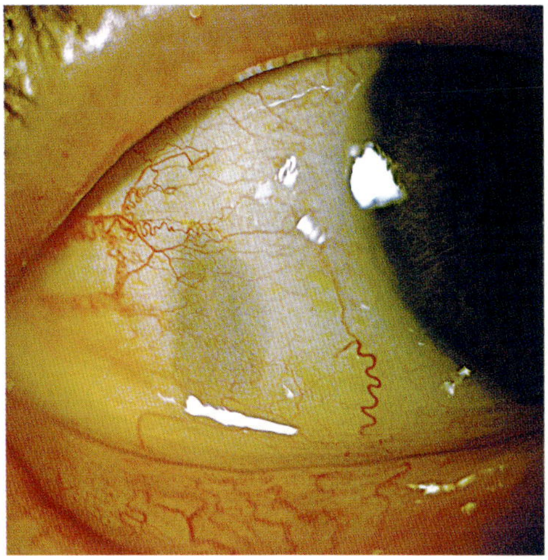

Figure 7-23 Senile scleral plaque (Cogan plaque), typically anterior to the horizontal rectus muscle insertions. *(Courtesy of Cornea Service, Paulista School of Medicine, Federal University of São Paulo.)*

either diffusely among the scleral collagen fibers in granular or crystalline form or focally in a plaque anterior to the horizontal rectus muscle insertions. This senile plaque *(Cogan plaque)* is visible as an ovoid or rectangular zone of grayish translucency (Fig 7-23) and is sometimes mistaken for a pigmented tumor. Histologic examination reveals that the midportion of the involved sclera contains a focal calcified plaque surrounded by relatively acellular collagen. This plaque does not elicit inflammation and rarely extrudes. If sufficiently dense, it may be visualized on a computed tomography scan.

Drug-Induced Depositions and Pigmentations

Ocular medications deposit within the cornea as a result of their concentration within the tear film, limbal vasculature, or aqueous humor or because of the specific affinity of their chemical properties to corneal tissue. Certain drugs deposit in a characteristic fashion and a particular corneal layer. The deposition of the drug may reduce vision, induce photosensitivity, or cause ocular irritation. Cessation of the drug often eliminates the symptoms and leads to resolution of the drug deposits. Most patients with drug-induced deposition are asymptomatic and do not require drug cessation.

Cornea Verticillata

Cornea verticillata, or *vortex keratopathy,* manifests as a whorl-like pattern of golden-brown or gray deposits in the inferior interpalpebral portion of the cornea (Fig 7-24). Various medications bind with the cellular lipids of the basal epithelial layer of the cornea.

Common drug-induced causes of cornea verticillata include

- amiodarone (most common)
- chloroquine
- hydroxychloroquine

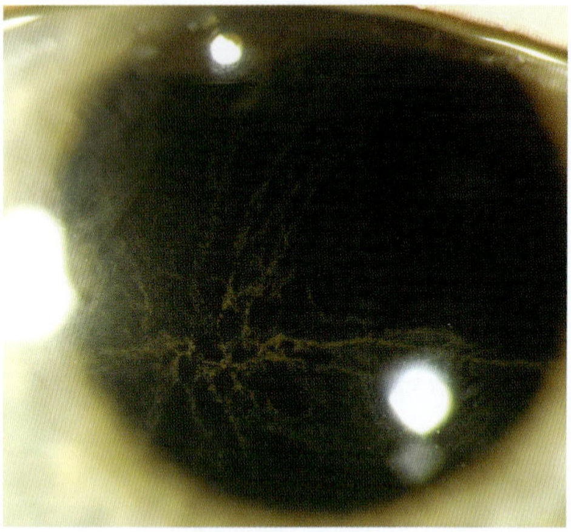

Figure 7-24 Cornea verticillata. A whorl-like pattern of golden-brown deposits are visible in the inferior interpalpebral portion of the cornea. *(Courtesy of Robert S. Feder, MD.)*

- indomethacin
- phenothiazines (eg, chlorpromazine)
- tamoxifen

See Table 7-7 for a comprehensive list of systemic drugs associated with cornea verticillata.

It is unusual for these deposits to cause reduced vision or ocular symptoms, although this has occurred in some patients. The deposits typically clear with discontinuation of the medication. Reduced vision associated with the use of amiodarone or tamoxifen prompts consideration of the possibility of optic neuropathy. Retinal toxicity associated with the use of drugs belonging to the aminoquinoline family can also reduce vision (see BCSC Section 12, *Retina and Vitreous,* for more on retinal toxicity). The differential diagnosis of cornea verticillata includes Fabry disease, a disorder of sphingolipid metabolism. See Chapter 10 for a discussion of corneal depositions associated with systemic diseases.

Table 7-7 Systemic Drugs Associated With Cornea Verticillata

Aminoquinolines (amodiaquine, chloroquine, hydroxychloroquine)	Mepacrine
Amiodarone	Monobenzone (topical skin ointment)
Antacids	Naproxen
Atovaquone	Perhexiline maleate
Clarithromycin	Phenothiazines (eg, chlorpromazine)
Clofazimine	Phenylbutazone
Gentamicin (subconjunctival)	Practolol
Gold	Retinoids (eg, isotretinoin)
Ibuprofen	Silver
Immunoglobulins	Suramin
Indomethacin	Tamoxifen
	Thioxanthenes (eg, chlorprothixene, thiothixene)

Data from Hollander DA, Aldave AJ. Drug-induced corneal complications. *Curr Opin Ophthalmol.* 2004;15(6):541–548; and Tyagi AK, Kayarkar VV, McDonnell PJ. An unreported side effect of topical clarithromycin when used successfully to treat *Mycobacterium avium*-intracellulare keratitis. *Cornea.* 1999;18(5):606–607.

Other Drug-Induced Corneal Deposits

Other drug-induced depositions include the following:

- *Ciprofloxacin therapy* applied topically (and, less often, other fluoroquinolones) can result in the deposition of a chalky white precipitate composed of ciprofloxacin crystals within an epithelial defect (Fig 7-25). Although white plaques predominate, a crystalline pattern may also be seen. The deposits resolve after the medication is discontinued.
- *Chlorpromazine,* a member of the phenothiazine family, may cause corneal pigmentation in up to one-third of patients on long-term therapy. It probably enters the cornea through the aqueous; therefore, the brown opacities are first found in the posterior stroma, Descemet membrane, and endothelium. The drug later spreads to the anterior stroma and epithelium. Chlorpromazine can also deposit on the anterior lens capsule.
- *Clofazimine* may produce anterior stromal opacities or crystalline deposits.
- *Isotretinoin* is typically associated with fine, diffuse, gray deposits in the central and peripheral cornea.
- *Gold salts* can be used in the treatment of rheumatoid arthritis. With long-term use and cumulative doses exceeding 1 gram, posterior stromal deposits that spare Descemet membrane and the endothelium develop in a high percentage of patients.
- Rifabutin, an antibiotic used to treat tuberculosis and prevent and treat *Mycobacterium avium* complex, has been described as causing stellate, refractile corneal endothelial deposits. These appear initially in the periphery but over time can extend to the central cornea.

See Table 7-3 for a list of corneal deposits that may be of diagnostic importance. Corneal deposits related to intraocular metallic foreign bodies are discussed in Chapter 15.

Palay DA. Corneal deposits. In: Mannis MJ, Holland EJ, eds. *Cornea.* Vol 1. 4th ed. Elsevier; 2017:251–264.

Raizman MB, Hamrah P, Holland EJ, et al. Drug-induced corneal epithelial changes. *Surv Ophthalmol.* 2017;62(3):286–301.

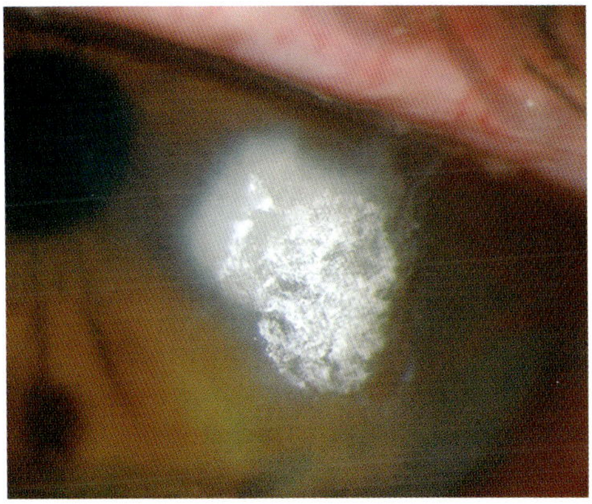

Figure 7-25 Ciprofloxacin deposit in the cornea. *(Courtesy of Robert W. Weisenthal, MD.)*

CHAPTER 8

Diagnosis and Management of Corneal Dystrophies

This chapter includes related videos. Go to www.aao.org/bcscvideo_section08 or scan the QR codes in the text to access this content.

Indicates selected key points within the chapter.

Highlights

- Genetic analysis has dramatically reshaped our understanding of corneal dystrophies.
- Recurrent erosions are typical of the transforming growth factor beta–induced *(TGFBI)* dystrophies because the deposited material, keratoepithelin, disrupts the epithelial basement membrane complex.
- *TGFBI* dystrophies can significantly worsen following excimer laser keratorefractive surgery.
- Deep anterior lamellar keratoplasty, when used to treat stromal dystrophy patients with vision impairment, eliminates the risk of endothelial rejection and reduces the risk of globe rupture after trauma.
- Endothelial keratoplasty is the preferred surgical approach for the management of corneal edema due to Fuchs dystrophy.

General Considerations

Corneal dystrophies typically

- are bilateral, with symmetrical involvement (asymmetry does occur)
- are inherited conditions that appear to have little or no relationship to environmental or systemic disease (epithelial basement membrane dystrophy may not be inherited)
- are first detectable early in life (late-onset Fuchs dystrophy is an exception)
- progress slowly, increase with age, and are often not symptomatic until later in life
- arise from genetic mutations that result in deposition of aberrant proteins (eg, mutations in the transforming growth factor beta–induced gene *[TGFBI]*, which leads to production of the keratoepithelin protein that is deposited in the anterior stroma)

- can be associated with recurrent erosion as a result of involvement of the epithelial basement membrane or Bowman layer
- present with blurred vision as a result of irregular astigmatism, stromal opacity, or corneal edema

In 2008, the International Committee for the Classification of Corneal Dystrophies (IC3D) revised the dystrophy nomenclature to more accurately reflect the evolving genetic, clinical, and histologic characteristics of the dystrophies. In this reclassification, updated in 2015, the dystrophies are classified into 4 groups:

- epithelial and subepithelial dystrophies
- epithelial–stromal *TGFBI* dystrophies
- stromal dystrophies
- endothelial dystrophies

The dystrophies are described according to a template consisting of clinical, pathologic, and genetic information. Within this system, a given dystrophy can be reclassified as more information about it becomes available. The classification is, therefore, upgradable. The updated version of the IC3D can be accessed at www.corneasociety.org.

The IC3D classification of major corneal dystrophies is summarized in Table 8-1. A comprehensive description of most corneal dystrophies is available in the IC3D publication but is beyond the scope of this volume. This chapter provides a basic discussion of the more representative dystrophies for which there is the best evidence.

The genetics of major corneal dystrophies is summarized in Table 8-2. A basic understanding of these diseases can be acquired without learning the specific genetic mutation of each dystrophy; however, it is important to appreciate the significance of particular genetic mutations. For example, mutations in the *TGFBI* gene lead to most of the stromal corneal dystrophies associated with recurrent corneal erosions. In addition, some dystrophies may appear the same phenotypically but differ genetically; conversely, dystrophies due to mutations in the same gene may have different phenotypes.

KEY QUESTIONS TO HELP DIAGNOSE AND DIFFERENTIATE THE CORNEAL DYSTROPHIES

During the clinical examination, the ophthalmologist is encouraged to consider the following questions to determine whether a dystrophy is present and to differentiate between the corneal dystrophies:

- Are other family members affected? (Note: It is often helpful to examine any blood relatives accompanying the patient.)
- Are there signs of inflammation? (Note: The presence of redness, stromal inflammatory cells, anterior chamber reaction, or neovascularization may indicate the condition is not a dystrophy.)
- Are the corneal opacities present in both eyes? (Note: Dystrophies are usually bilateral but can be asymmetrical.)
- In which corneal layer(s) do the opacities appear?

- Are there clear zones between the lesions? (Note: Clear zones may become less defined in the elderly.)
- Do the lesions extend to the limbus? (Note: Most dystrophies do not, but macular dystrophy is an exception.)
- Is the cornea abnormally thick, thin, or of normal thickness?
- Is the morphology of the lesions suggestive of a corneal dystrophy?

For further discussion of genetics, see the genetics section in BCSC Section 2, *Fundamentals and Principles of Ophthalmology.* See also Section 4, *Ophthalmic Pathology and Intraocular Tumors,* Chapter 6.

Weiss JS, Møller HU, Aldave AJ, et al. IC3D classification of corneal dystrophies—edition 2. *Cornea.* 2015;34(2):117–159.

Table 8-1 Major Corneal Dystrophies in the IC3D Classification

Epithelial and subepithelial dystrophies

1. Epithelial basement membrane dystrophy (EBMD): may be degenerative
2. Meesmann epithelial corneal dystrophy (MECD)
3. Gelatinous droplike corneal dystrophy (GDLD)
4. Epithelial recurrent erosion dystrophies (ERED)
5. Lisch epithelial corneal dystrophy (LECD)
6. Subepithelial mucinous corneal dystrophy (SMCD)

Epithelial–stromal *TGFBI* (keratoepithelin-associated) dystrophies

1. Reis-Bücklers corneal dystrophy (RBCD), atypical granular corneal dystrophy
2. Thiel-Behnke corneal dystrophy (TBCD)
3. Lattice corneal dystrophy
    a. Lattice corneal dystrophy type 1 (LCD1)
    b. Lattice corneal dystrophy variants (III, IIIA, I/IIIA, and IV)
4. Granular corneal dystrophy
    a. Granular corneal dystrophy type 1 (GCD1)
    b. Granular corneal dystrophy type 2 (GCD2)

Stromal dystrophies

1. Macular corneal dystrophy (MCD)
2. Schnyder corneal dystrophy (SCD)
3. Congenital stromal corneal dystrophy (CSCD)
4. Fleck corneal dystrophy (FCD)
5. Posterior amorphous corneal dystrophy (PACD)
6. Pre-Descemet corneal dystrophy (PDCD)

Endothelial dystrophies

1. Fuchs endothelial corneal dystrophy (FECD)
2. Posterior polymorphous corneal dystrophy (PPCD)
3. Congenital hereditary endothelial dystrophy (CHED)

TGFBI=transforming growth factor beta–induced.

Data from Weiss JS, Møller HU, Aldave A, et al. IC3D classification of corneal dystrophies—edition 2. *Cornea.* 2015;34(2):120.

Table 8-2 The Genetics of Major Corneal Dystrophies

Dystrophy	Gene Locus	Gene
Epithelial and subepithelial dystrophies		
Epithelial basement membrane dystrophy	Sporadic in most cases 5q31 in some cases	Transforming growth factor beta–induced *(TGFBI)* in 2 families
Meesmann epithelial corneal dystrophy (MECD)	12q13	Keratin K3 *(KRT3)*
MECD Stocker-Holt variant	17q12	Keratin K12 *(KRT12)*
Lisch epithelial corneal dystrophy	Xp22.3	Unknown
Gelatinous droplike corneal dystrophy	1p32	Tumor-associated calcium signal transducer 2 *(TACSTD2)*
Epithelial–stromal *TGFBI* (keratoepithelin-associated) dystrophies		
Reis-Bücklers corneal dystrophy	5q31	*TGFBI*
Thiel-Behnke corneal dystrophy	5q31	*TGFBI*
Lattice corneal dystrophy type 1	5q31	*TGFBI*
Granular corneal dystrophy type 1	5q31	*TGFBI*
Granular corneal dystrophy type 2	5q31	*TGFBI*
Stromal dystrophies		
Macular corneal dystrophy	16q22	Carbohydrate sulfotransferase 6 *(CHST6)*
Schnyder corneal dystrophy	1p36	UbiA prenyltransferase domain-containing protein 1 *(UBIAD1)*
Congenital stromal corneal dystrophy	12q21.33	Decorin *(DCN)*
Fleck corneal dystrophy	2q34	Phosphoinositide kinase, FYVE finger containing–*PIKFYVE (PIKFYVE)*
Posterior amorphous corneal dystrophy	12q21.33	Deletion of keratocan *(KERA)*, lumican *(LUM)*, decorin *(DCN)*, and epiphycan *(EPYC)*
Pre-Descemet corneal dystrophy	Unknown	Unknown
Endothelial dystrophies		
Late-onset Fuchs endothelial corneal dystrophy (FECD)	None (most commonly) 13pter–q12.13 (FECD2), 18q21.2–q21.3 (FECD3), 20p13–p12 (FECD4), 5q33.1–q35.2 (FECD5), 10p11.2 (FECD6), 9p24.1–p22.1 (FECD7), 15q25 (FECD8)	None (most commonly) Unknown, transcription factor 4 *(TCF4)* on chromosome 18
Early-onset variant FECD	1p34.3–p32	Collagen, type VIII, alpha-2 *(COL8A2)*
Posterior polymorphous corneal dystrophy: PPCD1	20p11.2–q11.2	Unknown
PPCD2	1p34.3–p32.3	Collagen, type VIII, alpha-2 *(COL8A2)*
PPCD3	10p11.22	Zinc finger E box–binding homeobox 1 *(ZEB1)*
Congenital hereditary endothelial dystrophy[a]	20p13 (telomeric portion)	Solute carrier family 4, sodium borate transporter, member 11 *(SLC4A11)*

[a] Formerly divided into CHED1 and CHED2; no convincing evidence of autosomal dominant form.

Data from Weiss JS, Møller HU, Lisch W, et al. The IC3D classification of the corneal dystrophies. *Cornea.* 2008;27(Suppl 2):S1–S83.

Major Corneal Dystrophies

Epithelial and Subepithelial Dystrophies

Epithelial basement membrane dystrophy

Alternative names Map-dot-fingerprint dystrophy, anterior basement membrane dystrophy, Cogan microcystic epithelial dystrophy

Inheritance No well-documented inheritance; may be degenerative

CLINICAL PRESENTATION Epithelial basement membrane dystrophy (EBMD) occurs in 6%–18% of the US population, more commonly in women, with increasing frequency in patients older than 50 years. The typical findings in the corneal epithelium are best seen by using a broad oblique slit-lamp beam or with retroillumination. (See Chapter 2 for a discussion of slit-lamp biomicroscopy.) The clinician can also identify EBMD by using the sclerotic scatter illumination technique. Using these techniques, the clinician can observe 4 typical patterns:

- maps
- fingerprint lines
- dots
- bleb pattern

These abnormalities occur in varying combinations and can change in number and distribution over time. *Fingerprint lines* are thin, parallel, hairlike lines that can be arranged in a concentric pattern resembling fingerprints or a horse's tail (Fig 8-1). *Maps* are geographic, irregular patterns or islands of thickened, gray, hazy epithelium with scalloped, circumscribed borders resembling coastlines (Fig 8-2). *Dots* are irregular round, oval, or comma-shaped intraepithelial opacities with discrete edges that contain the debris

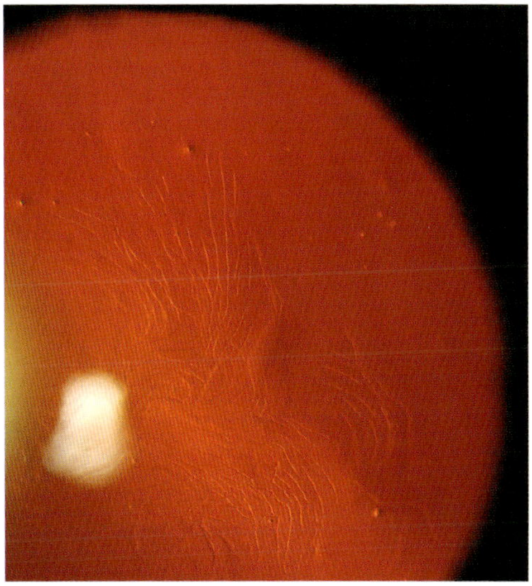

Figure 8-1 Epithelial basement membrane dystrophy (EBMD) can appear as fingerprint lines or as a horse's tail and is best seen with retroillumination, as seen here, or with indirect illumination. *(Courtesy of Robert S. Feder, MD.)*

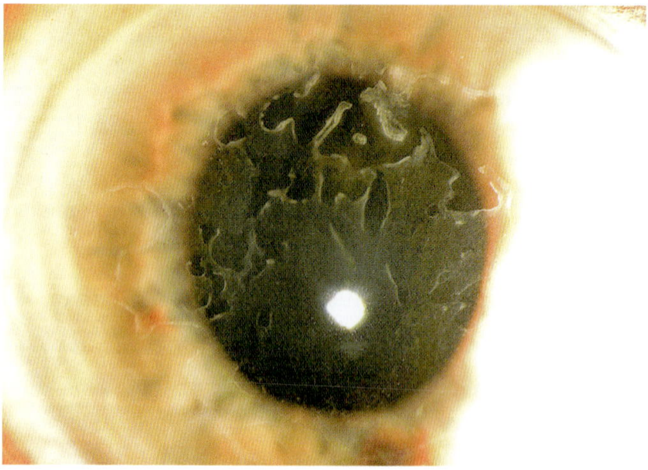

Figure 8-2 EBMD, seen using sclerotic scatter, demonstrates characteristic geographic maps. *(Courtesy of Robert S. Feder, MD.)*

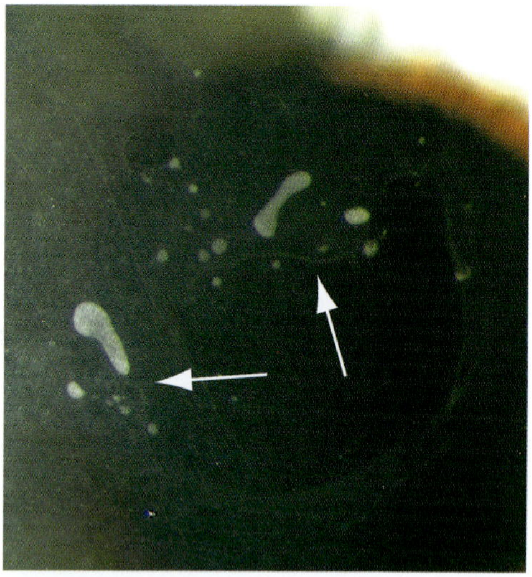

Figure 8-3 EBMD (seen using a broad, oblique slit beam) demonstrates geographic map areas and dots and putty-gray opacities *(arrows).* *(Courtesy of Robert S. Feder, MD.)*

of epithelial cells that collapsed and degenerated before reaching the epithelial surface (Fig 8-3). The *bleb pattern* resembles pebbled glass and is best seen with retroillumination.

Symptoms are typically related to recurrent epithelial erosions and/or blurred vision, ghosting, or monocular diplopia, occurring most commonly in patients older than 30 years. The impact of EBMD on vision correlates with the degree of surface disruption in proximity to the visual axis. The surface disruption appears as an irregularity (ie, negative staining) with instillation of topical fluorescein; the irregular astigmatism is confirmed on keratometry as irregular mires or on placido imaging as irregular rings (Fig 8-4).

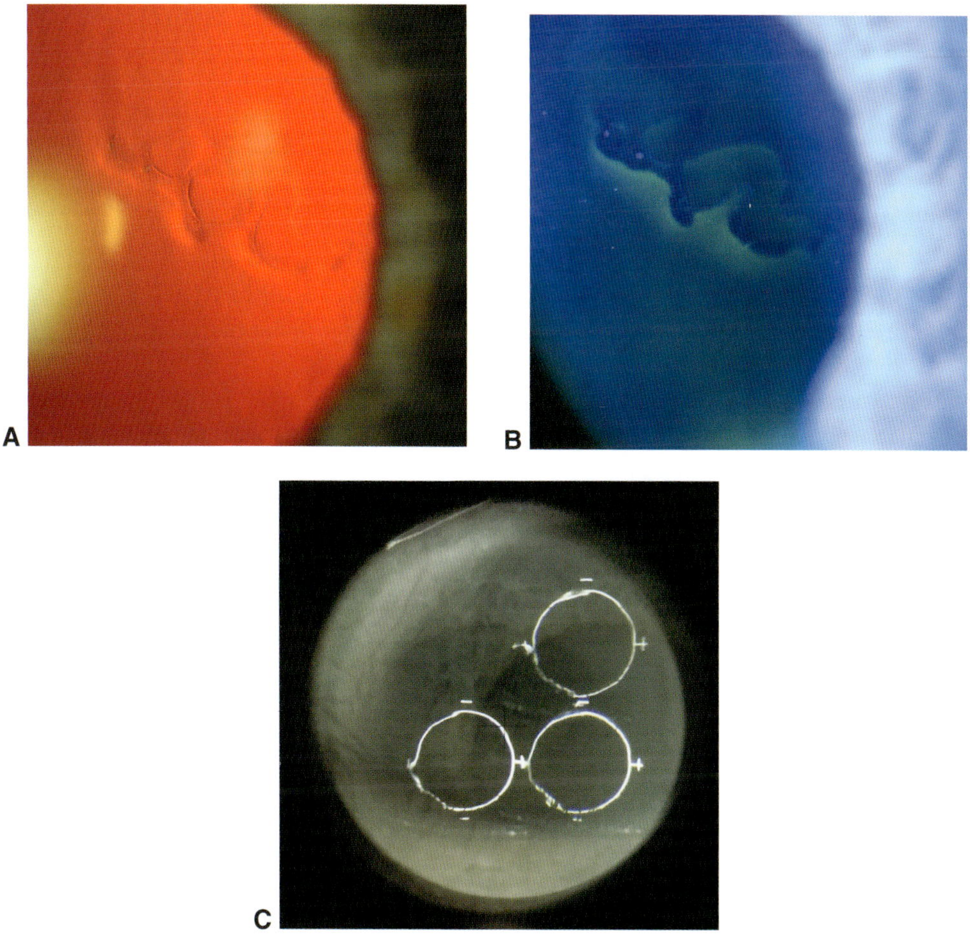

Figure 8-4 EBMD identification and impact. **A,** Maps can also be observed with a broad oblique slit beam or with retroillumination, as seen here. **B,** EBMD is more easily identified after instilling fluorescein. **C,** Keratometry reveals irregular mires that indicate the degree of irregular astigmatism within the central 3 mm; this information can help predict the impact on vision. Inferotemporal irregularity of the mires correlates with superotemporal EBMD. *(Courtesy of Robert S. Feder, MD.)*

> **CLINICAL PEARL**
>
> A rigid gas-permeable (RGP) contact lens overrefraction can help determine the visual impact of an irregular surface depending on the degree of vision improvement. This can be helpful when other causes of vision loss, such as cataract, are present.

Symptoms of recurrent erosion typically occur in the morning; however, discomfort in the morning may also occur in patients with nighttime lagophthalmos. Punctate erosions are usually noted in the inferior cornea in the latter. It is estimated that 10% of EBMD patients have corneal erosions, but 50% of patients with recurrent corneal erosions have EBMD. Therefore, it can be helpful to examine the fellow eye.

Unilateral dystrophic changes may be related to focal trauma rather than a dystrophy. In some cases, clinical findings may mimic corneal intraepithelial dysplasia; therefore, submitting removed material for histologic study may be warranted.

PATHOLOGY EBMD is an abnormality of epithelial turnover, maturation, and production of basement membrane. Histologic findings include the following:

- sheets of intraepithelial, multilamellar basal lamina material (maps)
- intraepithelial extension of basal laminar material (fingerprint lines)
- intraepithelial pseudocysts containing cytoplasmic debris (dots)
- irregular, subepithelial accumulation of fibrogranular material (bleb)

MANAGEMENT Asymptomatic patients usually do not require treatment. In patients with irregular astigmatism and blurred vision, epithelial debridement may be helpful. Chronic recurrent erosions can be managed medically with hypertonic sodium chloride ointment at night and/or drops during the day or a bandage soft contact lens. Use of a protective shield during sleep can also be helpful. Surgical management of recurrent erosions includes epithelial debridement, anterior stromal puncture, and phototherapeutic keratectomy (PTK). See Chapter 4 for a more detailed discussion of recurrent corneal erosion.

Meesmann epithelial corneal dystrophy

Inheritance Autosomal dominant (AD)

CLINICAL PRESENTATION Meesmann epithelial corneal dystrophy (MECD) appears very early in life. Tiny intraepithelial vesicles that extend to the limbus are seen most easily at the slit lamp with indirect illumination or retroillumination. The vesicles appear as minute bubble-like blebs (Fig 8-5). In 85% of eyes, the entire epithelium is affected. The epithelium

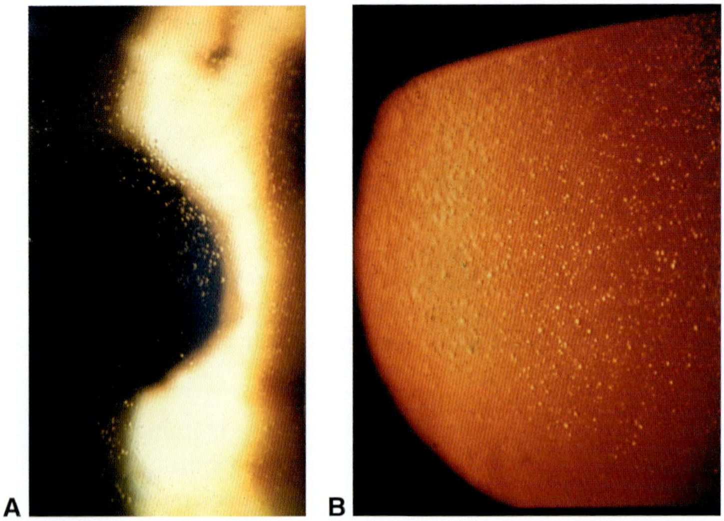

Figure 8-5 Meesmann corneal dystrophy. **A,** Indirect slit-lamp illumination reveals tiny bubble-like blebs. **B,** Blebs can also be observed against the red reflex. *(Part A courtesy of Robert S. Feder, MD; part B courtesy of Richard Abbott, MD.)*

surrounding the cyst is clear. Whorled and wedge-shaped epithelial patterns may be observed. The cornea may be slightly thinned, and corneal sensation may be reduced. Symptoms are usually limited to mild ocular irritation and a slight decrease in vision. Some patients report glare and light sensitivity. Painful recurrent erosions may occur.

The *Stocker-Holt variant,* which maps to a different gene (see Table 8-2), may have an earlier onset and demonstrate more severe signs and symptoms. The Stocker-Holt variant is an example of how genetic testing can help identify a more serious disease variant.

PATHOLOGY Intraepithelial cysts consisting of degenerated epithelial cell products, which stain positively with periodic acid–Schiff [PAS], are present. The epithelial cells contain an electron-dense accumulation of fibrogranular material surrounded by tangles of cytoplasmic filaments ("peculiar substance"). There are frequent mitoses and a thickened basement membrane with projections into the basal epithelium. On confocal microscopy, hyporeflective areas ranging in diameter from 40 µm to 150 µm are generally observed in the basal epithelium; however, some scattered hyperreflective circular spots may also be observed within these areas.

MANAGEMENT Most patients require no treatment, but if symptoms are frequent, soft contact lens wear may be helpful.

Gelatinous droplike corneal dystrophy

Alternative names Subepithelial amyloidosis, primary familial amyloidosis

Inheritance Autosomal recessive (AR)

CLINICAL PRESENTATION Onset of gelatinous droplike corneal dystrophy (GDLD) occurs in the first to second decade of life. Groups of multiple small nodules (mulberry configuration; Fig 8-6A) or lesions that appear similar to those of band keratopathy (Fig 8-6B) can be observed just beneath the epithelial layer. The lesions are visible on fluorescein staining. Superficial vascularization is often present. Stromal opacification or larger nodular lesions (kumquat-like lesions) may develop as the condition progresses (Fig 8-6C). Individuals with GDLD typically experience a significant decrease in vision, with photophobia, irritation, and tearing.

PATHOLOGY Light microscopy reveals subepithelial and stromal amyloid deposits. Disruption of epithelial tight junctions leads to abnormally high epithelial permeability. Confocal microscopy shows irregular, elongated epithelial cells with large accumulations of brightly reflective material (amyloid) noted within or beneath the epithelium and within the anterior stroma. Amyloid deposition can be noted in the basal epithelial layer on transmission electron microscopy. See also Chapter 10 for discussion of amyloidosis.

MANAGEMENT Surgical treatment options include superficial keratectomy, lamellar keratoplasty (LK), or penetrating keratoplasty (PK). However, there is a high recurrence rate within a few years. Soft contact lens use may help reduce postoperative recurrences.

Ide T, Nishida K, Maeda N, et al. A spectrum of clinical manifestations of gelatinous drop-like corneal dystrophy in Japan. *Am J Ophthalmol.* 2004;137(6):1081–1084.

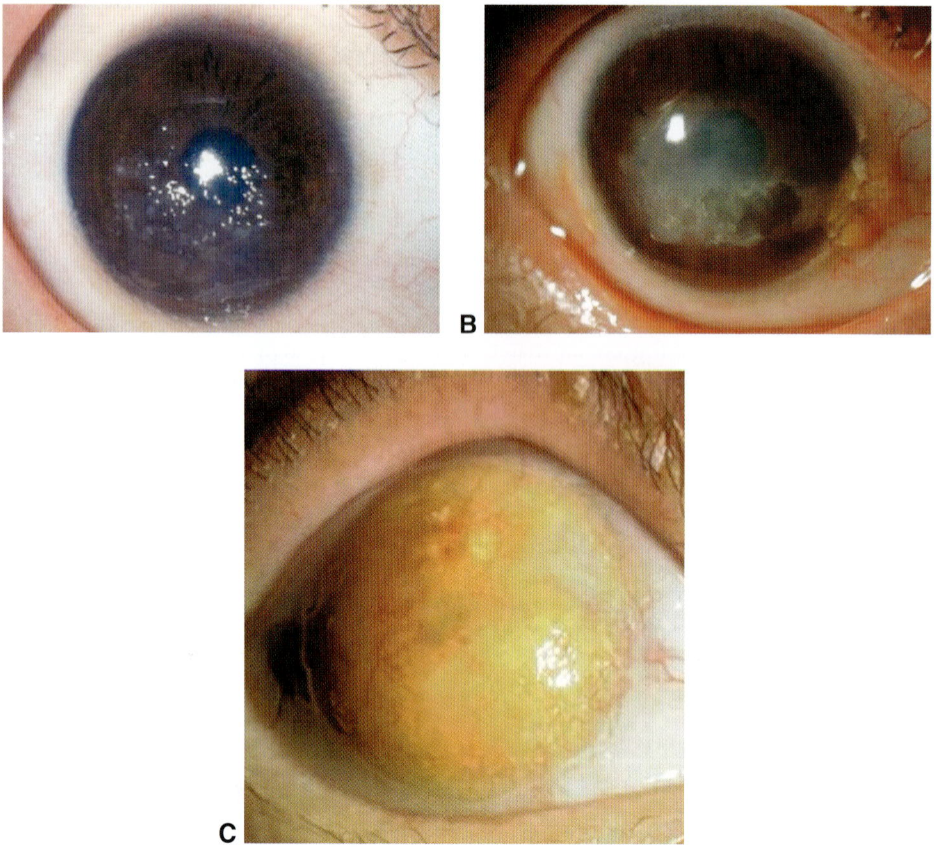

A B C

Figure 8-6 Gelatinous droplike corneal dystrophy. **A,** Mulberry type. **B,** Band keratopathy type. **C,** Kumquat-like type. *(Reproduced with permission from Weiss JS, Møller HU, Lisch W, et al. The IC3D classification of the corneal dystrophies.* Cornea. *2008;27(Suppl 2): S1–S42.)*

Epithelial–Stromal *TGFBI* Dystrophies

Reis-Bücklers corneal dystrophy

Alternative names Corneal dystrophy of Bowman layer type 1 (CDB1), atypical granular corneal dystrophy

Inheritance AD

CLINICAL PRESENTATION Reis-Bücklers corneal dystrophy (RBCD) appears in the first few years of life and mainly affects Bowman layer. Confluent, irregular, and coarse geographic opacities with varying densities develop primarily in the central cornea at both the level of Bowman layer and the superficial stroma (Fig 8-7A). Over time, the opacities may extend to the limbus and deeper stroma (Fig 8-7B).

The posterior cornea appears normal (Fig 8-7C). In moderate to advanced cases, stromal scarring can lead to surface irregularity. Symptoms often begin in the first or second

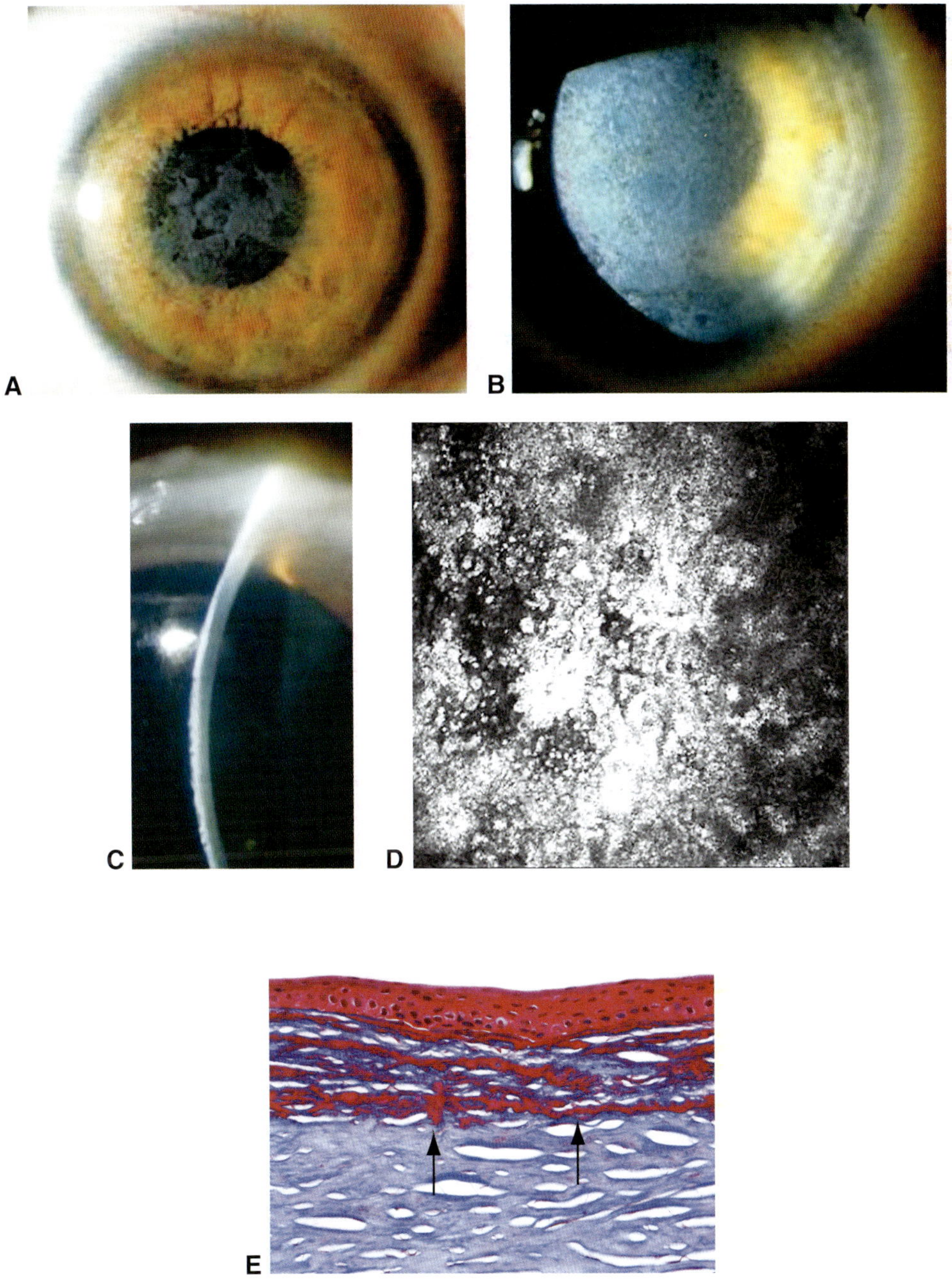

Figure 8-7 Reis-Bücklers corneal dystrophy (RBCD). **A,** Coarse geographic opacity of the superficial cornea. **B,** Broad, oblique illumination shows a dense, reticular, superficial opacity extending toward the limbus. **C,** Slit-lamp photograph showing irregularities at the level of Bowman layer. **D,** Confocal microscopy reveals highly reflective material with minimal shadows in the basal epithelium. **E,** Light microscopy with Masson trichrome stain reveals replacement of Bowman layer *(arrows)* with hyaline. Note thinner epithelium overlying areas of increased stromal involvement and vice-versa. *(Parts A–C reproduced with permission from Weiss JS, Møller HU, Lisch W, et al. The IC3D classification of the corneal dystrophies.* Cornea. *2008;27(Suppl 2):S1–S42. Part D courtesy of Kobayashi A, Sugiyama K. In vivo laser confocal microscopy findings for Bowman's layer dystrophies (Thiel-Behnke and Reis-Bücklers corneal dystrophies).* Ophthalmology. *2007;114(1):69–75. © 2007 by the American Academy of Ophthalmology. Part E courtesy of Tatyana Milman, MD.)*

decade of life with painful recurrent epithelial erosions. The erosions in eyes with RBCD are usually more severe and more frequent than in those with Thiel-Behnke corneal dystrophy (TBCD), but they recur less often over time. Anterior scarring and associated surface irregularity both contribute to reduced vision.

PATHOLOGY Confocal microscopy (Fig 8-7D) shows distinct deposits in the epithelium and Bowman layer. The basal epithelial cell layer and Bowman layer show high reflectivity associated with small granular deposits in the absence of shadows, which are typical of TBCD. Greater hyperreflectivity is observed in Bowman layer in RBCD than in TBCD. Light microscopy (Fig 8-7E) reveals disruption or absence of Bowman layer and replacement with a sheet-like connective tissue layer. This layer contains granular deposits that stain red with Masson trichrome stain. Transmission electron microscopy shows subepithelial electron-dense, rod-shaped bodies, which are immunopositive for the TGFBI protein keratoepithelin. Electron microscopy is helpful in differentiating RBCD histologically from TBCD, which has curly fibers (see the next section).

MANAGEMENT Initial treatment is aimed at the recurrent erosions. Superficial keratectomy, PTK, LK, or, in rare instances, PK may be performed. Deep anterior lamellar keratoplasty (DALK), while technically more challenging, eliminates the risk of endothelial rejection and, compared to PK, has a reduced risk of corneal rupture associated with trauma. Recurrence in a graft is common in all forms of keratoplasty.

Meghpara B, Hammersmith KM. Anterior corneal dystrophies. In: Mannis MJ, Holland EJ, eds. *Cornea.* Vol 1. 5th ed. Elsevier; 2022:701–711.

Thiel-Behnke corneal dystrophy

Alternative names Corneal dystrophy of Bowman layer type 2 (CDB2), honeycomb-shaped corneal dystrophy, Waardenburg-Jonkers corneal dystrophy

Inheritance AD

CLINICAL PRESENTATION The onset of Thiel-Behnke corneal dystrophy (TBCD) occurs in the first or second decade of life, manifesting as solitary flecks at the level of Bowman layer. Over time, symmetric subepithelial reticular opacities develop in a honeycomb pattern, sparing the peripheral cornea (Fig 8-8A). The opacities may progress to the deep stromal layers and the corneal periphery. Distinguishing TBCD from RBCD clinically is difficult, but noninvasive optical coherence tomography (OCT) and confocal microscopy may help differentiate these entities. Recurrent erosions in TBCD are less frequent and less severe than those in RBCD. Vision decreases secondary to increased corneal opacification.

PATHOLOGY High-resolution anterior segment OCT (AS-OCT) demonstrates hyperreflective material at the level of Bowman layer in a characteristic sawtooth configuration that helps distinguish TBCD from RBCD (Fig 8-8B). Light microscopy (Fig 8-8C) shows irregular thickening and thinning of the epithelial layer, which offset the ridges and furrows in the underlying stroma and the focal absences of the epithelial basement membrane. This is even better illustrated in Figure 8-7E. Bowman layer is replaced with fibrocellular material in the same pathognomonic wavy or sawtooth pattern. On electron microscopy, curly

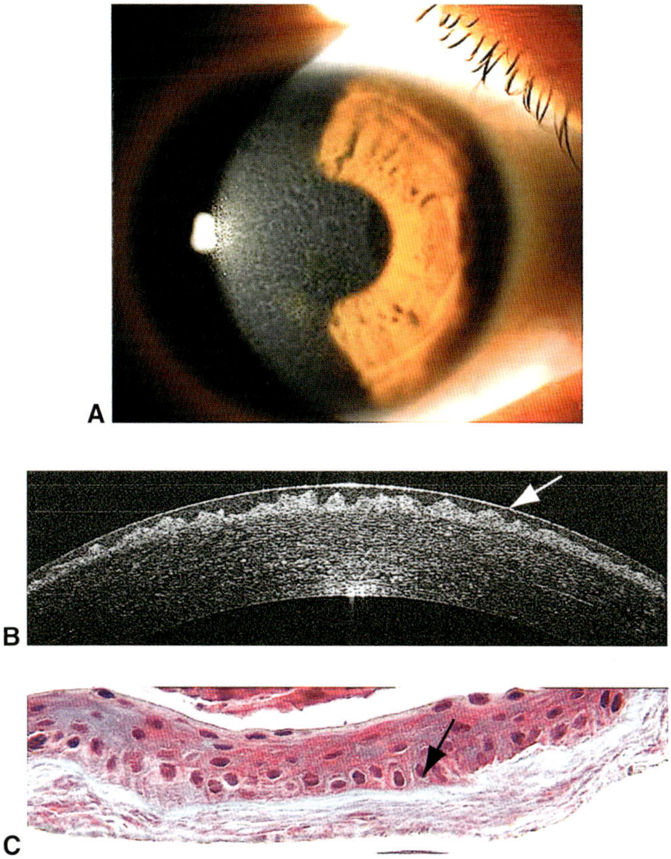

Figure 8-8 Thiel-Behnke corneal dystrophy (TBCD). **A,** Subepithelial reticular (honeycomb) opacities typical of this dystrophy. **B,** Anterior segment optical coherence tomography (AS-OCT) image shows extensive sawtooth pattern of hyperreflective material *(white arrow)* deposited at Bowman layer. **C,** Photomicrograph showing fibrocellular material *(black arrow)* that stained variably positive with Masson trichrome; (original magnification, 400×). *(Reproduced with permission from Vazjovic LM, Karp CL, Haft P, et al. Ultra-high-resolution anterior segment optical coherence tomography in the evaluation of anterior corneal dystrophies and degenerations.* Ophthalmology. *2011;118(7):1291–1296.)*

fibers (9–15 nm) rather than rod-shaped bodies are apparent, further distinguishing this dystrophy from RBCD. These curly fibers are immunopositive for the TGFBI protein, which is associated with the 5q31 locus. On confocal microscopy, distinct deposits are observed in the epithelium and Bowman layer. The deposits in the basal epithelial cell layer show reflectivity, with round edges and dark shadows not seen in RBCD. Bowman layer is replaced with irregular material that is reflective, but less reflective than in RBCD. The changes that differentiate RBCD from TBCD are summarized in Table 8-3.

MANAGEMENT Management is similar to the approach used for RBCD.

Kobayashi A, Sugiyama K. In vivo laser confocal microscopy findings for Bowman's layer dystrophies (Thiel-Behnke and Reis-Bücklers corneal dystrophies). *Ophthalmology.* 2007;114(1):69–75.

Table 8-3 Comparison of RBCD and TBCD

Point of differentiation	Reis-Bücklers corneal dystrophy (RBCD)	Thiel-Behnke corneal dystrophy (TBCD)
Corneal erosions	More frequent and more severe than TBCD	Less frequent and less severe than RBCD
Appearance	Coarse irregular geographic opacities	More regular delicate honeycomb appearance
Anterior segment OCT	Sawtooth pattern not prominent	Sawtooth pattern at Bowman layer
Confocal microscopy	Highly reflective material without shadows	Moderately reflective material with shadows
Transmission electron microscopy	Rod-shaped bodies immunopositive for TGFBI protein keratoepithelin	Curly fibers immunopositive for TGFBI protein keratoepithelin

OCT = optical coherence tomography; TGFBI = transforming growth factor beta–induced.

Lattice corneal dystrophy type 1 (classic) and variants

Alternative names Biber-Haab-Dimmer

Inheritance AD

CLINICAL PRESENTATION Lattice corneal dystrophy type 1 (LCD1) is relatively common and is characterized by refractile branching lines, so-called lattice lines, in the corneal stroma. The spectrum of corneal changes is broad, and the classic branching lattice lines may not be present in all cases. Subtle refractile lines, central and subepithelial ovoid white dots, and diffuse anterior stromal haze appear early in life and, in a corneal graft, these may be the first signs of recurrence. The typical branching refractile lines develop as the condition progresses and are best observed against a red reflex or with indirect illumination (Fig 8-9). These lines start centrally and superficially and spread centrifugally, becoming deeper. The stroma can take on a "ground-glass" appearance, but the peripheral cornea typically remains relatively clear. Epithelial erosions recur often and may occur as early as the first decade of life. Stromal haze and epithelial surface irregularity may decrease vision, typically in the fourth decade. Familial amyloidosis with lattice corneal changes (formerly lattice corneal dystrophy type II) is no longer considered a dystrophy (see Chapter 10). Variant lattice dystrophy type IIIA is associated with severe erosions that occur later in life. Thick, ropy lattice lines and heavy amyloid deposits are present (Fig 8-10). Because the findings in lattice dystrophy type IV occur more posteriorly than those in type IIIA, type IV is less likely to be associated with erosions.

CLINICAL PEARL

Crystalline deposits related to monoclonal gammopathy may resemble lattice lines. Polymorphic amyloid degeneration is often confused with lattice dystrophy; however, it presents in older individuals and occurs in the central and paracentral cornea, predominantly affecting the mid- and posterior stroma. (See Chapter 10, Table 10-6, for a summary of the ways in which amyloid occurs in the eye.)

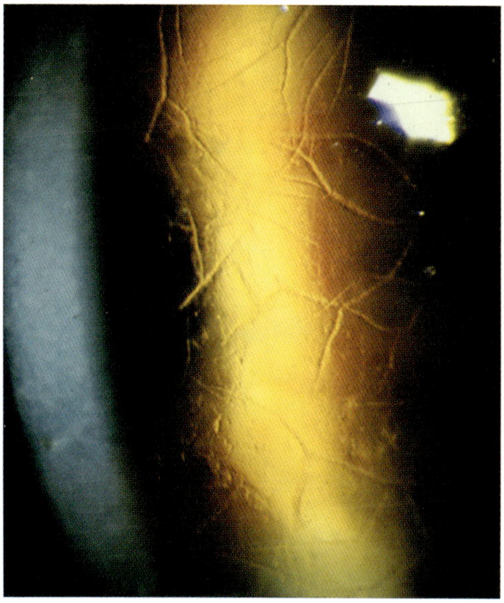

Figure 8-9 Classic lattice corneal dystrophy (LCD1).

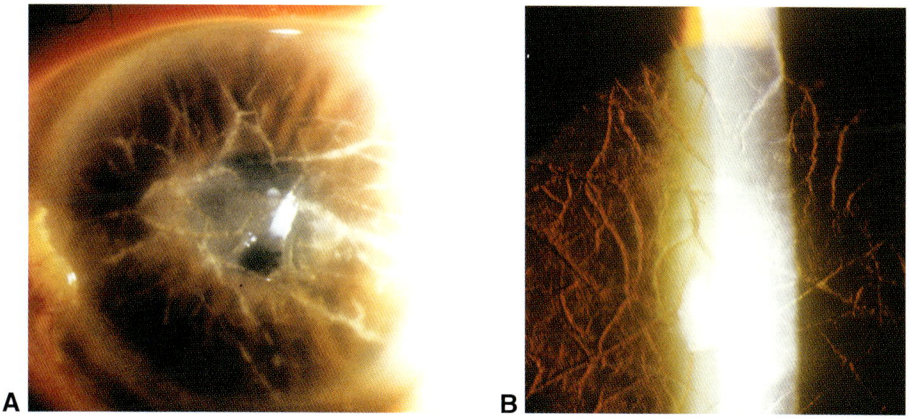

Figure 8-10 Variant lattice dystrophy type IIIA. **A,** Coarse linear opacities with central stromal haze. **B,** Retroillumination reveals thick lattice lines. *(Courtesy of Robert S. Feder, MD.)*

PATHOLOGY Light microscopy of classic lattice dystrophy reveals arborizing amyloid deposits concentrated most heavily in the anterior stroma. Amyloid may also accumulate in the subepithelial area, giving rise to poor epithelial–stromal adhesion, which results in corneal erosions. Epithelial atrophy and disruption, with degeneration of basal epithelial cells and focal thinning or absence of Bowman layer, progressively increase with age. An eosinophilic layer develops between the epithelial basement membrane and Bowman layer, with stromal deposition of the amyloid substance distorting the corneal lamellar architecture.

Amyloid stains rose to orange-red with Congo red dye (Fig 8-11A) and metachromatically with crystal violet dye (Table 8-4). Amyloid also exhibits birefringence, manifested as both dichroism (Fig 8-11B) and the ability to change the axis of polarized light. See BCSC Section 4, *Ophthalmic Pathology and Intraocular Tumors.*

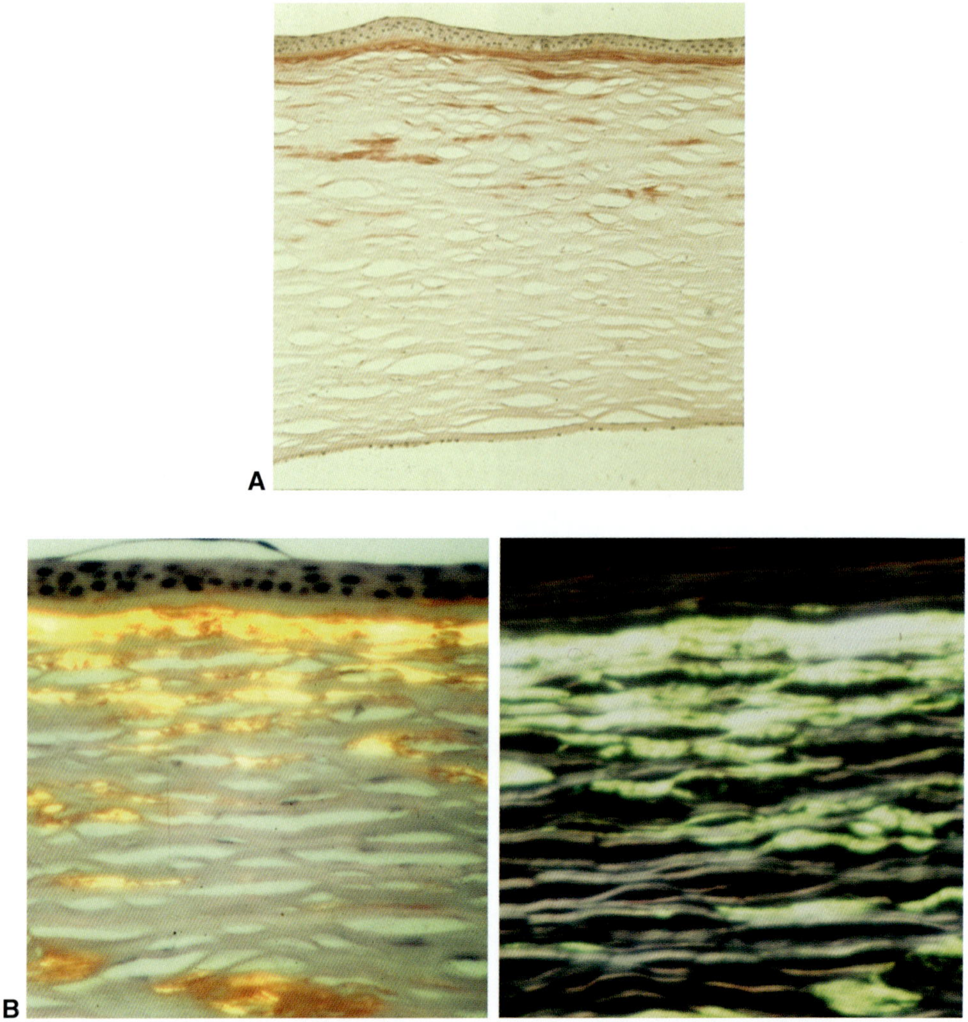

Figure 8-11 Histopathology of LCD1. **A,** Amyloid in lattice dystrophy stains positively with Congo red dye. **B,** When a polarizing filter is rotated, dichroism is demonstrated as the color changes from red-orange to apple green. *(Courtesy of Robert S. Feder, MD.)*

Electron microscopy reveals extracellular masses of fine 8–10-μm fibrils that are electron dense and randomly aligned. In vivo confocal microscopy reveals characteristic linear images (Fig 8-12) that should be differentiated from those associated with fungal hyphae.

MANAGEMENT Recurrent erosions are managed with therapeutic bandage soft contact lenses, superficial keratectomy, or PTK. Severe cases of lattice dystrophy with vision loss are treated with DALK or PK. Recurrence of lattice dystrophy in the corneal graft is common.

Aldave AJ, Bonnet C, de Sousa LB. The stromal dystrophies. In: Mannis MJ, Holland EJ, eds. *Cornea*. Vol 1. 5th ed. Elsevier; 2022:712–729.

Table 8-4 Histologic Differentiation of Granular, Lattice, Schnyder, and Macular Dystrophies

Dystrophy	Deposited Material	Masson Trichrome	Alcian Blue and Colloidal Iron	PAS	Oil red O and Sudan Black B	Congo Red
Granular type 1	Hyaline	+	–	–	–	–
Granular type 2 (granular-lattice)	Hyaline, amyloid[a]	+	–	–	–	+
Lattice type 1	Amyloid[a]	+	–	+	–	+
Schnyder	Phospholipid, cholesterol	–	–	–	+	–
Macular	Glycosaminoglycans (acid mucopolysaccharide)	–	+	–	–	–

PAS = periodic acid–Schiff.

[a] Amyloid also stains with thioflavine T and metachromatically with crystal violet. It demonstrates birefringence manifested as both dichroism and the polarization of light.

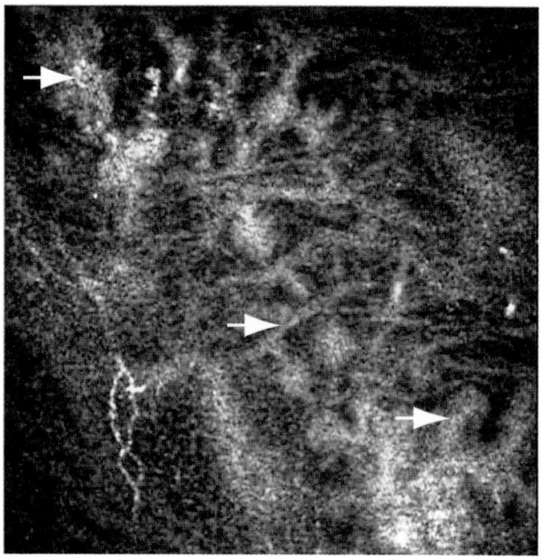

Figure 8-12 In vivo confocal microscopy image demonstrates branching lines *(arrows)* that correspond to lattice lines in the corneal stroma. *(Courtesy of Kailasanathan A, Maharajan S. In vivo confocal microscopy detects preclinical corneal lattice dystrophy.* Eye *(Lond). 2013;27(8):991–992.)*

Pradhan MA, Henderson RA, Patel D, McGhee CN, Vincent AL. Heavy chain amyloidosis in *TGFBI*-negative and gelsolin-negative atypical lattice corneal dystrophy. *Cornea.* 2011; 30(10):1163–1166.

Stock EL, Feder RS, O'Grady RB, Sugar J, Roth SI. Lattice corneal dystrophy type IIIA: clinical and histopathologic correlations. *Arch Ophthalmol.* 1991;109(3):354–358.

Granular corneal dystrophy type 1

Alternative names Groenouw corneal dystrophy type I, classic granular dystrophy

Inheritance AD

CLINICAL PRESENTATION The onset of granular corneal dystrophy type 1 (GCD1) occurs early in life with crumblike opacities in the superficial cornea. With direct illumination, the opacities appear white; however, indirect illumination reveals small translucent dots with vacuoles and a

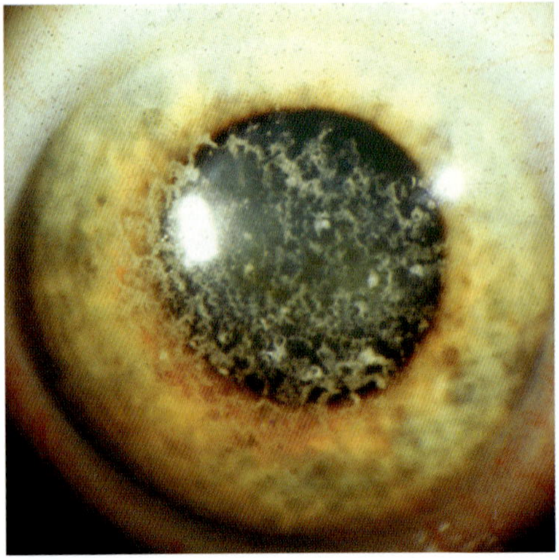

Figure 8-13 Granular corneal dystrophy type 1 (GCD1). *(Courtesy of Robert S. Feder, MD.)*

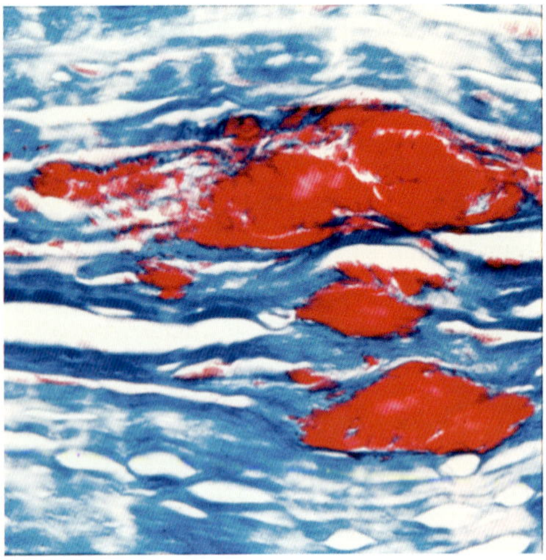

Figure 8-14 Hyaline in GCD1 stains red with Masson trichrome stain. *(Courtesy of Robert S. Feder, MD.)*

glassy splinter or "crushed bread crumb" appearance. Early in the disease process, the lesions are separated by clear spaces, but later they become more confluent. The lesions do not extend to the limbus but can extend anteriorly through focal breaks in Bowman layer (Fig 8-13). GCD1 is slowly progressive, with most patients maintaining good vision and visual acuity, only dropping to 20/200 after age 50 years in rare cases. Patients report glare and photophobia. Recurrent erosions occur and vision decreases as the opacities become more confluent.

Although the exact cause is unknown, a mutation different from that in RBCD, LCD1, and granular corneal dystrophy type 2 (GCD2; granular-lattice) has been identified in the *TGFBI* gene on 5q31.

PATHOLOGY The deposited granular material stains positively for hyaline as bright red with Masson trichrome (Fig 8-14; see Table 8-4). Electron microscopy reveals an electron-dense material made up of rod-shaped bodies immersed in an amorphous matrix. Histochemically, the deposits are noncollagenous protein that may derive from the corneal epithelium and/or keratocytes. Hyperreflective opacities are seen on confocal microscopy.

MANAGEMENT Early in the disease process, no treatment is needed. Recurrent erosions may be treated with therapeutic contact lenses and superficial keratectomy. PTK may be effective temporarily. When vision is affected, DALK or PK has a good prognosis. Recurrence is possible, presenting as fine subepithelial opacities anteriorly and peripherally in contrast to the original presentation.

CLINICAL PEARL

Laser refractive surgery is contraindicated in patients with *TGFBI* dystrophies such as granular dystrophy because of the risk of worsening the corneal opacity.

Granular corneal dystrophy type 2

Alternative names Avellino corneal dystrophy

Inheritance AD

CLINICAL PRESENTATION Patients with granular corneal dystrophy type 2 (GCD2) have a granular dystrophy both histologically and clinically, with shorter, whiter lattice lesions in addition to the granular lesions. Clinical findings in GCD2 differ from those in GCD1. Stellate-shaped, snowflake-like, and icicle-like opacities appear between the superficial stroma and midstroma (Fig 8-15). Lattice lines are also seen deeper than the snowflake opacities. Older patients have anterior stromal haze between deposits, which reduces vision. Pain may occur with mild corneal erosions.

PATHOLOGY Pathologically, both the hyaline deposits typical of granular dystrophy and the amyloid deposits typical of lattice dystrophy are present. These lesions extend from the basal epithelium to the deep corneal stroma. Individual opacities stain with the Masson trichrome or Congo red stain. The deposits appear as rod-shaped bodies on electron microscopy; randomly aligned fibrils of amyloid are also seen. Findings on confocal microscopy are a combination of those seen in GCD1 and LCD1.

MANAGEMENT Lamellar or penetrating keratoplasty may be useful, depending on the depth of the deposits. The dystrophy can recur in the graft. PTK is an alternative treatment and can be performed to reduce surface irregularity and increase corneal clarity. It can also result in a hyperopic refractive shift. Laser in situ keratomileusis (LASIK) and photorefractive keratectomy (PRK) are contraindicated because they may worsen the underlying disease.

Aldave AJ, Bonnet C, de Sousa LB. The stromal dystrophies. In: Mannis MJ, Holland EJ, eds. *Cornea*. Vol 1. 5th ed. Elsevier; 2022:712–729.

Holland EJ, Daya SM, Stone EM, et al. Avellino corneal dystrophy. Clinical manifestations and natural history. *Ophthalmology.* 1992;99(10):1564–1568.

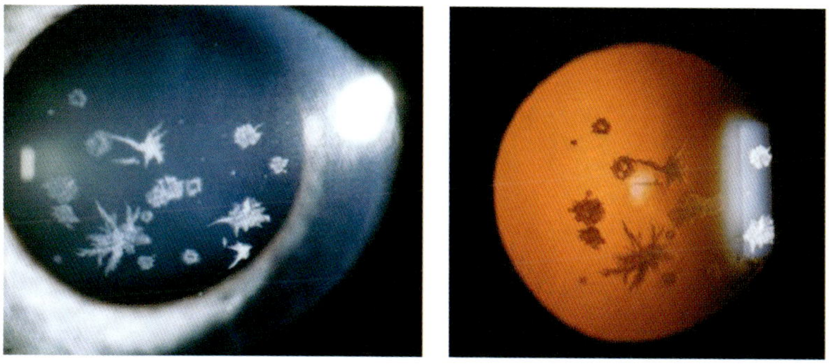

Figure 8-15 Granular corneal dystrophy type 2. Stellate-shaped opacities with intervening clear spaces can be seen in direct illumination *(left)* and in retroillumination *(right)*. *(Reproduced with permission from Weiss JS, Møller HU, Lisch W, et al. The IC3D classification of the corneal dystrophies.* Cornea. *2008;27(Suppl 2):S1–S42.)*

Kim TI, Hong JP, Ha BJ, Stulting RD, Kim EK. Determination of treatment strategies for granular corneal dystrophy type 2 using Fourier-domain optical coherence tomography. *Br J Ophthalmol.* 2010;94(3):341–345.

Stromal Dystrophies

Macular corneal dystrophy

Alternative names Groenouw corneal dystrophy type II

Inheritance AR

CLINICAL PRESENTATION Macular corneal dystrophy (MCD) occurs less frequently than the stromal dystrophies associated with *TGFBI* gene mutations. Unlike most corneal dystrophies, MCD has an autosomal recessive inheritance, involves the entire corneal stroma including the periphery, and may involve the corneal endothelium.

Individuals with MCD have clear corneas that begin to cloud between 3 and 9 years of age. Patients initially show superficial, irregular, whitish, flecklike opacities that evolve into focal, gray-white, superficial stromal opacities with intervening haze, in contrast to GCD. The opacities, which have indefinite edges (Fig 8-16), tend to be more superficial centrally and more posterior peripherally.

Involvement of Descemet membrane and endothelium is evidenced by the presence of guttate excrescences, but corneal edema does not occur. Dystrophic opacities in the periphery may also appear similar to keratic precipitates, but in contrast to inflammatory lesions, these occur in all quadrants of the posterior cornea. Epithelial erosions rarely develop, but a severe decrease in vision typically occurs between 10 and 30 years of age. Hypoesthesia has been noted.

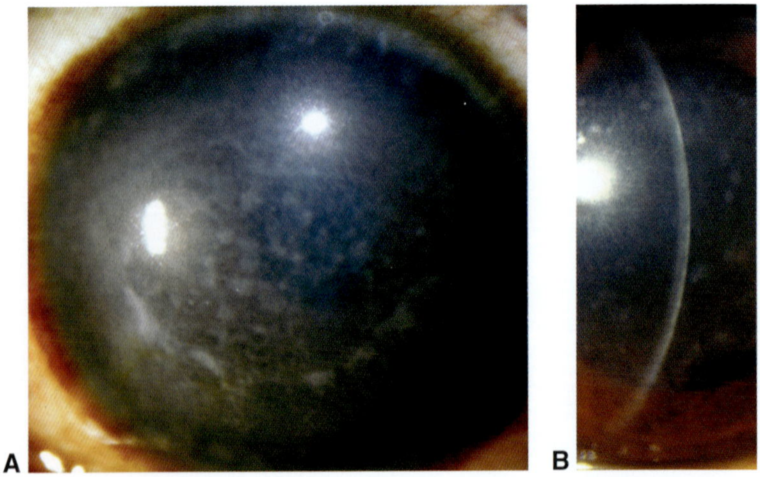

Figure 8-16 Macular corneal dystrophy (MCD). **A,** Diffuse illumination reveals involvement to the limbus with diffuse haze. **B,** Slit view. Typically, the cornea is thin with dense opacities that occur more posteriorly in the periphery and may resemble keratic precipitates *(Courtesy of Robert S. Feder, MD.)*

CLINICAL PEARL

Diffuse corneal thinning is common and may appear similar to long-standing interstitial keratitis (IK); however, patients with MCD lack the ghost vessels and thickened Descemet membrane seen in IK.

An enzyme-linked immunosorbent assay (ELISA) can be used to measure sulfated keratan sulfate in the serum. This test can help in the diagnosis of macular dystrophy, even in preclinical forms and carriers. The 3 variants of macular dystrophy are distinguished based on biochemical differences:

- *Type I:* In the most prevalent form, antigenic keratan sulfate (AgKS) is lacking in the cornea, serum, and cartilage. Errors occur in the synthesis of keratan sulfate and in the activity of specific sulfotransferases involved in the sulfation of the keratan sulfate lactose aminoglycan side chain.
- *Type IA:* Keratocytes show AgKS reactivity, but the extracellular material does not. There is no AgKS in the serum.
- *Type II:* All of the abnormal deposits react positively with AgKS, and the serum has low to normal levels of AgKS.

PATHOLOGY The deposits in MCD are glycosaminoglycans (GAGs); they stain with colloidal iron and alcian blue (Fig 8-17; see Table 8-4). These deposits accumulate in the endoplasmic reticulum and not in lysosomal vacuoles, as seen in systemic mucopolysaccharidoses. Electron microscopy reveals keratocytes and endothelial cells that stain positive for GAGs, as well as extracellular clumps of fibrogranular material that also stains for GAGs. On confocal microscopy, blurred accumulations of light-reflective material are seen in the anterior corneal stroma.

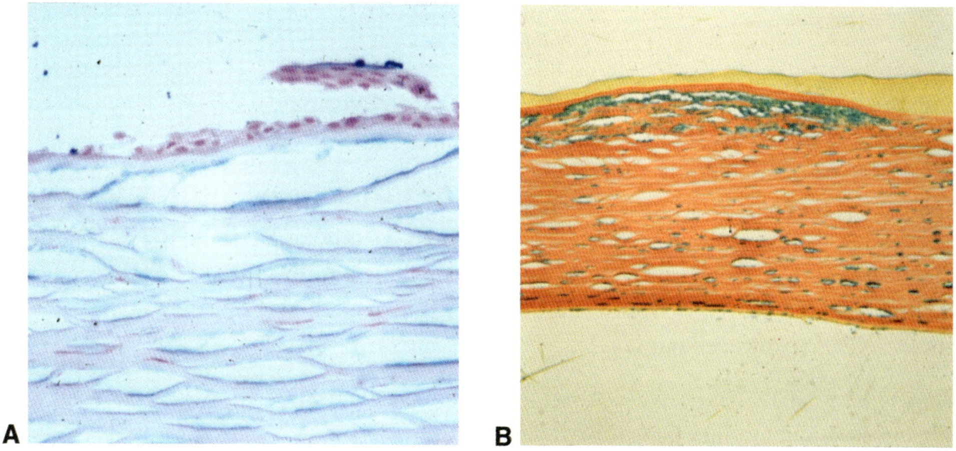

Figure 8-17 Glycosaminoglycan deposits in MCD stain positively with **(A)** alcian blue and **(B)** colloidal iron. *(Courtesy of Robert S. Feder, MD.)*

MANAGEMENT Recurrent erosions are rare and should be treated. Photophobia may be reduced with tinted contact lenses. PTK may be used for symptomatic anterior macular dystrophy. Definitive treatment requires PK or DALK, and recurrences are uncommon.

Aldave AJ, Bonnet C, de Sousa LB. The stromal dystrophies. In: Mannis MJ, Holland EJ, eds. *Cornea*. Vol 1. 5th ed. Elsevier; 2022:712–729.

Weiss JS, Møller HU, Aldave AJ, et al. IC3D classification of corneal dystrophies—edition 2. *Cornea*. 2015;34(2):117–159.

Schnyder corneal dystrophy

Inheritance AD

CLINICAL PRESENTATION Schnyder corneal dystrophy (SCD) is a rare, slowly progressive stromal dystrophy that may become apparent as early as the first year of life. Hypercholesterolemia occurs in two-thirds of affected individuals. The diagnosis is usually made by the second or third decade of life, although it may be further delayed in patients who have the crystalline form of the disease. Central subepithelial crystals are seen in only 50% of patients and do not involve the epithelium. For this reason, the name Schnyder crystalline dystrophy has been replaced.

SCD disproportionately reduces photopic vision despite maintenance of excellent scotopic vision. Vision and corneal sensation decrease with age. Glare increases because of progressive corneal haze. The spectrum of disease is shown in Figure 8-18.

Changes, which are progressive and predictable by age, include the following:

- ring or disclike central corneal opacification (can affect the full corneal stromal thickness) with or without subepithelial crystals; individuals younger than 23 years
- dense corneal arcus; third decade of life
- midperipheral corneal opacification (affects full thickness stroma); fourth decade of life
- corneal sensation decreases with age
- abnormal lipid profile

PATHOLOGY This condition is thought to be a local disorder of corneal lipid metabolism. Pathologically, the opacities are accumulations of unesterified and esterified cholesterol and phospholipids. Lipids stain with oil red O and Sudan black B (see Table 8-4). In the usual process of embedding tissue in paraffin, cholesterol and other fatty substances are dissolved; therefore, it is important to submit fresh tissue to the pathologist for special lipid stains. Electron microscopy shows abnormal accumulation of lipid and dissolved cholesterol in the corneal epithelium, in Bowman layer, and throughout the stroma. Confocal microscopy reveals disruption of the basal epithelial/subepithelial nerve plexus, with highly reflective intracellular and extracellular deposits.

MANAGEMENT PTK has been used to treat decreased vision resulting from subepithelial crystals, but it does not reduce panstromal haze. SCD patients older than 50 years usually require corneal transplant surgery to eliminate haze. The dystrophy can recur after PK or DALK.

A 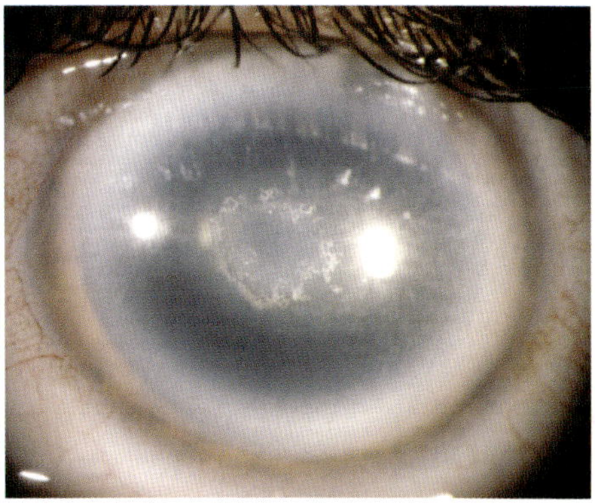

B 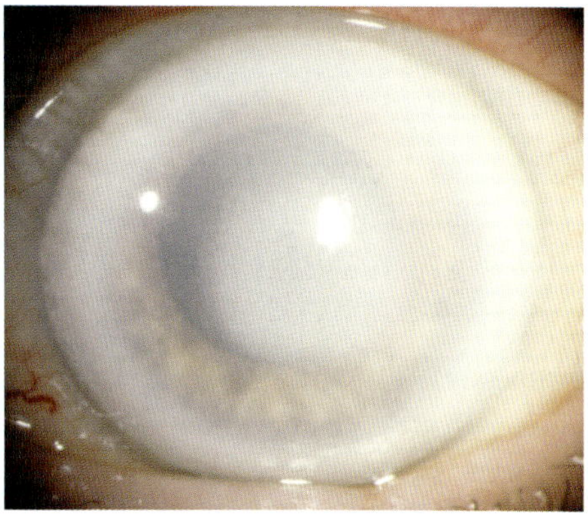

C 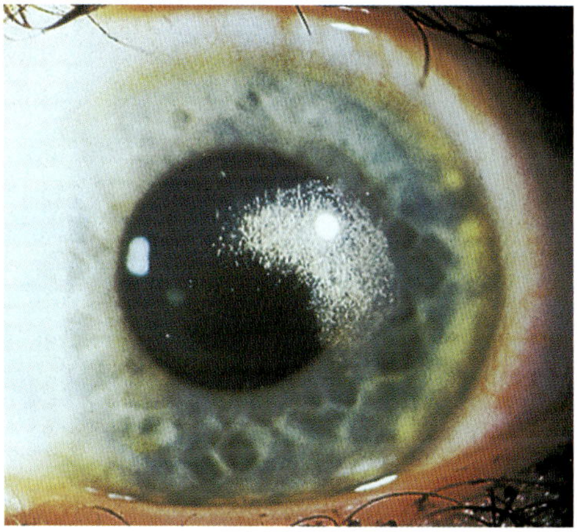

Figure 8-18 The spectrum of disease in Schnyder corneal dystrophy. **A,** Central subepithelial crystalline deposition and haze with corneal arcus. **B,** Central panstromal corneal opacity and arcus. No crystals are present. **C,** Paracentral anterior stromal crystals with minimal haze and no arcus. *(Courtesy of Jayne S. Weiss, MD.)*

CLINICAL PEARL

A fasting lipid profile should be done to detect possible hyperlipoproteinemia or hyperlipidemia. Patients with abnormal serum lipid levels are managed with dietary changes and/or medication, but despite this treatment progression of the corneal dystrophy is unaltered. Unaffected family members may also have an abnormal lipid profile and should be screened.

Weiss JS. Visual morbidity in thirty-four families with Schnyder crystalline corneal dystrophy (an American Ophthalmological Society thesis). *Trans Am Ophthalmol Soc.* 2007;105:616–648.

Congenital stromal corneal dystrophy

Inheritance AD

CLINICAL PRESENTATION In congenital stromal corneal dystrophy (CSCD), diffuse, bilateral corneal clouding with flakelike, whitish opacities is found throughout the stroma (Fig 8-19). The corneas are thickened. The course is either nonprogressive or slowly progressive, with moderate to severe vision loss.

PATHOLOGY The stromal lamellae are separated from each other in a regular manner, sometimes with areas of amorphous deposition. Electron microscopy reveals that the collagen fibril diameter is approximately half the normal size in all lamellae. Abnormal lamellar layers consisting of thin filaments arranged in an electron-lucent ground substance separate the lamellae of normal appearance. The keratocytes and endothelium are normal. Absence of the anterior banded zone of Descemet membrane has been reported. The epithelial cells are normal on confocal microscopy; however, evaluation is not possible because of increased reflectivity.

MANAGEMENT Refractive error is corrected with glasses or contact lens. Amblyopia therapy and/or strabismus surgery may be necessary. In advanced cases, PK is recommended. DALK can be considered if the diagnosis is certain.

Rødahl E, Knappskog PM, Bredrup C, Boman H. Congenital stromal corneal dystrophy. In: Adam MP, Ardinger HH, Pagon RA, et al, eds. *GeneReviews* [Internet]. University of Washington, Seattle; 1993–2021. Accessed November 13, 2021. www.ncbi.nlm.nih.gov/books/NBK2690

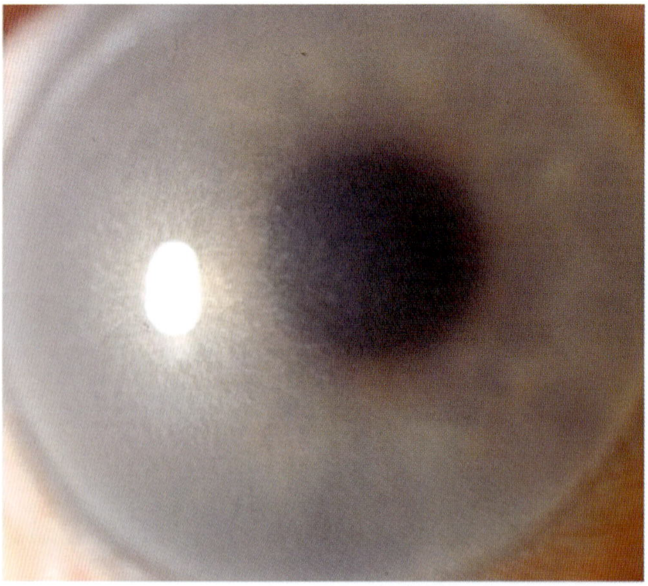

Figure 8-19 Congenital stromal corneal dystrophy: diffuse bilateral clouding with flakelike opacities throughout the stroma. *(Reproduced with permission from Weiss JS, Møller HU, Lisch W, et al. The IC3D classification of the corneal dystrophies.* Cornea. *2008;27(10:Suppl 2):S22.)*

Fleck corneal dystrophy

Alternative names François-Neetens speckled corneal dystrophy

Inheritance AD

CLINICAL PRESENTATION Fleck corneal dystrophy (FCD) is a nonprogressive condition that may be congenital or may present early in the first decade of life. Discrete, flat, gray-white, dandrufflike (sometimes ring-shaped) opacities appear throughout the corneal stroma extending to the periphery (Fig 8-20). The epithelium, Bowman layer, Descemet membrane, and endothelium are not involved. Fleck dystrophy may be unilateral or bilateral but asymmetric. Symptoms are minimal, and vision is usually not reduced. Fleck dystrophy may be associated with decreased corneal sensation, limbal dermoid, keratoconus, central cloudy dystrophy, punctate cortical lens changes, pseudoxanthoma elasticum, or atopy.

PATHOLOGY Affected keratocytes are vacuolated and contain 2 abnormal substances: excess glycosaminoglycan, which stains with alcian blue and colloidal iron; and lipids, which stain with Sudan black B and oil red O. Transmission electron microscopy reveals membrane-based inclusions with delicate granular material. Confocal microscopy shows an accumulation of pathologic material in stromal cells and inclusions in the basal nerves.

MANAGEMENT None is required.

Purcell JJ Jr, Krachmer JH, Weingeist TA. Fleck corneal dystrophy. *Arch Ophthalmol.* 1977; 95(3):440–444.

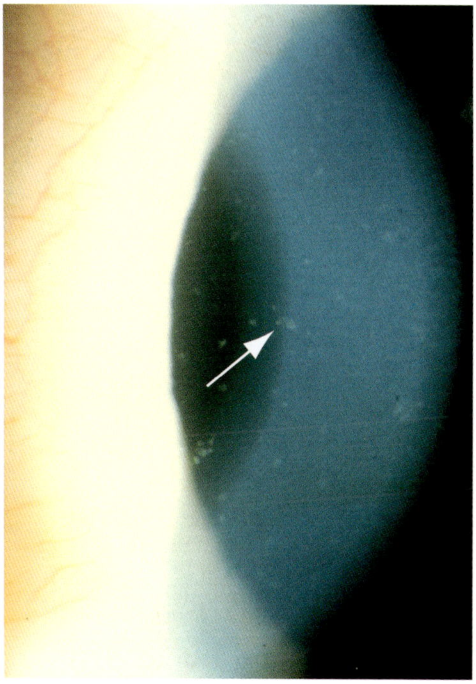

Figure 8-20 Dandrufflike opacities *(arrow)* seen in Fleck corneal dystrophy. *(Courtesy of Jay H. Krachmer, MD.)*

Posterior amorphous corneal dystrophy

Inheritance AD

CLINICAL PRESENTATION PACD presents in the first decade of life with a diffuse, sheetlike, gray-white opacity, usually in the posterior cornea (Fig 8-21). The condition is usually nonprogressive. The cornea is flat (<41.00 diopters) and thin (≥380 µm), and there is associated hyperopia. Cornea plana, a bilateral familial disease caused by a mutation in the *KERA* gene, is also associated with marked flattening of the cornea and is also stationary. In eyes affected by PACD, Descemet membrane and the corneal endothelium may be indented by opacities. Focal endothelial abnormalities, a prominent Schwalbe line, fine iris processes, pupillary remnant, iridocorneal adhesions, corectopia, pseudopolycoria, and anterior stromal tags have been noted. There is no associated glaucoma. Visual acuity is usually 20/40 or better. Posterior amorphous corneal dystrophy (PACD) may be an example of mesodermal dysgenesis rather than a true corneal dystrophy given the early onset, lack of progression, similarity to cornea plana, and iris abnormalities.

PATHOLOGY Focal attenuation of corneal endothelial cells and irregular stromal architecture anterior to Descemet membrane are observed on light microscopy. Electron microscopy reveals disorganization of the posterior stromal lamellae. A fibrillar layer interrupts Descemet membrane. On confocal microscopy, there are microfolds and a hyperreflective layer in the posterior stroma.

MANAGEMENT Typically no treatment is needed, but keratoplasty is sometimes performed.

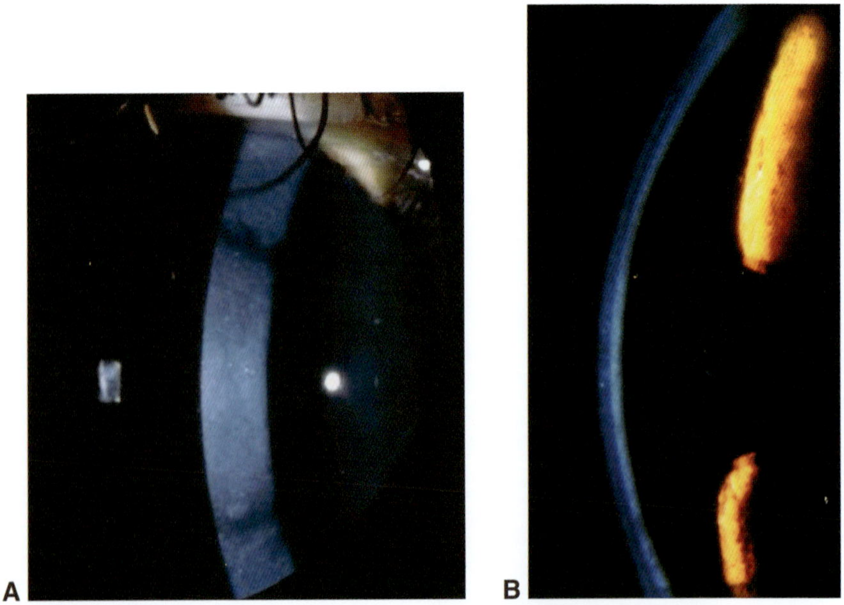

Figure 8-21 Posterior amorphous corneal dystrophy (PACD). **A,** Central, deep stromal pre-Descemet opacity. **B,** Slit-lamp photograph shows a diffusely thin, flat cornea with a posterior stromal opacity. *(Part A reproduced with permission from Weiss JS, Møller HU, Lisch W, et al. The IC3D classification of the corneal dystrophies.* Cornea. *2008;27(Suppl 2):S24; part B courtesy of Jay H. Krachmer, MD.)*

Aldave AJ, Rosenwasser GO, Yellore VS, et al. Linkage of posterior amorphous corneal dystrophy to chromosome 12q21.33 and exclusion of coding region mutations in *KERA, LUM, DCN,* and *EPYC. Invest Ophthalmol Vis Sci.* 2010, 51(8):4006–4012.

Dunn SP, Krachmer JH, Ching SS. New findings in posterior amorphous corneal dystrophy. *Arch Ophthalmol.* 1984;102(2):236–239.

Johnson AT, Folberg R, Vrabec MP, Florakis GJ, Stone EM, Krachmer JH. The pathology of posterior amorphous corneal dystrophy. *Ophthalmology.* 1990;97(1):104–109.

Pre-Descemet corneal dystrophy

Inheritance No definite pattern of inheritance, although pre-Descemet corneal dystrophy (PDCD) has been described in families through 2–4 generations

CLINICAL PRESENTATION Onset is usually after 30 years of age, but PDCD has been reported in children as young as 3 years old. Focal fine, polymorphic, gray opacities that may be central, annular, or diffuse are seen in the deep stroma just anterior to Descemet membrane (Fig 8-22). The rest of the cornea is unaffected. Vision is normal. Similar opacities have been described in pseudoxanthoma elasticum, X-linked and recessive ichthyosis, keratoconus, posterior polymorphous corneal dystrophy, and EBMD.

PATHOLOGY Large keratocytes are present in the posterior stroma, with vacuoles and intracytoplasmic inclusions containing lipidlike material. Electron microscopy reveals membrane-bound intracellular vacuoles containing electron-dense material suggestive of secondary lysosomes, and there are inclusions consistent with lipofuscin-like lipoprotein, suggesting a degenerative process.

MANAGEMENT None is indicated.

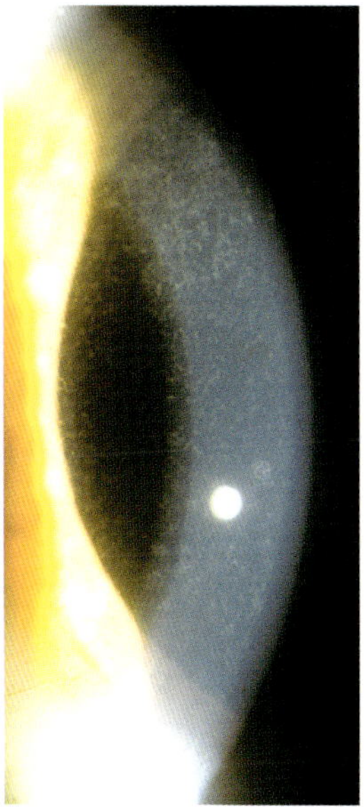

Figure 8-22 Punctate opacities just anterior to Descemet membrane in PDCD. *(Courtesy of Robert S. Feder, MD.)*

Endothelial Dystrophies

Fuchs endothelial corneal dystrophy

Alternative names Endothelial corneal dystrophy

Inheritance The gene for early-onset Fuchs endothelial corneal dystrophy (FECD) has been identified and mapped *(COL8A2)* and the specific mutation identified. Some forms of late-onset FECD have known genetic loci in which the gene has not yet been localized, but transcription factor 4 may be implicated. Most commonly, late-onset FECD presents with no known inheritance; however, cases with AD inheritance have been reported.

CLINICAL PRESENTATION Fuchs dystrophy usually presents in the fourth decade of life or later, although early-onset FECD may present as early as the first decade of life. Symptoms are rare before age 50 and are typically related to the edema, which causes a decrease in vision, contrast sensitivity, and/or glare. In some cases, symptoms of glare can occur with confluent central guttae in the absence of edema. Pain may result from ruptured bullae or microcystic edema. Symptoms are often worse upon awakening because of decreased surface evaporation during sleep. Painful episodes may subside once subepithelial fibrosis occurs.

Findings vary with the stage of the disease. Cornea guttae are first evident centrally and then spread toward the periphery (stage 1). In some patients, cornea guttae develop, but the disease never progresses beyond this stage (Fig 8-23). Cornea guttae may become confluent and take on a "beaten metal" appearance. In late-onset FECD, cornea guttae are larger than those observed in early-onset FECD. Stage 2 is characterized by endothelial decompensation and stromal edema (Fig 8-24). As the disease progresses, stromal edema may worsen, causing bullous keratopathy (stage 3). Descemet membrane may become thickened. Central corneal thickness may approach 1 mm (0.5–0.6 mm is typically considered normal). This can be associated with increased light scatter and symptoms of glare. Subepithelial fibrosis, scarring, and peripheral superficial vascularization secondary to chronic edema occur in end-stage disease (stage 4).

CLINICAL PEARL

Although it may be helpful in the initial evaluation of Fuchs dystrophy and in following the clinical course for loss of corneal endothelial cells, specular microscopy is not necessary in the presence of diffuse confluent guttae. Corneal thickness measurement with Scheimpflug tomography, OCT, ultrasound biomicroscopy, or ultrasonic pachymetry provides a better indicator of corneal endothelial function. Significant increase in corneal thickness in the morning or over time or an increase in posterior elevation over time may indicate endothelial dysfunction. See Chapter 2 for more detailed discussion of corneal pachymetry and specular microscopy.

PATHOLOGY The endothelial cells are noted to be more varied in size (polymegethism) and more irregular in shape (pleomorphism) than normal and are disrupted by excrescences

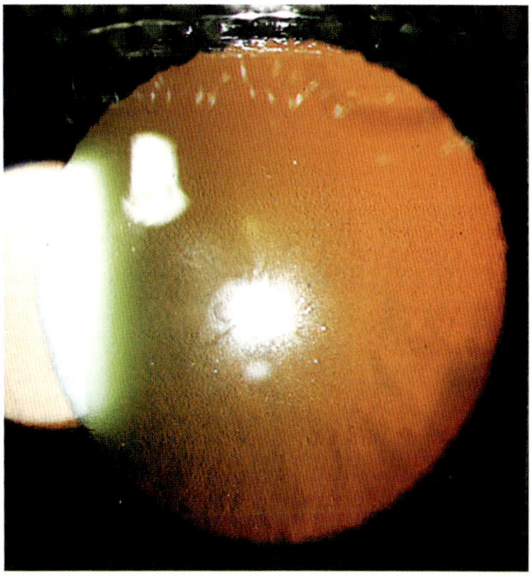

Figure 8-23 Fuchs endothelial corneal dystrophy (FECD). Cornea guttae are seen with retroillumination. *(Courtesy of Robert S. Feder, MD.)*

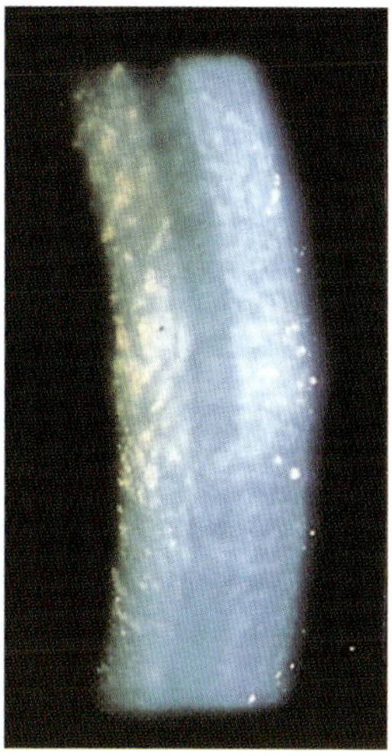

Figure 8-24 FECD showing the "beaten metal" appearance of the endothelium with mild stromal edema. *(Courtesy of Vincent P. deLuise, MD.)*

of collagen. See the section Endothelial Appearance and Function in Chapter 2. Primary dysfunction of the endothelial cells manifests as increased corneal swelling and deposition of collagen and extracellular matrix in a thickened Descemet membrane. It is not clear whether the reduction in the posterior nonbanded zone and the increase in thickness of the abnormal posterior collagenous layer are primary effects of endothelial dysfunction or are secondary to chronic corneal edema.

MANAGEMENT Early morning blurred vision or minor pain related to corneal edema can be reduced with hypertonic sodium chloride drops and ointment (5%) and/or measures taken to reduce intraocular pressure (IOP). Note that topical or oral carbonic anhydrase inhibitors may decrease endothelial pump function and increase corneal edema.

Restoration of vision generally requires keratoplasty. In the absence of significant scarring, PK has largely been replaced with EK (either DSAEK or DMEK). If significant stromal scarring is present, full-thickness keratoplasty should be considered. Refer to Chapter 16 for a more comprehensive discussion of keratoplasty.

In cases where the guttae are confined to the central cornea, Descemet stripping only (DSO), with the addition of a topical Rho kinase (ROCK) inhibitor to stimulate endothelial proliferation, is a keratoplasty alternative that eliminates the risk of rejection; however, it may have a prolonged postoperative course. This approach is under clinical investigation and has not yet been widely adopted.

If keratoplasty cannot be done, persistent or more severe pain can be managed with anterior stromal puncture, bandage soft contact lenses designed for extended wear, placement of amniotic tissue, or conjunctival flap surgery (see Chapter 5).

CATARACT SURGERY IN PATIENTS WITH FUCHS DYSTROPHY

When planning cataract surgery in a patient with Fuchs dystrophy, consider the following:

- A combined keratoplasty and phacoemulsification with intraocular lens (IOL) insertion is best performed
  - when corneal edema is present
  - if pachymetry readings are significantly greater in the morning
  - if the patient reports blurred vision in the morning
- Some surgeons prefer a combined approach even when edema is not present.
- If confluent guttae are present without edema, the patient may be satisfied with cataract surgery alone.
- If there are symptoms of glare due to extensive guttae and thickened Descemet membrane, the patient may benefit from endothelial keratoplasty (EK).

When cataract surgery alone is performed, it is important to warn patients with Fuchs dystrophy about the possibility of later corneal decompensation. When EK is combined with cataract surgery, and the IOL power is planned, the surgeon should anticipate a greater hyperopic shift for Descemet stripping automated endothelial keratoplasty (DSAEK) than for Descemet membrane endothelial keratoplasty (DMEK).

See BCSC Section 11, *Lens and Cataract,* and Videos 8-1 and 8-2.

VIDEO 8-1 Phacoemulsification with Fuchs dystrophy.
Courtesy of Edward J. Holland, MD.

VIDEO 8-2 Cornea debate: cataract surgery first or combined with endothelial keratoplasty?
Courtesy of Marian Sue Macsai-Kaplan, MD, and Francis W. Price Jr, MD.

Afshari NA, Igo RP Jr, Morris NJ, et al. Genome-wide association study identifies three novel loci in Fuchs endothelial corneal dystrophy. *Nat Commun.* 2017;8:14898.

Borkar DS, Veldman P, Colby KA. Treatment of Fuchs endothelial dystrophy by Descemet stripping without endothelial keratoplasty. *Cornea.* 2016;35(10):1267–1273.

Gottsch JD, Sundin OH, Liu SH, et al. Inheritance of a novel *COL8A2* mutation defines a distinct early-onset subtype of Fuchs corneal dystrophy. *Invest Ophthalmol Vis Sci.* 2005;46(6):1934–1939.

Li YJ, Minear MA, Rimmler J, et al. Replication of *TCF4* through association and linkage studies in late-onset Fuchs endothelial corneal dystrophy. *PLoS One.* 2011;6(4):e18044. Published April 20, 2011. Accessed November 13, 2021. http://journals.plos.org/plosone/article?id=10.1371/journal.pone.0018044

Patel SV, Hodge DO, Treichel EJ, Spiegel MR, Baratz KH. Predicting the prognosis of Fuchs endothelial corneal dystrophy by using Scheimpflug tomography. *Ophthalmology.* 2020;127(3):315–323.

Posterior polymorphous corneal dystrophy

Alternative names Posterior polymorphous dystrophy (PPMD), Schlichting dystrophy

Inheritance AD (isolated unilateral cases with similar phenotype but no heredity reported)

CLINICAL PRESENTATION Careful examination of the posterior corneal surface may show any or all of the following:

- isolated grouped endothelial vesicles (Fig 8-25A)
- geographic-shaped, discrete, gray lesions
- broad endothelial bands with scalloped edges (Fig 8-25B)

Various degrees of stromal edema, corectopia, and broad iridocorneal adhesions may also be seen (Fig 8-26). Fine iridocorneal adhesions may be seen on gonioscopy. Both chronic angle-closure and open-angle glaucoma can occur, and 14% of patients with posterior polymorphous corneal dystrophy (PPCD) have elevated IOP. PPCD is included in the differential diagnosis of congenital corneal opacity.

PATHOLOGY The most distinctive microscopic finding is the appearance of abnormal corneal endothelial cells that look and behave like epithelial cells or fibroblasts. These endothelial cells have the following features or characteristics that are typical of epithelial cells:

- microvilli
- multilayer growth in cell culture
- positive immunohistochemical staining for keratin
- rapid and easy growth in cell culture
- intercellular tight junctions
- proliferative tendencies

A diffuse abnormality of Descemet membrane is common, including thickening of the posterior nonbanded layer, a multilaminated appearance, and polymorphous alterations.

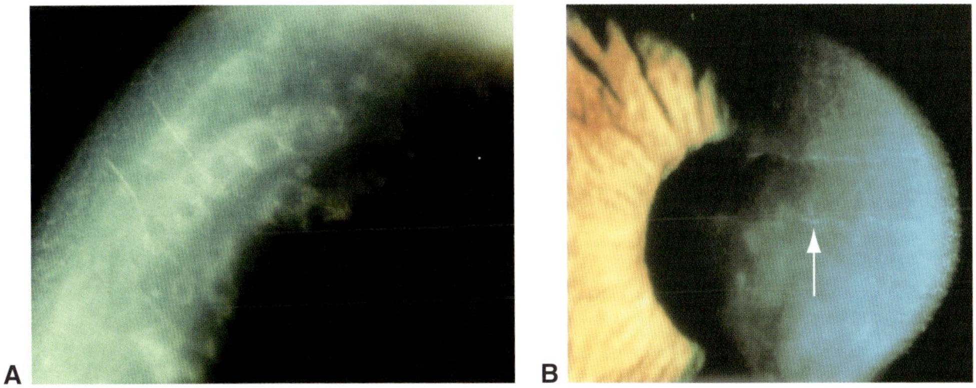

Figure 8-25 Findings in posterior polymorphous corneal dystrophy (PPCD). **A,** Broad, oblique view shows clusters of endothelial vesicles, which are commonly seen. **B,** Scallop-edged endothelial band *(arrow)*. *(Part A courtesy of Robert S. Feder, MD.)*

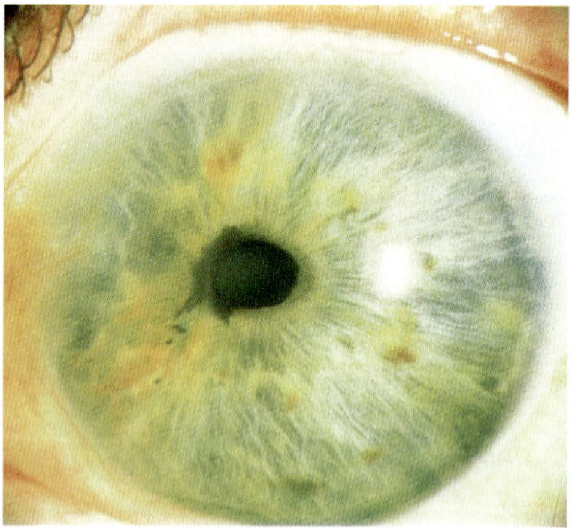

Figure 8-26 Iridocorneal adhesion and corectopia in PPCD.

Similar changes that are not limited to the cornea are seen in iridocorneal endothelial (ICE) syndrome (see Chapter 7). However, ICE is sporadic and almost always unilateral. Specular microscopy may reveal typical vesicles and bands, in contrast to the involved cells in ICE syndrome, which appear as dark areas with central highlights and light peripheral borders (see Fig 7-21 in this volume and BCSC Section 10, *Glaucoma*). Opinion is divided on the value of relying on specular microscopy alone in making the diagnosis. Confocal microscopy reveals vesicular lesions and railroad track, bandlike dark areas with irregular edges. Table 8-5 compares characteristics of PPCD with 2 other conditions in the differential diagnosis.

MANAGEMENT Most patients are asymptomatic. Mild corneal edema may be managed in the same manner as for early Fuchs dystrophy. In cases of localized swelling, anterior stromal puncture can be used to induce focal subepithelial fibrosis. With more severe disease, keratoplasty may be required and, if present, glaucoma must be managed. If peripheral anterior synechiae, glaucoma, or both are present preoperatively, the prognosis for successful corneal transplant is reduced. PPCD may recur in the graft. EK is the preferred approach in cases with limited stromal opacification.

Weiss JS, Weinstein JE. Descemet membrane and endothelial dystrophies. In: Mannis MJ, Holland EJ, eds. *Cornea*. Vol 1. 5th ed. Elsevier; 2022:730–748.

Congenital hereditary endothelial dystrophy

Alternative names Congenital hereditary endothelial dystrophy (CHED) was formerly divided into 2 forms, CHED1 (AD) and CHED2 (AR). However, a careful review of the findings from reported families suggests that CHED1 is actually indistinct from PPCD. There is now only a single form of CHED.

Inheritance AR

CLINICAL PRESENTATION CHED is a congenital, usually nonprogressive condition with asymmetric corneal clouding and edema that ranges from a diffuse haze to a ground-glass

Table 8-5 Comparison of PPCD, ICE, and Axenfeld-Rieger Syndrome

PPCD	ICE Syndrome[a]	Axenfeld-Rieger Syndrome[b]
Autosomal dominant	Sporadic; may be related to herpesvirus	Autosomal dominant in 75% of cases
Usually bilateral	Unilateral	Bilateral
May be stationary or slowly progressive	Progressive	Stationary
May be associated with broad PAS, corectopia	Broad PAS, corectopia, iris atrophy, iris nevi	Fine iris strands to posterior embryotoxon (anterior displaced Schwalbe line); iris hypoplasia; corectopia
Vesicles and bands on slit-lamp biomicroscopy and confocal microscopy; corneal edema uncommon	Dark areas with central highlights and light peripheral borders on specular microscopy; corneal edema possible	Normal corneal endothelium

ICE = iridocorneal endothelial; PAS = peripheral anterior synechiae; PPCD = posterior polymorphous corneal dystrophy.

[a] See Chapter 7.

[b] See Chapter 6.

appearance; focal gray spots are occasionally observed. Thickening of the cornea (2–3 times normal thickness) occurs (Fig 8-27), with rare subepithelial band keratopathy and IOP elevation. The presence of marked stromal edema helps distinguish CHED from CHSD and congenital glaucoma. Blurred vision and nystagmus occur with minimal to no tearing or photophobia.

PATHOLOGY There is diffuse thickening and lamination of Descemet membrane, with sparse atrophic corneal endothelial cells. On electron microscopy, multiple layers of basement membrane–like material are observed on the posterior part of Descemet membrane, along

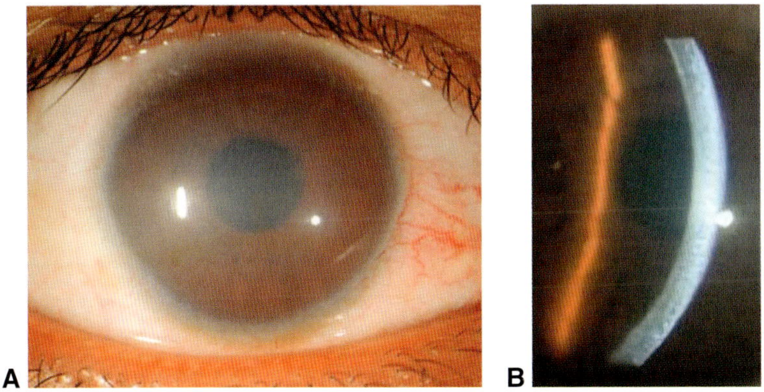

Figure 8-27 Congenital hereditary endothelial dystrophy. **A,** Milky appearance of the cornea with diffuse illumination. **B,** Slit view shows diffuse stromal thickening. *(Reproduced with permission from Weiss JS, Møller HU, Lisch W, et al. The IC3D classification of the corneal dystrophies.* Cornea. *2008;27(Suppl 2): S1–S42.)*

with degeneration of the endothelial cells, which show many vacuoles. Stromal thickening with severe disorganization and disruption of the lamellar pattern is evident.

MANAGEMENT Due to marked corneal edema present in more severe cases, corneal transplant (PK or EK) is required. Amblyopia may limit the visual outcome.

Aldave AJ, Han J, Frausto RF. Genetics of the corneal endothelial dystrophies: an evidence-based review. *Clin Genet.* 2013;84(2):109–119.

Weiss JS, Weinstein JE. Descemet membrane and endothelial dystrophies. In: Mannis MJ, Holland EJ, eds. *Cornea.* Vol 1. 5th ed. Elsevier; 2022:730–748.

CHAPTER 9

Clinical Approach to Corneal Ectatic Disease

This chapter includes related videos. Go to www.aao.org/bcscvideo_section08 or scan the QR codes in the text to access this content.

This chapter includes a case study. Go to www.aao.org/bcsccasestudy_section08 or scan the QR code in the text to access this content.

Indicates selected key points within the chapter.

Highlights

- The hallmark finding of keratoconus is corneal protrusion with thinning at the point of maximum protrusion, the apex of the cone.
- Keratoconus progresses rapidly in patients in their teens and twenties; thus, its development in young patients should be closely monitored. Corneal crosslinking may slow or arrest disease progression.
- Eye rubbing is a significant risk factor for the development of keratoconus, and patients should be cautioned against eye rubbing to reduce progression.
- In pellucid marginal degeneration (PMD), thinning occurs in a peripheral band, extending over several clock hours, with corneal protrusion on the central side of the band of thinning.

Keratoconus

Keratoconus (KC), a common disorder, occurs in approximately 1 in 2000 individuals. However, the incidence rate varies based on geographic location and the testing methodology. Typically, the central, inferior paracentral, or inferior midperipheral cornea undergoes progressive thinning and protrusion, resulting in a cone-shaped cornea (Figs 9-1, 9-2). There is a slight female preponderance, and a higher incidence has been reported in South Asian and the Middle Eastern countries. Although a hereditary pattern is not commonly observed, positive family histories have been reported in 6%–8% of cases. Considerable variations can occur in clinical findings within an affected family. The prevalence of KC in first-degree relatives is 3.34%. Clinically unaffected first-degree relatives have a higher chance of showing subclinical tomographic abnormalities associated with KC than the general population. Although multiple chromosomal loci for KC have been reported, the identification of specific

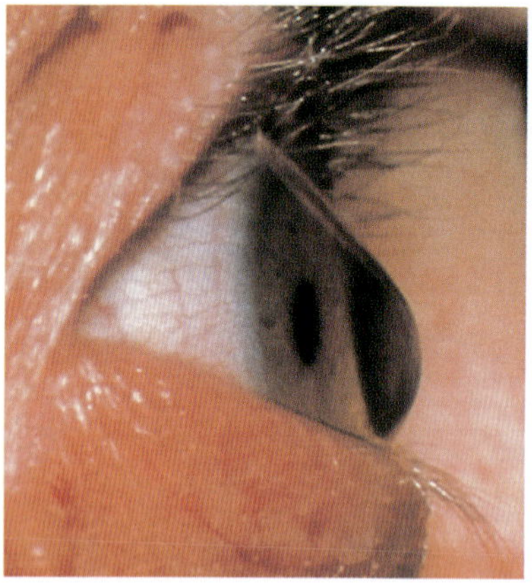

Figure 9-1 Clinical photo of keratoconus. Note the marked corneal protrusion, a hallmark of keratoconus.

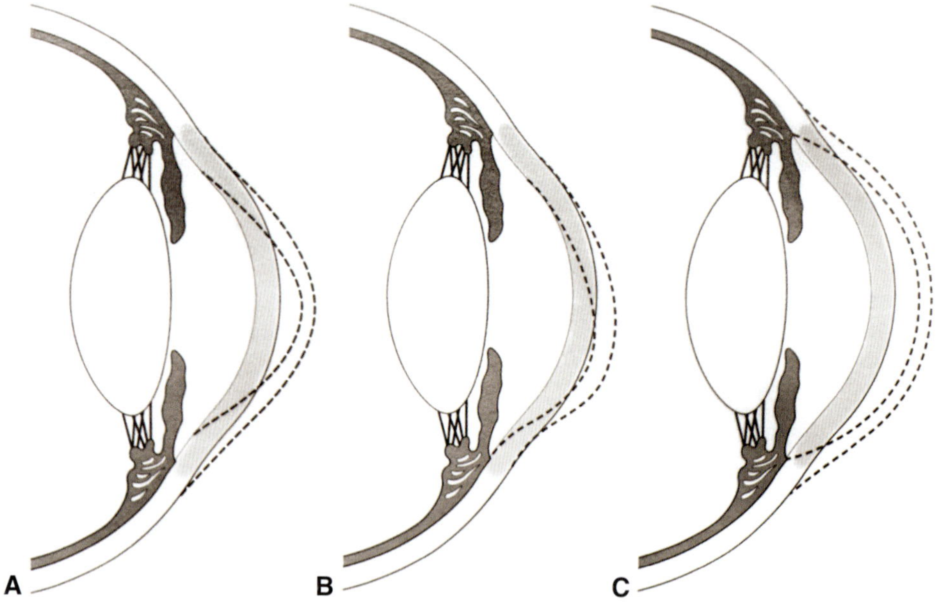

Figure 9-2 The presence of corneal thinning and the type of contour abnormality can help the clinician to identify the type of ectatic disorder. This illustration demonstrates the difference in the thinning pattern of various ectatic diseases. **A,** Keratoconus. **B,** Pellucid marginal degeneration. **C,** Keratoglobus. *(Modified with permission from Feder RS, Neems LC. Noninflammatory ectatic disorders. In: Mannis MJ, Holland EJ, eds.* Cornea. *Vol 1. 4th ed. Elsevier; 2017:821.)*

genes remains elusive. The development of sophisticated topographic (power mapping) and tomographic (elevation and thickness mapping) devices has dramatically improved the detection of corneal ectasia, particularly KC.

Factors that may play a role in the onset and progression of KC include

- genetic predisposition
- eye rubbing

- atopic disease and allergic keratoconjunctivitis
- contact lens wear
- abnormalities in collagen that result in hyperelastic joints
- ablative keratorefractive surgery in patients with preoperative high myopia or thin corneas
- oxidative stress

CLINICAL PEARL

Clinicians should consider the possibility of KC in young patients who require frequent changes in their eyeglass prescription due to increased myopia and astigmatism or whose refractive error cannot be fully corrected with spectacles.

KC onset occurs during puberty. The rate of progression of KC is highest in young individuals (in their teens and twenties); its development should be closely monitored in this subpopulation as vision may worsen and disease progression can be arrested or slowed with corneal crosslinking. Progression typically slows in the fourth decade of life and is unusual after the age of 40 years but can occur. Approximately 50% of patients with KC have hyperelastic joints. The association between atopic disease and KC is well established. The Dundee University Scottish Keratoconus Study (DUSK) reviewed 200 KC patients and found a high incidence of hay fever (30%), asthma (23%), and eczema (14%). Also, KC is commonly observed in patients with Down syndrome and other conditions associated with developmental delay as well as in patients with low vision, probably due to habitual eye rubbing. Table 9-1 presents common systemic and ocular associations with KC. The following references provide a comprehensive overview of these associations.

Feder RS, Neems LC. Noninflammatory ectatic disorders. In: Mannis MJ, Holland EJ, eds. *Cornea.* Vol 1. 4th ed. Elsevier; 2017:820–843.

Kiliç A, Colin J. Advances in the surgical treatment of keratoconus. *Focal Points: Clinical Modules for Ophthalmologists.* American Academy of Ophthalmology; 2012, module 2.

McMonnies CW. Abnormal rubbing and keratectasia. *Eye Contact Lens.* 2007; 33(6 Pt 1):265–271.

Saidel MA, Paik JY, Garcia C, Russo P, Cao D, Bouchard C. Prevalence of sleep apnea syndrome and high-risk characteristics among keratoconus patients. *Cornea.* 2012;31(6):600–603.

Sugar J, Macsai M. What causes keratoconus? *Cornea.* 2012;31(6):716–719.

Table 9-1 Conditions Commonly Associated With Keratoconus

Associated Systemic Conditions	Associated Ocular Diseases
Atopic disease	Aniridia
Down syndrome	Floppy eyelids
Ehlers-Danlos syndrome	Leber tapetoretinal degeneration[a]
Osteogenesis imperfecta	Retinitis pigmentosa
Mitral valve prolapse	Retinopathy of prematurity
Sleep apnea	Vernal keratoconjunctivitis

[a] Not to be confused with Leber hereditary optic atrophy.

Wang Y, Rabinowitz YS, Rotter JI, Yang H. Genetic epidemiological study of keratoconus: evidence for major gene determination. *Am J Med Genet.* 2000;93(5):403–409.

Weed KH, MacEwen CJ, Giles T, Low, J, McGhee CNJ. The Dundee University Scottish Keratoconus study: demographics, corneal signs, associated diseases, and eye rubbing. *Eye (Lond).* 2008;22(4):534–541.

CLINICAL PRESENTATION Although KC is typically bilateral, asymmetry is commonly observed. Apical thinning with protrusion or anterior bowing of the inferior paracentral or midperipheral cornea worsens with progression, as does the degree of irregular astigmatism. Generally, keratitis or corneal neovascularization is not observed; however, they may occur due to contact lens wear.

Common signs of KC include

- *scissoring of the light reflex on retinoscopy:* an early but nonspecific sign of KC; commonly associated with irregular astigmatism (Video 9-1)
- *Munson sign:* a late-stage nonspecific sign involving inferior deviation of the lower eyelid contour on downgaze (Fig 9-3)
- *Rizzuti sign:* focusing of the light within the nasal limbus when a penlight is shone from the temporal side; an early but nonspecific sign
- *Fleischer ring, partial or complete:* a brown-colored ring found at the base of the cone formed by the deposition of iron within the basal epithelium, which becomes narrower and increasingly well-defined with disease progression (Fig 9-4). It is best seen with the slit lamp using a broad, oblique beam or diffuse illumination with the cobalt blue filter.
- *Vogt striae:* fine, parallel lines observed in the posterior stroma at the apex of the cone, which may disappear with the application of external pressure (Fig 9-5)
- *apical scarring:* types commonly seen include
  - reticular scarring related to breaks in Bowman layer (Fig 9-6)
  - nummular scarring at cone apex related to contact lens wear
  - deep stromal scarring related to prior corneal hydrops

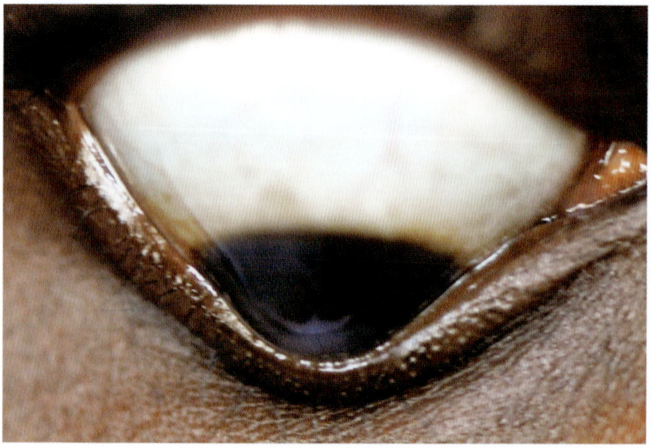

Figure 9-3 Clinical photo of Munson sign. Note the angulation of the lower eyelid with the eye in downgaze. *(Courtesy of Woodford S. Van Meter, MD.)*

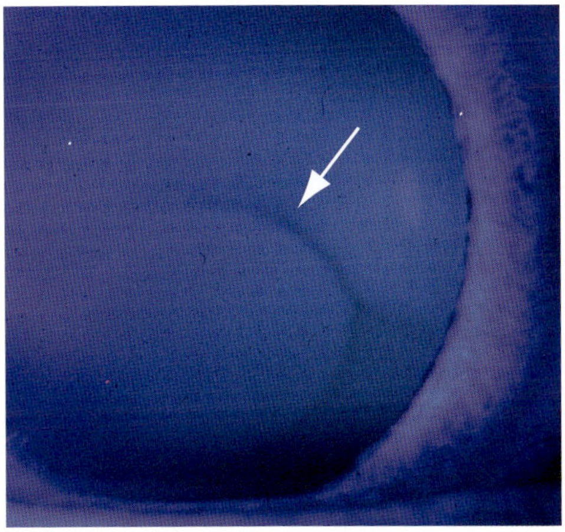

Figure 9-4 Fleischer ring *(arrow)*, iron deposited at the base of the cone, is best seen with cobalt blue light. *(Courtesy of Robert S. Feder, MD.)*

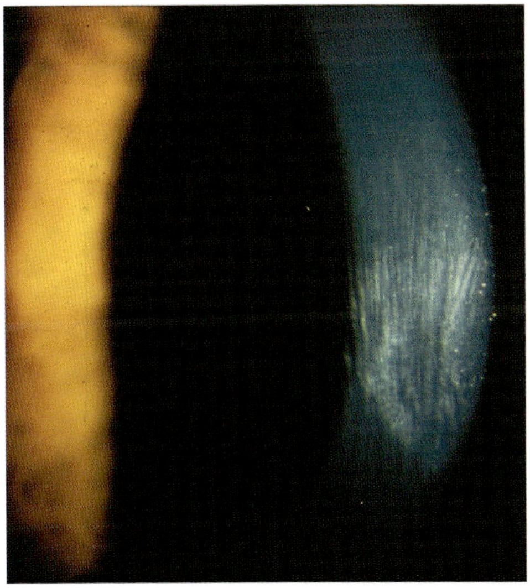

Figure 9-5 Broad oblique slit beam shows Vogt striae, fine folds in the posterior stroma at the cone apex; they become less apparent with the application of external pressure. *(Courtesy of Robert S. Feder, MD.)*

VIDEO 9-1 Scissoring seen with retinoscopy.
Original animation developed by Thomas F. Mauger, MD; retinoscopy scissoring by Robert S. Feder, MD.

Acute hydrops is a sudden onset of corneal edema that results from a tear in Descemet membrane (Fig 9-7) and is usually observed late in the disease course. Risk factors include allergy and eye rubbing. Acute hydrops is commonly observed in patients with Down syndrome. Spontaneous perforation in KC is rare.

Video 9-2 demonstrates how intensely KC patients rub their eyes. It is important to caution these patients against eye rubbing because it contributes to disease progression and increases the risk of hydrops in advanced cases. Corneal edema typically clears within 3 months but can lead to posterior stromal scarring. Occasionally, stromal clefts can be seen in association with hydrops; these clefts usually close but may result in corneal neovascularization.

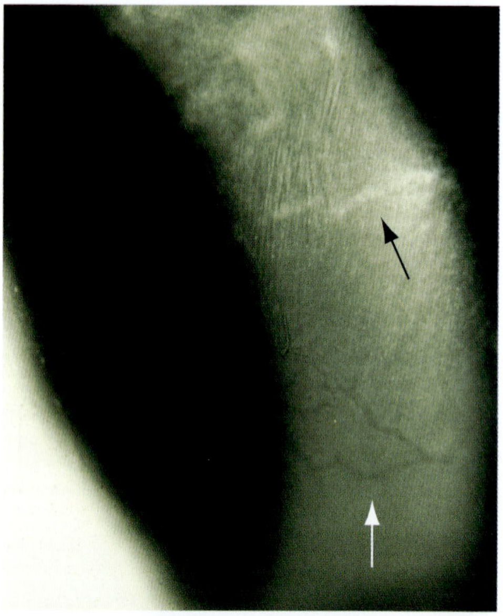

Figure 9-6 Broad, oblique slit-lamp image (high magnification) shows the mechanism of superficial reticular scarring in keratoconus. The *white arrow* indicates breaks in Bowman layer. The *black arrow* indicates where collagen has presumably filled in a previous break. Vogt striae can also be observed. *(Reprinted from Krachmer JH, Feder RS, Belin MW. Keratoconus and related noninflammatory corneal thinning disorders.* Surv Ophthalmol. *1984;28(4):293–322. Copyright 1984, with permission from Elsevier.)*

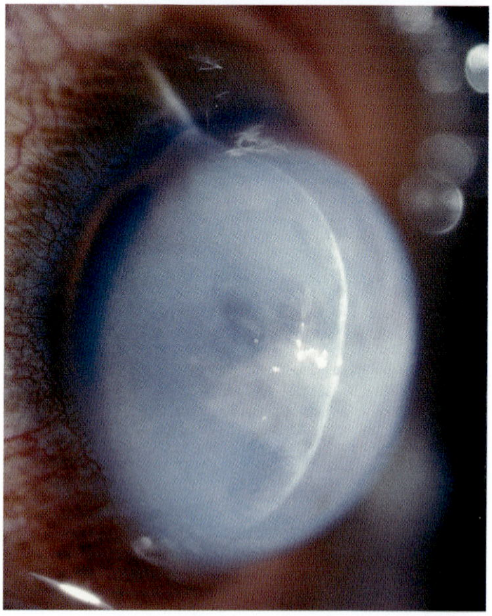

Figure 9-7 Clinical photo of acute hydrops. Corneal edema in keratoconus due to sudden rupture of Descemet membrane. *(Courtesy of Robert S. Feder, MD.)*

VIDEO 9-2 Vigorous eye rubbing in KC.
Courtesy of David D. Verdier, MD.

EVALUATION Although keratometry can be used to detect both irregular astigmatism and inferior steepening with upgaze, clinicians depend on more sophisticated techniques to evaluate corneal contour. Corneal topography and tomography have become indispensable for early diagnosis of KC, tracking its progression, fitting contact lenses, and managing the postoperative patient.

Topographic findings, obtained through Placido-based imaging (reflection of concentric rings), slit-scanning, or Scheimpflug-based devices (see Chapter 2), include

- increased overall steepening (>47.20 diopters [D])
- inferior steepening, especially when coincident with abnormal elevation and/or abnormal inferior thinning (Fig 9-8)
- superior flattening (see Fig 9-8)
- increase in inferior-superior (I-S) ratio (I/S >1.2 is considered significant)
- skewing of the radial axes (SRAX) >21° is considered suggestive of KC, while an orthogonal bow tie is typical of regular astigmatism (Fig 9-9)

Bow-tie asymmetry without skewing might be attributed to a decentered apex and thus, is not pathognomonic of KC. The bow tie pattern is ultimately lost as the disease progresses (see Fig 9-8). It is best not to rely solely on the power map when evaluating corneal contour (Fig 9-10).

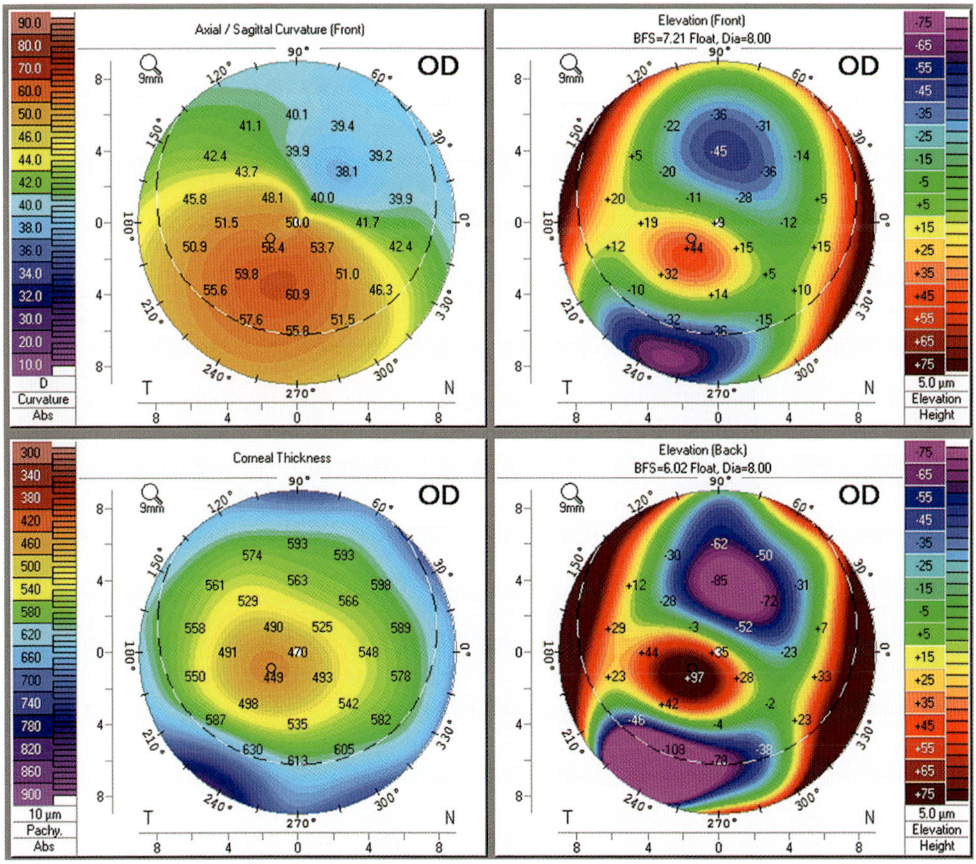

Figure 9-8 Scheimpflug-based corneal contour map. *Upper left:* Power map with inferior steepening and superior flattening. *Upper right:* An isolated island of anterior elevation above a best-fit sphere coincident with the maximum steepness. *Lower right:* An isolated island of posterior elevation. *Lower left:* Marked thinning in an area coincident with maximum steepening and elevation. *(Courtesy of Robert S. Feder, MD.)*

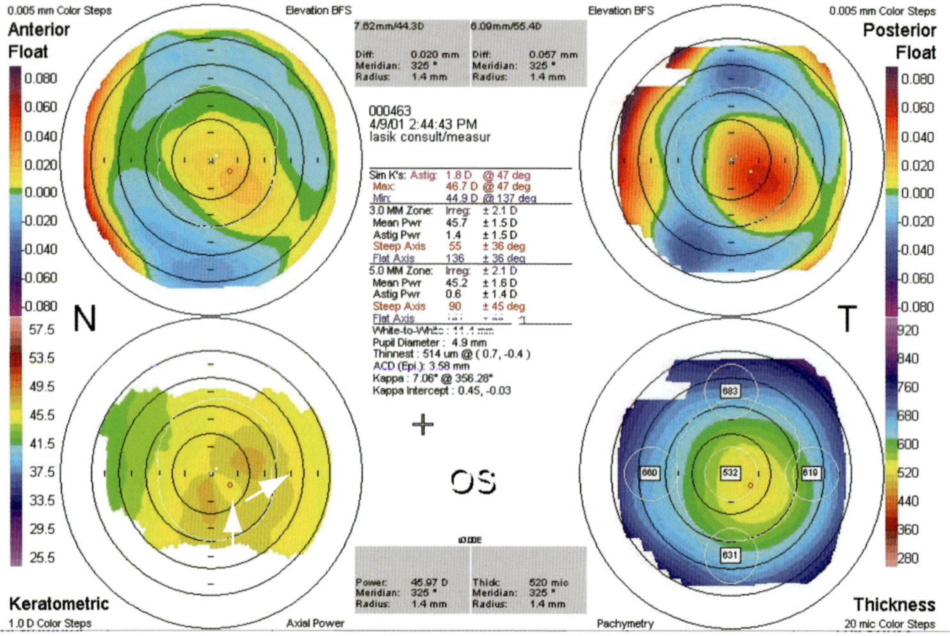

Figure 9-9 Slit-scanning images of early-stage keratoconus show skewing of the radial axes *(arrows)* in the power map *(lower left)*. Significant elevation above a best-fit sphere noted anteriorly *(upper left)* and posteriorly *(upper right)*. Decentration of the pachymetry map is shown *(lower right)*. This asymptomatic patient presented for laser in situ keratomileusis (LASIK) consultation. *(Courtesy of Robert S. Feder, MD.)*

Tomographic findings, obtained with slit-scanning devices, Scheimpflug imaging, or anterior segment optical coherence tomography (OCT; see Chapter 2), include

- isolated islands of elevation anteriorly and/or posteriorly: the elevation is relative to a computer-generated best fit sphere placed behind the anterior or posterior surface (see Figs 9-8, 9-9)
- asymptomatic posterior elevation: an early sign of subclinical KC (see Fig 9-10)
- abnormal thinning (<500 μm): typical in ectasia, especially if coincident with islands of elevation (see Fig 9-8)
- I-S difference of >30 μm in thickness at the 5 mm ring around the fixation
- difference of >30 μm between the 2 eyes in the thinnest pachymetric reading
- decentration of the thinnest part of the cornea on a pachymetry map (see Fig 9-8); normally, the thinnest cornea is centrally located
- enhanced ectasia risk, detected by comparing the difference between standard anterior and posterior elevation maps and maps in which the best-fit sphere is determined, excluding a 4-mm area around the thinnest cornea
- change in corneal thickness, evaluated from the area of minimum pachymetry to the limbus (occurs more dramatically in eyes with KC compared with eyes without)

Anterior segment OCT is used to map corneal epithelial thickness for early diagnosis and follow-up of KC. The normal corneal epithelium is thicker centrally and thinner

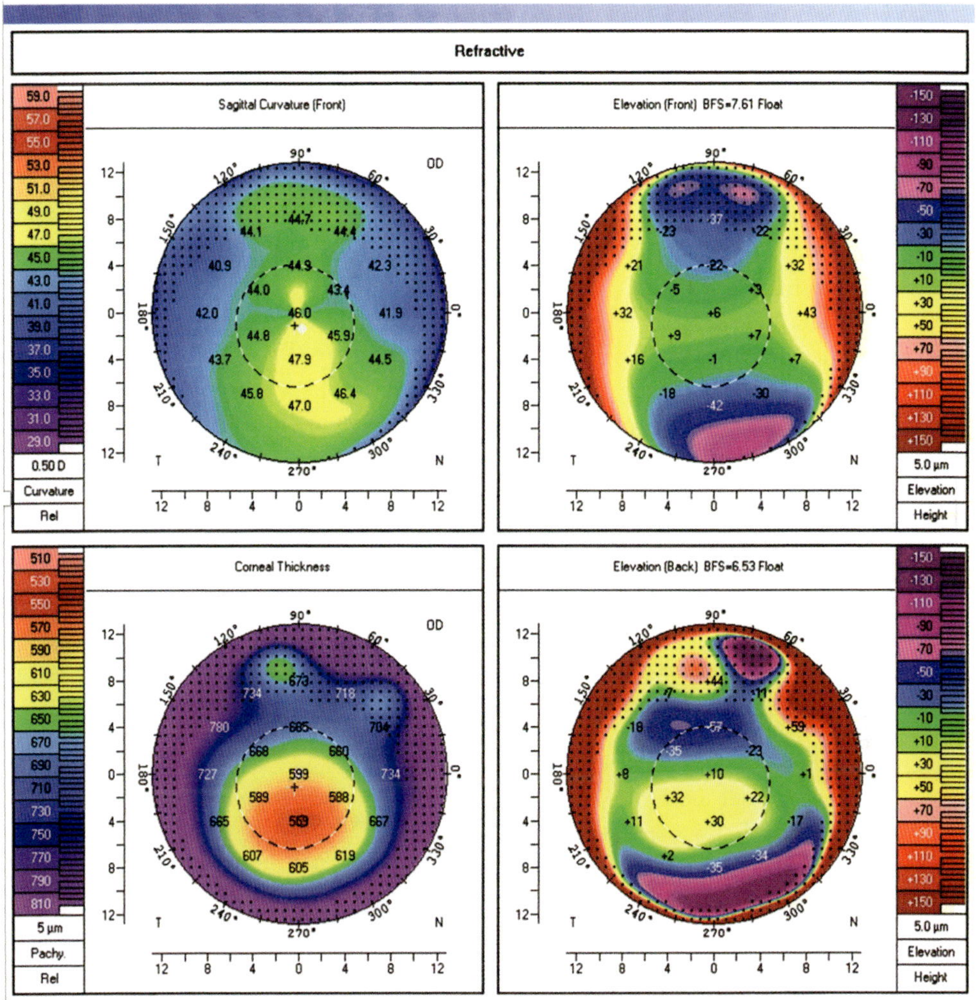

Figure 9-10 Scheimpflug-based images. *Upper left:* An asymmetric dumbbell with inferior steepening, but no skewing. *Lower left:* A decentered pachymetric map indicating normal corneal thickness. *Upper right:* Astigmatism without abnormal elevation. *Lower right:* Abnormal posterior elevation coincident with the point of maximal thinning. This analysis is suggestive of early ectasia rather than a decentered apex. *(Courtesy of Robert S. Feder, MD.)*

superiorly, while the keratoconic cornea is thinner at the apex of the cone, typically inferotemporally, and thicker superonasally. These findings correlate well with ectatic changes observed using other corneal tomography devices. In contact lens–induced warpage, an increase in the epithelial thickness of the central cornea is observed.

Wavefront aberrometry can detect the presence of corneal ectasia. Coma is the predominant form of higher-order aberration observed in KC. Other abnormal higher-order aberrations, such as trefoil and spherical aberrations, can also be detected. All these aberrations are more common in KC than in normal corneas.

Serial imaging is necessary to determine whether ectatic changes are stable or progressive or if subclinical or suspected KC has progressed and is likely to become symptomatic. These images can be used for *KC staging*. One of the staging methods is the Belin ABCD keratoconus grading system with progression display unique to Pentacam (Oculus). Other Scheimpflug systems can also be used for staging and progression analysis. The ABCD system uses the degree of anterior and posterior curvature around the thinnest part of the cornea along with pachymetry and best visual acuity. Once recorded, these values can be tracked over time. Older staging methods are less helpful since they predated modern corneal imaging technology.

Corneal ectasia can occur following ablative keratorefractive surgery such as laser in situ keratomileusis (LASIK) or photorefractive keratectomy (PRK). Risk factors include young age, high preoperative myopia, thin residual stromal bed, thin preoperative cornea, and abnormal preoperative contour (see Fig 9-9). A young patient with an unusual corneal contour who is considering refractive surgery should be observed over time to determine the possibility of progression toward KC.

Belin MW, Duncan JK. Keratoconus: The ABCD Grading System. *Klin Monatsbl Augenheilkd.* 2016; 233(06):701–707.

Feder RS. Corneal topography. In: Feder RS, ed. *The LASIK Handbook: A Case-based Approach.* 2nd ed. Wolters Kluwer; 2013:32–39.

Gomes JA, Tan D, Rapuano CJ, et al; Group of Panelists for the Global Delphi Panel of Keratoconus and Ectatic Diseases. Global consensus on keratoconus and ectatic diseases. *Cornea.* 2015;34(4):359–369.

Kanellopoulos AJ, Asimellis G. OCT corneal epithelial topographic asymmetry as a sensitive diagnostic tool for early and advancing keratoconus. *Clin Ophthalmol.* 2014;8:2277–2287.

Perez-Straziota CE, Schallhorn JM. *OCT epithelial mapping for refractive screening* [2017 American Academy of Ophthalmology Annual Meeting Video]. American Academy of Ophthalmology; 2017. www.aao.org

Weisenthal R. Optical coherence tomography. In: Feder RS, ed. *The LASIK Handbook: A Case-based Approach.* 2nd ed. Wolters Kluwer; 2013:40–46.

Yeu E, Belin MW, Khachikian SS. Topographic analysis in keratorefractive surgery. In: Mannis MJ, Holland EJ, eds. *Cornea.* Vol 1. 4th ed. Elsevier; 2017:1728–1735.

PATHOLOGY Histopathologic examination reveals the following characteristics of KC:

- iron deposition in the basal epithelium at the base of the cone
- fragmentation or breaks in Bowman layer with fibrous growth
- thinning of the corneal stroma and overlying epithelium
- folds or breaks in Descemet membrane
- variable amounts of apical scarring

MANAGEMENT Some cases of mild KC can be successfully managed with glasses. It is important to counsel patients regarding the risk of disease progression with continued eye rubbing, which in turn, can be reduced with optimal management of atopic diseases. As mentioned, KC progresses rapidly in young patients (in their teens and twenties), and thus, they should be examined more frequently. The disease is more likely to be stable in patients over age 40, but progression can still occur. Contact lenses can mask the associated irregular corneal astigmatism (Fig 9-11), and most affected patients report a dramatic improvement in vision with use. As the disease progresses, scarring and contour distortion can reduce the contact lens–corrected vision and make it more difficult to achieve a stable fit. Contact lens wear does not prevent KC progression. Although most patients will require rigid gas-permeable (RGP) lenses, some patients, particularly those with mild disease, may achieve improved vision and comfortable wear with soft lenses.

Contact lens options include

- soft toric lens
- RGP hard lens
- bicurved hard lens
- hybrid lens (hard center and soft skirt)
- piggyback system (hard lens on top of a soft lens)

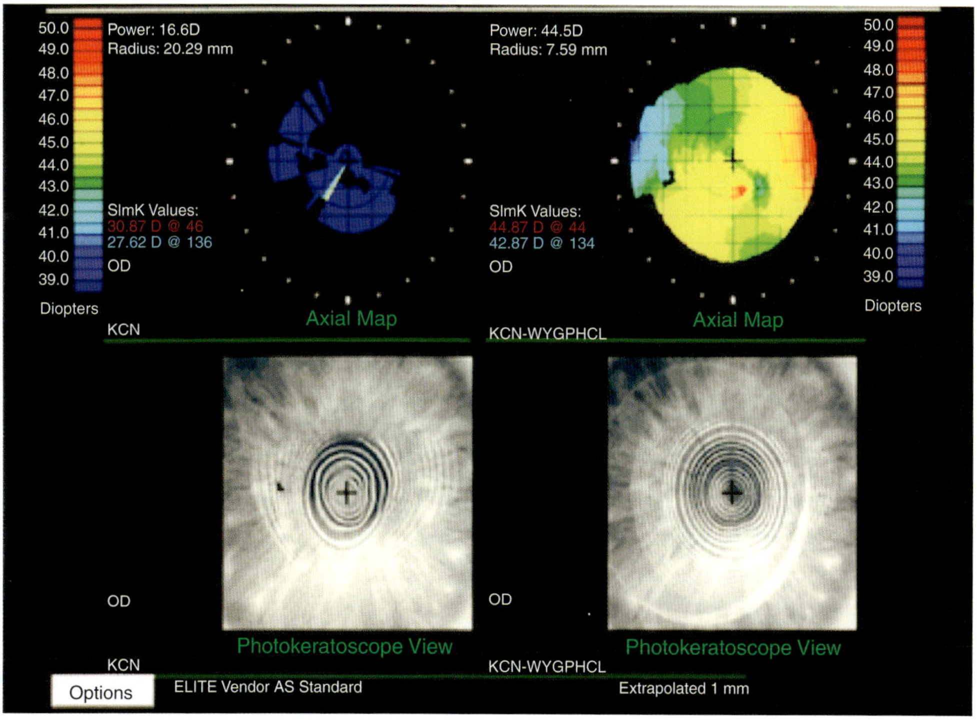

Figure 9-11 The effects of hard contact lenses on the keratoconus power map; without the lens *(left side)* and with the lens *(right side)*. *Upper left:* The power map shows flattening due to apical scarring. *Lower left:* The corresponding videokeratoscopic image is irregular with widely spaced rings centrally and narrowly spaced rings in the paracentral area. *Upper right:* The power map is much more regular when acquired from a patient wearing contact lenses. *Lower right:* The videokeratoscopic image is relatively normal, with rings more appropriately spaced. *(Reproduced with permission from Feder RS, Neems LC. Noninflammatory ectatic disorders. In: Mannis MJ, Holland EJ, eds.* Cornea. *Vol 1. 4th ed. Elsevier; 2017:820–843.)*

- mini-scleral lens with high oxygen permeability
- scleral lens with high oxygen permeability; this lens is becoming increasingly popular for patients unable to wear the standard RGP lens
- custom lathed scleral lens with high oxygen permeability

Surgical treatment for apical subepithelial scarring, a common cause of contact lens intolerance, includes mechanical debridement and phototherapeutic keratectomy. Treatment can improve patient comfort, but scarring may recur. Intrastromal corneal ring segments can be implanted to center the cone and facilitate successful contact lens wear. The procedure may not prevent disease progression, however, and is not intended to reduce dependence on glasses or contact lenses. Corneal crosslinking is used in patients who demonstrate progressive disease or are at a significant risk of progression, particularly adolescents. Older patients may benefit as well if they show signs of progression. Corneal crosslinking is most effective in mild to moderate cases and may not work as well in cases of post-LASIK ectasia or patients with advanced KC. It may be performed in combination with intrastromal ring insertion. For a more detailed discussion of intrastromal ring segments and corneal crosslinking, see the appendices at the end of this chapter.

Keratoplasty becomes an important option under the following circumstances:

- poor vision even with a comfortable stable fitting contact lens (usually due to scarring)
- contact lens intolerance despite the good vision achieved with the lens
- unstable contact lens fit (even with good vision and lens tolerance)
- progressive thinning toward the corneal periphery approaching the limbus, which requires a very large graft (associated with increased risk of rejection)
- corneal hydrops that fails to clear after several months

Penetrating keratoplasty (PK) is currently the preferred cornea transplant procedure for the treatment of KC in the United States and is associated with an excellent prognosis. Alternatively, many surgeons prefer deep anterior lamellar keratoplasty (DALK) for KC. This is particularly true in places where high-quality donor tissue is not readily available. Although technically more challenging, there are several advantages of DALK over PK. At 6 months post–DALK, the endothelial cell counts are significantly higher compared with PK. Although endothelial rejection does not occur with DALK, stromal rejection is still possible. Stromal scarring can result in reduced vision and symptoms of glare. In the event of trauma, postoperative wound integrity is better with DALK than with PK. (See Chapter 16 for further discussion of PK and DALK.)

Corneal hydrops is treated conservatively with topical hypertonic agents and/or a soft contact lens for several months. A cycloplegic agent and topical steroid may provide short-term relief by reducing inflammation and pain. Aqueous suppressants may decrease the flow of fluid into the cornea. Intracameral injection of air or a nonexpansile concentration of gas (SF_6 or C_3F_8) may help accelerate the resolution of hydrops. Pupil dilation and/or inferior peripheral iridectomy may reduce the risk of pupillary block after intracameral gas injection. Hydrops is not an indication for emergent keratoplasty.

AAO PPP Cornea/External Disease Committee, Hoskins Center for Quality Eye Care. Preferred Practice Pattern Guidelines. *Corneal Ectasia.* American Academy of Ophthalmology; 2018. www.aao.org/ppp

Feder RS, Neems LC. Noninflammatory ectatic disorders. In: Mannis MJ, Holland EJ, eds. *Cornea.* Vol 1. 4th ed. Elsevier; 2017:820–843.

Kiliç A, Colin J. Advances in the surgical treatment of keratoconus. *Focal Points: Clinical Modules for Ophthalmologists.* American Academy of Ophthalmology; 2012, module 2.

Panda A, Aggarwal A, Madhavi P, et al. Management of acute corneal hydrops secondary to keratoconus with intracameral injection of sulfur hexafluoride (SF6). *Cornea.* 2007;26(9):1067–1069.

Raiskup-Wolf F, Hoyer A, Spoerl E, Pillunat L. Collagen crosslinking with riboflavin and ultraviolet-A light in keratoconus: long-term results. *J Cataract Refract Surg.* 2008;34(5):796–801.

Pellucid Marginal Degeneration

Pellucid marginal degeneration (PMD) is an uncommon, usually nonhereditary, and bilateral corneal disorder with an unknown etiology. It is associated with peripheral corneal thinning without inflammation. PMD and KC can occur in more than 1 individual in a family. In rare instances, both diseases may be present in the same eye. PMD may be part of an ectasia continuum that includes KC (Case Study 9-1).

CASE STUDY 9-1 Corneal ectasia.
Courtesy of Robert S. Feder, MD.

CLINICAL PRESENTATION PMD is diagnosed in patients aged 20 to 40 years and affects men and women equally. The high, irregular astigmatism, characteristic of PMD, causes decreased vision. Typically, a 1–2-mm wide band of inferior corneal thinning (Fig 9-12), which occurs 1–2 mm from the limbus and extends up to 4 clock-hours (usually 4–8 o'clock), is observed. In rare cases, PMD may occur in the superior cornea. Corneal protrusion occurs at the central edge of the thinned area (Fig 9-13), resulting in a contour resembling a "beer belly." In contrast, the keratoconic cornea protrudes at the point of maximal thinning, which is typically just below the center (see Fig 9-2). At times, a clear distinction between PMD and KC is not possible. PMD is not associated with vascularization or lipid deposition, but posterior stromal scarring has been noted in the thinned area. These observations help differentiate PMD from other peripheral thinning disorders (Table 9-2). Studies have reported the occurrence of acute corneal hydrops as well as rare, spontaneous corneal perforation. Although the "crab claw" pattern is characteristic of the topographic map of PMD (Fig 9-14), a similar configuration can be found in inferior KC as well. Clinical correlation and review of elevation and pachymetric maps provide more accurate differentiation between these 2 disorders.

PATHOLOGY Pathologic examination reveals the following characteristics of PMD:

- normal-appearing epithelium, Descemet membrane, and endothelium
- stromal thinning with focal disruption of Bowman layer
- absence of lipid deposits, typical of Terrien marginal degeneration

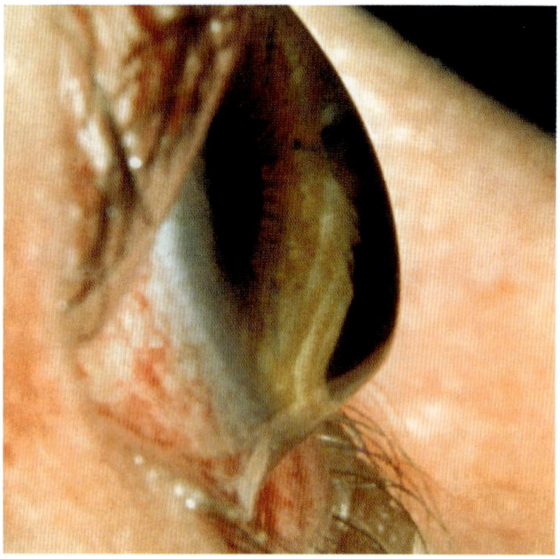

Figure 9-12 Clinical photo of pellucid marginal degeneration, which is characterized by inferior corneal protrusion above the band of thinning, which occurs 1–2 mm from the limbus and extends up to 4 clock-hours. *(Courtesy of Vincent P. deLuise, MD.)*

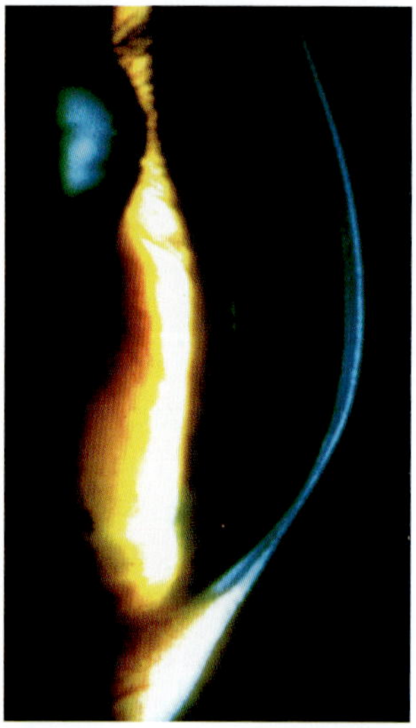

Figure 9-13 Slit view demonstrates corneal protrusion above a band of stromal thinning in pellucid marginal degeneration. *(Reprinted from Krachmer JH, Feder RS, Belin MW. Keratoconus and related noninflammatory corneal thinning disorders.* Surv Ophthalmol. *1984;28(4):293–322. Copyright 1984, with permission from Elsevier.)*

MANAGEMENT Early-stage PMD is treated with contact lenses, although the fit is more difficult to achieve in PMD than in KC. Although hybrid lenses are occasionally prescribed, scleral lenses are more commonly used in the treatment of PMD. Eventually, PK or DALK may be required to restore vision. Due to the location of the thinning, the grafts tend to be large and close to the limbus, making surgery technically more difficult and the graft more prone to rejection. Wedge resection and lamellar grafts are advocated as alternative or adjunctive procedures. Corneal crosslinking may also be considered for some of these patients.

AAO PPP Cornea/External Disease Committee, Hoskins Center for Quality Eye Care. Preferred Practice Pattern Guidelines. *Corneal Ectasia.* American Academy of Ophthalmology; 2018. www.aao.org/ppp

Table 9-2 Comparison of Pellucid Marginal Degeneration With Other Peripheral Corneal Thinning Disorders

	PMD	Terrien Marginal Degeneration[a]	Mooren Ulcer[b]	Furrow Degeneration[a]
Symptom	Blurred vision due to astigmatism; noninflammatory	Blurred vision due to astigmatism Typically noninflammatory, but a subset is associated with inflammation	Pain, redness, and blurred vision due to inflammation early; scarring late	None
Associated systemic disease	Typically none	None	May be associated with hepatitis C or Helminthic disease; unlike more typical PUK, which is often associated with systemic disease[c]	None
Age	20–40 years	Typically older than 40 years	Young individuals: more severe form; older individuals: milder form	Older adults
Sex	No predilection	Male predominance	No predilection	No predilection
Laterality	Bilateral with asymmetry possible	Often bilateral	Bilateral in younger individuals Unilateral in older individuals	Bilateral
Epithelial defects	None	Usually none	Typical	None
Location of thinning	Usually inferior	Usually superior; can be inferior	Typical onset is nasal or temporal, progresses circumferentially and then centrally with undermining of central edge	Circumlimbal thinning within the arcus
Vessels	None	Cross the area of thinning	Stop at the peripheral edge of defect	Not typical
Lipid	None	Lipid deposits at the central edge	None	None except the arcus
Arcus	None	None	None	Always

PUK = peripheral ulcerative keratitis.

[a] See Chapter 7.

[b] See Chapter 13.

[c] See Table 13-5.

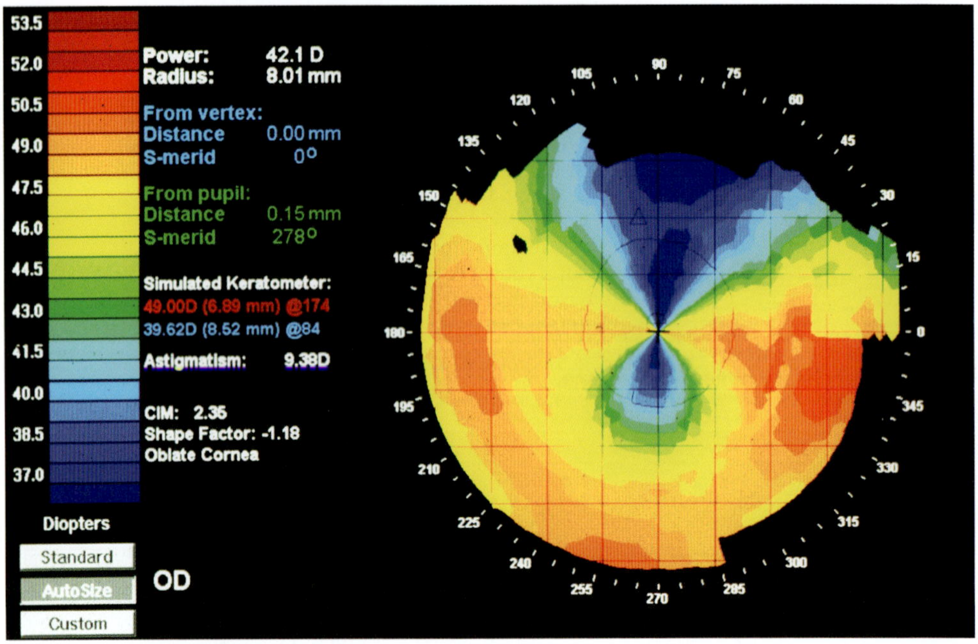

Figure 9-14 Power map shows the typical "crab claw" pattern seen in pellucid marginal degeneration, which is also observed in keratoconus with an inferiorly located apex. *(Courtesy of Robert S. Feder, MD.)*

Belin MW, Asota IM, Ambrosio R Jr, Khachikian SS. What's in a name: keratoconus, pellucid marginal degeneration, and related thinning disorders. *Am J Ophthalmol.* 2011;152(2):157–162.

Feder RS, Neems LC. Noninflammatory ectatic disorders. In: Mannis MJ, Holland EJ, eds. *Cornea.* Vol 1. 4th ed. Elsevier; 2017:820–843.

Keratoglobus

Keratoglobus is a rare, bilateral, noninflammatory condition that is typically present at birth, unlike keratoconus and PMD. It is usually not inherited. See Chapter 6.

CLINICAL PRESENTATION The corneas have a globular shape with a deep anterior chamber and a slightly increased diameter (Fig 9-15). Keratoglobus can be confused with other conditions in the differential diagnosis (Table 9-3). Patients generally present with diffuse corneal steepening and diffuse thinning worse in the periphery. This is in contrast to KC, which presents with inferior paracentral thinning at the cone apex (Fig 9-16; also see Fig 9-2). Spontaneous rupture of Descemet membrane with corneal hydrops can occur, but iron lines, stress lines, and anterior scarring are not typically observed. Prominent folds and areas of thickening in Descemet membrane are common. Unlike KC, keratoglobus is not associated with atopy or hard contact lens wear. Keratoglobus is strongly associated with blue sclerae and Ehlers-Danlos syndrome type VI (see Chapter 10).

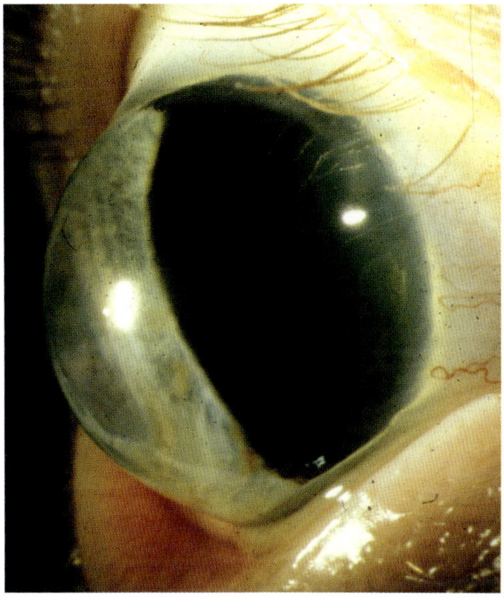

Figure 9-15 Clinical photo of keratoglobus, which is associated with a globular cornea and marked peripheral thinning. *(Courtesy of Robert S. Feder, MD.)*

Table 9-3 Comparison of Keratoglobus to Other Conditions in the Differential Diagnosis

	Keratoglobus	Anterior Megalocornea[a]	Congenital Glaucoma[a]
Thinning	Marked, greatest in the periphery	Normal thickness	Normal to increased thickness
Steepening	Marked; diffuse	Normal contour	Normal contour
Edema	None unless hydrops	None	Usually none
Haab striae	None	None	Common
Increased axial length	May be present	Usually not	Common
Increased IOP	No	No	Possible
Optic nerve head cupping	None	None	Common

IOP = intraocular pressure.

[a] See Chapter 6.

PATHOLOGY Keratoglobus may represent a defect in collagen synthesis. Histopathologic examination reveals the following characteristics:

- absent or fragmented Bowman layer
- thinned stroma with normal lamellar organization
- thin Descemet membrane

MANAGEMENT Contact lenses, especially scleral lenses, may be beneficial. The prognosis for PK is much poorer in keratoglobus than in the other corneal ectasias. Lamellar keratoplasty, followed by PK, could be considered in cases requiring intervention to maintain functional vision. Due to the possibility of spontaneous corneal rupture, patients must

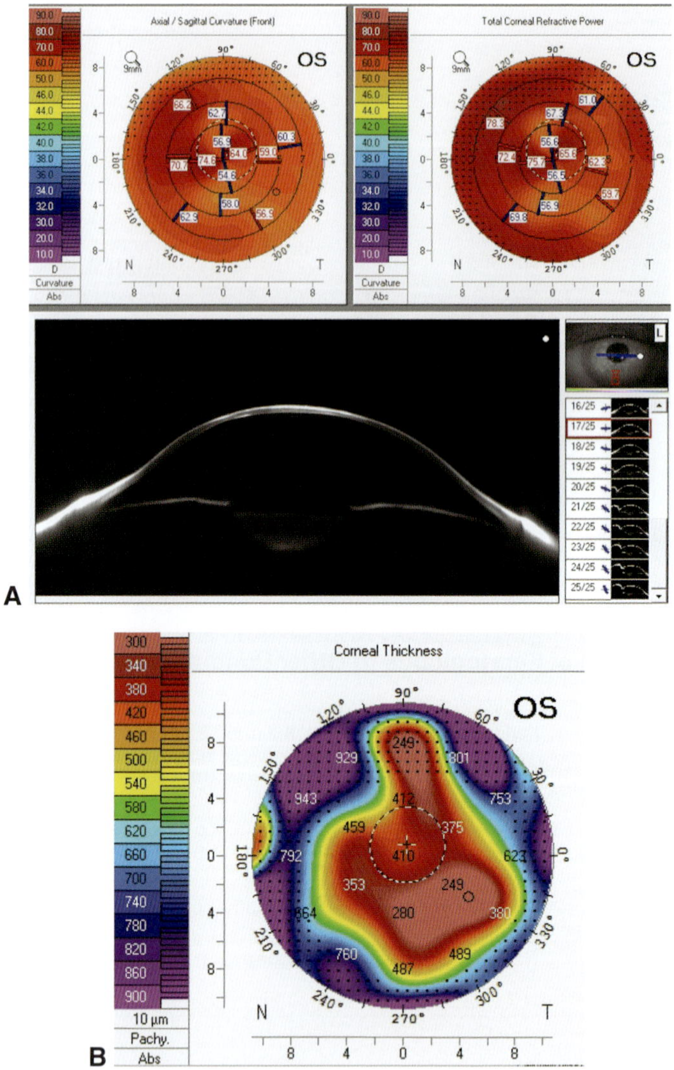

Figure 9-16 Keratoglobus. **A,** Scheimpflug-based power maps demonstrate marked diffuse corneal steepening *(above);* marked thinning and protrusion are seen in the Scheimpflug image *(below).* **B,** Thickness map shows marked thinning in a wide area. The dots indicate areas of poor reliability. *(Courtesy of Robert S. Feder, MD.)*

be counseled regarding the importance of protective eyewear. In children, high myopia is treated with spectacles to prevent amblyopia.

AAO PPP Cornea/External Disease Committee, Hoskins Center for Quality Eye Care. Preferred Practice Pattern Guidelines. *Corneal Ectasia.* American Academy of Ophthalmology; 2018. www.aao.org/ppp

Feder RS, Neems LC. Noninflammatory ectatic disorders. In: Mannis MJ, Holland EJ, eds. *Cornea.* Vol 1. 4th ed. Elsevier; 2017:820–843.

Appendix 9.1

Intrastromal Corneal Ring Segments for Treatment of Ectasia

Background

Intrastromal corneal ring segments (ICRSs) are circular arcs, made of polymethyl methacrylate (PMMA), which are surgically implanted in the posterior midperipheral corneal stroma (Figs 9-A1, 9-A2) through a lamellar channel to treat mild to moderate KC associated with contact lens intolerance. The thicker the segment and the closer the placement to the visual axis, the greater the effect. They can also treat low myopia. ICRSs are not indicated for the treatment of subclinical ectatic disease. Although unapproved, they are occasionally used to treat PMD. Implantation may result in a significant reduction in disease progression but does not cure the disease. Improved vision results from reduced astigmatism, flattened central cornea, and improved contact lens wear. Some of the ICRS options, including Ferrara rings (Ferrara Ophthalmics) or Kerarings (Mediphacos), have a smaller optical zone and a greater flattening effect than Intacs (Oasis Medical). Adverse effects resulting from ICRS implantation can be stopped and potentially reversed by removing the ring segments. If keratoplasty is planned, the ring segments should be removed approximately 1 month before the procedure. This appendix focuses on the US Food and Drug Administration (FDA)-approved Intacs. Ferrara rings and Kerarings are widely used outside the United States.

Indications and contraindications The labeled indications for Intacs in KC are

- progressive deterioration in vision, indicating gradual loss of functional vision, which cannot be corrected through contact lenses or glasses
- age 21 years or older
- clear central corneas

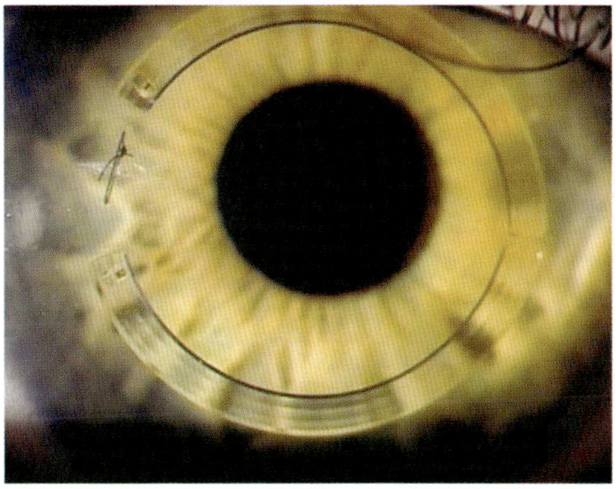

Figure 9-A1 Diffuse slit-lamp image shows two intrastromal ring segments. The nylon suture on the *left* indicates the radial incision. *(Courtesy of Colin J, Velou S. Current surgical options for keratoconus.* J Cataract Refract Surg. *2003;29(2):384.)*

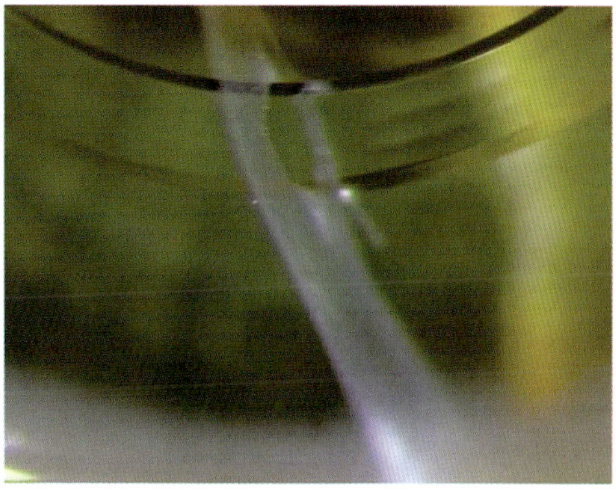

Figure 9-A2 Slit view of the ring segment at 70% depth (recommended). *(Courtesy of Colin J, Velou S. Current surgical options for keratoconus.* J Cataract Refract Surg. *2003;29(2):384.)*

- corneal thickness ≥450 μm at the proposed incision site
- lack of options other than corneal transplantation for improving functional vision

Although these are FDA labeling parameters, many surgeons perform Intacs insertion as exceptions to these criteria. Intacs are typically not recommended for patients

- who expect to be free from wearing glasses and contact lens postoperatively
- with mean keratometry readings >58.00 D
- with central corneal scarring
- who have corneal thickness <450 μm at the proposed incision site
- with collagen vascular, autoimmune, or immunodeficiency diseases
- who may be predisposed to future complications due to ocular conditions, such as herpetic keratitis, recurrent corneal erosion syndrome, or corneal dystrophy
- who are taking isotretinoin

Instrumentation

The Intacs segments have a 150° arc with a fixed inner diameter (6.8 mm) and outer diameter (8.1 mm) and have variable thicknesses, ranging from 0.25 to 0.45 mm in 0.05 mm increments. The degree of correction achieved is directly proportional to the thickness of the ring segments. A diamond knife is used to make a radial incision superiorly. Then, manually operated surgical equipment, including a suction ring and custom-designed lamellar dissector and suction ring, is used to create the channels. Alternatively, a femtosecond laser can be used to create both the radial incision and the corneal channels. Scheimpflug or OCT-generated pachymetry maps are used to measure thickness along the entire course of the channel dissection to reduce the risk of intraoperative perforation.

Technique

The procedure involves creating a lamellar channel at approximately 60%–70% stromal depth, followed by the insertion of the ring segments. The geometric center of the cornea is marked with a blunt hook. Next, the corneal thickness at the entry incision is measured using an ultrasonic pachymeter. A diamond knife, set to 60%–70% of the stromal thickness, is then used to create a 1.0 mm radial incision. Then, the custom-designed suction ring and lamellar dissector are used to create the channels at a 7 mm optical zone by blunt separation of the collagen lamellae. Video 9-A1 demonstrates the use of a femtosecond laser to create the channels. The channels are created in an arcuate pattern at the desired inner and outer diameters (inner diameter: 6.6 mm and outer diameter: 7.4 mm). The creation of narrow channels results in a greater therapeutic effect; however, it increases the difficulty of ring segment insertion. After the channels are created, specialized forceps are used to insert the first ring segment and rotate it into position, followed by the insertion and rotation of the second segment. Tissue glue or sutures are used to close the radial incision at the corneal surface.

VIDEO 9-A1 Implantation of asymmetric corneal ring segments for the surgical management of keratoconus.
Courtesy of George O. Waring IV, MD.

Some surgeons advocate the benefits of using two 0.35 mm ring segments, some promote a thicker inferior ring (see Video 9A-1), and some prefer a single ring inserted through a standard channel oriented to the steepest part of the cornea based on topographic measurements. When a single segment is placed inferiorly, it flattens the adjacent cornea but steepens the superior cornea (Fig 9-A3). This "beanbag effect" (ie, flattening 1 area and steepening another area) may yield a more physiologic improvement than the double segment-induced global flattening effect.

When combining ICRS with corneal crosslinking, it is best to implant the ICRS first and perform crosslinking later (see Appendix 9.2). Channel creation may be more difficult after crosslinking has been performed.

Outcomes

Ring segment insertion can improve uncorrected distance visual acuity (UDVA, formerly called *uncorrected visual acuity, UCVA*) and best-corrected visual acuity (BCVA; also called *corrected distance visual acuity, CDVA*) as well as contact lens tolerance. However, most patients still require optical correction to achieve their BCVA. ICRSs provide similar visual and refractive outcomes for KC patients by using either mechanical or femtosecond methods of channel creation. Most studies suggest that ICRS is most effective in patients with moderate KC (keratometry values <58.00 D). Topographic images show a reduction

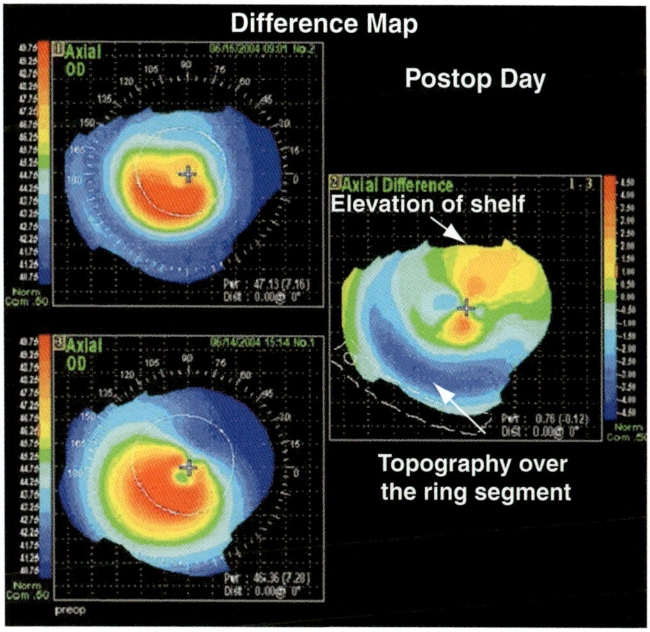

Figure 9-A3 Corneal topography analysis before and after single-segment Intacs implantation. The preoperative topography *(lower left)* shows oblique steepening, and the postoperative topography *(upper left)* shows contraction of a steep cone after the placement of single-segment Intacs outside the cone. The difference map (subtraction of preoperative and postoperative topography) *(right)* shows flattening over the ring segment *(blue)* and steepening in the overly flat area *(red)*. The apex of the cornea has moved toward the center. *(Courtesy of Brian S. Boxer Wachler, MD.)*

in inferior steepening as well as coma (spherical aberration common in KC) and the I-S ratio (see the "Evaluation" subsection under Kerataconus, earlier in this chapter).

A study evaluating the long-term stability of the cornea after Intacs insertion in 85 KC patients found that in patients with documented progression of KC, approximately 93% had no further progression (defined as <1.00 D astigmatism) between 1 and 5 years after Intacs implantation. In addition, no statistically significant differences were noted in the mean steep, flat, and average keratometry readings; manifest refraction spherical equivalent; and UDVA and BCVA ($P > .05$) between 1 and 5 years after ICRS insertion.

In limited early trials that used Intacs to treat post-LASIK ectasia, reduced myopia and improved UDVA were observed. However, the long-term effects of this approach for managing post-LASIK ectasia need further investigation. Use of Intacs for post-LASIK ectasia is an off-label treatment, and care should be taken with implantation in the presence of a lamellar interface.

Complications

Approximately 1% of the patients experience the loss of BCVA (≥2 lines of vision) after ICRS insertion, 1 year postoperatively. However, there may be issues related to the quality of vision.

Visual symptoms Approximately 14% of patients have reported the presence of severe and permanent visual symptoms probably related to large pupil diameter. These symptoms include

- difficulty with night vision (4.8%)
- blurred vision (2.9%)
- diplopia (1.6%)
- glare (1.3%)
- halos (1.3%)
- fluctuating distance vision (1.0%)
- fluctuating near vision (0.3%)
- photophobia (0.3%)

Adverse events The occurrence of adverse events (events that, if untreated, could be serious or result in permanent sequelae) has been reported in approximately 1% of patients. Reported adverse events include

- anterior chamber perforation
- anterior corneal perforation
- microbial keratitis
- implant migration or extrusion (Fig 9-A4)
- shallow ring segment placement
- corneal thinning over ring segment (Fig 9-A5)

Ocular complications At 12 months postoperatively, the occurrence of ocular complications has been reported in approximately 11% of patients (clinically significant events that do not result in permanent sequelae). These complications include

- reduced corneal sensitivity (5.5%)
- induced astigmatism between 1.00 and 2.00 D (3.7%)

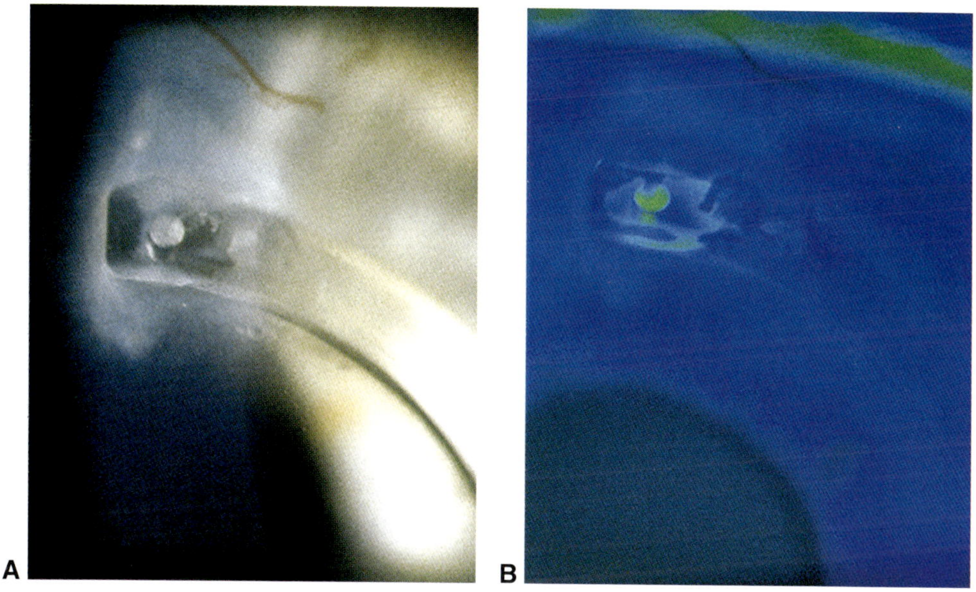

Figure 9-A4 Slit-lamp images show extrusion of a ring segment. **A,** Ring tip extrusion. **B,** Extrusion is easily seen with fluorescein dye. *(Courtesy of Brian S. Boxer Wachler, MD.)*

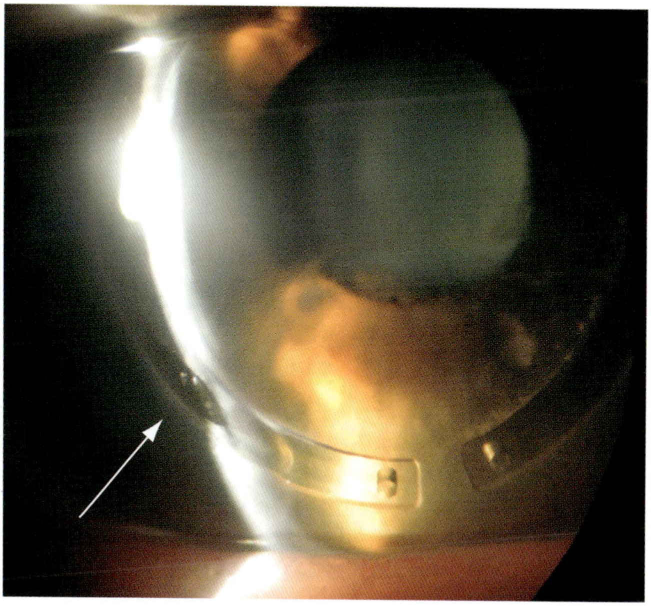

Figure 9-A5 Clinical photo shows corneal thinning over a ring segment *(arrow)* after the excessive use of a nonsteroidal anti-inflammatory drugs. *(Courtesy of Brian S. Boxer Wachler, MD.)*

- deep neovascularization at the incision site (1.2%) (can also occur over the segment; Fig 9-A6)
- persistent epithelial defect (0.2%)
- iritis/uveitis (0.2%)

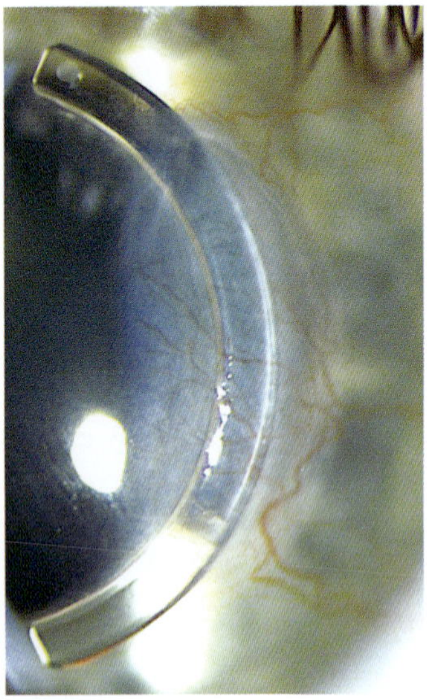

Figure 9-A6 Clinical photo shows intense vascularization over a ring segment. *(Courtesy of David D. Verdier, MD.)*

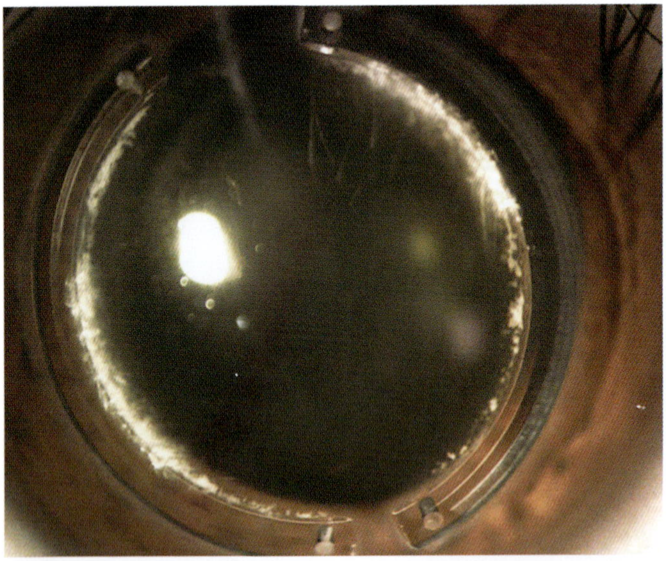

Figure 9-A7 Clinical photograph shows grade 4 deposits around the ring segments. The deposits can be graded on a scale from 0 (no deposits) to 4 (confluent deposits). These channel deposits are typically not apparent until weeks or months after surgery. Although the corneal opacities may cause cosmetic concerns, they are usually not problematic. *(Courtesy of Audrey Talley-Rostov, MD.)*

The presence of postoperative lamellar intrastromal channel deposits (Fig 9-A7) is found in up to 74% of cases. These deposits probably occur in response to corneal injury and activation of keratocytes; however, they do not appear to impact the functional outcomes of ICRS implantation.

AAO PPP Cornea/External Disease Committee, Hoskins Center for Quality Eye Care. Preferred Practice Pattern Guidelines. *Corneal Ectasia.* American Academy of Ophthalmology; 2018. www.aao.org/ppp

Alfonso JF, Lisa C, Fernández-Vega L, Madrid-Costa D, Montés-Micó R. Intrastromal corneal ring segment implantation in 219 keratoconic eyes at different stages. *Graefes Arch Clin Exp Ophthalmol.* 2011;249(11):1705–1712.

Bedi R, Touboul D, Pinsard L, Colin J. Refractive and topographic stability of Intacs in eyes with progressive keratoconus: five-year follow-up. *J Refract Surg.* 2012;28(6):392–396.

Kymionis GD, Tsiklis NS, Pallikaris AI, et al. Long-term follow-up of Intacs for post-LASIK corneal ectasia. *Ophthalmology.* 2006;113(11):1909–1917.

Rabinowitz YS. INTACS for keratoconus and ectasia after LASIK. *Int Ophthalmol Clin.* 2013; 53(1):27–39.

Sharma M, Boxer Wachler BS. Comparison of single-segment and double-segment Intacs for keratoconus and post-LASIK ectasia. *Am J Ophthalmol.* 2006;141(5):891–895.

Appendix 9.2

Corneal Crosslinking for Corneal Ectasia

Background

Corneal crosslinking (CXL) was first described by Spoerl and colleagues in 1997 as the "Dresden protocol." This crosslinking technique is commonly referred to as "epithelium-off" or "epi-off." CXL involves the saturation of the cornea with topical riboflavin (vitamin B_2) solution, followed by exposure to ultraviolet A (UVA) light to form strong chemical bonds between adjacent collagen fibrils, thereby increasing corneal rigidity. The crosslinking occurs due to the interaction between the oxygen free radicals generated by the combination of riboflavin, oxygen, and UVA light. The application of a hypotonic riboflavin solution prior to UVA treatment can be used to temporarily thicken a thinner cornea. In the presence of riboflavin, approximately 95% of the UVA light is absorbed in the anterior corneal stroma to a depth of 300 µm. A minimal stromal thickness of 400 µm after epithelial removal is recommended to avoid UVA-induced corneal endothelial damage. Safety studies, based on these thickness guidelines, have shown that CXL does not damage the endothelium.

CXL is performed to arrest or slow the progression of corneal ectasia in its earlier stages to preserve visual function. The patients will still require glasses or contact lenses; thus, surgeons need to counsel the patients and set realistic expectations regarding the surgical outcomes. CXL is the first-line treatment for mild to moderate corneal ectasia. Although crosslinking has been used globally for 2 decades, "epi-off" CXL received US FDA approval in 2016 for patients aged 14–65 years with progressive KC or postrefractive surgery ectasia. There are no well-defined criteria for disease progression, but the proposed metrics for evaluation are

- mean and/or maximum keratometry
- steepening of the anterior and posterior corneal surface
- thinnest pachymetry reading
- rate of change in thickness from the thinnest part of the cornea to the periphery
- refractive astigmatism

Anecdotal reports have suggested that CXL can be used to treat infectious keratitis that does not respond to traditional treatment; however, the benefit is questionable and further investigation is needed.

Surgical technique

The FDA-approved technique for the Dresden protocol is as follows:

- central corneal epithelium (9 mm) is removed following the technique used in PRK
- topical riboflavin (0.1% diluted in 20% dextran) is instilled every 2 minutes for 30 minutes
- the slit lamp is used to check the riboflavin fluorescence in the anterior chamber of the eye (Fig 9-A8)
- corneal thickness is checked with ultrasonic pachymetry
  - if the exposed stroma ≥400 µm, 30-minute UVA treatment (365 nm; 3 mW/cm^2 irradiation) with concomitant application of topical riboflavin every 2 minutes (Fig 9-A9)
  - if the exposed stroma <400 µm, a hypotonic riboflavin solution is applied every 15 seconds and pachymetry rechecked every 2 minutes until the measurement is ≥400 µm, followed by 30-minute UVA treatment
- a topical cycloplegic agent, an antibiotic, and a topical steroid are applied and a bandage soft contact lens is placed. Some clinicians also add a topical NSAID twice daily for 2 days to help control postoperative discomfort

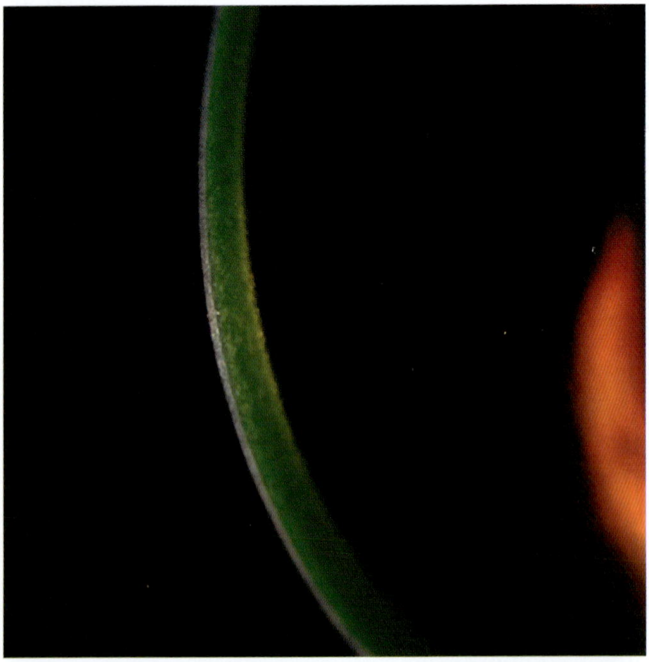

Figure 9-A8 Full-thickness, homogeneous stromal penetration of riboflavin during epithelium-on ("epi-on") corneal crosslinking (CXL). Riboflavin is not visible in the anterior chamber. Adequate riboflavin penetration is of paramount clinical importance prior to ultraviolet A (UVA) exposure. *(Courtesy of Roy S. Rubinfeld, MD, MA.)*

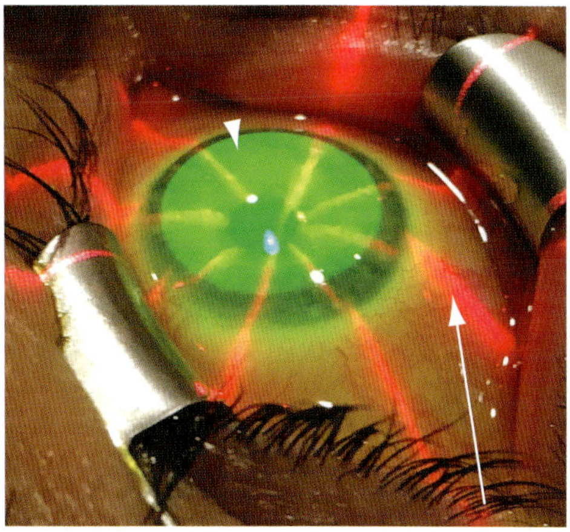

Figure 9-A9 CXL. Radial red lines *(arrow)* help the surgeon to adjust the distance between the UVA source and the eye. Green area *(arrowhead)* is the 9-mm irradiation zone. *(Courtesy of Robert S. Feder, MD.)*

Outcomes

Long-term studies have confirmed that the Dresden protocol stops the deterioration and progression of KC. The meta-analysis of 75 publications, with greater than 36-month follow-up period, showed a greater improvement in UDVA than CDVA, along with reduction in keratometric (corneal topography) values. Although a minor reduction in astigmatism was observed, there was no change in the spherical equivalent.

Another study analyzed data for 241 eyes that were treated with the "epi-off" protocol and had a minimum 6-month follow-up period. The results showed a significant reduction in corneal steepening of 2.68 D in the first year and of 4.84 D by the third year. The BCVA improved significantly by at least 1 line in 75 eyes in the first year and 19 eyes in the third year.

Several European studies have demonstrated a reduction in the number of keratoplasty surgeries for KC since the advent of CXL. However, this reduction could also be attributed to the advancements in contact lens technology.

Patients with mild to moderate KC have a better prognosis than patients with more severe disease. Young patients tend to progress more rapidly than older patients and therefore should be examined more frequently to detect progression and intervene with CXL. Patients with post-LASIK ectasia may not do as well as patients with KC, perhaps because the flap provides less biomechanical stability than an untreated cornea.

AAO PPP Cornea/External Disease Committee, Hoskins Center for Quality Eye Care. Preferred Practice Pattern Guidelines. *Corneal Ectasia.* American Academy of Ophthalmology; 2018. www.aao.org/ppp

Caporossi A, Mazzotta C, Baiocchi S, Caporossi T. Long-term results of riboflavin ultraviolet A corneal collagen cross-linking for keratoconus in Italy: the Siena eye cross study. *Am J Ophthalmol.* 2010;149(4):585–593.

Godefrooij DA, Gans R, Imhof SM, Wisse RP. Nationwide reduction in the number of corneal transplantations for keratoconus following the implementation of cross-linking. *Acta Ophthalmol.* 2016;94(7):675–678.

Hersh PS, Stulting RD, Muller D, Durrie DS, Rajpal RK, US Crosslinking Study Group. US multicenter clinical trial of corneal collagen crosslinking for treatment of corneal ectasia after refractive surgery. *Ophthalmology.* 2017;124(10):1475–1484.

Raiskup-Wolf F, Hoyer A, Spoerl E, Pillunat L. Collagen crosslinking with riboflavin and ultraviolet-A light in keratoconus: long-term results. *J Cataract Refract Surg.* 2008;34(5):796–801.

Wollensak G, Spoerl E, Seiler T. Riboflavin/ultraviolet A–induced collagen crosslinking for the treatment of keratoconus. *Am J Ophthalmol.* 2003;135(5):620–627.

Contraindications

CXL is relatively contraindicated in the following cases:

- corneal thickness <400 μm (some protocols may allow for treatment of corneas thicker than 300 μm)
- prior herpetic infection (due to possibility of viral reactivation with UV irradiation)
- severe corneal scarring or opacification
- history of poor epithelial wound healing
- severe ocular surface disease (eg, dry eye)
- autoimmune disorders

Complications

Possible complications of CXL may include

- photophobia
- delayed epithelial healing
- corneal stromal haze (which may be visually significant)
- decreased corneal sensitivity
- infectious keratitis
- sterile infiltrates
- corneal melting
- persistent corneal edema due to endothelial cell damage

Table 9-A1 lists the incidence of complications related to CXL. Complications seem to occur more frequently in patients older than 35 years and preoperative maximum steepening greater than 58.00 D.

Koller T, Mrochen M, Seiler T. Complication and failure rates after corneal crosslinking. *J Cataract Refract Surg.* 2009;35(8):1358–1362.

Table 9-A1 Complications Associated with Epi-Off CXL

	117 Eyes	1-year Follow-up
Loss ≥2 lines	2.9%	
Progression	7.6%	3% if K <58.00 D
Sterile infiltrates	7.6%	
Central stromal scar	2.8%	
Overall complication rate	1% if patient <35yrs	

CXL = corneal crosslinking; D = diopters; K = keratometry reading.

Data from Koller T, Mrochen M, Seiler T. Complication and failure rates after corneal crosslinking. *J Cataract Refract Surg.* 2009;35(8):1358–1362.

Alternative techniques

Transepithelial corneal crosslinking The complications of "epi-off" CXL mainly arise from the removal of the epithelium. Thus, some clinicians advocate the "epi-on" or transepithelial CXL procedure, which has had promising clinical outcomes. However, experimental studies have shown a significantly lower efficacy of transepithelial CXL compared with the standard epi-off approach due to the low epithelial permeability of riboflavin. Partial disruption of the superficial epithelial layers can enhance riboflavin penetration through the epithelium. Some researchers claim that even with adequate stromal concentration of riboflavin, decreased efficiency of the transepithelial CXL might be attributed to the attenuation of UVA radiation by the epithelium. This would imply that UVA energy may need to be increased or otherwise modulated beyond the current level of 5.4 J/cm^2 when the epithelium is kept intact.

Baiocchi S, Mazzotta C, Cerretani D, Caporossi T, Caporossi A. Corneal crosslinking: riboflavin concentration in corneal stroma exposed with and without epithelium. *J Cataract Refract Surg.* 2009;35(5):893–899.

Filippello M, Stagni E, O'Brart D. Transepithelial corneal collagen crosslinking: bilateral study. *J Cataract Refract Surg.* 2012;38(2):283–291.

Kanellopoulos AJ. Long term results of a prospective randomized bilateral eye comparison trial of higher fluence, shorter duration ultraviolet A radiation, and riboflavin collagen cross linking for progressive keratoconus. *Clin Ophthalmol.* 2012;6:97–101.

Stojanovic A, Zhou W, Utheim TP. Corneal collagen cross-linking with and without epithelial removal: a contralateral study with 0.5% hypotonic riboflavin solution. *Biomed Res Int.* 2014;2014:619398.

Accelerated corneal crosslinking New-generation lamps have been developed to shorten the duration of exposure to UVA radiation. Some offer fixed treatment times of 5 and 10 minutes at 18 and 10 mW/cm^2, respectively. Other systems allow a wide range of variation in time (1–30 minutes) and power (3 to 45 mW) and increased maximum irradiance to 10 J/cm^2. Kanellopoulos reported that the use of high-fluence UVA for a shorter time (7 mW/cm^2 for 15 minutes) was safe and effective and could achieve clinical results similar to the Dresden protocol in terms of stabilizing corneal ectasia.

Kanellopoulos AJ. Collagen cross-linking in early keratoconus with riboflavin in a femtosecond laser–created pocket: initial clinical results. *J Refract Surg.* 2009; 25(11):1034–1037.

Combined techniques Sometimes CXL treatment does not improve visual acuity enough to provide functional vision. Thus, ophthalmologists have attempted to combine CXL with various refractive surgical techniques. The implantation of ICRSs with sequential or subsequent CXL treatment has proven effective. It is recommended that the ring segment insertion be performed prior to CXL. Studies have shown that the limited use of topography-guided transepithelial PRK, followed by CXL, can improve visual acuity and stabilize KC. Same-day PRK, followed by CXL appears to be superior to sequential PRK after CXL. It is important to counsel patients regarding the risk of progressive ectasia following PRK prior to surgery. These combined techniques have not been widely adopted in the United States.

Kanellopoulos AJ. Comparison of sequential vs same-day simultaneous collagen cross-linking and topography-guided PRK for treatment of keratoconus. *J Refract Surg.* 2009;25(9):S812–818.

Stojanovic A, Zhang J, Chen X, Nitter TA, Chen S, Wang Q. Topography-guided transepithelial surface ablation followed by corneal collagen cross-linking performed in a single combined procedure for the treatment of keratoconus and pellucid marginal degeneration. *J Refract Surg.* 2010;26(2):145–152.

CHAPTER 10

Systemic Disorders With Corneal and Other Anterior Segment Manifestations

This chapter includes a related video. Go to www.aao.org/bcscvideo_section08 or scan the QR code in the text to access this content.

Indicates selected key points within the chapter.

Highlights

- Crystals in the cornea are often related to amyloid deposition but may also be related to cystinosis and dysproteinemia.
- A Kayser-Fleischer ring is found not only in Wilson disease but also in primary biliary cirrhosis, chronic active hepatitis, and exogenous chalcosis. It should not be confused with a Fleischer ring, an iron ring seen in keratoconus.
- Patients with diabetes may have problems with epithelial healing after debridement and are at risk for recurrent corneal erosion.
- The differential diagnosis for prominent corneal nerves includes multiple endocrine neoplasia and keratoconus.

Introduction

Corneal clarity can be affected by the accumulation of a variety of substances, such as carbohydrates, lipids, proteins, and amino or nucleic acids. The anterior segment can be affected by autoimmune, dermatologic, musculoskeletal, and other systemic diseases. Recognition of the manifestations of these disorders requires prompt medical intervention. This chapter reviews common systemic conditions affecting the anterior segment, particularly the cornea. See also BCSC Section 2, *Fundamentals and Principles of Ophthalmology,* and Section 6, *Pediatric Ophthalmology and Strabismus.*

Poll-The BT, Maillette de Buy Wenniger-Prick CJ. The eye in metabolic disease: clues to diagnosis. *Eur J Paediatr Neurol.* 2011;15(3):197–204.

Srinivasan S, Shehadeh-Mashor R, Slomovic AR. Corneal manifestations of metabolic diseases. In: Mannis MJ, Holland EJ, eds. *Cornea*. Vol 1. 4th ed. Elsevier; 2017:620–644.

Inherited Metabolic Diseases

Lysosomal Storage Diseases

Lysosomes are cellular organelles containing acid hydrolase enzymes that break down waste materials and cellular debris, including proteins, carbohydrates, lipids, and nucleic acids. Mutations in the genes that synthesize the lysosomal enzymes are responsible for more than 30 different human genetic diseases, collectively known as lysosomal storage diseases. Each of these disorders results from deficiency of a single lysosomal enzyme that prevents the normal breakdown of target molecules.

Systemic mucopolysaccharidoses

Systemic mucopolysaccharidoses (MPSs) are rare, inherited lysosomal storage diseases that occur in approximately 1 in 10,000 births (Table 10-1). They can cause corneal clouding as a result of the accumulation of incompletely degraded glycosaminoglycans (GAGs; previously called *mucopolysaccharides*) within the keratocytes, corneal epithelium, and endothelium as well as the extracellular matrix of the cornea. Diseases in this class include

- Hurler syndrome (MPS IH)
- Hurler-Scheie syndrome (MPS IH/S)
- Scheie syndrome (MPS IS)
- Hunter syndrome (MPS II)
- Sanfilippo syndrome (MPS III)
- Morquio syndrome (MPS IV)
- Maroteaux-Lamy syndrome (MPS VI)
- Sly syndrome (MPS VII)
- Natowicz syndrome (MPS IX)

MPS syndromes are autosomal recessive, except for Hunter syndrome, which is X-linked recessive. These disorders result from defects in various lysosomal enzymes and are associated with other ophthalmic and systemic manifestations.

CLINICAL PRESENTATION Of the MPS I disorders, Hurler syndrome (MPS IH) is the most serious; severe cognitive impairment and corneal clouding appear by 1 year of age (Fig 10-1). The life span of patients with Hurler syndrome is very limited unless a bone marrow transplant is performed. In contrast, symptoms of Scheie syndrome (MPS IS) do not appear until age 5–15 years. As in Hurler syndrome, corneal clouding occurs in Scheie syndrome and may or may not be present at birth. It is often slowly progressive from the periphery toward the center and can cause serious reduction in vision. Children with Scheie syndrome generally have ordinary intelligence and a typical life span. Ophthalmic manifestations of MPSs also include retinopathy and optic atrophy.

Table 10-1 Summary of Mucopolysaccharidosis Syndromes

MPS Syndrome	Inheritance	Enzyme Defect	Accumulated Material	Screening Test	Diagnostic Test	Corneal Changes	Other Ophthalmic Changes
MPS IH (Hurler syndrome)	Autosomal recessive	α-L-Iduronidase	Dermatan and heparan sulfate	Urine GAG	WBC enzyme assay	Severe clouding within first few years of life; diffuse punctate stromal opacities; epithelium and endothelium not affected	Pigmentary retinopathy, glaucoma, optic nerve swelling and atrophy, hypertelorism
MPS IS (Scheie syndrome)	Autosomal recessive	α-L-Iduronidase	Dermatan and heparan sulfate	Urine GAG	WBC enzyme assay	Slowly progressive corneal opacification causing decreased vision by second decade of life; corneal edema; corneal changes may be more prominent in periphery	Glaucoma may occur
MPS IH/S (Hurler-Scheie syndrome)	Autosomal recessive	α-L-Iduronidase	Dermatan and heparan sulfate	Urine GAG	WBC enzyme assay	Diffuse corneal opacification	Retinopathy
MPS II (Hunter syndrome)	X-linked recessive	Iduronate-2-sulfatase	Dermatan and heparan sulfate	Urine GAG	Plasma enzyme assay	Does not present as a congenital corneal opacity; corneal opacity may occur later in life in milder phenotypes	Exophthalmos, hypertelorism, optic nerve swelling and atrophy, retinopathy
MPS III A–D (Sanfilippo syndrome)	Autosomal recessive	Multiple enzyme defects	Heparan sulfate	Urine GAG	WBC enzyme assay Plasma enzyme assay	Uncommon	Moderate to severe pigmentary retinopathy with abnormal ERG response

(Continued)

Table 10-1 *(continued)*

MPS Syndrome	Inheritance	Enzyme Defect	Accumulated Material	Screening Test	Diagnostic Test	Corneal Changes	Other Ophthalmic Changes
MPS IV A–B (Morquio syndrome)	Autosomal recessive	Galactose-6-sulfatase (MPS IV A) β-Galactosidase (MPS IV B)	Keratan sulfate (MPS IV A and IV B) Chondroitin sulfate (MPS IV A)	Urine GAG	WBC enzyme assay	Opacities after age 10 years in 10% of patients; usually mild	Retinopathy, shallow orbits
MPS VI (Maroteaux-Lamy syndrome)	Autosomal recessive	*N*-Acetylgalactosamine-4-sulfatase	Dermatan sulfate	Urine GAG	WBC enzyme assay	Severe corneal clouding within first years of life; corneal edema	Narrow-angle glaucoma, optic neuropathy
MPS VII (Sly syndrome)	Autosomal recessive	β-Glucuronidase	Dermatan sulfate, keratan sulfate, chondroitin sulfate	Urine GAG	WBC enzyme assay	Corneal clouding	None
MPS IX (Natowicz syndrome)	Autosomal recessive	Hyaluronidase 1	Chondroitin sulfate	None	Cultured cells	None reported	None

ERG = electroretinogram; GAG = glycosaminoglycan; MPS = mucopolysaccharidosis; WBC = white blood cell.

Adapted from Srinivasan S, Shehadeh-Mashor R, Slomovic AR. Corneal manifestations of metabolic diseases. In: Mannis MJ, Holland EJ, eds. *Cornea.* Vol 1. 4th ed. Elsevier; 2017:620–644.

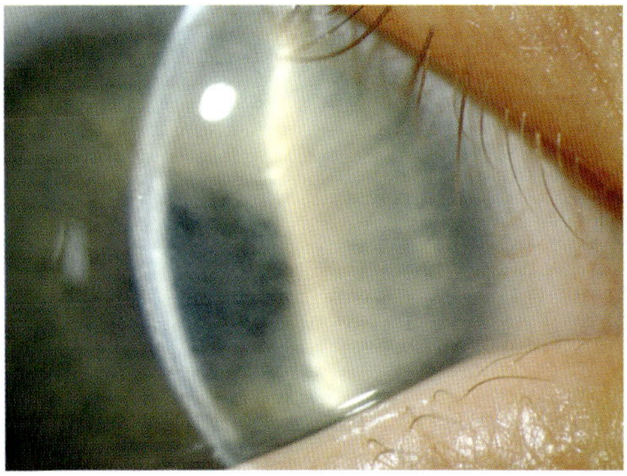

Figure 10-1 Slit-lamp photograph from a patient with Hurler syndrome, showing diffuse, patchy corneal clouding. *(Courtesy of Stephen E. Orlin, MD.)*

PATHOGENESIS Specific enzyme defects and genetic mutations have been identified for each of the MPSs. There is variation in phenotypic expression. For example, Hurler, Scheie, and Hurler-Scheie syndromes arise from different amino acid substitutions that result in a deficiency of α-L-iduronidase, which classifies them all as MPS I diseases. Hurler-Scheie is thought to result from the transmission of 1 Hurler gene and 1 Scheie gene.

LABORATORY EVALUATION Urine can be screened for the presence of GAGs, but the most precise method of diagnosing the various MPSs is through a leukocyte or plasma enzyme assay.

MANAGEMENT Penetrating keratoplasty (PK) or deep anterior lamellar keratoplasty (DALK) may be considered in the management of corneal clouding in the MPSs, although the patient's mental status or retinal and optic nerve abnormalities may limit visual improvement. The visual prognosis for patients with an MPS who have undergone PK is considered guarded, because the abnormal storage material may accumulate in the graft. Some regression of corneal clouding occurs in approximately one-third of patients following successful allogeneic bone marrow transplant. Enzyme replacement therapy is being used for several types of MPSs, and gene transfer therapy is under investigation.

Ashworth JL, Biswas S, Wraith E, Lloyd IC. Mucopolysaccharidoses and the eye. *Surv Ophthalmol.* 2006;51(1):1–17.

Sphingolipidoses

Sphingolipidoses (Table 10-2) are rare, inherited lysosomal storage diseases that cause deposits due to a buildup of complex lipids (gangliosides and sphingomyelin) in the corneal epithelium. This group includes 4 conditions:

1. Fabry disease (angiokeratoma corporis diffusum)
2. multiple sulfatase deficiency
3. generalized gangliosidosis (GM_1 gangliosidosis type I)
4. Tay-Sachs disease (GM_2 gangliosidosis type I)

CLINICAL PRESENTATION In the sphingolipidoses, the cornea exhibits distinctive changes consisting of whorl-like lines *(cornea verticillata)* originating in the basal layers of the epithelium located at the inferior central cornea (Fig 10-2; also see Chapter 7, Fig 7-24).

Table 10-2 Summary of Sphingolipidoses

Syndrome	Enzyme Defect	Accumulated Material	Screening Test	Diagnostic Test
Fabry disease	α-Galactosidase A	Globotriaosylceramide and blood group B substances	None	WBC enzyme assay
Farber lipogranulomatosis	Ceramidase	Ceramide	None	WBC enzyme assay
Gaucher disease	β-Glucosidase, saposin C activator	Glucosylceramide	None	WBC enzyme assay
Niemann-Pick A and B	Sphingomyelinase	Sphingomyelin	None	WBC enzyme assay
GM_1 gangliosidosis type I (generalized gangliosidosis)	β-Glucosidase	GM_1 ganglioside	Urine oligosaccharides	WBC enzyme assay
GM_2 gangliosidosis type I (Tay-Sachs disease)	β-Hexosaminidase A	GM_2 ganglioside and related glycolipids	None	WBC enzyme assay
GM_2 gangliosidosis type II (Sandhoff disease)	β-Hexosaminidase A and B	GM_2 ganglioside and related glycolipids	None	WBC enzyme assay
GM_2 gangliosidosis (GM_2 activator deficiency)	GM_2 activator protein	GM_2 ganglioside and related glycolipids	None	Cultured cells and natural substrate
Globoid cell leukodystrophy (Krabbe disease)	Galactocerebrosidase	Galactosylceramides	None	WBC enzyme assay

WBC = white blood cell.

Adapted from Srinivasan S, Shehadeh-Mashor R, Slomovic AR. Corneal manifestations of metabolic diseases. In: Mannis MJ, Holland EJ, eds. *Cornea.* Vol 1. 4th ed. Elsevier; 2017:620–644.

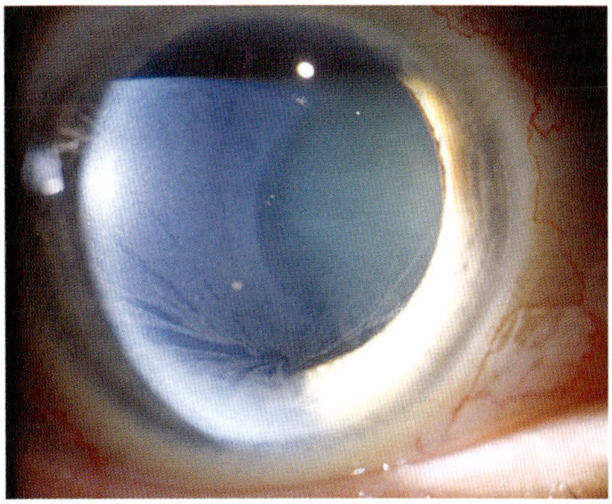

Figure 10-2 Slit-lamp photograph from a patient with Fabry disease, showing cornea verticillata, which are in the basal layers of the epithelium. *(Courtesy of Stephen E. Orlin, MD.)*

Periorbital edema occurs in 25% of cases, posterior spokelike cataracts in 50%, and conjunctival aneurysms in 60%. Other ocular signs include papilledema, retinal or macular edema, optic atrophy, and retinal vascular dilation. The corneal changes resemble those noted in patients after long-term oral chloroquine or amiodarone therapy and topical Rho kinase inhibitors or nitric oxide used in treating glaucoma.

Hemizygous males with X-linked Fabry disease are more seriously affected than heterozygous females and show the typical corneal changes. Fabry disease is also characterized by renal failure, peripheral neuropathy with painful dysesthesias in the lower extremities, and skin lesions (angiokeratomas). The skin lesions are small, round, vascular eruptions that later become hyperkeratotic. They consist of an accumulation of sphingolipid within the vascular endothelium.

Children with multiple sulfatase deficiency have subtle diffuse corneal opacities, macular changes in the retina, optic atrophy, and progressive psychomotor retardation. They die in the first decade of life.

The ocular findings in Tay-Sachs disease involve primarily the retina (eg, cherry red spot in the macula); however, the corneal endothelial cells can appear distended and filled with single membrane–bound vacuoles.

PATHOGENESIS Fabry disease is caused by a deficiency of α-galactosidase A, which leads to the accumulation of ceramide trihexoside in the renal and cardiovascular systems. Generalized gangliosidosis is characterized by deficiencies of β-galactosidases and the resultant accumulation of ganglioside GM_1 in the central nervous system and of keratan sulfate in somatic tissues. It has been linked to chromosome 3p12–p13. Tay-Sachs disease is related to the generalized gangliosidoses but results from β-hexosaminidase A deficiency, which causes accumulation of ganglioside GM_2.

LABORATORY EVALUATION In patients with Fabry disease, levels of α-galactosidase A are markedly decreased in urine and plasma. The conjunctival biopsy result may be positive before cornea verticillata is apparent. In Tay-Sachs disease, inclusion bodies can be seen in a conjunctival biopsy or in circulating blood leukocyte cells. Prenatal diagnosis can be performed with chorionic villus sampling. Gene sequencing may help in diagnosing

Fabry disease in suspected female carriers; enzyme levels may be close to normal in heterozygotes.

MANAGEMENT If a female patient is found to be an asymptomatic heterozygous carrier of Fabry disease, genetic counseling should be considered. Enzyme replacement with infusion of α-galactosidase A is a therapeutic option, but long-term benefit has not been proven. Corneal deposits have been cleared with enzyme replacement therapy. The addition of agents that help stabilize native enzymes may improve the efficacy of enzyme replacement therapy. There is an increased incidence of Tay-Sachs disease in people of Ashkenazi Jewish heritage. Genetic screening can be helpful in identifying carriers.

Fledelius HC, Sandfeld L, Rasmussen ÅK, Madsen CV, Feldt-Rasmussen U. Ophthalmic experience over 10 years in an observational nationwide Danish cohort of Fabry patients with access to enzyme replacement. *Acta Ophthalmol.* 2015;93(3):258–264.

Samiy N. Ocular features of Fabry disease: diagnosis of a treatable life-threatening disorder. *Surv Ophthalmol.* 2008;53(4):416–423.

Mucolipidoses

The mucolipidoses (MLs) are inherited disorders of carbohydrate and lipid metabolism combined. They are autosomal recessive conditions and have features common to both MPSs and lipidoses. The 4 currently recognized diseases (Table 10-3) in this class are

1. ML I (dysmorphic sialidosis)
2. ML II (inclusion cell disease)
3. ML III (pseudo-Hurler polydystrophy)
4. ML IV

CLINICAL PRESENTATION All of the MLs are characterized by varying degrees of corneal clouding, which is often progressive. A retinal cherry-red spot and retinal degeneration are also associated with many of these disorders.

Table 10-3 Summary of Mucolipidoses

Disease	Enzyme Defect	Accumulated Material	Screening Test	Diagnostic Test
ML I (dysmorphic sialidosis)	Neuraminidase	Sialic add	Urine sialic acid	Cultured cells
ML II (inclusion cell disease)	Transferase	Many	Urine oligosaccharides	Plasma enzyme assay
ML III (pseudo-Hurler polydystrophy)	Transferase	Many	Urine oligosaccharides	Plasma enzyme assay
ML IV	Mucolipin-1	Lipids and mucopolysaccharides	Urine oligosaccharides	Histology

ML = mucolipidosis.

Adapted from Srinivasan S, Shehadeh-Mashor R, Slomovic AR. Corneal manifestations of metabolic diseases. In: Mannis MJ, Holland EJ, eds. *Cornea.* Vol 1. 4th ed. Elsevier; 2017:620–644.

PATHOGENESIS Incompletely degraded GAGs accumulate in the cornea and viscera, and sphingolipids are deposited in the retina and central nervous system.

The ML IV gene has been mapped to the short arm of chromosome 19. Histologic examination of corneal scrapings has revealed the accumulation of intracytoplasmic storage material in the corneal epithelium. All MLs are caused by a defect in lysosomal acid hydrolase enzymes.

LABORATORY EVALUATION Plasma cells are vacuolated, and levels of plasma lysosomal hydrolases are elevated. In ML IV, in which corneal clouding is present from birth, conjunctival biopsy shows intralysosomal inclusion bodies that are

- single membrane–limited cytoplasmic vacuoles containing both fibrillogranular and membranous lamellar materials
- lamellar and concentric bodies resembling those of Tay-Sachs disease

There is no evidence of mucopolysacchariduria or cellular metachromasia. Chorionic villus sampling has been used for prenatal diagnosis of ML II.

MANAGEMENT Both PK and lamellar keratoplasty (LK) have been associated with generally poor results because resurfacing is impaired by the abnormal epithelial cells. Allograft limbal stem cell transplantation may be an option.

Srinivasan S, Shehadeh-Mashor R, Slomovic AR. Corneal manifestations of metabolic diseases. In: Mannis MJ, Holland EJ, eds. *Cornea.* Vol 1. 4th ed. Elsevier; 2017:620–644.

Miscellaneous lysosomal storage diseases

Several autosomal recessive lysosomal storage diseases do not fit into a specific category. These include

- galactosialidosis (Goldberg syndrome)
- mannosidosis
- fucosidosis

PATHOGENESIS Goldberg syndrome is a cathepsin-related disorder with features similar to those of β-galactosidase and sialidase deficiencies. Mannosidosis is caused by deficient activity of the enzyme mannosidase. There are 2 subtypes: α-mannosidosis and β-mannosidosis. Both galactosialidosis and mannosidosis are associated with corneal clouding.

Fucosidosis is due to mutations in the *FUCA1* gene, which result in reduction in activity of the α-L-fucosidase enzyme. Histologic studies have revealed that even when the cornea appears clinically normal in patients with fucosidosis, corneal endothelial cells show the presence of cytoplasmic, membrane-bound, confluent areas of fibrillar, granular, and multilaminated deposits.

Hypolipoproteinemias

Abnormal reductions in serum lipoprotein levels occur in 5 autosomal recessive disorders:

1. lecithin-cholesterol acyltransferase (LCAT) deficiency
2. fish eye disease
3. Tangier disease

4. familial hypobetalipoproteinemia
5. Bassen-Kornzweig syndrome

The last 2 disorders do not result in corneal disease; the discussion in this section focuses on the other 3 disorders.

CLINICAL PRESENTATION Familial LCAT deficiency is characterized by peripheral arcus and stromal haze made up of myriad minute focal deposits of lipid that appear early in childhood but do not interfere with vision (Fig 10-3). Corneas affected by fish eye disease show obvious clouding from minute gray-white-yellow dots that progress from the periphery to the central cornea resulting in decreased vision. Tangier disease is characterized by findings of large orange tonsils and enlarged liver, spleen, and lymph nodes. Affected corneas show diffuse clouding and posterior focal stromal opacities but no arcus. Neuropathy leads to lagophthalmos and corneal sequelae.

PATHOGENESIS LCAT promotes transfer of excess cholesterol from peripheral tissues to the liver; a deficiency of this enzyme results in accumulation of unesterified cholesterol in the plasma and tissues. This cholesterol accumulation, in turn, leads to atherosclerosis, renal insufficiency, early corneal arcus, and corneal clouding composed of minute focal lipid deposits.

LCAT deficiency and fish eye disease are allelic variants of the same genetic locus on chromosome 16q22.1. In fish eye disease, LCAT levels are normal, but the enzyme does not function properly. Tangier disease is characterized by a complete absence of serum high-density lipoproteins (HDLs) with atherosclerosis and an accumulation of cholesterol in tissues, including the cornea. The gene responsible for this disease maps to chromosome 9q22–q31.

LABORATORY EVALUATION AND MANAGEMENT The serum lipid profile shows characteristic low levels of HDL (almost absent in Tangier disease). A pathognomonic finding of all these conditions is hypocholesterolemia. Recognition of hypolipoproteinemia can allow the clinician to make appropriate referrals and encourage the patient to seek genetic counseling.

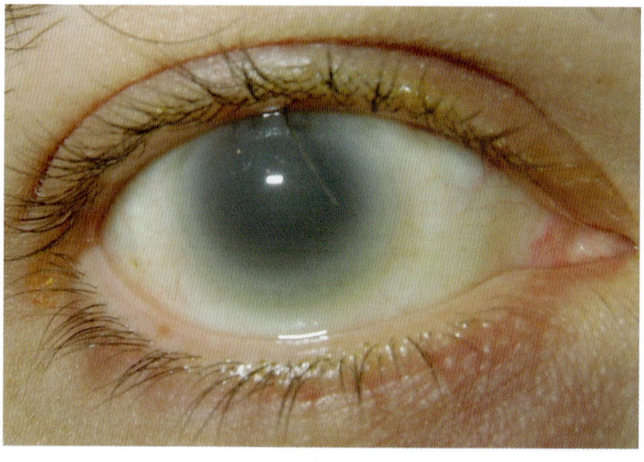

Figure 10-3 Clinical photograph from a patient with familial lecithin-cholesterol acyltransferase (LCAT) deficiency, showing peripheral arcus and stromal haze. *(Courtesy of Gerald Zaidman, MD.)*

Disorders of Amino Acid, Nucleic Acid, Protein, and Mineral Metabolism

Cystinosis

Cystinosis is a rare autosomal recessive metabolic disorder affecting 35 infants per 10 million births. The disease is characterized by the accumulation of the amino acid cystine within lysosomes. Table 10-4 summarizes the ocular and systemic findings in this and other disorders of amino acid metabolism. See also BCSC Section 6, *Pediatric Ophthalmology and Strabismus.*

Table 10-4 Disorders of Amino Acid Metabolism

Type	Heredity	Enzyme Defect	Accumulated Material	Ocular Findings	Associated Nonocular Conditions
Cystinosis	Rare autosomal recessive	Defect in cystinosin	Cystine	Polychromatic cystine crystals in conjunctiva, trabecular meshwork, corneal stroma, and iris	Dwarfism
				Photophobia (usually)	Renal dysfunction
				Retinal depigmentation	
Tyrosinemia	Autosomal recessive	Type I: fumarylacetoacetate deficiency	Tyrosine	Photophobia, tearing, conjunctival injection, tarsal papillary hypertrophy, pseudodendrites	Hyperkeratotic lesions of palms, soles, and elbows
		Type II: tyrosine aminotransferase		Epithelial breakdown with secondary corneal neovascularization and scarring	Cognitive impairment
Alkaptonuria	Rare autosomal recessive	Homogentisic acid oxidase	Homogentisic acid	Ochronotic (brownish) deposits of alkapton in corneal epithelium or in Bowman layer near limbus	Arthropathy
				Rectus muscle tendons and adjacent sclera develop blue-black discoloration of the conjunctiva and sclera	Renal calculi Pigmentation of cartilaginous structures, including earlobes, trachea, nose, and tendons

CLINICAL PRESENTATION Cystinosis is categorized on the basis of the patient's age at diagnosis and the severity of symptoms. *Nephropathic cystinosis* is divided into infantile (classic) and intermediate (juvenile or adolescent) forms. Dwarfism and progressive renal dysfunction are prominent in infantile cystinosis and less severe in the juvenile disease. Life expectancy is normal in *nonnephropathic cystinosis* (formerly called *adult cystinosis*). All 3 types are characterized by the deposition of fine iridescent and polychromatic cystine crystals in the conjunctiva, cornea, iris, and other parts of the eye. The crystals are densest in the peripheral cornea but are present throughout the anterior stroma, even within the central cornea (Fig 10-4), and can be observed in the trabecular meshwork with gonioscopy. Patients with cystinosis often have photophobia, and the crystals can recur following PK. Table 10-5 lists other causes of corneal crystals.

Liang H, Baudouin C, Hassani RTJ, Brignole-Baudouin F, Labbe A. Photophobia and corneal crystal density in nephropathic cystinosis: an in vivo confocal microscopy and anterior segment optical coherence tomography study. *Invest Ophthalmol Vis Sci.* 2015;56(5):3218–3225.

PATHOGENESIS A defect in cystine transport across the lysosomal membrane leads to intracellular accumulation of cystine and to crystal formation in tissues of the body, mainly the kidney and the eye. The defective gene in cystinosis, *CTNS,* has been mapped to chromosome 17p13.

LABORATORY EVALUATION Cystine crystals may be seen in conjunctiva, blood leukocytes, and bone marrow. Conjunctival biopsy should be submitted in glutaraldehyde solution to avoid dissolving the crystals.

MANAGEMENT Topical cysteamine 0.44% is a commercially available agent used to reduce the density of the crystals and diminish corneal pain, possibly by reducing the frequency of corneal erosions. Cysteamine is thought to react with intracellular cystine, forming a cysteine–cysteamine disulfide that is transported through the lysosome by the normal lysine transport system, thereby depleting the cystinotic cells of cystine. Posterior segment manifestations

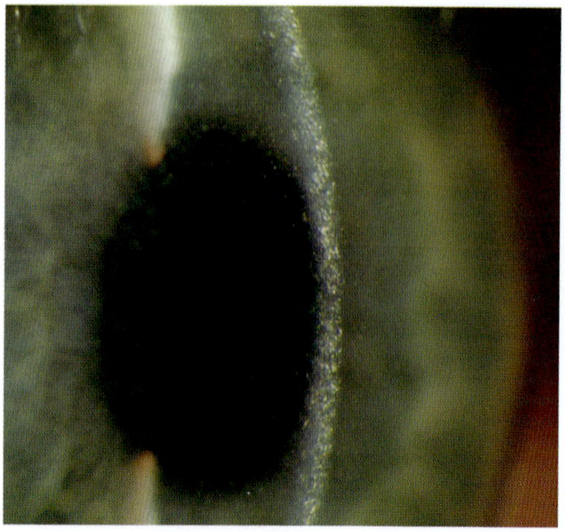

Figure 10-4 Nonnephropathic cystinosis. Slit-lamp photograph shows diffuse stromal refractile crystals. *(Courtesy of Stephen E. Orlin, MD.)*

Table 10-5 Corneal Crystals Associated With Systemic Disease

Medical Disorders	Specific Conditions and Medications [a]
Lipid keratopathies	Familial lipoprotein disorders LCAT deficiency Schnyder corneal dystrophy Tangier disease
Disorders of protein metabolism	Cystinosis Gout Hyperuricemia Tyrosinemia
Immunoglobulin disorders	Benign monoclonal gammopathy Cryoglobulinemia Multiple myeloma Rheumatoid arthritis Waldenström macroglobulinemia
Miscellaneous causes	Calcium deposits Oxalosis Porphyria

LCAT = lecithin-cholesterol acyltransferase.

[a] Medications that cause corneal crystal formation.

such as pigmentary retinopathy and optic nerve involvement may be treated with oral cysteamine, which may also prevent or stabilize renal function.

Tyrosinemia

Tyrosinemia encompasses a group of inborn errors in the metabolism of the amino acid tyrosine.

CLINICAL PRESENTATION Ocular changes seen in tyrosinemia type II include marked photophobia, tearing, conjunctival injection, and tarsal papillary hypertrophy. Patients with tyrosinemia type II may show hyperkeratotic lesions of the palms, soles, and elbows, as well as cognitive impairment.

> **CLINICAL PEARL**
>
> Affected patients experience recurrent episodes of corneal erosions and pseudodendrites (Fig 10-5), which usually do not stain well with fluorescein or rose bengal. Continued episodes of epithelial breakdown can result in corneal vascularization and scarring. It is important to consider this disorder in young children who may carry a diagnosis of bilateral recurrent herpes simplex virus keratitis.

PATHOGENESIS Tyrosinemia type I, an autosomal recessive disease caused by fumarylacetoacetate deficiency, is not associated with corneal pathology. Tyrosinemia type II (Richner-Hanhart syndrome) is an autosomal recessive disorder resulting from defective tyrosine aminotransferase, which leads to excess tyrosine in the blood and urine. The

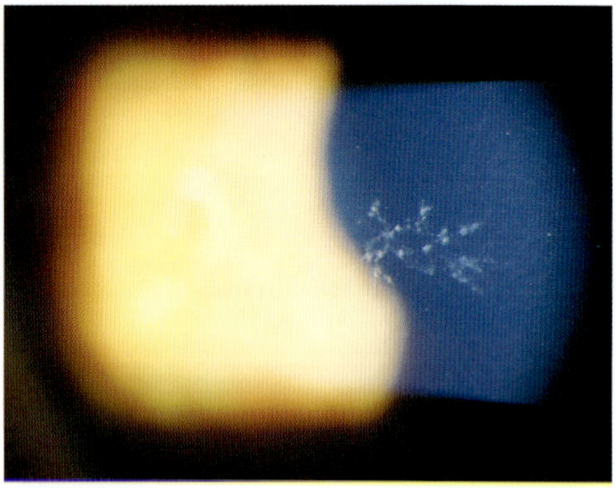

Figure 10-5 Slit-lamp photograph shows a pseudodendrite in a patient with tyrosinemia. *(Courtesy of Robert W. Weisenthal, MD.)*

elevated tyrosine level likely has a direct effect on lysosomal membranes, leading to enzyme release. The gene defect is located on chromosome 16q22.1–22.3.

LABORATORY EVALUATION Hypertyrosinemia and tyrosinuria with normal phenylalanine levels and conjunctival biopsy showing soluble tyrosine aminotransferase deficiency are diagnostic.

MANAGEMENT Restriction of dietary intake of tyrosine and phenylalanine can reduce the severity of both the corneal and systemic changes, including cognitive impairment. Institution of appropriate dietary restrictions, even later in life, can improve mental status.

Alkaptonuria

Alkaptonuria is a rare autosomal recessive disorder caused by deficiency of the enzyme homogentisic acid oxidase (also known as homogentisate 1,2-dioxygenase), which leads to an accumulation of homogentisic acid.

CLINICAL PRESENTATION Darkly pigmented, dotlike opacities, similar to those seen in spheroidal degeneration, may appear in the corneal epithelium or in Bowman layer, near the limbus. The medial and lateral rectus muscle tendons and the sclera adjacent to the tendon insertions develop a smudgelike bluish-black pigmentation (Fig 10-6). Systemic findings include arthropathy; renal calculi; and pigmentation of cartilaginous structures, including earlobes, trachea, nose, tendons, dura mater, heart valves, and prostate.

PATHOGENESIS The enzyme involved in the degradation pathway of tyrosine and phenylalanine, homogentisic acid oxidase, is deficient in patients with this disorder. The defect is caused by mutations in the *HGD* gene, which maps to chromosome 3q13.33. The enzyme deficiency leads to a buildup of homogentisic acid, which is oxidized and polymerized into alkapton, a brown-black material similar to melanin. Alkapton binds to collagen and is then deposited in connective tissues as a dark pigment; this process is known as *ochronosis.*

LABORATORY EVALUATION Elevated levels of homogentisic acid in the urine are diagnostic for alkaptonuria. The urine of affected patients turns dark on standing.

MANAGEMENT No specific therapy is available, but high-dose ascorbic acid may reduce arthropathy in young patients. Gene therapy may be a future treatment.

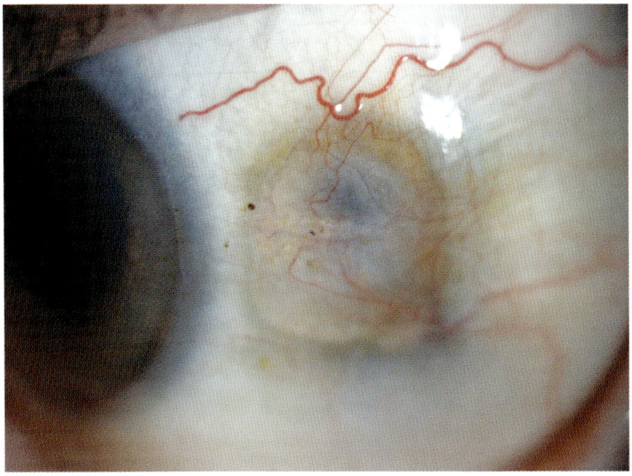

Figure 10-6 Slit-lamp photograph from a female patient with alkaptonuria shows ochronosis (scleral pigmentation) at the insertion of the lateral rectus muscle. *(Courtesy of Irving M. Raber, MD.)*

Amyloidosis

The amyloidoses are a heterogeneous group of diseases characterized by the extracellular accumulation of amyloid in various tissues and organs, including the cornea and conjunctiva. Amyloid deposits may be composed of many different types of proteins, including immunoglobulin fragments. The deposits are insoluble and inert, but they interfere with the normal structure and function of tissues and organs.

Amyloid has the following staining characteristics:

- positive staining with Congo red dye (see Fig 8-11A)
- dichroism and apple-green birefringence (see Fig 8-11B)
- metachromasia with crystal violet dye
- fluorescence in ultraviolet light with thioflavin T stain

CLASSIFICATION AND CLINICAL PRESENTATION Ocular amyloidosis is classified as either primary (idiopathic) or secondary (associated with a chronic disease) and as either localized or systemic. A useful classification of the amyloidoses considers these 4 types. Each type is summarized in Table 10-6.

Primary localized amyloidosis is the most common form of ocular amyloidosis. Conjunctival amyloid plaques occur in the absence of systemic involvement (Fig 10-7). Gelatinous droplike corneal dystrophy (formerly primary familial amyloidosis), classic lattice corneal dystrophy type 1 (LCD1), and lattice variants are special forms of primary localized amyloidosis and are discussed in Chapter 8. Polymorphic amyloid degeneration is discussed in Chapter 7.

Primary systemic amyloidosis is a heterogeneous group of diseases in which waxy, ecchymotic eyelid papules occur in association with vitreous veils and opacities as well as with pupillary anomalies such as light–near dissociation. Orbital involvement, extraocular muscle involvement with ophthalmoplegia, and scleral infiltration with uveal effusion

Table 10-6 Amyloid in the Eye

Type	Heredity	Ocular Distribution and Findings	Other Associated Ocular and Systemic Conditions
Primary localized amyloidosis	Nonfamilial	Conjunctival plaque Polymorphic amyloid degeneration	None
	Familial	Lattice corneal dystrophy and lattice variants Granular corneal dystrophy type 2 (Avellino) Gelatinous droplike dystrophy	
Primary systemic amyloidosis	Nonfamilial	Eyelid skin and conjunctiva (very rare)	Occult plasma cell dyscrasias
	Familial	Ophthalmoplegia (orbital and muscle infiltrates), ptosis, vitreous veils, dry eye, pupillary abnormalities	Cardiomyopathy, peripheral neuropathy, gastrointestinal disease Skin involvement
		Meretoja syndrome, cranial neuropathies	Meretoja syndrome (facial palsies, skin nodules, rarely renal involvement)
Secondary localized amyloidosis	Nonfamilial Familial	Conjunctiva, eyelid skin, cornea None	Trachoma, psoriasis, trauma, phlyctenulosis, retinopathy of prematurity, keratoconus, bullous keratopathy, interstitial keratitis, leprosy, trichiasis, tertiary syphilis, uveitis, climatic droplet keratopathy
Secondary systemic amyloidosis	Nonfamilial	Vitreous body (rare) (corneal deposits are not amyloid)	Multiple myeloma
		Conjunctiva, eyelid skin (rare)	Infectious diseases (tuberculosis, leprosy, syphilis) Inflammatory diseases (rheumatoid arthritis, other connective tissue disorders) Hodgkin disease
	Familial	Corneal nerve enlargement is not due to amyloid	Multiple endocrine neoplasia type 2A

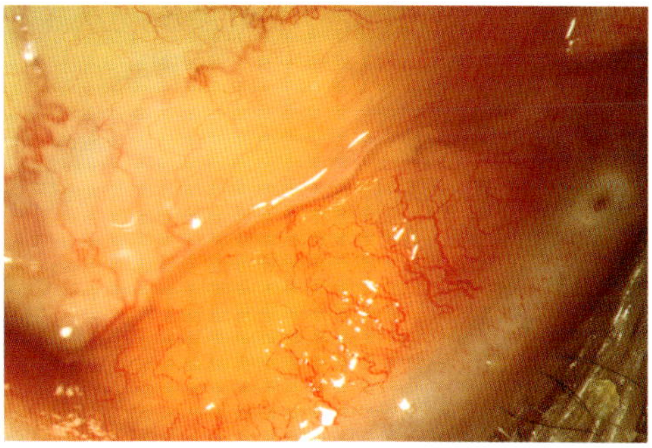

Figure 10-7 Clinical photograph shows yellowish amyloid deposition in the inferior palpebral conjunctiva. *(Courtesy of Robert S. Feder, MD.)*

have been reported. The most common form of primary systemic amyloidosis is an autosomal dominant group of diseases linked to mutations in the transthyretin gene (*TTR*, prealbumin) on chromosome 18 (18q11.2–q12.1); more than 40 mutations in this gene have been described.

Familial amyloidosis (Meretoja syndrome) is a primary systemic amyloidosis that presents in the third to fourth decade of life. Affected patients have a characteristic facies; dermatochalasis; lagophthalmos; pendulous ears; cranial and peripheral nerve palsies; and dry, lax skin with amyloid deposition (Fig 10-8). The ophthalmologist is often the first physician to see patients with this condition, who typically present with corneal findings. The findings are similar to those in LCD. Typical corneal lattice lines are heavier in the periphery and spread centripetally from the limbus. The central cornea is relatively spared. Corneal sensation is reduced. The risk of open-angle glaucoma may be increased, and dry eye and recurrent erosions may occur late in life.

PATHOLOGY OF FAMILIAL AMYLOIDOSIS Light microscopy shows amyloid in the lattice lines as a discontinuous band under Bowman layer and within the sclera. The amyloid in this condition is related to gelsolin and is observed to be deposited in the conjunctiva, sclera, and ciliary body; along the choriocapillaris; in the ciliary nerves and vessels; and in the optic nerve. On confocal microscopy, deposits are observed along the basal epithelial cells and

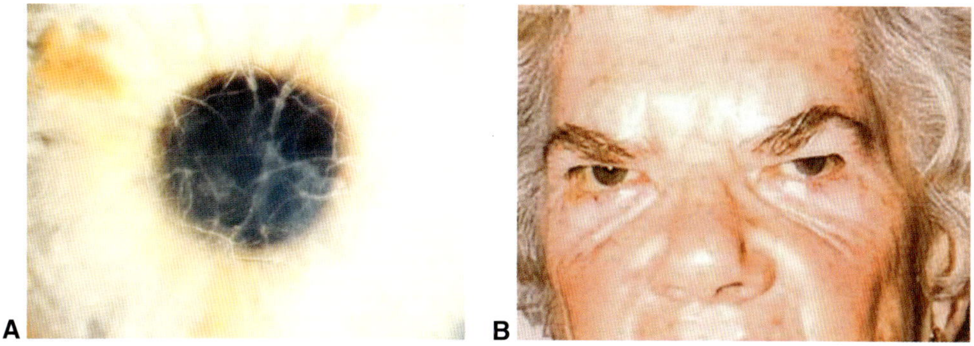

Figure 10-8 Familial amyloidosis (Meretoja syndrome). **A,** Diffuse lattice lines. **B,** Typical facies. *(Reproduced with permission from Weiss JS, Møller H, Lisch W, et al. The ICD3 classification of the corneal dystrophies.* Cornea. *2008; 27(10 Suppl 2):S16.)*

stromal nerves. On electron microscopy, amyloid has a typical filamentous appearance. Outside the eye, amyloid is detected in arterial walls, peripheral nerves, and glomeruli.

MANAGEMENT Treating the systemic manifestations requires a team approach. The ophthalmologic involvement also requires collaboration of ocular subspecialists in order to manage diplopia due to cranial nerve dysfunction, vitreous involvement, and glaucoma, should they occur. Conjunctival involvement usually does not require treatment. Management of recurrent erosions due to corneal involvement is discussed in Chapter 8. Superficial corneal disease associated with significant visual dysfunction can be managed with phototherapeutic keratectomy or with PK or LK in patients who exhibit marked stromal disease. However, the underlying condition may recur.

Reidy JJ. Corneal and conjunctival degenerations. In: Mannis MJ, Holland EJ, eds. *Cornea.* Vol 1. 4th ed. Elsevier; 2017:856–874.

Gout

Disorders of purine metabolism cause *hyperuricemia* (increased serum uric acid). *Gout* results from deposition of urate crystals in the joints or kidney.

CLINICAL PRESENTATION Acute inflammation of the sclera, episclera, or conjunctiva can occur. Fine corneal epithelial and stromal deposits may appear in the absence of inflammation. Either an orange-brown band keratopathy or a typical whitish band keratopathy is seen in rare cases.

PATHOGENESIS Hyperuricemia may be familial, arising from an enzyme deficiency, for example, hypoxanthine phosphoribosyltransferase as occurs in Lesch-Nyhan syndrome. More commonly, gout is polygenic or secondary to obesity, cytotoxic chemotherapy, myeloproliferative disease, diuretic therapy, or excessive alcohol consumption.

LABORATORY EVALUATION Serum uric acid level is typically elevated. However, in urate keratopathy, the uric acid level may be normal in the presence of keratopathy if there is no concurrent inflammation.

MANAGEMENT Indomethacin, colchicine, or phenylbutazone is used for acute treatment; long-term reduction in uric acid levels should be pursued with medications such as allopurinol. Superficial corneal deposits can be removed mechanically with scraping or keratectomy.

Wilson disease

Wilson disease *(hepatolenticular degeneration)* is an autosomal recessive disorder that results in copper deposition in multiple organs of the body, including ocular structures.

CLINICAL PRESENTATION Muscular rigidity increases, and tremor and involuntary movement gradually occur in a fluctuating course resembling Parkinsonism. Unintelligible speech and mild dementia usually occur concomitantly. Hepatic or nervous system symptoms each occur in 40% of patients. In the cornea, a golden-brown, ruby-red, or green pigment ring (Kayser-Fleischer ring) consisting of copper deposits appears in peripheral Descemet membrane (Fig 10-9), although not all patients with Wilson disease manifest this ring. The Kayser-Fleischer ring can occur in association with other conditions (eg,

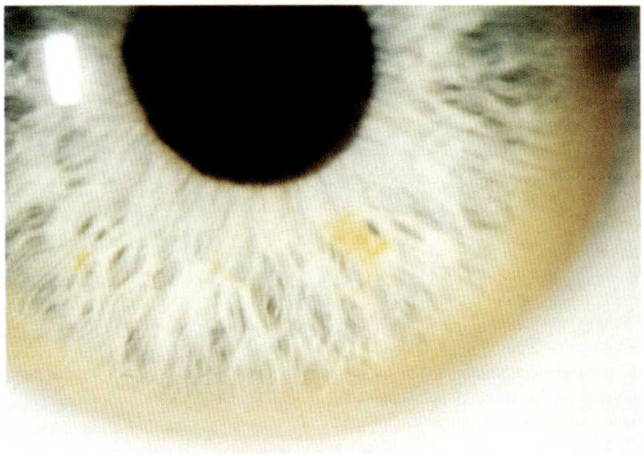

Figure 10-9 Wilson hepatolenticular degeneration. Deposits of copper in Descemet membrane (Kayser-Fleischer ring). *(Reproduced with permission from Krachmer JH, Mannis MJ, Holland EJ, eds.* Cornea. *Vol 1. 3rd ed. Elsevier/Mosby; 2011:299.)*

primary biliary cirrhosis, chronic active hepatitis, multiple myeloma, and chalcosis) and should not be confused with the iron ring seen in keratoconus (ie, Fleischer ring). Gonioscopy may assist in visualizing the ring. A "sunflower" cataract may be present. Retinal dysfunction with associated electrophysiologic abnormalities may occur.

PATHOGENESIS Wilson disease occurs as a result of multiple allelic substitutions or deletions in a Cu^{2+}-ATPase-transporting β-polypeptide, linked to mutations in the *ATP7B* gene on chromosome 13q14.3–q21. Because of these enzyme defects, copper is deposited first in the liver, then in the kidneys, and eventually in the brain and the cornea at the level of Descemet membrane (see Fig 10-9).

LABORATORY EVALUATION Patients with Wilson disease are unable to incorporate radioactive copper into ceruloplasmin. Low serum ceruloplasmin, high non-ceruloplasmin-bound serum copper, and high urinary copper are findings suggestive of the diagnosis, which can be confirmed with liver biopsy. Nonspecific findings of proteinuria, aminoaciduria, glycosuria, uricaciduria, hyperphosphaturia, and hypercalciuria are observed.

MANAGEMENT Wilson disease can be treated with penicillamine. Liver transplantation is reserved for patients with fulminant liver failure. The Kayser-Fleischer ring disappears gradually with therapy, including liver transplant, and the disappearance of the rings can be used to help monitor therapy. Electrophysiologic abnormalities from retinal dysfunction typically improve after treatment of the disease.

Porphyria

The porphyrias are a group of disorders characterized by excess production and excretion of porphyrins, which are pigments involved in the synthesis of heme, specifically in forming the nonprotein part of hemoglobin and some other biological molecules. Porphyria cutanea tarda, the form most commonly associated with ocular surface disease, is either sporadic or inherited in an autosomal dominant pattern (chromosome band 1p34).

CLINICAL PRESENTATION Hyperpigmentation, erythema, scleroderma-like changes, increased fragility, and vesicular and ulcerative lesions occur on sun-exposed surfaces of the body, including the conjunctiva and cornea. There is interpalpebral injection, and the conjunctiva may develop vesicles, scarring, and symblepharon mimicking bullous pemphigoid; conjunctival necrosis may also occur. Necrotizing scleritis has been reported. The cornea may be affected by exposure or by thinning and perforation at the limbus. Skin and ocular lesions may fluoresce.

PATHOGENESIS The enzyme uroporphyrinogen decarboxylase is deficient, resulting in an accumulation of porphyrins in the liver and in the circulation. Typically, a second insult to the liver, such as alcoholism or drug metabolism, triggers the condition in late middle age.

A severe form of porphyria, called *hepatoerythropoietic porphyria (HEP),* is a rare homozygous presentation of the same enzymatic defect, but onset of the disease is in infancy.

LABORATORY EVALUATION Reduced liver and red cell uroporphyrinogen decarboxylase confirms the diagnosis. Hepatic biopsy shows liver parenchymal cells filled with porphyrins that fluoresce bright red in ultraviolet light. Urine turns dark on standing in light.

MANAGEMENT Protection from ultraviolet light and reduction of iron by phlebotomy or subcutaneous deferoxamine are the principal treatments. No specific ocular treatment is available, although artificial tears may help wash away porphyrins. Corneal thinning and perforation are treated in standard ways.

Skeletal and Connective Tissue Disorders

Many musculoskeletal and connective tissue diseases affect the cornea. The corneal manifestations of these diseases are outlined in Table 10-7. Only the most common conditions will be discussed in this chapter.

Ehlers-Danlos Syndrome

Ehlers-Danlos syndrome (EDS), a heterogeneous group of diseases, is characterized by hyperextensibility of joints and skin, tendency to bruise easily, and formation of "cigarette paper" scars. There are more than 20 known types of EDS, which are classified as autosomal dominant, autosomal recessive, or X-linked recessive.

CLINICAL PRESENTATION Ehlers-Danlos syndrome type VI (EDS VI), or the ocular–scoliotic type, is autosomal recessive and associated with moderate joint and skin extensibility, as well as severe scoliosis. Corneal findings include keratoconus, keratoglobus, and a brittle cornea that can be easily ruptured with minor trauma. Other ocular findings include epicanthal folds, blue sclera, glaucoma, ectopia lentis, retinal detachment, and angioid streaks.

PATHOGENESIS Multiple genetic loci have been identified. Specific defects occur in collagen type I and III synthesis; lysyl hydroxylase deficiency may occur as well.

LABORATORY EVALUATION Traditionally, clinical diagnosis of EDS VI is confirmed by an insufficiency of hydroxylysine on analysis of hydrolyzed dermis and/or reduced enzyme activity in cultured skin fibroblasts. However, the diagnosis can also be confirmed by an altered urinary ratio of lysyl pyridinoline to hydroxylysyl pyridinoline, which is characteristic of EDS VI.

MANAGEMENT Recognition of EDS VI is essential. In addition, the clinician must be aware of the association with mitral valve prolapse, spontaneous bowel rupture, and strabismus

Table 10-7 Skeletal and Connective Tissue Disorders With Ocular Involvement

Name	Corneal Findings	Other Ocular Findings
Albright hereditary osteodystrophy	None	Zonular cataracts with multicolored flecks in 25% of affected patients
Apert syndrome	Exposure keratitis with severe proptosis Keratoconus (very rare) Megalocornea (very rare)	Strabismus (exotropia with V pattern) Absence of extraocular muscles; proptosis, ocular hypopigmentation, optic atrophy Rare: nystagmus, ptosis, cataract, ectopia lentis, coloboma of iris
Carpenter syndrome; acrocephalopolysyndactyly type II	Exposure keratitis secondary to severe proptosis Microcornea (rare) Corneal leukoma (rare)	Epicanthal folds, downward slant, hypertelorism or hypotelorism, optic atrophy, strabismus Rare: coloboma of the iris and choroid, congenital cataract, lens subluxation, nystagmus, retinal detachment
Cockayne syndrome Type A Type B	Raised inferior corneal lesion, band keratopathy, recurrent erosions	Cataracts, retinal dystrophy, nystagmus, iris atrophy, hyperopia, enophthalmos, strabismus
Crouzon syndrome	Exposure keratitis with severe proptosis Keratoconus (very rare) Microcornea (very rare)	Strabismus (exotropia with V pattern) Exophthalmos, hypertelorism, optic atrophy in 30% of affected patients Rare: nystagmus, glaucoma, cataract, ectopia lentis, aniridia, anisocoria, myelinated nerve fibers
Ehlers-Danlos syndrome (EDS) EDS I EDS II EDS III EDS IV EDS V EDS VI EDS VII–AD EDS VII–AR EDS VIII	Brittle cornea in type VI Keratoconus in types I and VI Keratoglobus in type VI	Epicanthal folds, blue sclera, retinal detachment, glaucoma, ectopia lentis, angioid streaks (rare)
Goldenhar-Gorlin syndrome; oculoauriculovertebral syndrome; hemifacial microsomia	Limbal dermoid	Coloboma most commonly in the upper eyelid, strabismus (25% of affected patients), Duane retraction syndrome, microphthalmos, anophthalmos, lacrimal system dysfunction, optic nerve hypoplasia, tortuous retinal vessels, macular hypoplasia and heterotropia, choroidal hyperpigmentation, iris and retinal colobomas
Hallermann-Streiff-François syndrome; oculomandibulodyscephaly	1 case of sclerocornea	Congenital cataracts, spontaneous resorption of lens cortex with secondary membranous cataract formation, glaucoma, uveitis, retinal folds, optic nerve dysplasia, microphthalmos

(Continued)

Table 10-7 *(continued)*

Name	Corneal Findings	Other Ocular Findings
Hypophosphatasia Infantile Childhood Adult	Band keratopathy with conjunctival calcifications in infantile form	Blue sclera, cataracts, optic atrophy secondary to craniostenosis, atypical retinitis pigmentosa; ocular complications present only in infantile and childhood forms, not in adult form
Marfan syndrome	Megalocornea (uncommon) Flat cornea Keratoconus (uncommon)	Ectopia lentis, strabismus, cataracts, myopia, retinal detachment, glaucoma, blue sclera
Nail–patella syndrome; onycho-osteodysplasia	Microcornea	Cataracts, microphthalmos
Oculodento-osseous dysplasia AD AR	Microcornea	Hypotelorism, convergent strabismus, anterior segment dysgenesis, glaucoma, cataracts, remnants of the hyaloid system
Osteogenesis imperfecta Type I Type II Type III Type IV	Decreased central corneal thickness Keratoconus (rare) Megalocornea (rare) Posterior embryotoxon (rare)	Blue sclera Rare: congenital glaucoma, cataract, choroidal sclerosis, subhyaloid hemorrhage, hyperopia, ectopia lentis
Parry-Romberg syndrome; progressive facial hemiatrophy	Neuroparalytic keratitis	Enophthalmos, oculomotor palsies, pupillary abnormalities, Horner syndrome, heterochromia, intraocular inflammation, optic nerve hypoplasia, choroidal atrophy
Pierre Robin malformation	Megalocornea (rare)	Congenital glaucoma, high myopia, vitreoretinal degeneration, retinal detachment, esotropia, congenital cataracts, microphthalmos
Rothmund-Thomson syndrome	Degenerative lesions of cornea	Cataracts
Treacher Collins syndrome; mandibulofacial dysostosis	Microcornea	Lower eyelid coloboma, bony orbit dysplasia, absent lower eyelid cilia, absent lower eyelid lacrimal puncta, iris coloboma, microphthalmos, strabismus, downward slant
Werner syndrome	Corneal edema secondary to endothelial decompensation following cataract surgery Poor wound healing	Presenile posterior subcapsular cataracts (age 20–30 years), proptosis, blue sclera Rare: nystagmus, astigmatism, telangiectasia of iris, macular degeneration, pigmentary retinopathy

AD = autosomal dominant; AR = autosomal recessive.

Adapted from Al-Shamekh S, Traboulsi EI. Skeletal and connective tissue disorders with anterior segment manifestations. In: Mannis MJ, Holland EJ, eds. *Cornea*. Vol 1. 4th ed. Elsevier; 2017:647–648. With permission from Elsevier.

surgery complications, as well as the potential to confuse the brittle cornea with injury due to child abuse. Use of patch grafts for repair of corneoscleral ruptures has been successful. Genetic counseling should be considered.

Marfan Syndrome

Marfan syndrome is a common autosomal dominant disorder associated with disorders of the eye (ectopia lentis) (Fig 10-10), heart (dilation of the aortic root and aneurysms of the aorta), and skeletal system (arachnodactyly, pectus excavatum, and kyphoscoliosis).

CLINICAL PRESENTATION Abnormal fibrillin synthesis leads to thinning of the sclera (blue sclera), subluxation of the lens, and flattening of the cornea. Open-angle glaucoma and cataract occur at a higher incidence and at an earlier age compared with the unaffected population. Megalocornea is uncommon, but excessive flattening, in the range of 35.00 diopters (D), may occur.

PATHOGENESIS Fibrillin and glycoprotein make up the microfibrillar system of the extracellular matrix. Fibrillin is found in corneal basement membrane, zonular fibers of the lens and capsule, and sclera. Abnormalities are caused by defects in fibrillin synthesis; Marfan syndrome is caused by mutations in the *FBN1* gene, which encodes fibrillin-1 and maps to chromosome 15q21.1.

MANAGEMENT Cardiac evaluation is important, given that premature mortality is associated with aortic complications. Treatment of lens subluxation may require the use of advanced cataract surgery techniques such as capsular tension rings or scleral fixation. In severe cases of subluxation, a pars plana approach may be a safer method to remove the lens. BCSC Section 11, *Lens and Cataract,* discusses the lens subluxation caused by Marfan syndrome and its treatment.

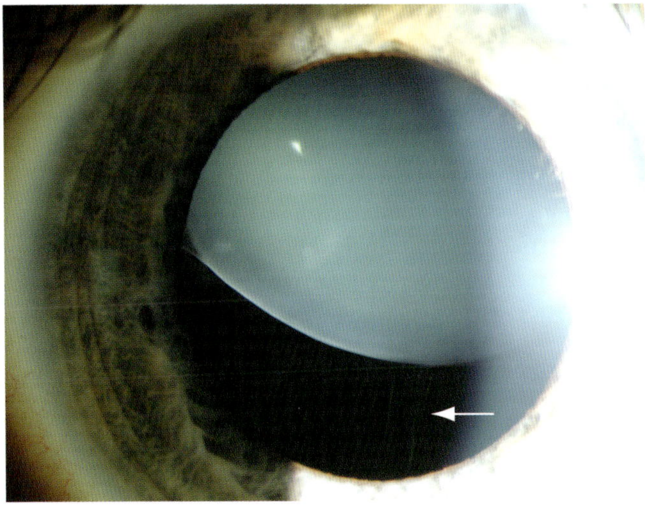

Figure 10-10 Slit-lamp photograph from a patient with Marfan syndrome, showing superior displacement of the lens. Note the stretched zonular fibers *(arrow)*. *(Courtesy of Stephen E. Orlin, MD.)*

Osteogenesis Imperfecta

Osteogenesis imperfecta (OI) is a rare, dominantly inherited condition occurring in 1 in 20,000 live births. There are 4 clinical types of OI resulting from mutations in the *COL1A1* and *COL1A2* genes. The disease causes defects in the skeleton and teeth, skin, and joints; hearing deficits; and ocular anomalies.

CLINICAL PRESENTATION Due to abnormal collagen, patients with OI are susceptible to brittle bones and multiple skeletal fractures. Conductive or sensorineural hearing loss is present in the majority of patients and usually begins in adolescence. Patients are predisposed to brittle teeth. Ocular manifestations include blue sclera (Fig 10-11), which is present throughout life in type I OI but fades within the first few years of life in the other types, and optic nerve damage due to fractures in the skull. Corneal findings include reduced central corneal thickness (average of 450 μm), keratoconus, and megalocornea. Table 10-8 summarizes other conditions associated with blue sclera. In infants and children referred for nonaccidental trauma with multiple fractures (formerly called shaken baby syndrome), OI should be considered in the differential diagnosis.

PATHOGENESIS The genetic mutation causes abnormalities of the α1 or α2 chain of type I collagen. As a result, the collagen fibrils fail to mature to their normal diameters.

MANAGEMENT Treatment with oral bisphosphonates reduces bone resorption, and aggressive orthopedic management of fractures is indicated. Low-impact exercise might help preserve bone and muscle integrity.

Goldenhar-Gorlin Syndrome

Goldenhar-Gorlin syndrome, also known as *oculoauriculovertebral (OAV) syndrome,* is a rare congenital condition characterized by incomplete development of the ear, nose, soft palate, lip, and mandible. It is associated with anomalous development of the first and second branchial arches. See Chapter 6.

CLINICAL PRESENTATION The most common corneal manifestation is a limbal dermoid (Fig 10-12A). Other ocular findings include preauricular appendages (Fig 10-12B); colobomas of the eyelids, most commonly in the upper eyelid; and strabismus. Affected patients may have hemifacial microsomia (underdevelopment), hearing difficulties, and aural fistulae. In addition, scoliosis can develop secondary to incomplete development of the vertebrae. See Table 10-7 for additional clinical findings.

Corneal dermoids can occur independently of Goldenhar-Gorlin syndrome. They are choristomas (ie, normal tissue in an atypical location) and are composed of fibrous and fatty

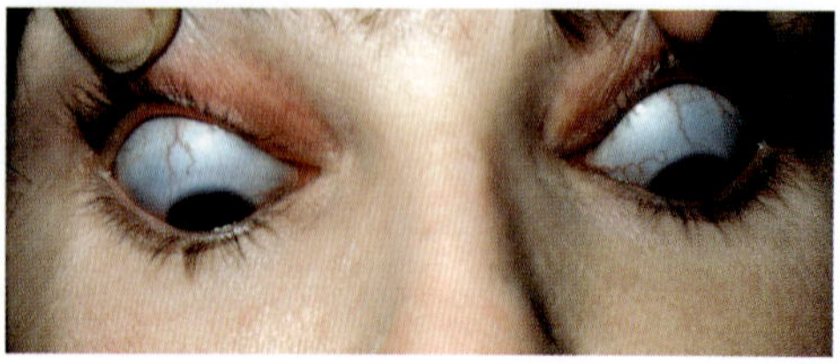

Figure 10-11 Clinical photograph shows blue sclera in a patient with osteogenesis imperfecta. *(Courtesy of Stephen E. Orlin, MD.)*

Table 10-8 Conditions and Medications Associated With Blue Sclera

Local	Systemic	Medications
High myopia	Alkaptonuria	Amiodarone
Prior necrotizing scleritis	Brittle cornea syndrome	Antimalarials
Oculodermal melanocytosis (nevus of Ota)	Ehlers-Danlos syndrome type VI	Minocycline
Previous eye surgeries	Hypophosphatasia	Phenothiazines
Thin sclerae in neonates	Marfan syndrome	
	Osteogenesis imperfecta	
	Primary adrenal insufficiency (Addison disease)	

tissue and occasionally hair and sebaceous gland material. Limbal dermoids are covered by conjunctiva and often have an arcus-like deposition of lipid along their anterior corneal border. A dermoid can involve the entire cornea and even the entire anterior segment.

PATHOGENESIS The cause of Goldenhar-Gorlin syndrome is uncertain, but it may have a genetic component.

MANAGEMENT Corneal dermoids can be associated with amblyopia as a result of significant corneal astigmatism. As an affected child grows, the dermoid may enlarge, but it will have no malignant potential. The elevated portion of the dermoid can be surgically shaved down to improve cosmetic appearance, but the lesion often extends deep into the corneal and scleral tissues. Even after surgical debulking, corneal astigmatism may remain; however, use of a rigid contact lens or a mini scleral design (MSD) lens can improve vision. LK can also improve the cosmetic appearance. Excision alone may result in significant scarring.

Al-Shamekh S, Traboulsi EI. Skeletal and connective tissue disorders with anterior segment manifestations. In: Mannis MJ, Holland EJ, eds. *Cornea.* Vol 1. 4th ed. Elsevier; 2017:645–664.

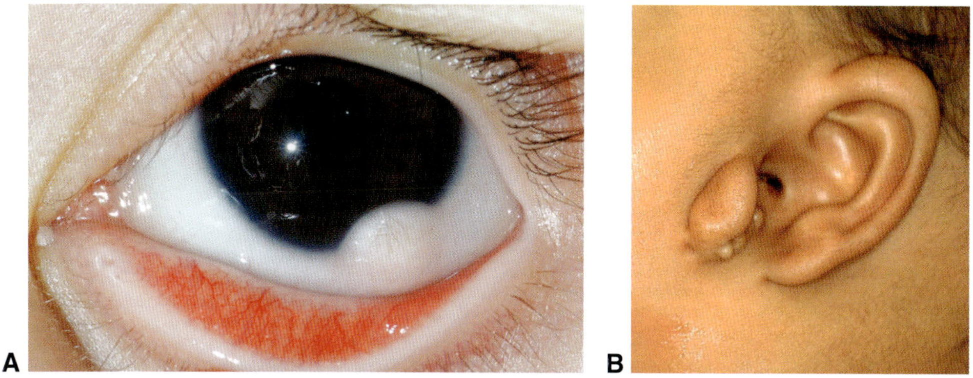

Figure 10-12 Goldenhar-Gorlin syndrome. **A,** Clinical photograph shows an inferotemporal limbal dermoid. Note the multiple hair follicles. **B,** External photograph shows preauricular appendages. *(Courtesy of Stephen E. Orlin, MD.)*

Nutritional Disorder: Vitamin A Deficiency

Vitamin A deficiency is a leading cause of blindness in countries with high rates of malnutrition and is responsible for at least 20,000–100,000 new cases of blindness worldwide each year. It is estimated that approximately 140 million children are vitamin A deficient worldwide. The earliest manifestation of vision impairment due to vitamin A deficiency is night blindness, or *nyctalopia.* At greatest risk are malnourished infants and babies born to vitamin A–deficient mothers. Concurrent corneal infections due to herpes simplex virus, measles virus, or bacteria predispose these children to keratomalacia and blindness. Although xerophthalmia usually results from low dietary intake of vitamin A, decreased absorption of vitamin A may also be responsible. In cases of vitamin A deficiency and xerophthalmia occurring in countries with a low rate of malnutrition, the condition is usually caused by unusual self-imposed dietary practices, chronic alcoholism, or lipid malabsorption (observed in cystic fibrosis, biliary cirrhosis, and bowel resection). The increase in gastric bypass surgical procedures may be expected to result in an increased incidence of vitamin A deficiency.

CLINICAL PRESENTATION A common ocular finding is the Bitôt spot (Fig 10-13), a superficial foamy, gray, triangular lesion on the bulbar conjunctiva that appears near the limbus within the palpebral aperture. This spot consists of keratinized epithelium, inflammatory cells, debris, and *Corynebacterium xerosis. Corynebacterium* bacilli metabolize the debris, producing the foamy appearance. Prolonged vitamin A deficiency may lead to corneal xerosis with corneal ulceration and scarring and may eventually cause diffuse corneal necrosis or keratomalacia. The World Health Organization classifies the ocular surface changes of xerophthalmia (X) into 3 stages:

1. conjunctival xerosis, without (stage X1A) or with (stage X1B) Bitôt spots
2. corneal xerosis (stage X2)
3. corneal ulceration, with keratomalacia involving less than one-third (stage X3A) or more than one-third (stage X3B) of the corneal surface

PATHOGENESIS Vitamin A deficiency causes blindness by inhibiting the production of rhodopsin. Xerosis (abnormal dryness) of the conjunctiva and cornea due to vitamin A

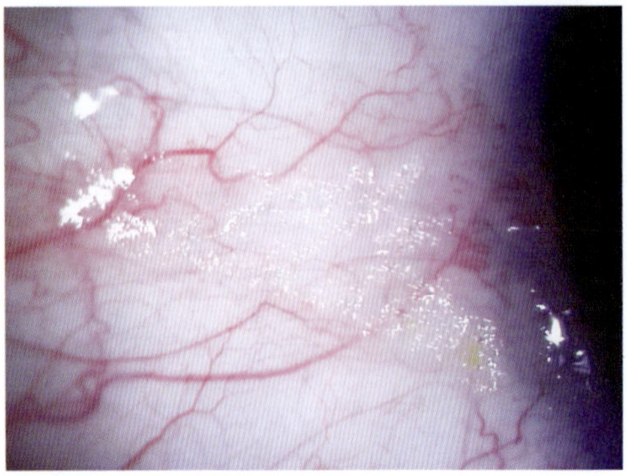

Figure 10-13 Slit-lamp photograph shows a foamy Bitôt spot in the temporal bulbar conjunctiva. *(Courtesy of Joseph D. Iuorno, MD.)*

deficiency is associated with loss of mucus production by the goblet cells. Similar changes can occur in epithelial cells of the gastrointestinal, genitourinary, and respiratory tracts.

MANAGEMENT Systemic vitamin A deficiency, associated with keratomalacia, is a medical emergency with a mortality rate of 50% if left untreated. Although administration of oral vitamin A will address the acute manifestations of keratomalacia, patients with this condition are usually affected by much broader protein-energy malnutrition and should be treated with both vitamin and protein-calorie supplements. Malabsorption may render oral administration ineffective in patients with acute vitamin A deficiency. Maintaining adequate corneal lubrication, preventing secondary infection, and protecting the cornea from keratolysis are essential steps in treating keratomalacia. More importantly, identifying and treating the underlying causes of vitamin A deficiency are vital to successful clinical management of the ocular complications.

Mannis T, Mannis MJ, Paranjpe DR, Kirkness CM. Nutritional disorders. In: Mannis MJ, Holland EJ, eds. *Cornea.* Vol 1. 4th ed. Elsevier; 2017:676–687.

Sommer A. Vitamin A deficiency and clinical disease: an historical overview. *J Nutr.* 2008;138(10):1835–1839.

Hematologic Disorders

The excess synthesis of immunoglobulins by plasma cells in multiple myeloma, Waldenström macroglobulinemia, and benign monoclonal gammopathy may be associated with crystalline corneal deposits.

CLINICAL PRESENTATION Ocular findings may include

- crystalline deposition in all layers of the cornea or in the conjunctiva
- copper deposition in the cornea (Kayser-Fleischer ring)
- sunflower cataract
- "sludging" of blood flow in the conjunctiva and retina
- pars plana proteinaceous cysts
- infiltration of the sclera
- orbital bony invasion with proptosis

Multiple myeloma is characterized by the proliferation of a single clone of plasma cells with altered immunoglobulin (Ig) production. Corneal crystalline deposits are numerous, scintillating, and polychromatic (Fig 10-14). Copper deposition has been reported at Descemet membrane and the anterior lens capsule. The deposits are typical of IgG κ-chain deposition and may be related to the size of the paraprotein and the chronicity of the disease (Video 10-1).

VIDEO 10-1 Slit-lamp view of corneal stromal crystals in a case of multiple myeloma.
Courtesy of Joseph D. Iuorno, MD.

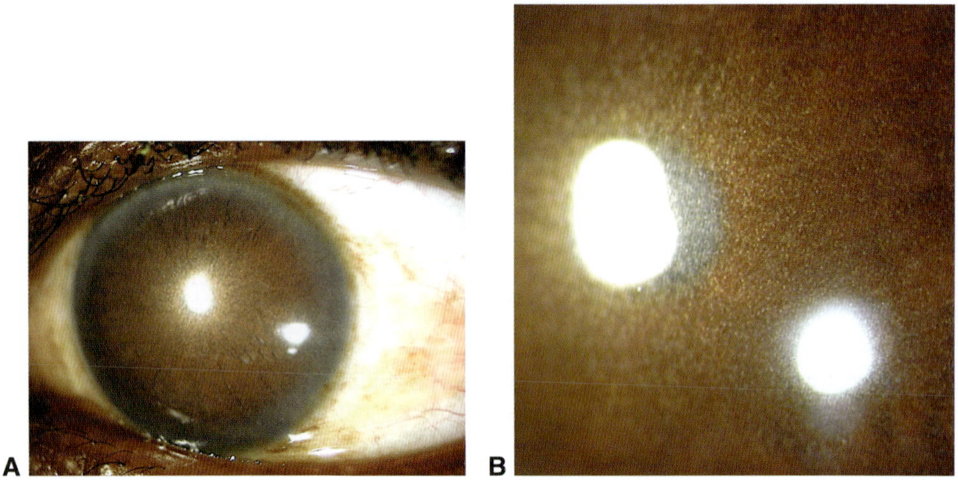

Figure 10-14 Multiple myeloma. **A,** Slit-lamp photograph shows stromal crystals. **B,** Close-up image of the same eye. *(Courtesy of Joseph D. Iuorno, MD.)*

Waldenström macroglobulinemia is characterized by malignant proliferation of plasma cells generating IgM, causing hyperviscosity syndrome, principally in older men. It has been associated with deposition of needlelike crystals in the subepithelial and deep stromal layers of the cornea (Fig 10-15).

Benign monoclonal gammopathy is a frequent (up to 6%) finding in individuals older than 60 years. Results of the systemic evaluation in these cases are negative, but a mild increase in paraprotein (<3 g/dL) is detected. Slit-lamp findings of iridescent crystals resemble those of multiple myeloma but are very infrequent (ie, occur in approximately 1%–2% of affected patients).

Cryoglobulins, proteins that precipitate upon exposure to cold, occur nonspecifically in autoimmune disorders, immunoproliferative disorders, and hepatitis B viral infection. Ophthalmic findings include occasional crystalline corneal deposits, amorphous limbal masses, and signs of retinal hyperviscosity.

PATHOGENESIS Monoclonal proliferation of plasma cells (B lymphocytes) leads to overproduction of both light (κ or λ) chains and heavy (α, γ, ε, δ, or μ) chains (collectively

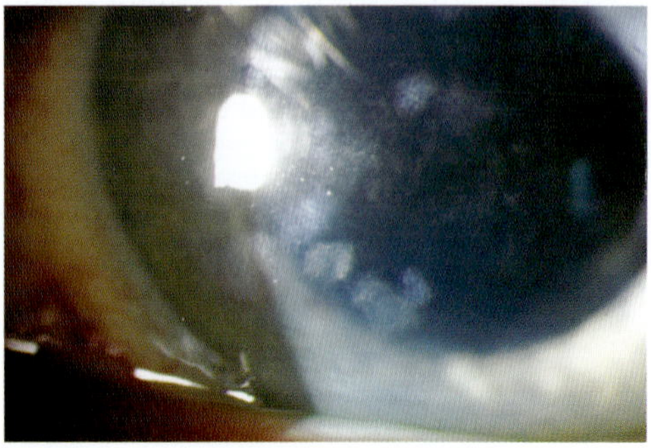

Figure 10-15 Clinical photograph from a patient with Waldenström macroglobulinemia, showing amorphous deposits in the stroma. *(Courtesy of Robert W. Weisenthal, MD.)*

termed M proteins), overproduction of light chains with or without production of heavy chains (Bence Jones proteins), or overproduction of heavy chains without light chains (ie, heavy-chain disease). Pathogenesis is related either to direct tissue invasion, particularly of the bone marrow, or to hyperviscosity syndrome. Secondary hypercalcemia may occur. Deposition of paraproteins in the cornea is very rare and is related to diffusion of the proteins—probably from the limbal vessels or, alternatively, from the tears or aqueous humor—followed by precipitation that may be related to corneal temperature or local tissue factors. There are many causes of corneal crystalline deposits; the appearance and location of the deposits can help distinguish the underlying etiology. Table 10-5 lists potential causes of corneal crystals.

LABORATORY EVALUATION Serum protein electrophoresis, complete blood count (CBC), and general screening for albumin/globulin and calcium levels are performed when clinical suspicion of immunoglobulin excess arises. Further testing for systemic evaluation depends on clinical suspicion and the initial findings.

MANAGEMENT No ophthalmic treatment is necessary unless the amorphous deposits interfere with vision and need to be removed with LK. Crystals resolve slowly after successful treatment of the underlying malignancy.

Choulakian MY. Hematologic diseases and malignancies. In: Mannis MJ, Holland EJ, eds. *Cornea*. Vol 1. 4th ed. Elsevier; 2017:688–695.

Endocrine Diseases

Diabetes

The most common disorder of carbohydrate metabolism, diabetes, has nonspecific corneal manifestations. See BCSC Section 1, *Update on General Medicine,* for detailed discussion of diabetes.

CLINICAL PRESENTATION Diabetic keratopathy includes superficial punctate epitheliopathy, epithelial erosions, hypoesthesia, persistent epithelial defects, and corneal edema. These changes occur with increasing frequency and severity in patients with long-standing disease. Surgical removal of the epithelium in patients with diabetes may result in the loss of the basal cells and basement membrane and lead to prolonged healing difficulties. Faint vertical folds in Descemet membrane and deep stroma (Waite-Beetham lines) are not specific to diabetes but may represent early corneal endothelial dysfunction and increased stromal hydration.

LABORATORY EVALUATION An increase in glycosylated hemoglobin is related to poor control of diabetes and may correlate with poor corneal healing due to recurrent erosion, wound healing, or epitheliopathy, as well as progressive retinopathy.

MANAGEMENT Diabetes is not a contraindication to cataract or PK surgery if the patient is medically stable. However, if the patient has decreased corneal sensation or a history of recurrent erosion secondary to poor epithelial adherence, laser in situ keratomileusis (LASIK) may be contraindicated. Measures that can improve diabetic epitheliopathy include the following:

- improving treatment of meibomian gland dysfunction
- increasing lubrication
- avoiding toxic medications
- minimizing epithelial debridement during retinal surgery
- using therapeutic contact lenses, exercising caution because of the risk of infection

Multiple Endocrine Neoplasia

Multiple endocrine neoplasia (MEN) represents a group of disorders that affect the endocrine system. MEN typically involves tumors in at least 2 endocrine glands; these growths can be benign or malignant. The condition is classified as MEN 1, MEN 2A, or MEN 2B, depending on the glands involved.

CLINICAL PRESENTATION MEN 1 is a disorder that involves the pituitary gland, parathyroid glands, and the islet cells of the pancreas. Visual field defects due to pituitary gland tumors may be observed. Patients with MEN 2A may have enlarged corneal nerves. MEN 2B is characterized by medullary carcinoma of the thyroid gland, pheochromocytoma, and mucosal neuromas. Patients with MEN 2B also have enlarged corneal nerves. In addition, they often have a marfanoid body habitus. Conjunctival and eyelid neuromas and keratoconjunctivitis sicca may occur. Table 10-9 lists other causes of prominent corneal nerves (Fig 10-16) from either true enlargement or increased visibility.

PATHOGENESIS MEN 2 either results from a spontaneous mutation of the *RET* gene or is inherited in an autosomal dominant fashion.

MANAGEMENT Patients with MEN should be followed by an endocrinologist to manage the multiple hormonal deficiencies that occur. In MEN 1, patients who demonstrate visual field defects require neuroradiologic testing and a team approach that includes a neurosurgeon. In MEN 2, patients with hypertension should have a workup for pheochromocytoma, and those with anterior neck masses should be evaluated for medullary carcinoma of the thyroid.

Parathyroid Disease

Parathyroid hormone and calcitonin (1 of the hormones produced by the thyroid gland) play key roles in regulating the amount of calcium in the blood and within the bones.

Table 10-9 Conditions Associated With Prominent Corneal Nerves

Systemic Diseases	Ocular Diseases
Multiple endocrine neoplasia type 2B	Keratoconus
Phytanic acid storage disease (Refsum syndrome)	Ichthyosis
Hansen disease (leprosy, beading of nerves)	Fuchs endothelial corneal dystrophy
Familial dysautonomia (Riley-Day syndrome)	Corneal edema
Neurofibromatosis	Congenital glaucoma
	Acanthamoeba perineuritis

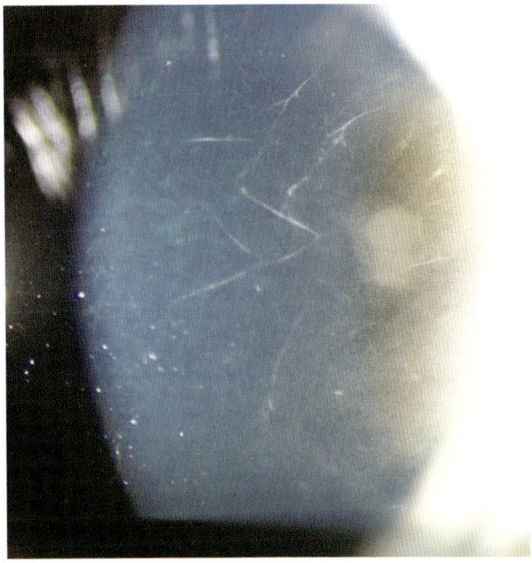

Figure 10-16 Prominent corneal nerves. *(Courtesy of Robert W. Weisenthal, MD.)*

CLINICAL PRESENTATION *Band keratopathy* can result from calcium deposition in the superficial layers of the cornea and Bowman layer within the interpalpebral fissure.

PATHOGENESIS Primary hyperparathyroidism is most commonly associated with benign proliferation of chief cells within a single parathyroid gland and, in rare cases, with MEN. Secondary hyperparathyroidism can be caused by renal disease in which excessive amounts of calcium are lost and the glands release a compensatory amount of parathyroid hormone. Parathyroid hyperplasia can occur in the presence of hypercalcemia and hypophosphatemia associated with milk-alkali syndrome, sarcoidosis, and excessive intake of vitamin D. Calcium deposition can occur despite normal parathyroid function and normal levels of systemic serum calcium. See Chapter 7 for further discussion.

MANAGEMENT If the patient is symptomatic with decreased vision or discomfort, the calcium can be removed with ethylenediaminetetraacetic acid (EDTA). See Chapter 7 for further discussion.

Darvish-Zargar M, Bartow RM. Endocrine disease and the cornea. In: Mannis MJ, Holland EJ, eds. *Cornea.* Vol 1. 4th ed. Elsevier; 2017:696–704.

Dermatologic Diseases

Dermatologic disorders, particularly those involving the eyelids, commonly have associated ophthalmic findings.

Ichthyosis

Ichthyosis represents a diverse group of hereditary skin disorders characterized by excessively dry skin and accumulation of scales. These diseases are usually diagnosed during the first year of life.

Ichthyosis vulgaris, an autosomal dominant trait, is the most common hereditary scaling disorder, affecting 1 in 250–300 people. Ocular involvement varies with this form of ichthyosis.

CLINICAL PRESENTATION Eyelid scaling, cicatricial ectropion, and conjunctival thickening are common in ichthyosis. Corneal opacities occurring independently of eyelid and conjunctival disease are noted in 50% of patients with X-linked ichthyosis but are rarely seen in patients with ichthyosis vulgaris. Dotlike opacities resembling punctuation marks appear diffusely just anterior to Descemet membrane or in deep stroma and become more apparent with age without affecting vision. (See Chapter 8 for a discussion of pre-Descemet corneal dystrophy.) Nodular corneal degeneration and band keratopathy have been described. Secondary corneal changes such as vascularization and scarring from severe ectropion-related exposure can develop.

MANAGEMENT The goal of treatment in all ichthyosis disorders is to hydrate the skin and eyelids, remove scales, and slow the turnover of epidermis, when appropriate. These disorders are not responsive to corticosteroids.

Ectodermal Dysplasia

Ectodermal dysplasia is a rare hereditary condition that displays variable defects in the morphogenesis of ectodermal structures. It is a component of at least 150 distinct hereditary syndromes. Ectodermal dysplasia represents a heterogeneous group of conditions characterized by the following:

- presence of abnormalities at birth
- nonprogressive course
- diffuse involvement of the epidermis plus at least 1 of its appendages (hair, nails, teeth, sweat glands)
- various inheritance patterns

CLINICAL PRESENTATION Many ocular abnormalities have been described in the ectodermal dysplasias, including sparse eyelashes and eyebrows, blepharitis, ankyloblepharon, hypoplastic lacrimal ducts, diminished tear production, abnormal meibomian glands, dry conjunctivae, pterygia, corneal scarring and neovascularization, cataract, and glaucoma. The ocular surface changes may be due to limbal stem cell deficiency. Although the dermatologic manifestations are nonprogressive, the corneal conditions can worsen with time.

MANAGEMENT The ocular surface changes and blepharitis can be managed with tear replacement and preservation, together with eyelid hygiene. Keratolimbal autograft transplantation in combination with PK can be considered.

Xeroderma Pigmentosum

Xeroderma pigmentosum is a rare autosomal recessive disease characterized by extreme skin photosensitivity resulting from an impaired ability to repair sunlight-induced damage to DNA.

CLINICAL PRESENTATION During the first or second decade of life, the sun-exposed skin develops areas of focal hyperpigmentation, atrophy, actinic keratosis, and telangiectasia—as if the patient had received a heavy dose of radiation. Later, many cutaneous neoplasms appear; these include squamous cell carcinoma, basal cell carcinoma, and melanoma.

Corneal findings include exposure keratopathy, ulceration, neovascularization, scarring, and even perforation. Keratoconus and gelatinous droplike corneal dystrophy have also been reported. Ocular manifestations include photophobia, tearing, blepharospasm, and signs and symptoms of keratoconjunctivitis sicca. The conjunctiva can become dry and inflamed with telangiectasia and hyperpigmentation. Pingueculae and pterygia often occur. The eyelids can be involved, with progressive atrophy, madarosis, trichiasis, scarring, symblepharon, entropion, ectropion, and sometimes even loss of the entire lower eyelid. Ocular neoplasms occur in 11% of affected patients, most frequently at the limbus. Squamous cell carcinoma is the most frequent histologic type, followed by basal cell carcinoma and melanoma.

Other dermatologic disorders that have ocular manifestations include seborrhea, staphylococcal hypersensitivity, rosacea, and atopic disease. The cornea may show marginal ulceration, neovascularization, and pannus formation. These topics are discussed in depth in Chapter 3.

MANAGEMENT Skin protection from ultraviolet radiation, including use of sunscreen and protective clothing, is the mainstay of therapy. In addition, patients with xeroderma pigmentosum should be monitored for skin and eyelid malignancies.

Mannis MJ, Macsai MS, Huntley AC, eds. *Eye and Skin Disease.* Lippincott-Raven; 1996.

Sadowsky AE. Dermatologic disorders and the cornea. In: Mannis MJ, Holland EJ, eds. *Cornea.* Vol 1. 4th ed. Elsevier; 2017:705–718.

CHAPTER 11

Infectious Diseases of the Cornea and External Eye: Viral Infections

This chapter includes a related video. Go to www.aao.org/bcscvideo_section08 or scan the QR code in the text to access this content.

Indicates selected key points within the chapter.

Highlights

- Most organisms are eventually cleared from the site of an acute infection, but some persist in the host indefinitely; for example, herpes simplex virus (HSV) and varicella-zoster virus (VZV) establish latency in trigeminal ganglion cells after primary infection.
- Topical antiviral medications for herpes simplex keratitis are rarely needed for longer than 7–10 days. Persistent disease despite topical antiviral therapy suggests misdiagnosis, medication toxicity, or immune dysfunction.
- A recombinant zoster vaccine is recommended for all immunocompetent patients 50 years and older to prevent herpes zoster and associated postherpetic neuralgia.
- Sterilizing the tonometer with alcohol does not prevent transmission of adenovirus.
- Severe acute respiratory syndrome coronavirus 2 (SARS-CoV-2), the virus that causes coronavirus disease 2019 (COVID-19), may present with conjunctivitis, and transmission is possible through ocular secretions. Thus, ophthalmologists should wear proper personal protective equipment (PPE) when examining patients.

Virology

Viruses are small (10–400 nm in diameter) obligate intracellular parasites consisting of a single- or double-stranded RNA or DNA genome surrounded by a protective protein shell, or capsid, with or without an external lipid envelope (viruses are referred to as enveloped or nonenveloped). The envelope contains an outer layer of glycoproteins or spike projections (Fig 11-1). The host cell–derived lipid bilayer or envelope is vulnerable to damage by ultraviolet (UV) light, detergents, alcohols, and general-use antiseptics.

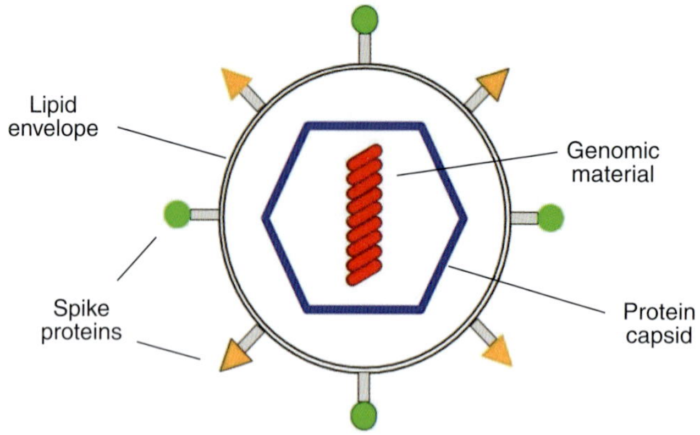

Figure 11-1 Components of virus structure. *(Courtesy of Shahzad I. Mian, MD.)*

Characteristics of *enveloped viruses* (eg, herpes simplex virus [HSV], HIV, and severe acute respiratory syndrome coronavirus 2 [SARS-CoV-2]) include the following:

- They are susceptible to the external environment.
- Their infectivity is short-lived outside the host.
- They are difficult to transmit via fomites or medical instruments.
- The use of alcohol to sterilize medical instruments is generally sufficient to prevent transmission of infection.

Characteristics of *nonenveloped viruses* (eg, adenoviruses) include the following:

- They are relatively resistant to environmental insult.
- They can persist for weeks outside the human host.
- The use of alcohol to sterilize medical instruments is not sufficient to prevent transmission of infection.

The Baltimore classification groups viruses on the basis of how messenger RNA (mRNA) is produced during viral replication (Fig 11-2). Unlike DNA viruses, which direct the host cell to replicate, RNA viruses can either direct the host cell or encode RNA polymerase enzymes to replicate RNA into DNA. While antiviral vaccines work by targeting structural proteins such as the glycoproteins bound to the membrane envelope, antiviral medications typically target viral replication. The additional step in RNA replication commonly results in mutations in the RNA viruses, leading to increased adaptability in host cells and challenges in prevention and treatment.

Viral infections are diagnosed and treated primarily on the basis of clinical evaluation. Diagnostic testing may be necessary in atypical cases, in cases slow to improve, and in order to collect objective data in public health and surveillance programs. Table 11-1 summarizes the benefits and limitations of various diagnostic techniques.

For further discussion of infectious diseases, see BCSC Section 1, *Update on General Medicine.*

King AMQ, Lefkowitz E, Adams MJ, Carstens EB. *Virus Taxonomy: Ninth Report of the International Committee on Taxonomy of Viruses.* Elsevier; 2012.

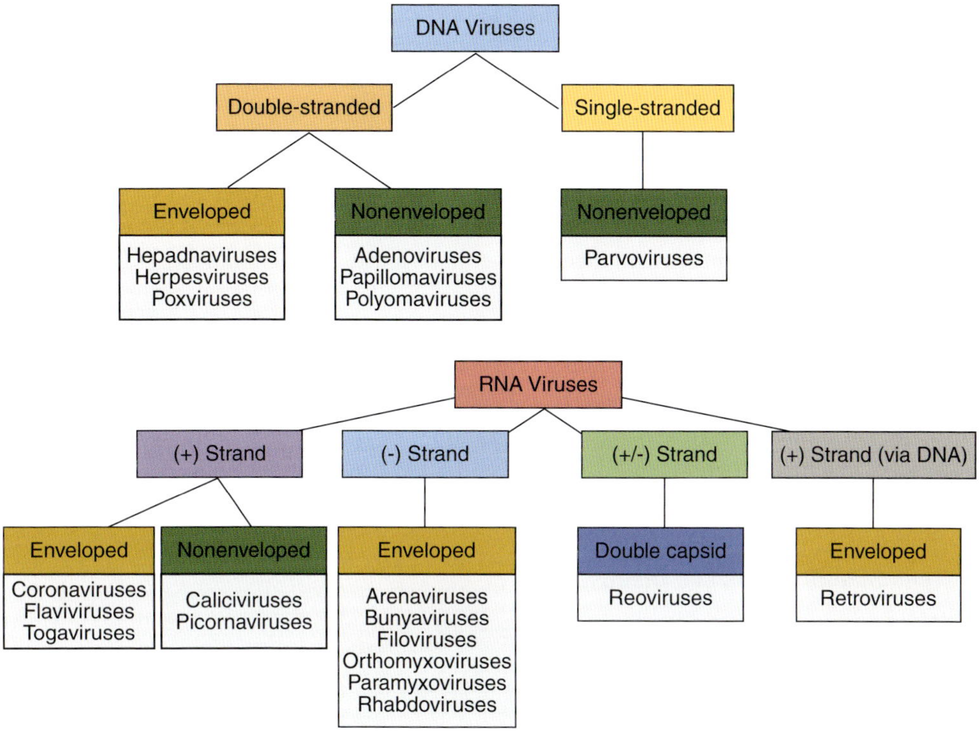

Figure 11-2 Baltimore classification of viruses. *(Courtesy of Shahzad I. Mian, MD.)*

Table 11-1 Benefits and Limitations of Diagnostic Techniques for Viral Infections

Diagnostic Techniques	Benefits	Limitations
Cell culture	Gold standard for confirmation of infections such as adenovirus and HSV	Limited survival of virus after collection; delay in getting results; cost
Serology	Increase in specific humoral antibodies is suggestive of acute infection	Negative serology result does not exclude infection; IgM detection is not always possible; there may be cross-reactivity with related pathogens
PCR	Improved accuracy in diagnosis	High cost; inefficient method for most cases, including HSV and HZV
Immunostaining	Antigen detection methods (eg, immunofluorescence, immunochromatography) do not require viable organism; can provide rapid results; point-of-care adenovirus test has high sensitivity and specificity	Variable cost

HSV = herpes simplex virus; HZV = herpes zoster virus; IgM = immunoglobulin M; PCR = polymerase chain reaction.

Rutala WA, Weber DJ; Healthcare Infection Control Practices Advisory Committee (HICPAC). Guideline for disinfection and sterilization in healthcare facilities, 2008. Centers for Disease Control and Prevention website. Updated May 2019. Accessed November 13, 2021. www.cdc.gov/infectioncontrol/guidelines/disinfection/index.html

DNA Viruses: Herpesviruses

The structure of all herpesviruses includes a core of linear double-stranded DNA genome, surrounded by an icosahedral protein capsid, which is contained in an envelope studded with viral glycoproteins. Of the 8 known human herpesviruses, those that affect the eye include herpes simplex virus types 1 and 2 (HSV-1 and HSV-2), varicella-zoster virus (VZV), Epstein-Barr virus (EBV), cytomegalovirus (CMV), and Kaposi sarcoma–associated herpesvirus (KSHV). All herpesviruses establish latency in their natural hosts, but the site of latency varies. For example, whereas HSV-1, HSV-2, and VZV establish latent infections in neurons of the sensory ganglia such as the trigeminal ganglion, EBV latency occurs in B lymphocytes.

Herpes Simplex Virus Eye Diseases

HSV infections are a worldwide public health problem, affecting an estimated one-third of the global population. Most primary exposure to HSV occurs early in life; however, primary exposure is becoming increasingly delayed.

Primary ocular infection

CLINICAL PRESENTATION Primary ocular HSV infection typically manifests as a blepharoconjunctivitis. The conjunctival inflammatory response is follicular and accompanied by a palpable preauricular lymph node. Vesicles on the skin (Fig 11-3) or eyelid margin (Fig 11-4) are important for diagnosis. Epithelial keratitis can develop in patients with primary ocular HSV infection (Fig 11-5), but stromal keratitis and uveitis are uncommon.

Signs that can help the clinician distinguish acute primary ocular HSV infection from acute primary infection associated with adenovirus include

- vesicles on the skin or eyelid margin or ulcers on the bulbar conjunctiva (common in primary ocular HSV)
- dendritic epithelial keratitis (common in HSV)
- conjunctival membranes or pseudomembranes (typical of adenovirus)

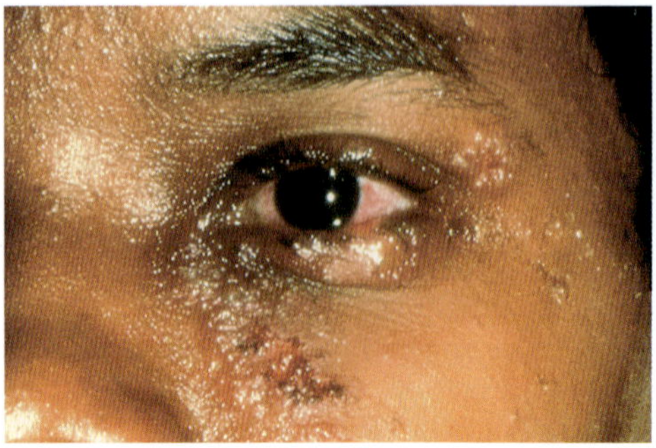

Figure 11-3 Skin vesicles of herpes simplex virus (HSV) dermatoblepharitis. *(Courtesy of James Chodosh, MD, MPH.)*

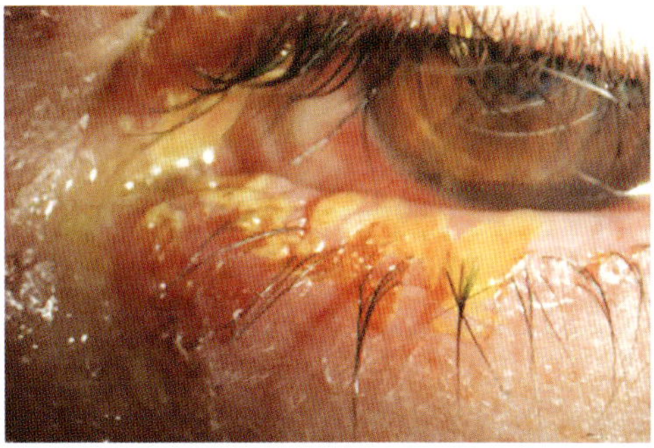

Figure 11-4 Eyelid margin ulcers characteristic of primary ocular HSV infection after vesicular rupture. *(Courtesy of Cornea Service, Paulista School of Medicine, Federal University of São Paulo.)*

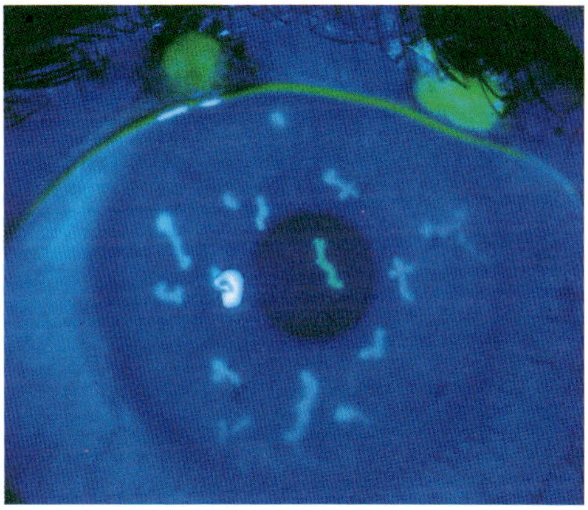

Figure 11-5 Fluorescein staining of an eye with primary HSV infection demonstrates characteristic upper eyelid margin ulcers and a coarse epithelial keratitis, which can coalesce into arborizing dendrites. *(Courtesy of James Chodosh, MD, MPH.)*

In contrast to recurrent disease, laterality is not a reliable distinguishing feature. Primary HSV infections are usually unilateral but can be bilateral. In contrast, adenoviral infections are more commonly bilateral; they can be unilateral, bilateral but asymmetric, or bilateral with delayed involvement of the second eye.

PATHOGENESIS HSV-1 and HSV-2 are antigenically related. HSV-1 more commonly causes infection above the waist (orofacial and ocular infection) and HSV-2, below the waist (genital infection); but either virus can cause disease in either location. Primary infection with HSV-1 frequently manifests as a nonspecific upper respiratory tract infection and is recognized as HSV less than 5% of the time. In industrialized societies, the age at which individuals undergo serologic conversion is increasing; HSV is now more commonly acquired in adolescence than in childhood. HSV infection is spread by direct contact with infected lesions or their secretions, usually as a result of exposure to viruses shed without clinical symptoms. HSV can be transmitted to the neonate during passage through the birth canal of a mother with active genital infection. In the newborn, HSV can cause systemic infection, including encephalitis or disease confined to the skin and mucous membranes. BCSC Section 6, *Pediatric Ophthalmology and Strabismus,* discusses congenital herpes infection in greater detail.

HSV spreads from infected skin and mucosal epithelium via sensory nerve axons to establish latent infection in associated sensory nerve ganglia, most commonly the trigeminal ganglion. Latent infection of the trigeminal ganglion may occur in the absence of recognized primary infection, and reactivation of the virus may follow in any of the 3 branches of cranial nerve V (CN V; ophthalmic nerve [V_1], maxillary nerve [V_2], and mandibular nerve [V_3]), despite primary disease in the area of innervation of a particular branch. Approximately 0.15% of the US population has a history of external ocular HSV infection. Stromal keratitis, the most common blinding manifestation associated with HSV, develops in approximately one-fifth of these individuals.

Liesegang TJ. Herpes simplex virus epidemiology and ocular importance. *Cornea.* 2001;20(1):1–13.

Pepose JS, Keadle TL, Morrison LA. Ocular herpes simplex: changing epidemiology, emerging disease patterns, and the potential of vaccine prevention and therapy. *Am J Ophthalmol.* 2006;141(3):547–557.e2.

LABORATORY EVALUATION Demonstration of HSV is possible in active epithelial infection with viral culture or antigen or DNA detection methodologies. Results of serologic tests for neutralizing or complement-fixing immunoglobulins may show a rising antibody titer during primary infection, but these tests are of no diagnostic assistance during recurrent episodes. As most adults are latently infected with HSV, serologic testing generally is helpful only when the results are negative. Laboratory tests are indicated in complicated cases when the clinical diagnosis is uncertain and in all cases of suspected neonatal herpes infection. Specimen acquisition is discussed in the online Appendix for this volume at www.aao.org/bcscappendix_section08.

MANAGEMENT Primary ocular HSV infection is a self-limited condition. Oral antiviral therapy speeds resolution of signs and symptoms. Table 11-2 summarizes the antiviral agents that are effective against ocular HSV infections. For discussion about their use, see the subsections on the respective clinical syndromes later in this chapter.

Recurrent ocular infection

CLINICAL PRESENTATION Recurrent HSV infection can affect almost any ocular tissue, including the eyelid, conjunctiva, cornea, iris, uveal tract, trabecular meshwork, retina, and optic nerve. Recurrent infection is typically unilateral, with only 3% of patients demonstrating bilateral disease. The presence of bilateral disease should increase concern for immune dysfunction (eg, atopic dermatitis).

PATHOGENESIS Recurrent HSV infection is caused by reactivation of the virus from a latently infected sensory ganglion, transport of the virus down the nerve axon to sensory nerve endings, and subsequent infection of the ocular surface. HSV latency within the cornea as a cause of recurrent disease remains a controversial concept.

Although psychological stress, systemic infection, UV light exposure, the patient's menstrual cycle, and contact lens wear are thought to act as triggers for the recurrence of HSV ocular disease, this hypothesis was not confirmed by the Herpetic Eye Disease Study (HEDS). However, there have been reports of UV light–induced reactivation of herpes labialis and keratitis. HSV keratitis recurs more frequently in patients with HIV infection, but the severity of the keratitis is equal to that occurring in immunocompetent persons.

Table 11-2 Antiviral Agents in External/Corneal Infections With Herpes Simplex Virus

Agent	Mechanism of Action	Administration	Dosage for Acute Disease
Ganciclovir	Incorporates into viral DNA preventing DNA synthesis	0.15% ophthalmic gel	Topical 5×/day until healed, then 3×/day for 1 week
Penciclovir	Inhibits viral DNA polymerase	1% dermatologic cream[a]	Topical 8×/day for 4 days
Trifluridine	Pyrimidine analogue Blocks DNA synthesis	1% ophthalmic solution	Topical 8–9×/day until healed, then 4×/day for 1 week
Vidarabine	Purine analogue Inhibits DNA polymerase	3% ophthalmic ointment[b]	Topical 5×/day for 10 days
Acyclovir	Activated by herpes simplex virus thymidine kinase to inhibit viral DNA polymerase	3% ophthalmic ointment[c] 5% dermatologic ointment[a] 200, 400, 800 mg tablet; 200-mg/5-mL suspension	Topical 5×/day for 10 days Topical 6×/day for 7 days Oral 400 mg 5×/day for 10 days
Famciclovir[d]	Prodrug of penciclovir	125, 250, 500 mg tablet	Oral 250 mg 3×/day for 10 days
Valacyclovir[d]	L-valyl ester of acyclovir	500, 1000 mg tablet	Oral 1000 mg 2×/day for 10 days
Valganciclovir	L-valyl ester of ganciclovir	450 mg tablet	Oral induction: 900 mg (2) 450-mg tablets 2×/day for 21 days Oral maintenance: 900 mg (2) 450-mg tablets once daily

[a] Not for ophthalmic use.

[b] No longer manufactured; can be obtained through compounding pharmacies.

[c] Not commercially available in the United States.

[d] Optimal dose for ocular disease not determined.

Herpetic Eye Disease Study Group. Psychological stress and other potential triggers for recurrences of herpes simplex virus eye infections. *Arch Ophthalmol.* 2000;118(12):1617–1625.

White ML, Chodosh J. Reviewed and endorsed by the Ocular Microbiology and Immunology Group. *Herpes simplex virus keratitis: a treatment guideline—2014.* American Academy of Ophthalmology; 2014. www.aao.org/clinical-statement/herpes-simplex-virus-keratitis-treatment-guideline

Blepharoconjunctivitis Eyelid and/or conjunctival involvement can occur in patients with recurrent ocular HSV infection, although it may be clinically indistinguishable from primary infection. The condition is self-limited, but it can be treated with antiviral agents to shorten the course of illness and thus reduce the exposure of the cornea to viral infection.

Epithelial keratitis One of the most common presentations of clinically recognizable recurrent ocular HSV infection is epithelial keratitis.

CLINICAL PRESENTATION Patients with epithelial keratitis may experience foreign-body sensation, light sensitivity, redness, and blurred vision. HSV infection of the corneal epithelium manifests as areas of punctate epithelial keratitis (Fig 11-6) that may coalesce into 1 or more arborizing dendritic epithelial ulcers with branches that have terminal bulbs. The swollen corneal epithelium at the edge of the ulcer stains with rose bengal (Fig 11-7) or lissamine green dye. The epithelial defect within the bed of the ulcer stains with fluorescein (Fig 11-8). (See Chapter 2 for a review of the different stains.) Areas of dendritic keratitis may coalesce further, enlarging into a more expansive geographic epithelial ulcer (Figs 11-9, 11-10), particularly when topical corticosteroids have been used.

Patients with HSV epithelial keratitis exhibit a ciliary flush and mild conjunctival injection. Mild stromal edema and subepithelial inflammatory cell infiltration may occur beneath the epithelial keratitis. Following resolution of dendritic epithelial keratitis treated with topical antiviral agents, nonsuppurative subepithelial infiltration and scarring may be seen just posterior to the area of prior epithelial ulceration, resulting in a ghost opacity, or *footprint* (Fig 11-11), which reflects the position and shape of the prior epithelial involvement. This is less likely to occur after epithelial debridement.

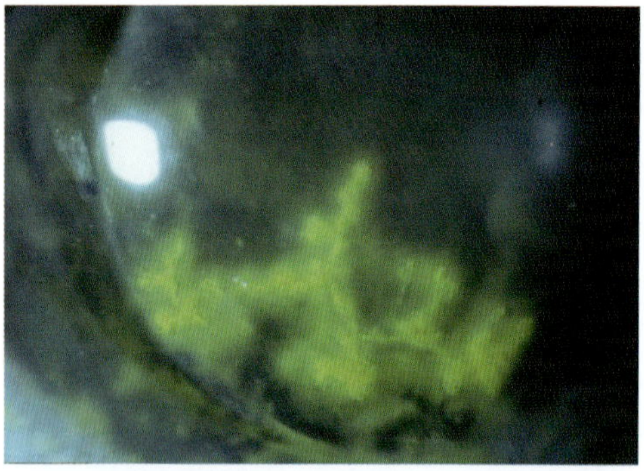

Figure 11-6 Fluorescein staining of an HSV epithelial dendrite. *(Courtesy of Terry Bergstrom, MD.)*

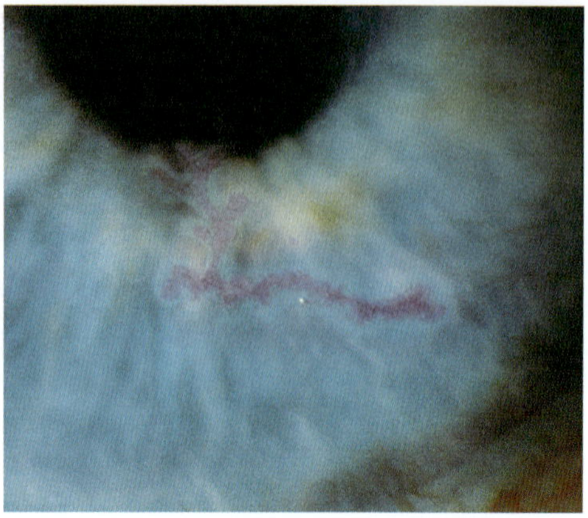

Figure 11-7 Rose bengal staining of herpetic epithelial keratitis outlines a typical dendrite. *(Courtesy of James Chodosh, MD, MPH.)*

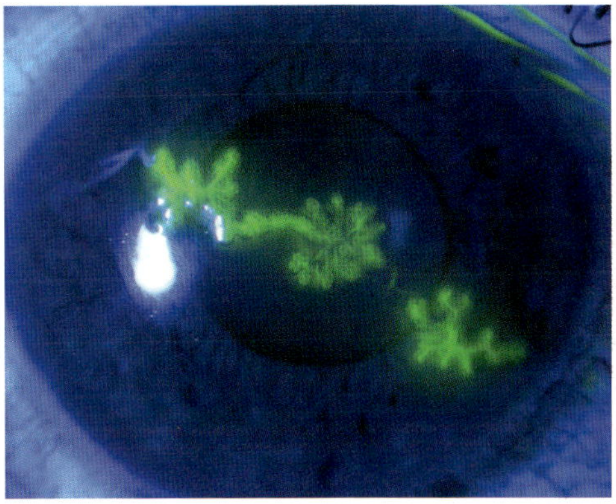

Figure 11-8 Fluorescein brightly stains the base of the HSV epithelial dendritic lesions in a cornea following laser in situ keratomileusis (LASIK). *(Courtesy of Arie L. Marcovich, MD, PhD.)*

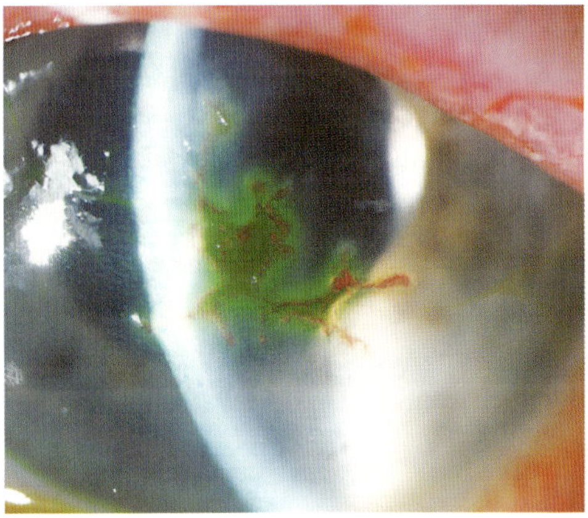

Figure 11-9 Combined fluorescein and rose bengal staining of geographic HSV keratitis. *(Courtesy of Cornea Service, Paulista School of Medicine, Federal University of São Paulo.)*

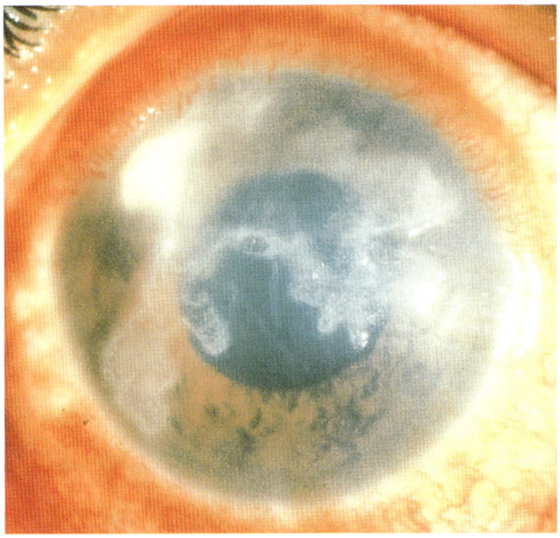

Figure 11-10 Herpetic geographic epithelial keratitis. *(Reprinted with permission from Chodosh J. Viral keratitis. In: Parrish RK, ed.* The University of Miami Bascom Palmer Eye Institute Atlas of Ophthalmology. *Current Medicine; 1999.)*

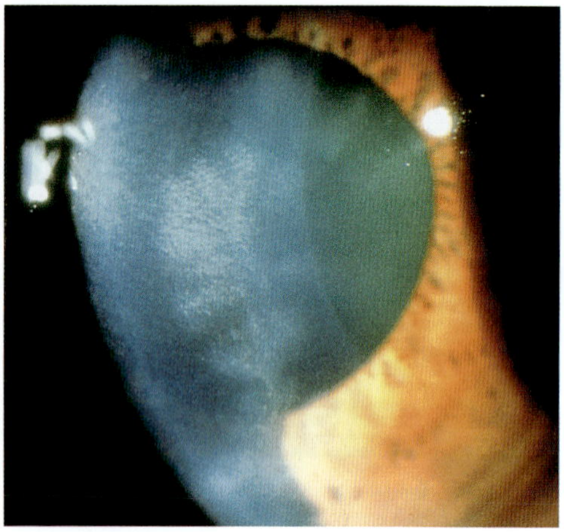

Figure 11-11 Residual stromal inflammation following dendritic epithelial keratitis may leave a ghost opacity or footprint of the dendrite. *(Reprinted with permission from Chodosh J. Viral keratitis. In: Parrish RK, ed.* The University of Miami Bascom Palmer Eye Institute Atlas of Ophthalmology. *Current Medicine; 1999.)*

Focal or diffuse reduction in corneal sensation occurs during and following HSV epithelial keratitis. The distribution of corneal hypoesthesia is related to the extent, duration, severity, and number of recurrences of herpetic keratitis. See Chapter 4 for a more detailed description of neurotrophic keratopathy.

Dendriform epithelial lesions that may be confused with epithelial keratitis may develop in various settings (Table 11-3).

LABORATORY EVALUATION A specific clinical diagnosis of HSV as the cause of dendritic keratitis can usually be made on the basis of characteristic clinical features. Multinucleated giant cells (nonspecific) and intranuclear inclusions (more typical of herpesviruses) may be seen on corneal scrapings. Tissue culture, antigen detection techniques (eg, enzyme-linked immunosorbent assay [ELISA]), and polymerase chain reaction (PCR) may be helpful in establishing the diagnosis in atypical cases.

MANAGEMENT Most cases of HSV epithelial keratitis resolve spontaneously, and there is no evidence to suggest that topical antiviral therapy influences the subsequent development of stromal keratitis or recurrent epithelial disease. However, treatment shortens the clinical course and could conceivably reduce the magnitude of any associated herpetic neuropathy, subepithelial scarring, or the potential risk of immune-mediated diseases of

Table 11-3 Differential Diagnosis of Dendriform Epithelial Lesions

Acanthamoeba epithelial keratitis	Neurotrophic keratopathy (postherpetic, diabetes)
Adenovirus (uncommon)	Soft contact lens wear (due to solutions containing thimerosal)
EBV (rare)	Topical medication use (antivirals, β-blockers)
Epithelial deposits (eg, iron lines, Fabry disease, tyrosinemia type II, systemic drug use)	VZV
Epithelial regeneration line following erosion	

EBV = Epstein-Barr virus; VZV = varicella-zoster virus.

the cornea. The following antiviral agents can be used alone or in combination with epithelial debridement:

- Trifluridine 1% solution 8 to 9 times daily is efficacious for both dendritic and geographic epithelial keratitis. Exacerbation of neurotrophic keratopathy and punctal stenosis may occur, especially with prolonged use.
- Ganciclovir 0.15% gel every 2 hours seems to have similar efficacy and may be less toxic than trifluridine.
- Acyclovir 3% ophthalmic ointment 5 times daily has been reported to be as effective as and less toxic than trifluridine, but in the United States, the ophthalmic form is available only through compounding pharmacies.
- Oral acyclovir 400 mg 5 times daily is effective and is not associated with ocular toxicity.

Frequent topical treatment is generally recommended until the epithelium is healed. The frequency is then reduced for the next week and stopped rather than tapered. Treatment of the disease with topical antivirals is generally discontinued within 10 days to avoid unnecessary toxicity to the ocular surface. Gentle epithelial debridement with a dry cotton-tipped applicator or cellulose sponge speeds resolution and may be helpful as adjunctive therapy in patients with large dendrites or drug-resistant HSV keratitis.

Oral acyclovir is commonly used because it is as effective as topical antivirals for the treatment of epithelial keratitis and does not cause ocular toxicity. Valacyclovir, a prodrug of acyclovir, is just as effective for ocular HSV disease but can cause thrombotic thrombocytopenic purpura/hemolytic uremic syndrome in severely immunocompromised patients such as those with AIDS. Caution is warranted when using valacyclovir in patients with compromised liver or kidney function or unknown immune status. Alternative systemic antiviral drugs are listed in Table 11-2.

CLINICAL PEARL

Because topical corticosteroids can potentiate dendritic keratitis, they are generally contraindicated. They should be used with great caution in the presence of active herpetic epithelial keratitis because of the risk of prolonged viral shedding and worsening of keratitis.

Patients with epithelial keratitis taking systemic corticosteroids for other indications should be treated with systemic antiviral therapy.

Stromal keratitis HSV stromal keratitis is the form of recurrent herpetic external disease associated with the greatest visual morbidity. Stromal involvement results from immunologic activity generated by the host against the virus. Each episode of active stromal keratitis increases the risk of future episodes and reduced visual function. Live virus may also be present with stromal keratitis.

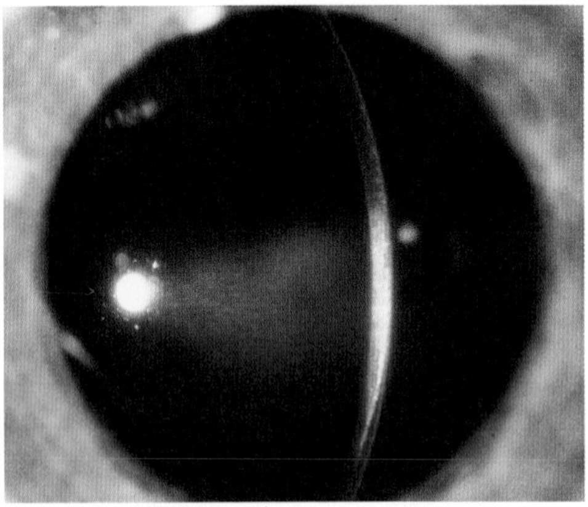

Figure 11-12 Herpetic interstitial keratitis (nonnecrotizing). *(Reprinted with permission from Chodosh J. Viral keratitis. In: Parrish RK, ed.* The University of Miami Bascom Palmer Eye Institute Atlas of Ophthalmology. *Current Medicine; 1999.)*

Table 11-4 Differential Diagnosis of Herpetic Interstitial Keratitis[a]

Acanthamoeba keratitis	Mumps keratitis
Atopic keratitis	Sarcoidosis
Cogan syndrome	Syphilis
EBV keratitis	Tuberculosis
Lyme disease	Vernal keratitis
	VZV keratitis

EBV = Epstein-Barr virus; VZV = varicella-zoster virus.
[a] See Chapter 13 for discussion of immune-mediated keratitis.

CLINICAL PRESENTATION *Herpetic stromal keratitis* can be nonnecrotizing (interstitial or disciform) or necrotizing, and different forms may present simultaneously. *Herpetic interstitial keratitis* presents as unifocal or multifocal interstitial haze or whitening of the stroma in the absence of epithelial ulceration (Fig 11-12). Mild stromal edema may accompany the haze, but epithelial edema is not typical. In the absence of significant conjunctival injection or anterior chamber cells, it may be difficult to identify active disease in an area of previous scarring and thinning. Long-standing or recurrent HSV interstitial keratitis may be associated with corneal vascularization. The differential diagnosis of herpetic interstitial keratitis is presented in Table 11-4.

Herpetic disciform keratitis is a primary endotheliitis that presents as corneal stromal and epithelial edema in a round or oval distribution, associated with keratic precipitates underlying the zone of edema (Fig 11-13). Disciform keratitis may be confused with secondary corneal endothelial decompensation due to uveitis resulting from the presence of iridocyclitis. In disciform keratitis, however, disc-shaped stromal edema and keratic precipitates appear out of proportion to the degree of anterior chamber reaction. Disciform keratitis due to HSV and that due to VZV are clinically indistinguishable.

Necrotizing herpetic keratitis appears as a suppurative corneal inflammation (Fig 11-14). It may be severe, progress rapidly, and appear clinically indistinguishable from fulminant bacterial or fungal keratitis. Overlying epithelial erosion is common, but the epithelial defect may be eccentric to the infiltrate, and the edges of the epithelial ulcer do not stain with

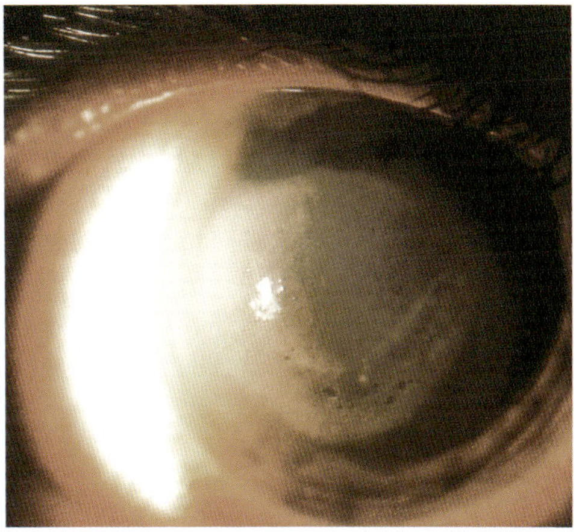

Figure 11-13 Herpetic disciform keratitis (non-necrotizing) seen with sclerotic scatter illumination. *(Reprinted with permission from Chodosh J. Viral keratitis. In: Parrish RK, ed.* The University of Miami Bascom Palmer Eye Institute Atlas of Ophthalmology. *Current Medicine; 1999.)*

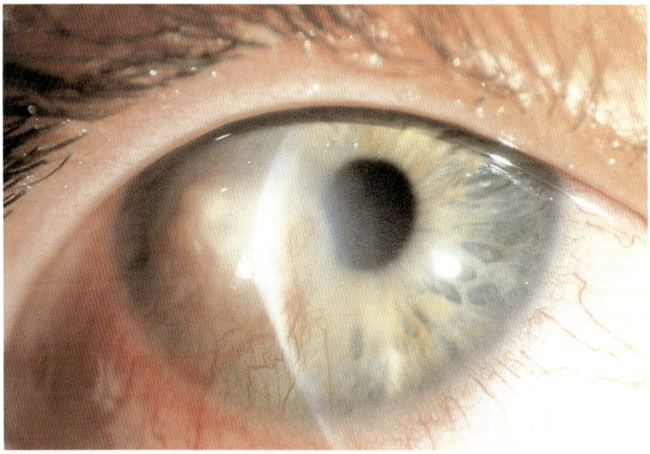

Figure 11-14 Necrotizing herpetic stromal keratitis.

rose bengal dye. Corneal stromal vascularization is common. The differential diagnosis for necrotizing herpetic keratitis includes

- microbial keratitis
  - bacterial
  - fungal
  - *Acanthamoeba*
- retained foreign body
- topical anesthetic abuse

Farooq AV, Shukla D. Corneal latency and transmission of herpes simplex virus-1. *Future Virol.* 2011;6(1):101–108.

Liesegang TJ. Herpes simplex virus epidemiology and ocular importance. *Cornea.* 2001;20(1):1–13.

Young RC, Hodge DO, Liesegang TJ, Baratz KH. Incidence, recurrence, and outcomes of herpes simplex virus eye disease in Olmsted County, Minnesota, 1976–2007: the effect of oral antiviral prophylaxis. *Arch Ophthalmol.* 2010;128(9):1178–1183.

MANAGEMENT Many past controversies regarding the optimal management of HSV stromal keratitis were resolved by the landmark HEDS (Table 11-5). Most importantly, HEDS findings showed that topical corticosteroids given with a prophylactic antiviral reduce persistence or progression of stromal inflammation and shorten the duration of HSV stromal keratitis. Long-term suppressive oral acyclovir therapy also reduces the rate of recurrent HSV keratitis and helps preserve vision. Lifelong antiviral prophylaxis is recommended for patients with multiple recurrences of HSV stromal keratitis or sight-threatening involvement.

Table 11-5 The Herpetic Eye Disease Study

Question	Study Design	Findings	Comment
Does acyclovir prophylaxis minimize HSV recurrences?	703 patients with inactive disease and off medications randomized to oral acyclovir (400 mg 2×/day) vs placebo for 12 months; followed for 18 months.	Recurrent ocular disease was less (about 50%) in acyclovir prophylaxis group, especially in patients with recurrent stromal keratitis.	Long-term prophylaxis recommended for patients with recurrent HSV stromal keratitis.
Do topical corticosteroids effectively treat stromal keratitis?	106 patients with stromal keratitis randomized to topical corticosteroids or placebo for 10 weeks. Treatment started with prednisolone 1% 8×/day and tapered to prednisolone 1/8% 1×/day. Both groups received topical trifluridine.	Yes. Topical corticosteroids significantly decreased stromal inflammation and shortened duration of keratitis.	The optimal corticosteroid regimen was not evaluated. Some patients respond to less corticosteroid and some may need a shorter/longer taper. Delaying corticosteroids for several weeks had no detrimental effect on vision.
Is oral acyclovir, in addition to treatment with trifluridine and corticosteroids, helpful in treating stromal keratitis?	104 patients with stromal keratitis randomized to oral acyclovir (400 mg 5×/day) vs placebo for a 10-week course. Both groups also received topical prednisolone and trifluridine.	No. Treatment of nonnecrotizing stromal keratitis with oral acyclovir was not beneficial.	Insufficient patients with necrotizing stromal keratitis to comment on effectiveness of acyclovir.
Is treatment-dose oral acyclovir helpful in treating HSV anterior uveitis?	50 patients with anterior uveitis treated with oral acyclovir (400 mg 5×/day) vs placebo for 10-week course.	Too few patients. A non–statistically significant trend favoring the use of oral acyclovir.	Many clinicians favor use of oral acyclovir for treatment of HSV iridocyclitis.

Table 11-5 *(continued)*

Question	Study Design	Findings	Comment
Does oral acyclovir prevent stromal keratitis and anterior uveitis from developing in patients with epithelial keratitis?	287 patients with epithelial keratitis received 3-week oral acyclovir (400 mg 5×/day) vs placebo; followed for 12 months.	No. No difference in development of stromal keratitis or anterior uveitis.	Best predictor for stromal keratitis is history of previous stromal keratitis.
What triggers HSV recurrences?	308 patients kept weekly log of stress, systemic infections, sunlight exposure, menstruation, contact lens wear, and eye injury.	No factors confirmed as triggers for recurrence.[a]	

[a] With 33 valid recurrences, none of these factors were associated with a recurrence of ocular herpes simplex virus (HSV) infection. When the 26 recurrences excluded for being reported late were examined, high stress and systemic infection were found to have been reported significantly more frequently than in the 33 valid responses.

Data from Kip KE, Cohen F, Cole SR, et al; Herpetic Eye Disease Study Group. Recall bias in a prospective cohort study of acute time-varying exposures: example from the Herpetic Eye Disease Study. *J Clin Epidemiol.* 2001;54(5):482–487.

The experimental protocol applied by HEDS investigators for patients with herpetic stromal keratitis is a useful starting point for a treatment algorithm. Initial treatment of visually significant herpetic interstitial keratitis is as follows:

- prednisolone 1% drops every 2 hours
- one of the following prophylactic antiviral drugs:
  - topical trifluridine 4 times daily
  - an oral agent such as acyclovir 400 mg twice daily
  - valacyclovir 500 mg once daily

Subsequent treatment is as follows:

- prednisolone drops, which are tapered every 1–2 weeks depending on degree of clinical improvement to the lowest possible dosage that controls the inflammation.
- an antiviral, given to prevent severe epithelial keratitis should the patient shed HSV while using corticosteroid. This is continued until the patient has completely stopped the corticosteroids, or until the use is <1 drop of prednisolone 1% per day.

Currently available topical antiviral medications are not absorbed by the cornea through an intact epithelium; in contrast, orally administered acyclovir penetrates an intact cornea and anterior chamber. In this context, anecdotal evidence suggests that the patient might benefit from oral acyclovir to treat the deep corneal inflammation of disciform keratitis. The HEDS showed no additional benefit when acyclovir was added to trifluridine and prednisolone for the treatment of herpetic stromal keratitis, but disciform keratitis was not analyzed separately. Some cornea specialists routinely substitute oral acyclovir for topical trifluridine in treating disciform keratitis.

Necrotizing stromal keratitis is probably the least common but most destructive form of herpetic keratitis. The diagnosis is frequently one of exclusion following negative cultures for fungal and bacterial pathogens, but it is suggested by a history of facial, conjunctival, and/or corneal HSV infection. The toxicity of topical antiviral agents may be undesirable in patients with necrotizing inflammation and can confuse the clinical picture. Therefore, an oral antiviral such as acyclovir is preferred. Fortunately, necrotizing herpetic keratitis seems to be very sensitive to topical corticosteroids, and twice-daily dosing may be sufficient to control inflammation in many patients.

Iridocyclitis A history or clinical evidence of prior HSV ocular disease supports a diagnosis of HSV iridocyclitis. Granulomatous or nongranulomatous iridocyclitis may accompany necrotizing stromal keratitis or occur independently of corneal disease. Elevated intraocular pressure (IOP) caused by trabeculitis, pigmentary dispersion, and/or patchy iris atrophy presenting as transillumination defects may be found in patients with HSV iridocyclitis. Viral antigen has been cultured from the anterior chamber of such patients and its presence positively correlated with ocular hypertension. Therefore, the diagnosis of HSV iridocyclitis is supported by the unilateral presentation associated with an elevated IOP, with or without prominent pigment dispersion and focal iris atrophy.

See BCSC Section 1, *Update on General Medicine,* for additional discussion of viral therapeutics and Section 2, *Fundamentals and Principles of Ophthalmology,* for discussion of specific antiviral agents.

Barron BA, Gee L, Hauck WW, et al. Herpetic Eye Disease Study. A controlled trial of oral acyclovir for herpes simplex stromal keratitis. *Ophthalmology.* 1994;101(12):1871–1882.

Herpetic Eye Disease Study Group. A controlled trial of oral acyclovir for iridocyclitis caused by herpes simplex virus. *Arch Ophthalmol.* 1996;114(9):1065–1072.

Herpetic Eye Disease Study Group. A controlled trial of oral acyclovir for the prevention of stromal keratitis or iritis in patients with herpes simplex virus epithelial keratitis. The Epithelial Keratitis Trial. *Arch Ophthalmol.* 1997;115(6):703–712.

Herpetic Eye Disease Study Group. Acyclovir for the prevention of recurrent herpes simplex virus eye disease. *N Engl J Med.* 1998;339(5):300–306.

Herpetic Eye Disease Study Group. Oral acyclovir for herpes simplex virus eye disease: effect on prevention of epithelial keratitis and stromal keratitis. *Arch Ophthalmol.* 2000;118(8):1030–1036.

Wilhelmus KR, Gee L, Hauck WW, et al. Herpetic Eye Disease Study. A controlled trial of topical corticosteroids for herpes simplex stromal keratitis. *Ophthalmology.* 1994;101(12):1883–1895.

Complications of herpetic eye disease

Complications of herpetic eye disease affect all layers of the cornea.

Epitheliopathy When topical antiviral treatment is prolonged, epitheliopathy is common, and its severity and duration are directly related to the duration of antiviral use. Topical antiviral toxicity presents most commonly as diffuse punctate corneal epithelial erosions with conjunctival injection. Limbal stem cell deficiency may result either from recurrent infection and inflammation or from the frequent use of topical antiviral drugs.

Neurotrophic keratopathy Neurotrophic keratopathy may develop in patients with reduced corneal sensation secondary to previous herpetic infection. (See the section on neurotrophic keratopathy and persistent corneal epithelial defects in Chapter 4.) Neurotrophic keratopathy is characterized by punctate epithelial erosions, sometimes with a vortex pattern of punctate fluorescein staining; chronic epithelial regeneration lines; and frank neurotrophic ulcers. These ulcers can be distinguished from herpetic epithelial keratitis by a relative absence of rose bengal staining. Neurotrophic ulcers (see Chapter 4, Fig 4-5) are typically round or oval and are located in the central, inferior, or inferonasal cornea. Corneal epithelium at the edges of a neurotrophic ulcer may appear to roll under itself and typically has a gray, elevated appearance.

Neurotrophic keratopathy may be exacerbated by topical antiviral trifluridine treatment. Mainstays of treatment include

- liberal use of nonpreserved lubricating drops, gels, and ointments
- punctal occlusion
- autologous serum

In cases of neurotrophic ulcers, treatment to prevent progressive stromal thinning and perforation includes

- bandage or scleral contact lenses
- amniotic membrane application, either self-retaining or surgical
- use of cenegermin (Oxervate), a topical recombinant human nerve growth factor, to aid corneal epithelialization
- lateral tarsorrhaphy

Metaherpetic ulcers Ulcers may also occur from neurotrophic mechanisms or a devitalized corneal stroma. Active or resolving interstitial stromal keratitis due to HSV is associated with a chronic epithelial defect that does not stain with rose bengal.

Persistent bullous keratopathy Severe or long-standing disciform keratitis may result in permanent endothelial cell deficiency with persistent bullous keratopathy. Pain and vision loss may require either endothelial keratoplasty or full thickness cornea transplantation.

Corneal scarring Stromal inflammation in general, whether interstitial or necrotizing, commonly leads to permanent corneal scarring and irregular astigmatism. Both scarring and astigmatism may improve with time in some patients. Fitting with a gas-permeable contact lens usually improves vision beyond that achieved with spectacle refraction. In patients with deep corneal stromal vascularization due to prior necrotizing herpetic inflammation, secondary lipid keratopathy may further impair vision. Topical corticosteroids may suppress new vessel growth and halt additional lipid deposition.

Surgical treatment of herpetic eye disease

Penetrating keratoplasty (PK) or deep anterior lamellar keratoplasty (DALK) is indicated in selected patients with visually significant stromal scarring not correctable with a spectacle or contact lens. Oral antiviral therapy may improve graft survival by reducing the risk of HSV recurrence, allowing more liberal use of topical corticosteroids. DALK has the advantage of eliminating the risk of endothelial rejection. Oral antiviral agents are not toxic to the corneal epithelium and are therefore generally preferable to topical antivirals in patients after keratoplasty. Optical PK is successful with respect to graft survival in nearly 80% of cases when performed in eyes without signs of active inflammation for at least 6 months prior to surgery. See Chapter 16 for additional discussion of PK and DALK.

PK is indicated in eyes with impending or frank corneal perforation due to necrotizing or neurotrophic ulcers, although stromal inflammation and ulceration may develop, and graft failure may occur. Therefore, small descemetoceles and perforations in inflamed eyes may best be treated by applying cyanoacrylate tissue adhesive and a bandage contact lens (see Chapter 5, Video 5-7) and delaying surgery until inflammation can be controlled. Amniotic membrane transplantation or conjunctival flaps may also be used for persistent epithelial defects with and without corneal thinning. After several failed keratoplasties, keratoprosthesis is an option, given the risk of subsequent graft failure due to rejection and/or recurrence in HSV corneal disease.

Varicella-Zoster Virus Dermatoblepharitis, Conjunctivitis, and Keratitis

As with other herpes viruses, VZV causes a primary infection (varicella, or chickenpox) and establishes a subsequent latent infection, occasionally followed by recurrent disease (zoster, or shingles, discussed later in this chapter). VZV infection of childhood, now uncommon in countries with widespread VZV vaccination programs, is usually a self-limited infection rarely associated with long-term sequelae. However, infection of adults or immunosuppressed individuals can be fatal. VZV infection, whether primary or recurrent, can usually be distinguished from HSV infection through a careful history and examination. Distinguishing features of each infection are listed in Table 11-6.

Primary infection

CLINICAL PRESENTATION In children, VZV infection manifests with fever, malaise, and a vesicular dermatitis that lasts 7–10 days. Except for eyelid vesicles and follicular conjunctivitis, ocular involvement is uncommon during primary infection.

Table 11-6 Differentiating Features of Eye Disease Caused by Herpes Simplex Virus and Reactivation of Varicella-Zoster Virus

	Herpes Simplex Virus	Varicella-Zoster Virus
Postherpetic neuralgia	No	Common
Pain	Moderate	Severe
Bilateral involvement	Uncommon	No
Dermatomal distribution	Incomplete	Complete
Skin scarring	No	Common
Corneal hypoesthesia	Focal or diffuse	May be severe
Recurrent epithelial keratitis	Common	Rare
Dendrite morphology	Central epithelial ulceration with terminal bulbs; geographic in presence of corticosteroids	Smaller without central ulceration or terminal bulbs; dendriform mucous plaques occur later
Iris atrophy	Patchy	Sectoral

The rash associated with chickenpox begins as macules and progresses to papules, vesicles, and then pustules that dry, crust over, and may leave individual scars. Ocular involvement may include follicular conjunctivitis, occasionally associated with a vesicular lesion on the bulbar conjunctiva or eyelid margins. Punctate or dendritic epithelial keratitis is uncommon. Although subepithelial infiltrates, microdendritic keratitis, stromal keratitis, disciform keratitis, uveitis, and elevated IOP are rare, recurrent varicella keratouveitis may cause significant morbidity in some patients.

PATHOGENESIS Primary VZV infection occurs upon direct contact with VZV skin lesions or respiratory secretions via airborne droplets and is highly contagious for previously uninfected individuals. As with HSV, the site of VZV latency is the sensory ganglia and, in approximately 20% of infected individuals, the virus reactivates later. Of all cases of VZV infection, 15% involve CN V, or the trigeminal nerve.

LABORATORY EVALUATION Acute or recurrent VZV infection can be confirmed in the laboratory by immunodiagnostic methods, viral culture, and PCR. Serologic testing is used primarily to identify adults who have not previously been infected and might benefit from prophylactic vaccination. As with HSV, scrapings from the base of a vesicle can be tested by cytology, PCR, or culture, or for the presence of VZV antigen. Conjunctival scrapings or corneal impression cytology specimens can be similarly analyzed by culture, antigen detection, or PCR.

MANAGEMENT Because infected individuals shed the virus in respiratory secretions before the onset of the characteristic rash, avoiding infected persons is not always possible. Vaccination against varicella is recommended for anyone older than 1 year without a history of chickenpox or with a negative serologic test result. The severity of signs and symptoms may be reduced in clinically ill patients by the administration of oral acyclovir. In contrast with HSV keratitis, significant VZV keratitis or uveitis can be treated with topical corticosteroids.

Recurrent infection

Although herpes zoster (shingles) in otherwise healthy children has been described in the literature, the majority of infected persons are healthy adults with no specific predisposing factors. Zoster tends to occur in patients under the conditions presented in Table 11-7.

CLINICAL PRESENTATION Zoster manifests as a painful vesicular dermatitis typically localized to a single dermatome on the thorax or face. Initially, affected patients may report fever and malaise and experience warmth, redness, and increased sensation in the affected dermatome. The most commonly affected dermatomes are on the thorax (vertebrae T3 through L3) and those supplied by CN V.

Table 11-7 Risk Factors for Herpes Zoster

Sixth to ninth decades of life	HIV infection
Use of immunosuppressive therapy	Major surgery
Systemic malignancy	Trauma
Debilitating disease	Radiation therapy

Herpes zoster ophthalmicus (HZO) (Fig 11-15) refers to involvement of the ophthalmic division (V_1) of CN V, which is affected more often than the maxillary and mandibular branches. A maculopapular rash, followed by vesicles and then pustules, is characteristic. Zoster dermatitis may result in large scabs that resolve slowly and leave significant scarring. Neurotrophic keratopathy and sectoral iris atrophy are characteristic. Inflammation of almost any ocular tissue can occur and recur in HZO.

Zoster dermatitis is accompanied by pain and dysesthesia. The pain usually decreases as lesions resolve; however, neuralgia in the affected dermatome can continue for months to years. The severity of pain ranges from mild to incapacitating. Ocular involvement occurs in more than 70% of patients with zoster of the ophthalmic division of CN V and may appear in association with the nasociliary, frontal, or lacrimal branch. Ophthalmic complications may also occur with zoster of the second (maxillary) division of CN V. In immunosuppressed patients, zoster may involve more than 1 division of the trigeminal nerve at the same time; after reactivation, disease may be chronic, and there may be multiple recurrences. See BCSC Section 2, *Fundamentals and Principles of Ophthalmology,* for discussion of the innervation of the eye and face.

Eyelid vesicular eruption can lead to secondary bacterial infection, eyelid scarring, marginal notching, loss of cilia, trichiasis, and cicatricial entropion or ectropion. Scarring and occlusion of the lacrimal puncta or canaliculi may occur resulting in dry eye disease or excessive tearing. Episcleritis or scleritis associated with zoster may be nodular, zonal, or diffuse.

Punctate and dendritic epithelial keratitis caused by viral replication in the corneal epithelium are common manifestations of ophthalmic zoster. Herpes zoster pseudodendrites

- do not have central epithelial ulceration (like HSV dendrites)
- form branching lesions
- resemble raised or "stuck-on" mucous plaques
- stain minimally with fluorescein and rose bengal dyes
- have blunt ends rather than terminal bulbs

The elevated dendriform mucous plaques may occur on the cornea weeks to months after resolution of the skin lesions. These may be chronically culture-positive for VZV in patients with AIDS. Diminished corneal sensation occurs in up to 50% of patients.

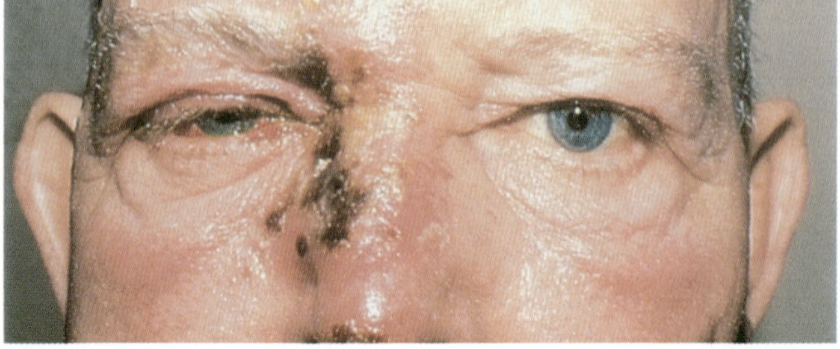

Figure 11-15 Herpes zoster ophthalmicus (HZO). *(Courtesy of Vincent P. deLuise, MD.)*

Nummular corneal infiltrates are said to be characteristic of zoster stromal keratitis (Fig 11-16), but the interstitial keratitis, disciform keratitis, and anterior uveitis with increased IOP in HZO are clinically indistinguishable from those caused by HSV infection. Chronic corneal stromal inflammation can lead to corneal vascularization, lipid keratopathy (Fig 11-17), and corneal opacity. Corneal anesthesia may be profound, and neurotrophic keratopathy due to HZO can be difficult to manage.

Focal choroiditis, occlusive retinal vasculitis, and retinal detachment have been reported. Ipsilateral acute retinal necrosis (ARN) temporally associated with HZO is uncommon. Dilated fundus examination is recommended in patients with HZO to rule out posterior segment involvement.

Orbital or central nervous system involvement resulting from an occlusive arteritis may lead to eyelid ptosis, orbital edema, and proptosis. Papillitis or retrobulbar optic neuritis may also develop. Cranial nerve palsies, when meticulously investigated, have been reported to occur in up to one-third of cases of HZO; CN III (oculomotor nerve) is the most commonly affected CN. Cranial nerve involvement may occur within the orbit or the cavernous sinus. Systemic dissemination is unusual in immunocompetent patients but can occur in up to 25% of those who are immunocompromised.

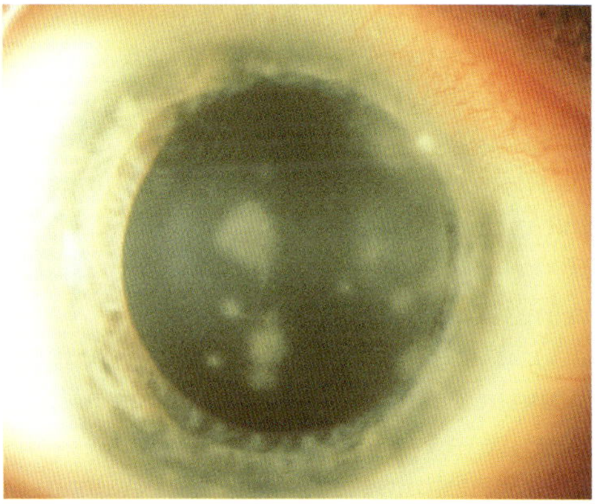

Figure 11-16 Nummular keratitis of HZO. *(Courtesy of Rhea L. Siatkowski, MD.)*

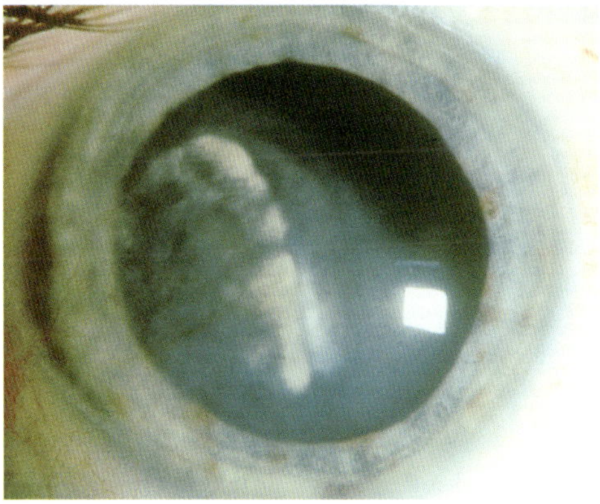

Figure 11-17 Lipid keratopathy following HZO. *(Reprinted with permission from Chodosh J. Viral keratitis. In: Parrish RK, ed.* The University of Miami Bascom Palmer Eye Institute Atlas of Ophthalmology. *Current Medicine; 1999.)*

PATHOGENESIS Following primary infection, VZV establishes latency in sensory ganglia. Zoster represents endogenous reactivation of latent virus in individuals with a waning level of immunity to infection.

MANAGEMENT The US Food and Drug Administration (FDA) has approved 2 varicella-zoster vaccines for the prevention of shingles. The live zoster vaccine (Zostavax) became available in 2006, but as of November 2020, it is unavailable in the United States. The Centers for Disease Control and Prevention (CDC) had recommended 1 dose of Zostavax for adults aged 60 years and older. The vaccine reduced the risk for developing zoster by 51.3% and was 66.5% effective for preventing postherpetic neuralgia (PHN).

CLINICAL PEARL

A recombinant zoster vaccine (Shingrix), available since 2017, is recommended by the CDC administered as 2 doses separated by 2 to 6 months for immunocompetent adults aged 50 years and older.

The efficacy of the Shingrix vaccine for the prevention of herpes zoster was 96.6% in persons aged 50–59 years and 97.4% in persons aged 60–69 years. Efficacy for PHN prevention was 91.2% in adults older than 50 years and 88.8% in those older than 70 years.

Studies indicate that the incidence of herpes zoster rises with increasing age, starting from age 50 years, suggesting that the vaccine should be recommended for persons younger than 60 years. Vaccines are generally less effective in patients with advanced age because their immune response to the vaccine is less robust. There are currently no clear recommendations concerning the use of the adult vaccine in patients with previous HZO, but the potential to reactivate or exacerbate HZO-related ocular inflammation exists. It is suggested that vaccinations be administered during an extensive quiet period.

Randomized clinical trials have found that oral antiviral therapy for HZO reduces viral shedding from vesicular skin lesions, reduces the chance of systemic dissemination of the virus, and decreases the incidence and severity of the most common ocular complications. If begun within 72 hours of the onset of symptoms, oral antiviral therapy may reduce the duration and severity if not the incidence of PHN. There are also reports to suggest that initiating antiviral therapy after 72 hours, especially in the presence of new vesicles, is beneficial.

The current treatment recommendation for HZO is oral valacyclovir 1 g 3 times per day, acyclovir 800 mg 5 times per day, or famciclovir 500 mg 3 times per day, for 7–10 days, best if started within 72 hours of the onset of skin lesions. Topical antiviral medications are not effective, except in the treatment of corneal epithelial mucoid plaques or more chronic epithelial disease. Intravenous acyclovir therapy (10 mg/kg every 8 hours) is indicated in patients at risk for disseminated zoster due to immunosuppression. Cutaneous lesions may be treated with warm, moist compresses and topical antibiotic ointment. Topical corticosteroids and cycloplegics are indicated for keratouveitis. The use of oral corticosteroids is controversial, as no clear impact has been shown on the incidence or duration of PHN. However, some clinicians use a tapering dosage for patients older than 60 years with HZO to reduce subsequent PHN. The Zoster Eye Disease Study (ZEDS) is currently evaluating whether prophylaxis with oral antivirals may be indicated to reduce risk of recurrent ocular complications, including epithelial and stromal keratitis and anterior uveitis, after HZO.

Postherpetic neuralgia may respond to capsaicin cream applied to the involved skin, but low doses of amitriptyline, desipramine, clomipramine, or carbamazepine may be necessary to control severe symptoms. Gabapentin and pregabalin can also be efficacious in managing PHN. For a patient with significant pain, early referral to a pain management specialist can be considered. Aggressive lubrication with nonpreserved artificial tears, gels, or ointments, as well as topical cenegermin (Oxervate), combined with punctal occlusion and tarsorrhaphy, if needed, are helpful in managing neurotrophic keratopathy.

CDC. Shingles (herpes zoster) vaccines. Centers for Disease Control and Prevention website. Reviewed September 9, 2020. Accessed November 13, 2021. www.cdc.gov/vaccinesafety/vaccines/shingles-herpes-vaccine.html

Liesegang TJ. Herpes zoster ophthalmicus: natural history, risk factors, clinical presentation, and morbidity. *Ophthalmology.* 2008;115(2 Suppl):S3–S12.

Liesegang TJ. Varicella zoster virus vaccines: effective, but concerns linger. *Can J Ophthalmol.* 2009;44(4):379–384.

Lo DM, Jeng BH, Gillespie C, Wu M, Cohen EJ. Current practice patterns and opinions on the management of recent-onset or chronic herpes zoster ophthalmicus of Zoster Eye Disease Study investigators. *Cornea* 2019;38(1):13–17.

Oxman MN, Levin MJ, Johnson GR, et al; Shingles Prevention Study Group. A vaccine to prevent herpes zoster and postherpetic neuralgia in older adults. *N Engl J Med.* 2005;352(22):2271–2284.

Schmader KE, Levin MJ, Gnann JW Jr, et al. Efficacy, safety, and tolerability of herpes zoster vaccine in persons aged 50–59 years. *Clin Infect Dis.* 2012;54(7):922–928.

Epstein-Barr Virus Dacryoadenitis, Conjunctivitis, and Keratitis

CLINICAL PRESENTATION Diagnosis of EBV dacryoadenitis, conjunctivitis, and keratitis is made on the basis of a history of recent infectious mononucleosis and/or persistently high EBV serologic titers. EBV is the most common cause of acute dacryoadenitis, characterized by inflammatory enlargement of 1 or both lacrimal glands. Acute follicular conjunctivitis, Parinaud oculoglandular syndrome, and bulbar conjunctival nodules have been reported in patients with acute infectious mononucleosis and may be the result of EBV infection. EBV-associated keratitis may be unilateral or bilateral and may, in select cases, appear similar to the interstitial keratitis induced by HSV, VZV, Lyme disease, adenovirus, or syphilis. There are 3 principal forms of EBV stromal keratitis:

- type 1: multifocal subepithelial infiltrates that resemble adenoviral keratitis
- type 2: multifocal, blotchy, pleomorphic infiltrates with active inflammation (Fig 11-18) or granular ring-shaped opacities (inactive form) in the anterior to midstroma
- type 3: multifocal deep or full-thickness peripheral infiltrates, with or without vascularization, that resemble interstitial keratitis due to syphilis

Because ocular disease resulting from EBV is rare, clinical suspicion for it is usually low; EBV should be considered in patients with disease refractory to conventional antiviral treatment.

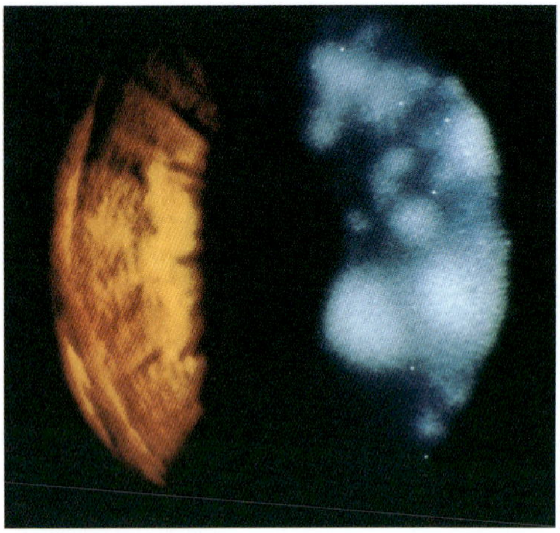

Figure 11-18 Type 2 stromal keratitis caused by Epstein-Barr virus. *(Reprinted with permission from Chodosh J. Viral keratitis. In: Parrish RK, ed.* The University of Miami Bascom Palmer Eye Institute Atlas of Ophthalmology. *Current Medicine; 1999.)*

PATHOGENESIS EBV is a common herpesvirus that infects most humans by early adulthood. Spread of EBV occurs through the sharing of saliva, and the virus results in subclinical infection in the first decade of life. If acquired later in life, it can cause infectious mononucleosis. The virus remains latent in B lymphocytes and pharyngeal mucosal epithelial cells throughout life.

LABORATORY EVALUATION Because it is difficult to isolate the virus, the diagnosis of EBV infection depends on the detection of antibodies to various viral components. During acute infection, first immunoglobulin (Ig) M and then IgG antibodies to viral capsid antigens (VCAs) appear. Anti-VCA IgG may persist throughout the patient's life. There is an increase in the level of antibodies to early antigens during the acute phases of the disease and a subsequent decrease to low or undetectable levels in most individuals. Antibodies to EBV nuclear antigens appear weeks to months later, providing serologic evidence of past infection. EBV PCR can increase the number of positive diagnoses by more than 16% by confirming a positive IgM VCA in the absence of heterophilic antibodies.

MANAGEMENT Acyclovir is not an effective treatment for the clinical signs and symptoms of infectious mononucleosis, but the impact of antiviral therapy on the corneal manifestations of EBV infection remains unknown. Corticosteroids may be effective in patients with reduced vision due to apparent EBV stromal keratitis, but they should not be administered without a prophylactic antiviral if HSV infection is a possibility.

Luderer R, Kok M, Niesters NGM, Schuurman R, de Weerdt O, Thijsen SFT. Real-time Epstein-Barr PCR for the diagnosis of primary EBV infections and EBV reactivation. *Mol Diagn.* 2005;9(4):195–200.

Cytomegalovirus Keratitis and Anterior Uveitis

CMV is a widespread herpesvirus that infects more than 90% of humans by 80 years of age.

CLINICAL PRESENTATION CMV has been most commonly associated with a sectoral, necrotizing retinitis that is found almost exclusively in patients with AIDS and other immunocompromised states. Few anterior segment complications were associated with CMV retinitis, with the exception of thin stellate keratic precipitates. In rare cases, epithelial and stromal CMV keratitis have been described, usually when CMV infection was undiagnosed prior to keratoplasty. However, CMV has been increasingly identified as a significant cause of anterior uveitis and corneal endotheliitis (Fig 11-19). It should be suspected in patients presenting with graft rejection that does not respond well to corticosteroids. The presence of keratic precipitates, endothelial cell loss, and diffuse or local corneal edema suggests CMV endotheliitis. The anterior uveitis is characterized by acute or chronic anterior chamber inflammation, with moderate to severe increases in IOP that are variably responsive to topical corticosteroids. These presentations are often misdiagnosed as HSV-related endotheliitis, trabeculitis, Posner-Schlossman syndrome, or endothelial graft rejection and can be distinguished only by their response to therapy and by results of laboratory investigation.

PATHOGENESIS Spread of CMV occurs through the sharing of saliva, ingestion of breast milk, or sexual contact. CMV causes subclinical infection in children and a nonspecific febrile illness lasting 1–3 weeks in adults. A viremia transmits the virus to the bone marrow, where it becomes latent until activated, which enables expression and shedding of the virus.

LABORATORY EVALUATION Laboratory confirmation of CMV-associated anterior segment disease is usually accomplished through PCR testing for CMV in the aqueous humor. Aqueous humor is obtained by an anterior chamber tap, which must be performed during an episode of active disease for greatest yield. Concurrent serum testing should also be performed to rule out a systemic viremia as a cause of intraocular detection. In addition, concomitant testing for other herpesviruses can be performed. CMV-associated

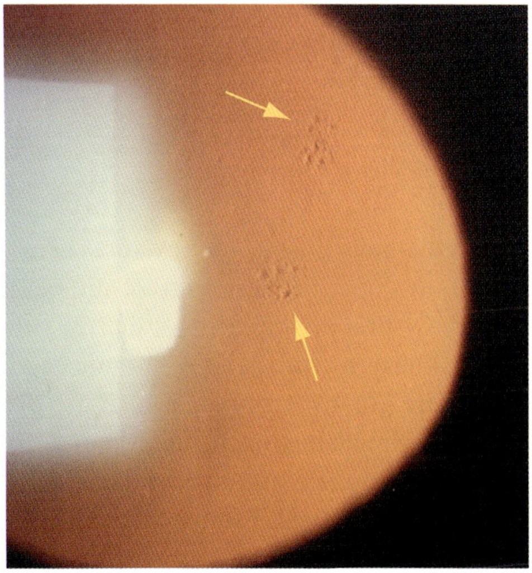

Figure 11-19 Clusters of keratic precipitates *(arrows)* in cytomegalovirus corneal endotheliitis. *(Courtesy of Cornea Service, Paulista School of Medicine, Federal University of São Paulo.)*

anterior segment disease may also be diagnosed through histologic examination of corneal biopsy or surgical specimens.

MANAGEMENT The optimal treatment of CMV-associated anterior segment disease is unknown, but treatment with oral valganciclovir 900 mg twice daily, with the possibility of lower maintenance dosing, is effective.

> **CLINICAL PEARL**
>
> CMV-associated anterior segment disease is treated with ganciclovir or its prodrugs and is not responsive to famciclovir or acyclovir or its derivatives. Resistance of a presumed HSV infection to these agents raises suspicion about the diagnosis of CMV.

Valganciclovir, a prodrug of ganciclovir, may be poorly tolerated, and recurrence of disease with withdrawal of the medication is common. Alternatives include ganciclovir implants and topical ganciclovir, which has demonstrated therapeutic effects when used as an adjunct to systemic therapy and when used in a maintenance role. Recurrence is possible after keratoplasty. The role of corticosteroids is unclear, as corticosteroid use may prolong or worsen CMV-associated anterior segment disease. Caution is warranted when using corticosteroids in these patients.

Carmichael A. Cytomegalovirus and the eye. *Eye (Lond).* 2012;26(2):237–240.

Chan ASY, Mehta JS, Al Jajeh I, Iqbal J, Anshu A, Tan DTH. Histological features of *Cytomegalovirus*-related corneal graft infections, its associated features and clinical significance. *Br J Ophthalmol.* 2016;100(5):601–606.

Chee SP, Bacsal K, Jap A, Se-Thoe SY, Cheng CL, Tan BH. Corneal endotheliitis associated with evidence of cytomegalovirus infection. *Ophthalmology.* 2007; 114(4):798–803.

Koizumi N, Suzuki T, Uno T, et al. Cytomegalovirus as an etiologic factor in corneal endotheliitis. *Ophthalmology.* 2008;115(2):292–297.e3.

Other DNA Viruses

Adenoviruses

The Adenoviridae are nonenveloped, double-stranded DNA viruses. Adenoviruses cause a broad spectrum of diseases, including infections of the upper respiratory tract and ocular surface, meningoencephalitis, acute hemorrhagic cystitis in young boys, diarrhea in children, acute respiratory disease in children and military recruits, and respiratory and hepatic failure in an immunocompromised host. There are 49 serotypes, which are divided into 6 distinct subgroups on the basis of genetic sequencing. Each subgroup (A–F) of adenoviruses and, to a lesser degree, each serotype has unique tissue affinity that results in the association of specific adenoviruses with distinct clinical syndromes.

Knipe DM, Howley PM, eds. *Fields Virology.* 7th ed. Wolters Kluwer; 2020.

CLINICAL PRESENTATION Most adenoviral eye disease presents clinically as 1 of 3 classic syndromes:

- simple follicular conjunctivitis (multiple serotypes)
- pharyngoconjunctival fever (most commonly serotype 3 or 7)
- epidemic keratoconjunctivitis (usually serotype 8, 19, or 37, subgroup D)

The different adenoviral syndromes are indistinguishable early in infection and may be unilateral or bilateral.

Adenoviral follicular conjunctivitis is self-limited, not associated with systemic disease, and often so transient that patients do not seek care. Epithelial keratitis, if present, is mild and fleeting.

Pharyngoconjunctival fever is characterized by fever, headache, pharyngitis, follicular conjunctivitis, and preauricular adenopathy. The systemic signs and symptoms may mimic those of influenza. Any associated epithelial keratitis is mild.

Epidemic keratoconjunctivitis (EKC) is the only adenoviral syndrome with significant corneal involvement and may be preceded by an upper respiratory tract infection. EKC is bilateral in most patients. One week to 10 days after inoculation, severe follicular conjunctivitis develops, associated with a punctate epithelial keratitis. The conjunctival morphology is follicular but may be obscured by chemosis. Petechial conjunctival hemorrhages and, occasionally, larger subconjunctival hemorrhages can occur. Preauricular adenopathy is prominent. Pseudomembranes or true membranes, which bleed upon removal (Fig 11-20) and consist of mucus, fibrin, and inflammatory cells, occur predominantly on the tarsal conjunctiva. It can therefore be helpful to evert the upper lid for evaluation if the diagnosis is not otherwise obvious. Patients report tearing, light sensitivity, and foreign-body sensation. Although both eyes are often involved, signs and symptoms are typically less pronounced in the second eye. Large central geographic corneal erosions can develop and may persist for several days despite patching and lubrication. Within 7–14 days after onset of ocular symptoms, multifocal, moderate-sized, subepithelial and anterior stromal corneal infiltrates become apparent on slit-lamp examination (Fig 11-21). Photophobia and

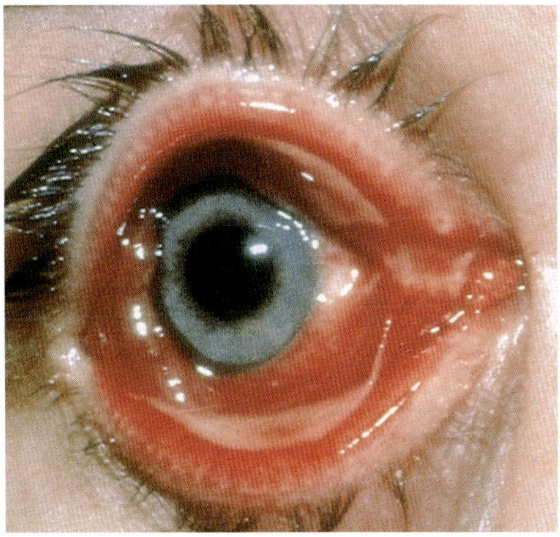

Figure 11-20 Conjunctival membranes in a patient with epidemic keratoconjunctivitis (EKC). *(Courtesy of James Chodosh, MD, MPH.)*

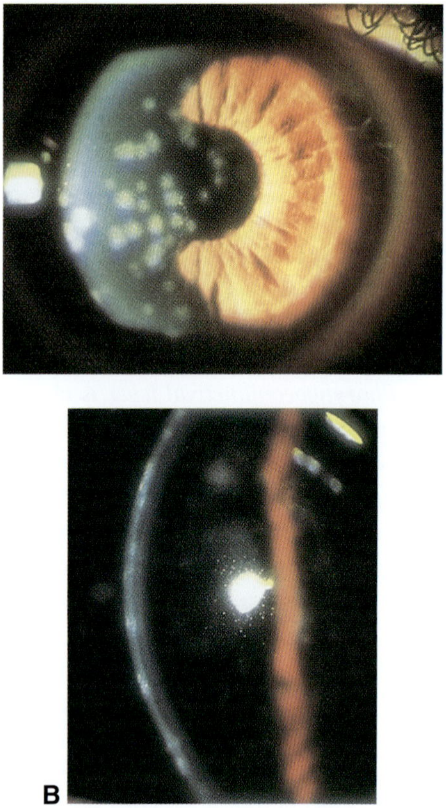

Figure 11-21 Subepithelial corneal infiltrates in a patient with EKC. **A,** Infiltrates are well visualized with a broad oblique slit beam. **B,** Slit beam demonstrates the superficial location of infiltrates. *(Courtesy of Vincent P. deLuise, MD.)*

reduced vision from adenoviral subepithelial infiltrates may persist for months to years. The evolution of keratitis in EKC is summarized in Figure 11-22. Long-term complications of conjunctival membranes include subepithelial conjunctival scarring, symblepharon formation, and dry eye due to alterations within the lacrimal glands or lacrimal ducts.

PATHOGENESIS Adenoviruses are transmitted by close contact with ocular or respiratory secretions, contaminated fomites, or contaminated swimming pools. Transmission occurs more readily in populations living in close quarters, such as schools, nursing homes, military housing, and summer camps.

Transmission of adenoviruses by contaminated instruments or eyedrops in physicians' offices may also occur. For this reason, IOP measurements should preferably be taken with an instrument that has a disposable cover.

TONOMETER TIP DISINFECTION

An alcohol prep pad does not eradicate adenovirus from the tonometer tip. Tonometer tip cleaning requires application of dilute bleach (1 part household bleach [containing 5.25%–6.15% sodium hypochlorite] and 9 parts water) for at least 10 minutes. Care must be taken to clean residual bleach from the tonometer tip before use to prevent corneal toxicity.

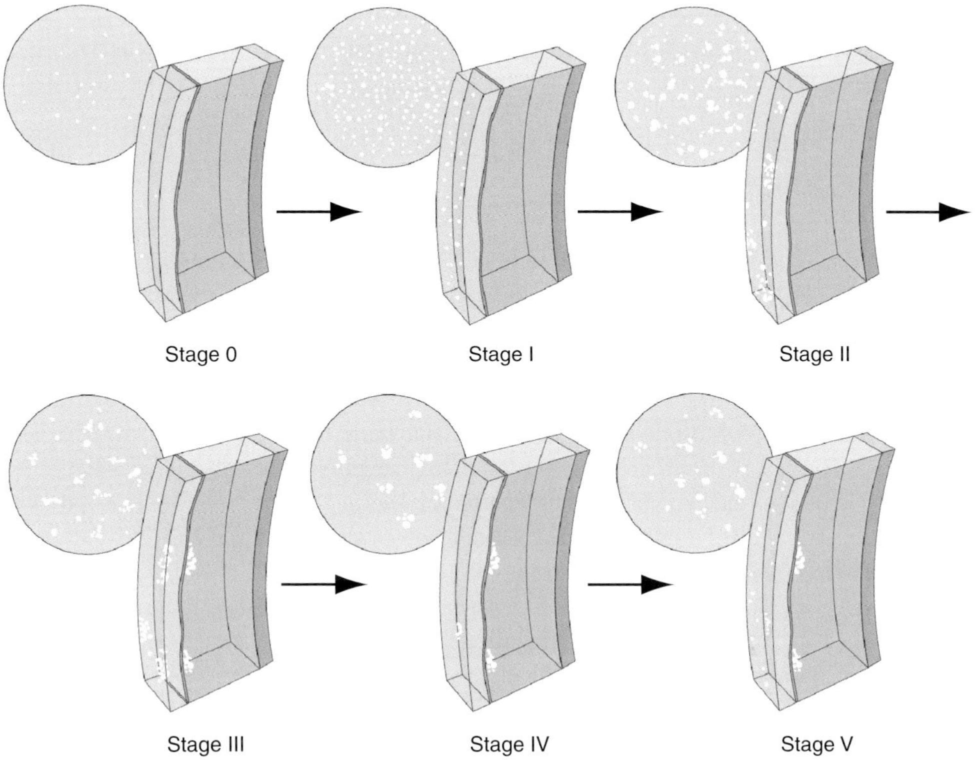

Figure 11-22 Schematic drawing illustrating the natural progression of specific corneal epithelial and stromal pathology in EKC. *Stage 0,* Poorly staining, minute punctate opacities within the corneal epithelium. *Stage I,* Fine punctate epithelial keratitis (PEK). *Stage II,* Fine and coarse PEK. Stains brightly with rose bengal. *Stage III,* Coarse granular infiltrates within deep epithelium, early subepithelial infiltrates, and diminished PEK. *Stage IV,* Classic subepithelial infiltrates without PEK. *Stage V,* Punctate epithelial granularity adjacent to and distinct from the subepithelial infiltrates. *(Adapted from Jones DB, Matoba AY, Wilhelmus KR.* Problem solving in corneal and external diseases. *Course 626, presented at the American Academy of Ophthalmology; 1995.)*

In EKC, epithelial keratitis occurs because of adenovirus replication within the corneal epithelium. Subepithelial infiltrates are likely caused by an immunopathologic response to viral infection of keratocytes in the superficial corneal stroma.

LABORATORY EVALUATION The diagnosis of EKC is suspected in patients with bilateral follicular conjunctivitis associated with petechial conjunctival hemorrhages, conjunctival membrane formation, or the subsequent presence of bilateral subepithelial infiltrates. Although viral cultures readily differentiate adenovirus from HSV infection, the clinical disease typically subsides or resolves before results become available. A rapid immunodetection assay to detect adenovirus antigens in the conjunctiva is commercially available.

MANAGEMENT Therapy for adenoviral ocular infection is primarily supportive. Cool compresses and artificial tears may provide symptomatic relief. Topical combination antibiotic-corticosteroid drops may be indicated only when the clinical signs, such as mucopurulent discharge, suggest an associated bacterial infection or when a viral cause is less certain. Some clinicians advocate peeling the pseudomembranes associated with acute adenoviral conjunctivitis (Video 11-1).

VIDEO 11-1 Peeling/stripping a pseudomembrane.
Courtesy of Joseph D. Iuorno, MD.

Topical corticosteroids also reduce photophobia and improve vision impaired by adenoviral subepithelial infiltrates. Corticosteroids may prolong adenovirus shedding. Their use should be reserved for patients with more severe symptoms and signs of adenovirus infection, including conjunctival membranes and reduced vision due to bilateral subepithelial infiltrates. Nonsteroidal anti-inflammatory drugs are ineffective for treating subepithelial infiltrates, but they may be helpful in preventing recurrence following tapering of the corticosteroids. Topical cyclosporine 1% or other immunomodulatory agents may be considered when other therapies fail. In addition, a combination of povidone-iodine 1.0% and dexamethasone 0.1% 4 times daily can reduce symptoms and expedite recovery in patients with EKC.

Actively infected persons readily transmit adenoviruses. Viral shedding may persist for 10–14 days after the onset of clinical signs and symptoms. Transmission can be prevented by personal hygiene measures, including frequent handwashing; avoiding the sharing of towels, pillowcases, and handkerchiefs; and disposal of contaminated facial tissues. Individuals who work with the public, in schools, or in health care facilities in particular should consider a temporary leave of absence from work to prevent infecting others. Patients are considered infectious if they are still injected and tearing. It is more difficult to assess transmissibility in patients treated with topical corticosteroids, who may still shed the virus even though the disease appears to be well controlled.

Kovalyuk N, Kaiserman I, Mimouni M, et al. Treatment of adenoviral keratoconjunctivitis with a combination of povidone-iodine 1.0% and dexamethasone 0.1% drops: a clinical prospective controlled randomized study. *Acta Ophthalmol.* 2017;95(8):e686–e692.

Poxviruses

The Poxviridae are a large family of enveloped, double-stranded DNA viruses, with a distinctive brick or ovoid shape and a complex capsid structure. The best-known poxviruses are molluscum contagiosum, vaccinia (cow pox), and variola (smallpox).

Molluscum contagiosum

CLINICAL PRESENTATION A molluscum nodule is smooth, with an umbilicated central core. In comparison to a keratoacanthoma, it is smaller and associated with less inflammation. The diagnosis is based on detection of the characteristic eyelid lesions in the presence of a follicular conjunctivitis. Punctate epithelial erosions and, in rare cases, a corneal pannus may occur. A careful search for eyelid margin molluscum lesions should be initiated in the presence of chronic follicular conjunctivitis (Fig 11-23). Extensive facial and eyelid lesions can be observed in cases of poorly controlled AIDS (Fig 11-24). It can also present in young girls as a result of sharing makeup.

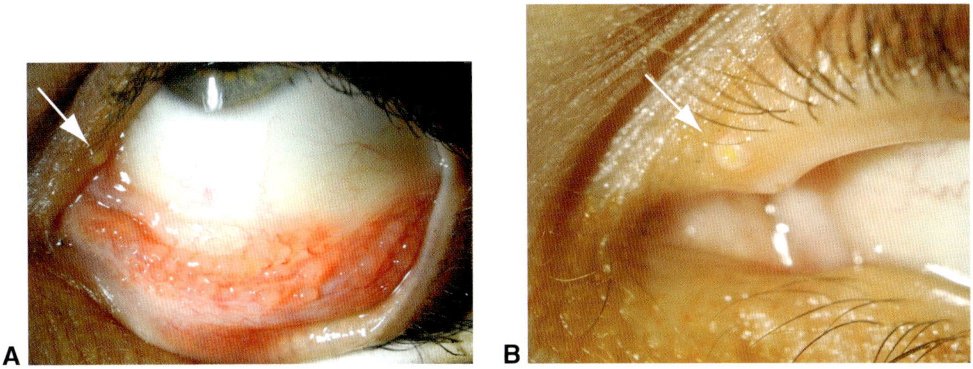

Figure 11-23 Molluscum contagiosum. **A,** Follicular conjunctivitis with a molluscum lesion *(arrow)*. **B,** Higher-magnification view of umbilicated lid lesion *(arrow)*. *(Courtesy of Christopher J. Rapuano, MD.)*

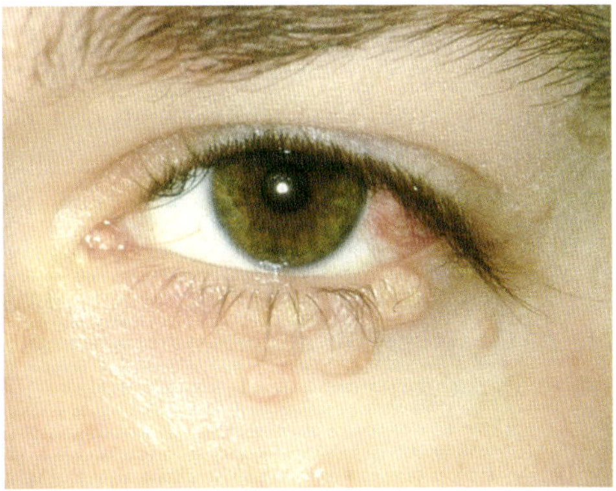

Figure 11-24 Multiple molluscum contagiosum lesions on the eyelid of a patient with AIDS. *(Courtesy of James Chodosh, MD, MPH.)*

PATHOGENESIS Molluscum contagiosum virus is spread by direct contact with infected individuals. Infection produces 1 or more nodules on the skin and eyelid margin and, less commonly, on the conjunctiva. Eyelid nodules release viral particles into the tear film, which leads to follicular conjunctivitis.

LABORATORY EVALUATION The molluscum contagiosum virus cannot be cultured using standard techniques. Histologic examination of an expressed or excised nodule shows eosinophilic, intracytoplasmic inclusions within epidermal cells.

MANAGEMENT Spontaneous resolution occurs but can take months to years. Treatment options include complete excision, cryotherapy, or incision and curettage of the central portion of the lesion.

Vaccinia

Concern that smallpox (variola) virus might be used as a biological weapon has prompted the reinstitution of a smallpox vaccination program, especially for military personnel, using live vaccinia virus. Ocular complications from self-inoculation have been reported, including potentially severe periorbital pustules, conjunctivitis, and keratitis. Treatment includes topical trifluridine. Use of vaccinia-immune globulin (VIG) is controversial but is indicated for severe ocular disease. Concern about the use of VIG stems from limited rabbit studies that have demonstrated a possible increase in corneal scarring. Individuals who are immunosuppressed, atopic, pregnant, breastfeeding, allergic to the vaccine, or living with a high-risk household contact should not receive the vaccine because of the risk of possibly fatal, progressive vaccinia.

Fillmore GL, Ward TP, Bower KS, et al. Ocular complications in the Department of Defense Smallpox Vaccination Program. *Ophthalmology.* 2004;111(11):2086–2093.

Neff JM, Lane JM, Fulginiti VA, Henderson DA. Contact vaccinia—transmission of vaccinia from smallpox vaccination. *JAMA.* 2002;288(15):1901–1905.

Papillomaviruses

Human papovaviruses, also called human papillomaviruses (HPVs), are small, nonenveloped, double-stranded DNA viruses with an icosahedral capsid. Persistent viral infection of susceptible epithelial cells induces cellular proliferation and can lead to malignant transformation. (See the section Tumors of Epithelial Origin in Chapter 14.) Early viral gene products stimulate cell growth and lead to a skin wart or a conjunctival papilloma. As HPV-containing basal epithelial cells mature and differentiate into superficial epithelial cells, they allow for complete viral gene expression and produce infectious virus. HPV-16 and HPV-18 stereotypically integrate their viral genome into host chromosomal DNA, which is associated with malignant transformation and squamous cell carcinoma. Immunization strategies designed to reduce the incidence of cervical cancer are specifically targeted against HPV oncogenes, which may result in a decreased incidence of these tumors in the future.

Verrucae and *papillomas* are caused by papillomavirus infection of the skin and conjunctival epithelium (Fig 11-25). Papillomavirus-associated conjunctival intraepithelial neoplasia and squamous cell carcinoma share many histologic features with similar lesions in the uterine cervix. Another neoplasm, Kaposi sarcoma of the skin or conjunctiva, is associated with infection with human herpesvirus-8, not HPV. (See Chapter 14.)

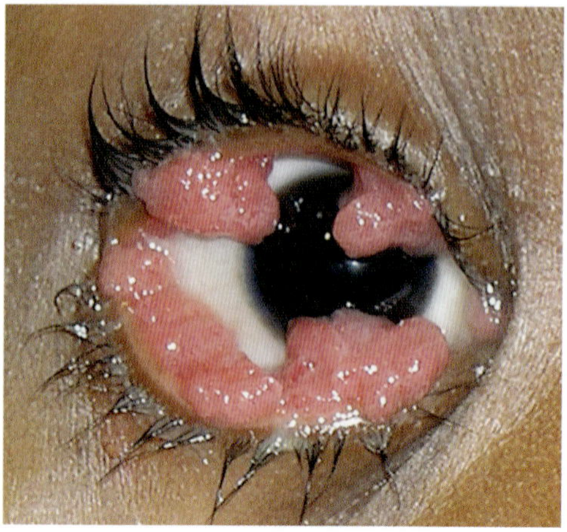

Figure 11-25 Conjunctival papillomas. *(Courtesy of Elmer Y. Tu, MD.)*

MANAGEMENT Medical therapeutic options include systemic cimetidine 30 mg/kg daily in 3 divided doses for 3 months or more, or topical interferon-α_{2b} 4 times daily for the same treatment period. "No-touch" surgical excision with adjuvant cryotherapy is the preferred surgical option and is followed by administration of oral cimetidine or topical interferon, as described above. Seeding of adjacent conjunctiva may occur following surgical excision, resulting in spread.

Kaliki S, Arepalli S, Shields CL, et al. Conjunctival papilloma: features and outcomes based on age at initial examination. *JAMA Ophthalmol.* 2013;131(5):585–593.

RNA Viruses

Eye infections due to RNA viruses are less common than those due to DNA viruses, and these infections usually manifest as follicular conjunctivitis associated with an upper respiratory tract infection (Table 11-8). Certain RNA virus infections may cause pathologic changes in virtually any ocular tissue; for example, influenza virus can affect the lacrimal gland, cornea, iris, retina, optic nerve, and other cranial nerves.

Coronaviruses

COVID-19

Coronavirus disease 2019 (COVID-19) is a multiorgan disease caused by severe acute respiratory syndrome coronavirus 2 (SARS-CoV-2), a single-stranded, enveloped RNA virus. In 2020, the disease rapidly spread worldwide, resulting in a pandemic. Patients with COVID-19 can also have ocular involvement; the most common manifestations are consistent with conjunctivitis. The incidence ranges from 0.8% to 31.6%.

Table 11-8 RNA Viruses Known to Cause Ocular Surface Disease

Virus Family	Virus	Clinical Syndrome
Coronaviridae	SARS-CoV-2	COVID-19
Orthomyxoviridae	Influenza	Follicular conjunctivitis Inflammation of the lacrimal gland, cornea, iris, retina, optic nerve, and other cranial nerves
Paramyxoviridae	Avulavirus	Newcastle disease
	Measles (rubeola)	Follicular conjunctivitis, measles keratopathy
	Mumps	Follicular conjunctivitis
Picornaviridae	Rhinovirus	Common cold Follicular conjunctivitis
Retroviridae	HIV	Seroconversion conjunctivitis
Rhabdoviridae	Rabies	Transmission via corneal transplant
	Enterovirus 70	Acute hemorrhagic conjunctivitis
	Coxsackievirus A24	Acute hemorrhagic conjunctivitis
Togaviridae	Rubella	Congenital rubella syndrome: salt-and-pepper retinopathy, microphthalmos, cataract, deafness, congenital heart disease, other systemic abnormalities

COVID-19 = coronavirus disease 2019; SARS-CoV-2 = severe acute respiratory syndrome coronavirus 2.

In addition to primary ocular infection directly related to COVID-19, patients who are critically ill can develop secondary ocular disease. Patients in the intensive care unit are at high risk for ocular surface diseases, such as exposure keratopathy, with rates of up to 40%. In ventilated patients who have acute respiratory distress syndrome, prone positioning is often used to improve gas exchange. This practice can not only cause ocular surface disease but can also be associated with increased IOP and ischemic optic neuropathy. A rare COVID-19–related inflammatory disease has been reported to develop in children; this condition has been named *pediatric multisystem inflammatory syndrome.* Children with this syndrome exhibit symptoms similar to those observed in Kawasaki disease and toxic shock syndrome (TSS), including fever, conjunctivitis, abdominal pain, and rash. To date, treatment has been primarily supportive. However, intravenous remdesivir has been shown to shorten the length of time patients stay in the hospital. Convalescent plasma from patients who have recovered is under evaluation for treatment of those with moderate to severe disease. The use of dexamethasone has shown efficacy in patients with severe respiratory disease. Several vaccines have shown a high degree of efficacy in large clinical trials. The vaccines appear to be safe when evaluated over the time period that complications would be expected to occur. Large-scale production and distribution are the current challenges.

Paramyxoviruses

The Paramyxoviridae are a family of single-stranded, enveloped RNA viruses that cause numerous human diseases. Historically, the most-recognized paramyxoviruses have been measles and mumps.

Measles

The classic triad of postnatally acquired measles (rubeola) consists of cough, coryza, and follicular conjunctivitis. Mild epithelial keratitis may be present. Optic neuritis, retinal vascular occlusion, and pigmentary retinopathy occur less commonly. Measles keratopathy, a major source of blindness in resource-limited regions globally, typically presents as corneal ulceration in malnourished, vitamin A–deficient children (see Chapter 10). A rare and fatal complication of infection with the measles virus, subacute sclerosing panencephalitis (SSPE), occurs in approximately 1 per 100,000 cases, often years after clinically apparent measles.

Mumps

Infection with the mumps virus may result in dacryoadenitis, sometimes concurrent with parotid gland involvement. Follicular conjunctivitis, epithelial and stromal keratitis, anterior uveitis trabeculitis, and scleritis have all been reported within the first 2 weeks after onset of parotitis.

Rubella

Rubella virus, when acquired in utero, may cause microphthalmos, corneal haze, cataracts, iris hypoplasia, iridocyclitis, glaucoma, and salt-and-pepper pigmentary retinopathy. Congenital ocular abnormalities due to rubella are much worse when maternal infection occurs early in pregnancy. Measles, mumps, and rubella are all uncommon in places where childhood vaccination is regularly performed.

Picornaviruses

Picornaviruses are single-stranded, nonenveloped viruses that can cause ocular disease.

Acute hemorrhagic conjunctivitis

Acute hemorrhagic conjunctivitis (AHC), caused by enterovirus 70, coxsackievirus A24 variant, and, less commonly, adenovirus 11, is one of the most dramatic ocular viral syndromes. It is characterized by sudden onset of follicular conjunctivitis in association with multiple petechial hemorrhages of bulbar and tarsal conjunctiva. The hemorrhages may become confluent and resemble those associated with trauma. Eyelid edema, preauricular adenopathy, chemosis, and punctate epithelial keratitis may be associated with infection. AHC is highly contagious and occurs in large and rapidly spreading epidemics. In approximately 1 out of 10,000 cases due to enterovirus 70, a polio-like paralysis follows; neurologic deficits are permanent in up to one-third of affected individuals.

Retroviruses

Retroviruses are single-stranded, enveloped RNA viruses that encode a viral enzyme, reverse transcriptase, that assists in conversion of the single-stranded RNA genome into a circular double-stranded DNA molecule.

Human immunodeficiency virus

The retrovirus of greatest medical importance is the etiologic agent of AIDS. HIV enters the human host via sexual contact at mucosal surfaces, through breastfeeding, or via blood-contaminated needles. Sexually transmitted infection is facilitated by uptake of HIV by dendritic cells at mucosal surfaces. $CD4^+$ T lymphocytes are a primary target of the virus, as are dendritic cells and monocyte-macrophages. Infection of these cell types induces predictable defects of innate and acquired (both humoral and cellular) immunity. Primary viremia results in an infectious mononucleosis–like HIV prodrome, followed by seeding of the peripheral lymphoid organs and development of a measurable immune response. Conjunctivitis may occur during this seroconversion prodrome in a small number of patients and is self-limited. Infected patients may remain otherwise asymptomatic for several years, but $CD4^+$ T lymphocytes are progressively depleted. Clinical immunodeficiency eventually develops.

AIDS-related ocular disorders include HZO; molluscum contagiosum; keratoconjunctivitis sicca; microsporidial keratoconjunctivitis; HIV neuropathy; cryptococcal optic neuritis; retinal microvasculopathy; choroiditis and retinitis due to syphilis; mycobacterial infection; pneumocystosis; toxoplasmosis; and CMV, HSV, and VZV infections. See BCSC Section 1, *Update on General Medicine,* and Section 9, *Uveitis and Ocular Inflammation.*

Rhabdoviruses

Rabies virus is a single-stranded, enveloped virus that can be transmitted via corneal transplant. Corneal biopsy and impression cytology have been useful in the early diagnosis of rabies virus infection.

Cunningham ET Jr, Margolis TP. Ocular manifestations of HIV infection. *N Engl J Med.* 1998;339(4):236–244.

Lai TY, Wong RL, Luk FO, Chow VW, Chan CK, Lam DS. Ophthalmic manifestations and risk factors for mortality of HIV patients in the post-highly active anti-retroviral therapy era. *Clin Exp Ophthalmol.* 2011;39(2):99–104.

Zaidman GW, Billingsley A. Corneal impression test for the diagnosis of acute rabies encephalitis. *Ophthalmology.* 1998;105(2):249–251.

CHAPTER 12

Infectious Diseases of the Cornea and External Eye: Bacterial, Fungal, and Parasitic Infections

Indicates selected key points within the chapter.

Highlights

- The incidence of bacterial conjunctivitis in children is similar to that of viral conjunctivitis; in contrast, 80% of infectious conjunctivitis cases in adults are viral in origin.
- Most cases of acute bacterial conjunctivitis resolve in 2 to 7 days without treatment. Delaying treatment 3 to 4 days might significantly reduce the unnecessary use of antibiotics without affecting outcomes. Treatment may be necessary in cases with persistent or worsening signs.
- Contact lens–related bacterial keratitis can be treated with topical fluoroquinolones. Topical fortified antibiotics should be reserved for ulcers that are large, sight threatening, poorly responsive, and/or atypical.
- Natamycin 5% suspension is recommended for the treatment of most cases of filamentous fungal keratitis, particularly those caused by *Fusarium* species, which are the most common causative agents of exogenous fungal keratitis in the southern United States.
- Corticosteroid exposure induces acanthamoebal excystment in vitro and may worsen clinical outcomes when used prior to effective anti-acanthamoebal therapy.

Normal Ocular Flora

Bacterial colonization of the eyelid margin and conjunctiva is normal and can be beneficial as long as normal flora competitively inhibit pathogenic strains. The spectrum of normal ocular flora varies with the age and geographic locale of the host. In the eye of an infant delivered vaginally, multiple bacterial species predominate, including *Staphylococcus aureus, S epidermidis,* streptococci, and *Escherichia coli.* Streptococci and pneumococci predominate during the first 2 decades of life. Although gram-negative bacteria occur more frequently in the external eye as an individual's age increases, *S epidermidis*, other coagulase-negative staphylococci, *S aureus,* and diphtheroids are common throughout life (Table 12-1). Nonpathogenic

Table 12-1 Relative Prevalence of the Normal Flora of the External Eye

Microorganisms	Normal Conjunctiva	Normal Eyelid Margin
Staphylococcus epidermidis	+++	+++
Staphylococcus aureus	++	++
Micrococcus spp	+	++
Corynebacterium spp (diphtheroids)	++	++
Propionibacterium acnes	++	++
Streptococcus spp[a]	+	±
Haemophilus influenzae[a]	±	–
Moraxella spp	±	–
Enteric gram-negative bacilli	±	–
Bacillus spp	±	–
Anaerobic bacteria	+	±
Yeasts (*Malassezia furfur, Candida* spp)	–	+
Filamentous fungi	±	–
Demodex spp	–	++

[a] More common in children.

colonization of the eyelid margin with *Demodex folliculorum* and *D brevis* increases with age. Any disturbance in the ocular surface (eg, contact lens wear, tear deficiency, or application of topical antibiotics or corticosteroids) can alter the flora of the eyelid and conjunctiva.

Fintelmann RE, Hoskins EN, Lietman TM, et al. Topical fluoroquinolone use as a risk factor for in vitro fluoroquinolone resistance in ocular cultures. *Arch Ophthalmol.* 2011;129(4):399–402.

Graham JE, Moore JE, Jiru X, et al. Ocular pathogen or commensal: a PCR-based study of surface bacterial flora in normal and dry eyes. *Invest Ophthalmol Vis Sci.* 2007;48(12):5616–5623.

Kemal M, Sümer Z, Toker MI, Erdoğan H, Topalkara A, Akbulut M. The prevalence of *Demodex folliculorum* in blepharitis patients and the normal population. *Ophthalmic Epidemiol.* 2005;12(4):287–290.

Pathogenesis of Ocular Infections

Many microorganisms are capable of causing infectious diseases of the external eye; the most common of these pathogens are listed in Table 12-2. Ocular infection can occur via exogenous inoculation or, in rare cases, by hematogenous seeding. Characteristics of an infection—including its onset and severity—are a function of multiple factors: the virulence of the pathogen, the inoculum size, and the competence and nature of host defense mechanisms. Virulence factors represent evolutionary adaptations in microorganisms that confer increased odds of infection and survival. Correspondingly, more virulent pathogens are more likely to cause infection than an equal number of less virulent pathogens. The status of host defense mechanisms also determines the inoculum amount at which infection is likely to occur.

In many species of microorganisms, ocular infection is established by characteristic pathogenic mechanisms. Following exogenous inoculation, adherence to the ocular surface is the first step. To facilitate this process, some microorganisms (eg, *Candida albicans* and *Acanthamoeba* trophozoites) express adhesins, proteins that bind with high affinity to molecules on the host cell surface. A few organisms can invade an intact epithelium

Table 12-2 Principal Causes of External Ocular Infections

Condition	Viruses	Bacteria	Fungi	Parasites
Dermatoblepharitis	HSV Varicella-zoster virus	*Staphylococcus aureus* *Streptococcus* spp	—	—
Blepharitis	HSV Molluscum contagiosum	*Staphylococcus* spp *Moraxella* spp	—	*Phthirus pubis* *Demodex* spp
Conjunctivitis	Adenovirus HSV Picornavirus	*Chlamydia trachomatis* *Staphylococcus aureus* *Streptococcus* spp *Neisseria gonorrhoeae* *Haemophilus influenzae* *Moraxella* spp	—	—
Keratitis	HSV	*Pseudomonas aeruginosa* *Staphylococcus aureus* *Staphylococcus epidermidis* *Streptococcus pneumoniae* *Moraxella* spp	*Fusarium* spp *Aspergillus* spp *Candida albicans*	*Acanthamoeba* spp
Dacryoadenitis	Epstein-Barr virus Mumps virus	*Staphylococcus aureus* *Streptococcus pneumoniae*	—	—
Canaliculitis	HSV	Actinomycetes *Streptococcus* spp *Staphylococcus* spp	*Candida* sp, *Aspergillus* sp	—
Dacryocystitis		*Staphylococcus* spp *Streptococcus* spp	*Candida* (rare)	—

HSV = herpes simplex virus.

Table 12-3 Organisms That Can Invade an Intact Epithelium

Corynebacterium diphtheriae
Fusarium spp
Haemophilus influenza
Listeria monocytogenes
Neisseria gonorrhoeae
Neisseria meningitidis
Shigella spp

(Table 12-3), but most must rely on a disrupted epithelial barrier. Microbial proteases facilitate host invasion by inducing cell lysis, degrading the extracellular matrix, and activating corneal matrix–derived metalloproteinases in the host cell to trigger autodigestion. Bacterial exotoxins, such as those produced by streptococci, staphylococci, and *Pseudomonas aeruginosa*, can induce corneal cell necrosis. *Acanthamoeba* species and certain fungi secrete collagenases. *P aeruginosa* secretes enzymes that destroy collagen and proteoglycan components of the cornea. These enzymes also degrade immunoglobulins, complement proteins, interleukins, and other inflammatory cytokines.

After adhering, certain bacterial species avoid host-cell phagocytosis by organizing into a biofilm. In most acute infections, pathogenic microorganisms are eventually cleared, but in some cases, the pathogen persists in the host indefinitely. For example, chlamydial organisms persist within intracellular phagosomes, yielding chronic localized disease. Further discussion of bacteriology, mycology, and parasitology pertinent to ocular infection is included in the online Appendix at www.aao.org/bcscappendix_section08.

McDougald D, Rice SA, Barraud N, Steinberg PD, Kjelleberg S. Should we stay or should we go: mechanisms and ecological consequences for biofilm dispersal. *Nat Rev Microbiol.* 2011;10(1):39–50.

Momburg F, Hengel H. Corking the bottleneck: the transporter associated with antigen processing as a target for immune subversion by viruses. *Curr Top Microbiol Immunol.* 2002;269:57–74.

Diagnostic Laboratory Techniques

The recent increase in atypical ocular infections and the emergence of antibiotic-resistant strains have underscored the importance of procedures for specific microbiologic diagnosis. However, an understanding of the normal flora and cytology of the ocular surface is needed in order to interpret infectious disease findings. Materials for specimen collection and evaluation are summarized in Tables 12-4 and 12-5.

Thompson PP, Kowalski RP. A 13-year retrospective review of polymerase chain reaction testing for infectious agents from ocular samples. *Ophthalmology.* 2011;118(7):1449–1453.

Table 12-4 Materials for Collecting Eyelid, Conjunctival, and Corneal Specimens for Ocular Microbiology

Viral Infections	Chlamydial Infections	Bacterial, Fungal, or Acanthamoebal Infections
Topical anesthetic	Topical anesthetic	Topical anesthetic
Dacron swabs	Dacron swabs	Calcium alginate or Dacron swabs
Spatula	Spatula	Spatula
Glass slides	Glass slides	Glass slides
Viral transport medium	Chlamydial transport medium	Bacterial transport medium
		Blood agar plate
		Chocolate agar plate
		Sabouraud dextrose agar plate or brain–heart infusion agar[a]
		Nonnutrient agar plate with *Escherichia coli* or *Enterobacter aerogenes* overlay[b]
		Thioglycollate or meat broth

[a] Fungal.
[b] Acanthamoebal.

Table 12-5 Commonly Used Stains and Culture Media for Infectious Keratitis

Suspected Organism	Stain	Media
Acanthamoeba	Acridine orange Calcofluor white Gram Giemsa Indirect immunofluorescence antibody	Nonnutrient agar with bacterial overlay *(Enterobacter aerogenes, Escherichia coli)* Blood agar Buffered charcoal–yeast extract agar
Aerobic bacteria	Gram Acridine orange	Blood agar Chocolate agar Thioglycollate broth
Anaerobic bacteria	Gram Acridine orange	Anaerobic blood agar Phenylethyl alcohol agar in anaerobic chamber Thioglycollate or chopped meat broth
Fungi	Gram Acridine orange Calcofluor white	Blood agar (25°C) Sabouraud agar (25°C) Brain–heart infusion agar (25°C)
Mycobacteria	Gram Acid-fast Lectin	Blood agar Löwenstein-Jensen agar

Specimen Collection

To maximize recovery of infectious agents, it is important to inoculate the specimen immediately into room-temperature culture media. Microscope slides may then be prepared for Gram, Giemsa, or other special stains. To avoid contamination and false-positive results, the specimen-collection tool should not be touched to any nonsterile surface. The C-shaped streak method of plate inoculation (Fig 12-1) is not the preferred method in every microbiology lab. However, when this is used, a separate sterile instrument or swab is required for each row of C-shaped streaks on the agar plate as well as for each type of culture broth. Culture transport tubes may be used if agar plates and broth are unavailable. Consultation and collaboration with the microbiology laboratory is key to avoiding errors in specimen preparation. When culture results are negative, a second culture in alternative media may be considered, especially in a case of an ocular ulcer that is nonresponsive to treatment. A medication washout period may be advisable to improve the chance of recovering a detectable amount of the disease agent.

Corneal biopsy may be performed in cases of apparent microbial infection for which repeated culture findings from corneal scrapings are negative (see Chapter 13). *Molecular diagnostics*, such as polymerase chain reaction (PCR), are the most sensitive of the existing rapid methods to detect microbial pathogens in clinical specimens. PCR can add diagnostic value for assessment of pathogens that are difficult to culture in vitro or require a long cultivation period, such as *Acanthamoeba*. See the online Appendix and BCSC Section 4, *Ophthalmic Pathology and Intraocular Tumors*, for additional discussion of specimen collection and handling, as well as assessment of microbiologic isolates in the laboratory.

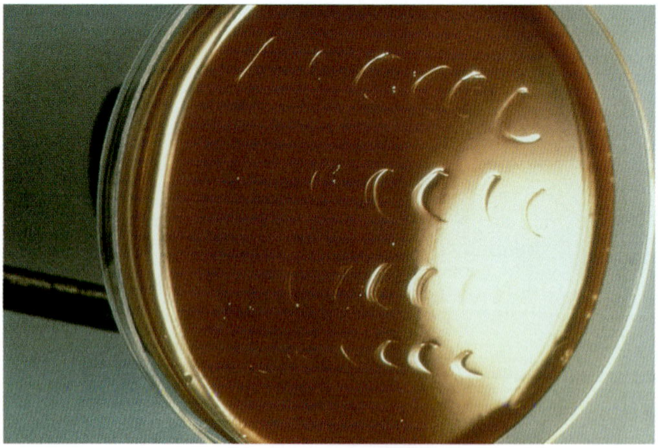

Figure 12-1 "C" streaks on a chocolate blood agar plate. *(Courtesy of James Chodosh, MD, MPH.)*

Alexandrakis G, Haimovici R, Miller D, Alfonso EC. Corneal biopsy in the management of progressive microbial keratitis. *Am J Ophthalmol.* 2000;129(5):571–576.

Kumar RL, Cruzat A, Hamrah P. Current state of in vivo confocal microscopy in management of microbial keratitis. *Semin Ophthalmol.* 2010;25(5–6):166–170.

Taravati P, Lam D, Van Gelder RN. Role of molecular diagnostics in ocular microbiology. *Curr Ophthalmol Rep.* 2013;1(4):10.

Younger JR, Johnson RD, Holland GN, et al. Microbiologic and histopathologic assessment of corneal biopsies in the evaluation of microbial keratitis. *Am J Ophthalmol.* 2012;154(3): 512–519.e2.

Infections of the Eyelid Margin and Conjunctiva

Staphylococcal Blepharitis

Staphylococcal bacteria on the anterior eyelid margin can cause blepharitis. Although this condition has an infectious etiology, inflammation plays a significant role and can result in bacterial overgrowth and a prolonged local immune response, despite antimicrobial therapy. Tears contain inhibitors of bacterial growth, and cases of tear deficiency often are accompanied by staphylococcal blepharitis. The inflammation associated with blepharitis also can lead to dry eye symptoms. (See Chapter 3.)

Fungal and Parasitic Infections of the Eyelid Margin

Demodex is a genus of mites that typically exists as commensal parasites of humans. Clinical diagnosis of *Demodex* colonization is based on the presence of waxy "sleeves" around the eyelashes (Fig 12-2) or cylinders extending from the eyelid margin. In some patients, *Demodex* infestation triggers an inflammatory response resulting in blepharitis, but the pathogenic role of these parasites is unclear. The infestation may be mitigated by applying diluted tea tree

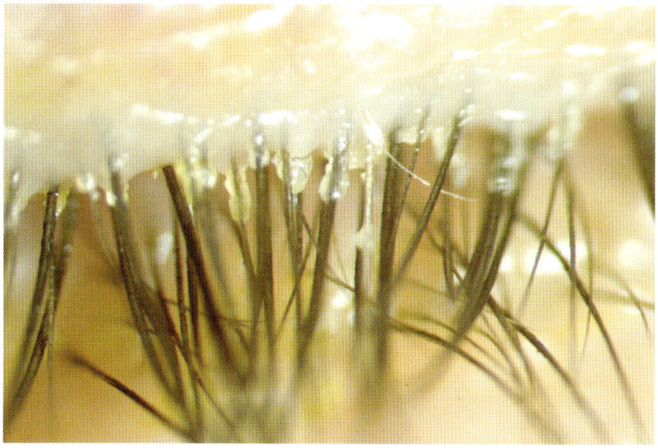

Figure 12-2 *Demodex*-associated "sleeves." *(Courtesy of Elmer Y. Tu, MD.)*

oil to the base of the eyelashes. Other organisms that survive by consuming lipids of the eyelid glands, such as *Malassezia furfur,* have also been implicated in certain types of blepharitis.

Lice infestation of the eyelids and eyelashes, also known as *phthiriasis palpebrum,* is an uncommon cause of conjunctivitis or blepharitis that affects adolescents and young adults secondary to infestation with pubic lice and ova. In rare instances, lice may extend to the ocular region after infesting the head or body (pediculosis; caused by *Pediculus humanus capitis* or *P humanus corporis,* respectively). The lice and nits (eggs) can be removed manually with jeweler's forceps, but pubic hairs are usually treated chemically with a pediculicide. To smother the lice, ointment can be applied to the eyelid margins twice daily for at least 10 days. (The incubation period of the nits is 7–10 days.) It is recommended that the area be periodically examined for 10 to 14 days to detect recurrence and remove any new nits. Bed linen, clothing, and any items of close contact should be washed and dried at the highest temperature setting (at least 50°C).

Bacterial Conjunctivitis in Children and Adults

CLINICAL PRESENTATION Bacterial conjunctivitis is likely in patients who present with conjunctival inflammation and purulent discharge. The rapidity of onset, severity of conjunctival inflammation, and presence of discharge can be helpful in determining the possible causative organism (Table 12-6). In children, conjunctivitis of bacterial and viral etiologies occur at similar rates, whereas 80% of cases of infectious conjunctivitis in adults is viral in origin. Though usually self-limited, bacterial conjunctivitis can occasionally be severe and sight-threatening, particularly when caused by virulent species, such as *Neisseria gonorrhoeae* or *Streptococcus pyogenes.* In rare cases, bacterial conjunctivitis may precede life-threatening systemic disease, such as in cases of *N meningitidis* infection.

PATHOGENESIS Bacterial conjunctivitis is characterized by bacterial overgrowth, infiltration of the conjunctival epithelial layer, and sometimes extension into the substantia propria.

Table 12-6 Clinical Classification of Bacterial Conjunctivitis

Course of Onset	Severity	Common Organisms	Ophthalmia Neonatorum Postpartum Onset and Associated Findings
Slow (days to weeks)	Mild to moderate	*Staphylococcus aureus* *Moraxella lacunata* *Proteus* spp Enterobacteriaceae	Variable onset
		Pseudomonas aeruginosa	Rare Keratitis, corneal perforation
		Chlamydia trachomatis	Onset: day 5–14 Absence of conjunctival follicles Pneumonitis, otitis media (50% of cases)
		Herpes simplex virus	Onset: in the first 2 weeks of life Nonspecific conjunctivitis
Acute or subacute (hours to days)	Moderate to severe	*Haemophilus influenzae* biotype III[a] *Haemophilus influenzae*	Variable onset
		Streptococcus pneumoniae	Variable onset
		Streptococcus viridans	Variable onset
		Staphylococcus aureus	Variable onset
Hyperacute (<24 hours)	Severe	*Neisseria gonorrhoeae* *Neisseria meningitidis*	Onset: day 1–13 (commonly day 3–5) Keratitis, endophthalmitis, systemic infection

[a] Previously referred to as *Haemophilus aegyptius.*

The infection is transmitted either by direct contact with an infected individual's secretions (usually, eye–hand contact) or from the patient's own nasal and sinus mucosa to the eye. In an adult with unilateral bacterial conjunctivitis, the nasolacrimal system should be examined; nasolacrimal duct obstruction, dacryocystitis, or canaliculitis may be the underlying cause.

Acute purulent conjunctivitis

CLINICAL PRESENTATION Acute purulent conjunctivitis is a self-limited infection of the conjunctiva characterized by an acute inflammatory response with purulent discharge of less than 3 weeks duration (Fig 12-3). Conjunctivitis caused by *Streptococcus pneumoniae* involves moderate purulent discharge, eyelid edema, chemosis, conjunctival hemorrhage,

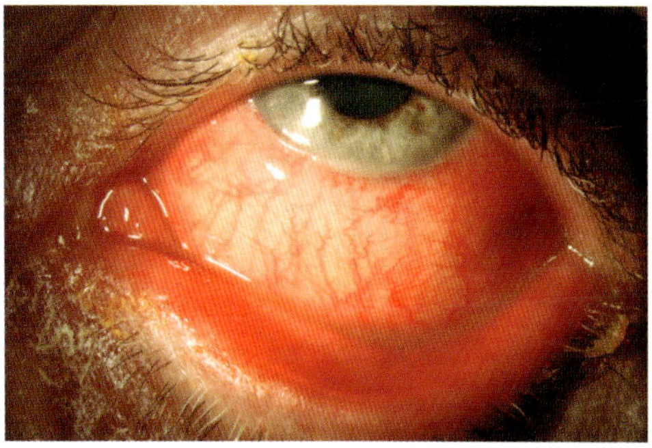

Figure 12-3 Acute bacterial conjunctivitis. *(Courtesy of Shahzad I. Mian, MD.)*

occasionally inflammatory membranes on the tarsal conjunctiva, and, in rare cases, corneal ulceration. In young children, conjunctivitis due to *Haemophilus influenzae* infection may occur alongside otitis media; in adults, conjunctivitis associated with chronic *H influenzae* infection is possible (eg, in smokers or patients with chronic bronchopulmonary disease). *H influenzae* biotype III (formerly *H aegyptius*) causes acute purulent conjunctivitis that resembles that caused by *S pneumoniae*. Distinguishing features of infection with *H influenzae* biotype III include absent conjunctival membranes and frequent peripheral corneal epithelial ulcers and stromal infiltrates. Preseptal cellulitis owing to *H influenzae* infection may result in fulminant *Haemophilus* meningitis, for which up to 20% of patients who recover experience long-term neurologic sequelae. The incidence of *H influenzae* infection has been reduced by a vigorous program of vaccination. Infection with *Staphylococcus aureus* may lead to acute blepharoconjunctivitis associated with discharge that, when compared with pneumococcal conjunctivitis, involves less purulent discharge and generally less severe signs of infection.

PATHOGENESIS Cases may occur spontaneously, with an associated infectious process elsewhere, or due to contagious spread. The most common etiologic pathogens, *Streptococcus pneumoniae, Streptococcus viridans, Haemophilus influenzae,* and *Staphylococcus aureus,* occur at frequencies dependent on patient age and geographic location.

LABORATORY EVALUATION Gram-stain smears and culture of the conjunctiva are usually not necessary in uncomplicated, predominantly self-limited cases of suspected bacterial conjunctivitis but are recommended for the following:

- patients who are immunocompromised—including neonates and debilitated individuals—to assess the risk of local and systemic complications
- patients with severe purulent conjunctivitis, to differentiate it from hyperpurulent conjunctivitis, which generally requires systemic therapy
- patients in whom the initial therapy failed

MANAGEMENT Most cases of acute bacterial conjunctivitis resolve in 2 to 7 days without treatment. Results of multiple prospective studies have suggested that delaying treatment until day 3 or 4 can significantly decrease the unnecessary use of antibiotics, without affecting outcomes. After this delay, initiating treatment only in patients with persistent or worsening signs would still be expected to shorten the disease course and improve symptoms. If the conjunctivitis is improving on day 4, antibiotics may not be necessary. Cases likely due to viral infection should *not* be treated routinely with antibiotics.

If further intervention is indicated, it can be directed by the results of the Gram stain of the conjunctival smear. However, it is preferable to base treatment on the findings of bacterial culture as smear results may be inconclusive. Cultures of the nose or throat may be obtained if an associated sinusitis or pharyngitis is present. In cases of relapsing conjunctivitis, even if no overt sinusitis, rhinitis, or pharyngitis is present, it is recommended that nasal or throat swabs be obtained because organisms in the respiratory tract mucosa may be the source of infection.

Empiric therapy with topical polymyxin B-trimethoprim, aminoglycoside, fluoroquinolone, or bacitracin may be initiated before results of the Gram stain or culture have been received. The dosing schedule is 4 to 6 times daily for approximately 5 to 7 days unless otherwise indicated. Gram-negative coccobacilli on stained smears are usually caused by *Haemophilus* species, and treatment with polymyxin B-trimethoprim is recommended. Supplemental oral antibiotics may be given to patients in the following groups:

- patients with acute purulent conjunctivitis associated with pharyngitis
- cases of conjunctivitis-otitis syndrome
- children with *Haemophilus* conjunctivitis

Topical ophthalmic corticosteroids and drops that combine corticosteroids with antibiotics for treatment of acute infectious conjunctivitis may be considered in cases of moderate to severe inflammation. Complications associated with topical steroid use, including increased intraocular pressure (IOP), glaucoma, and cataracts, can be minimized by administering a short course of treatment (<2 weeks).

Hyperacute gonococcal conjunctivitis

CLINICAL PRESENTATION Gonococcal conjunctivitis is a severe purulent form of conjunctivitis that presents with explosive onset and very rapid progression, with signs of massive exudation, severe chemosis, eyelid edema, marked conjunctival hyperemia, and, in untreated cases, corneal infiltrates, melting, and perforation (Figs 12-4, 12-5). Gonococcal conjunctivitis is one of the few bacterial diseases that is associated with preauricular lymphadenopathy and the formation of conjunctival membranes. Keratitis, the principal cause of sight-threatening complications, occurs in 15% to 40% of cases. Corneal

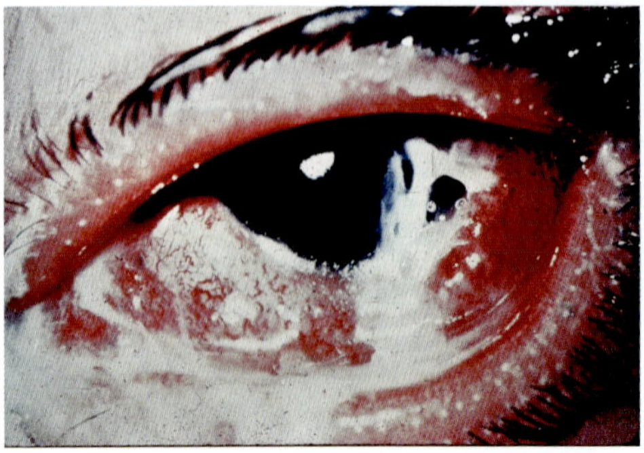

Figure 12-4 Hyperacute bacterial conjunctivitis. *(Courtesy of Robert S. Feder, MD.)*

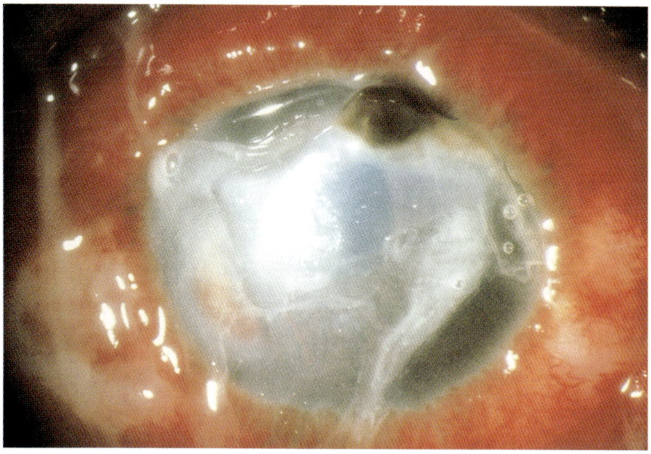

Figure 12-5 Peripheral corneal ulceration and perforation occurring several days after onset of hyperacute conjunctivitis caused by *Neisseria gonorrhoeae.*

involvement may consist of diffuse epithelial haze, epithelial defects, marginal infiltrates, and ulcerative keratitis that can progress rapidly to perforation.

PATHOGENESIS The organism most commonly responsible for hyperacute conjunctivitis is *Neisseria gonorrhoeae*. Gonococcal conjunctivitis is a sexually transmitted disease that results from direct transmission of the organism. Modes of transmission include from the genitalia to the hands and then to the eyes or from the mother to the neonate during vaginal delivery.

LABORATORY EVALUATION *Neisseria gonorrhoeae* grows well on chocolate agar and Thayer-Martin media.

MANAGEMENT For treatment of gonococcal conjunctivitis, systemic antibiotic therapy is indicated; topical ophthalmic antibiotics are given as adjunctive therapy only. Current treatment regimens for gonococcal conjunctivitis reflect the increasing prevalence of *penicillin-resistant N gonorrhoeae (PRNG)* in the United States. Ceftriaxone, a third-generation cephalosporin, is highly effective against PRNG. Patients with gonococcal conjunctivitis without corneal ulceration may be treated on an outpatient basis with 1 intramuscular (IM) injection of ceftriaxone (1 g); patients with corneal ulceration should be admitted to the hospital and treated intravenously (IV) with ceftriaxone (1 g IV every 12 hours) for 3 consecutive days. Patients with penicillin allergy may receive spectinomycin (2 g IM) or oral fluoroquinolones (ciprofloxacin 500 mg or ofloxacin 400 mg orally twice daily for 5 days). When possible, fluoroquinolones should be avoided in children because of potential adverse effects on joint cartilage.

Topical ointments containing erythromycin, bacitracin, or gentamicin as well as ciprofloxacin solution may be considered as supplemental therapeutic options. In severe cases, the recommended approach is copious, frequent (every 30–60 minutes) irrigation of the conjunctival sac with normal saline to remove inflammatory cells, proteases, and debris that may be toxic to the ocular surface and contribute to corneal melting.

Table 12-7 Sexually Transmitted Pathogens Associated With Conjunctivitis

Organism	Onset	Presentation
Neisseria gonorrhoeae	<24 hours	Hyperacute with copious discharge, conjunctival edema
HIV	Day 11–28	Conjunctival edema, watery discharge
Chlamydia trachomatis	Days to weeks	Follicular conjunctivitis
Herpes simplex virus	2 weeks	Follicular conjunctivitis
Treponema pallidum	Weeks to months	Granulomatous conjunctivitis

Evidence suggests that up to one-third of patients with gonococcal conjunctivitis have concurrent chlamydial venereal disease. Because of this, it is recommended that patients receive supplemental oral antibiotics for treatment of chlamydial infection. Patients should be advised to refer their sex partners for evaluation and treatment. Other sexually transmitted pathogens that cause conjunctivitis (Table 12-7) include *Treponema pallidum,* HIV, *Chlamydia trachomatis,* and herpes simplex virus (HSV). For further discussion of syphilis, see BCSC Section 1, *Update on General Medicine,* and Section 9, *Uveitis and Ocular Inflammation.*

American Academy of Ophthalmology Cornea/External Disease Committee, Hoskins Center for Quality Eye Care. Preferred Practice Pattern Guidelines. *Conjunctivitis.* American Academy of Ophthalmology; 2018. www.aao.org/ppp

Cortina MS, Tu EY. Antibiotic use in corneal and external eye infections. *Focal Points: Clinical Modules for Ophthalmologists.* American Academy of Ophthalmology; 2011, Module 6.

Holland EJ, Fingeret M, Mah FS. Use of topical steroids in conjunctivitis: a review of the evidence. *Cornea.* 2019;38(8):1062–1067.

Bacterial conjunctivitis in neonates

The etiology of bacterial conjunctivitis in neonates is reflective of the vaginal and nosocomial flora (see Table 12-6), with the most severe form caused by *Neisseria gonorrhoeae.* Ophthalmia neonatorum is discussed in more detail in BCSC Section 6, *Pediatric Ophthalmology and Strabismus.*

Neonatal gonococcal conjunctivitis typically presents as bilateral conjunctival discharge occurring 3 to 5 days after birth. The discharge may be serosanguineous during the first several days, with subsequent development of copious purulent exudate, severe corneal complications, and endophthalmitis. Infected infants may have additional localized gonococcal infections, including rhinitis and proctitis. A rare complication is disseminated gonococcal infection, in which arthritis, meningitis, pneumonia, and sepsis occur, resulting in death.

MANAGEMENT Prenatal screening for maternal gonococcal genital infection and neonatal antibiotic prophylaxis have reduced the rate of neonatal gonococcal conjunctivitis. Because of emerging resistance of *N gonorrhoeae* to various antibiotics—including penicillin, fluoroquinolones, and tetracycline—the currently recommended first-line treatment for neonatal gonococcal conjunctivitis is ceftriaxone.

For *nondisseminated infections,* a single IV or IM injection of ceftriaxone (up to 125 mg or a dose of 25–50 mg/kg) or cefotaxime (100 mg/kg) is recommended.

For *disseminated infection,* augmentation of the treatment regimen, based on consultation with an infectious disease specialist, is advised. Either approach should be combined with saline irrigation of the conjunctiva every hour until discharge is eliminated. If corneal involvement is suspected, application of topical erythromycin or gentamicin ointment or frequent application of topical fluoroquinolone and topical cycloplegia may be considered. Systemic treatment is advised for infants born to mothers with active gonorrhea, even in the absence of conjunctivitis.

American Academy of Pediatrics. Gonococcal infections. In: Pickering LK, Baker CJ, Kimberlin DW, Long SS, eds. *2009 Red Book: Report of the Committee on Infectious Diseases.* 28th ed. American Academy of Pediatrics; 2009:305–313.

Centers for Disease Control and Prevention; Workowski KA, Berman SM. Sexually transmitted diseases treatment guidelines 2006. *MMWR Recomm Rep.* 2006;55(RR-11):1–94.

Cortina MS, Tu EY. Antibiotic use in corneal and external eye infections. *Focal Points: Clinical Modules for Ophthalmologists.* American Academy of Ophthalmology; 2011, module 6.

Chlamydial conjunctivitis

Trachoma and adult inclusion conjunctivitis, caused by the bacterium *Chlamydia trachomatis*, are discussed individually in the following sections. Trachoma is caused by infection with *C trachomatis* serotypes A–C; serotypes D–K cause adult and neonatal inclusion conjunctivitis.

Trachoma Among countries in which clean water and sanitation are lacking or inadequate, trachoma is a leading cause of preventable blindness. Globally, trachoma is responsible for visual impairment in nearly 2.2 million people and for blindness in 1.2 million. Trachoma is endemic in the Middle East and in developing regions around the world. In the United States, trachoma occurs sporadically among Native American populations and in residents of mountainous areas of the Southeast. Most infections are transmitted from eye to eye, but transmission also is possible by flies or household fomites. Other bacteria can also be spread by these routes, and secondary bacterial infections are common in patients with trachoma.

Solomon AW, Holland MJ, Alexander ND, et al. Mass treatment with single-dose azithromycin for trachoma. *N Engl J Med.* 2004;351(19):1962–1971.

CLINICAL PRESENTATION The symptoms of trachoma include foreign-body sensation, redness, tearing, and mucopurulent discharge. These are followed by a severe follicular reaction, which occurs predominantly in the superior tarsal conjunctiva and sometimes in the superior and inferior fornices, inferior tarsal conjunctiva, semilunar fold, and limbus. In acute trachoma, follicles on the superior tarsus may be obscured by diffuse papillary hypertrophy and inflammatory cell infiltration. Large tarsal follicles in trachoma may become necrotic, eventually healing with significant scarring. Linear or stellate scarring of the superior tarsus *(Arlt line)* is common in these cases (Fig 12-6). Involution and necrosis of follicles may result in limbal depressions known as *Herbert pits* (Fig 12-7). Corneal findings in trachoma include the following:

- epithelial keratitis
- focal and multifocal peripheral and central stromal infiltrates
- superficial fibrovascular pannus, most prominent in the superior third of the cornea but possibly extending centrally into the visual axis (Fig 12-8)
- aqueous tear deficiency from severe scarring of the conjunctival and lacrimal gland ducts, resulting from chronic disease

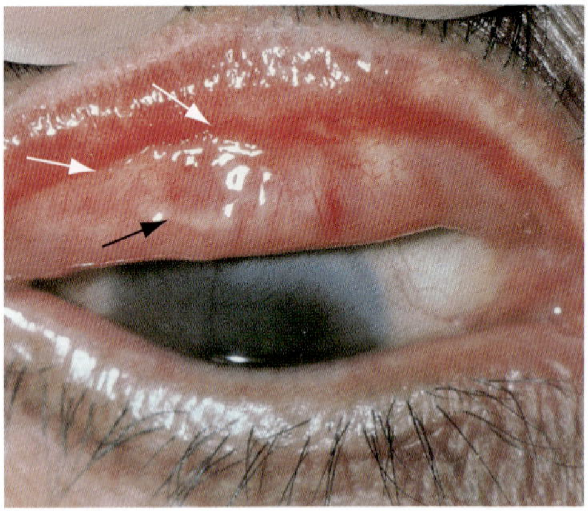

Figure 12-6 Linear scarring of the superior tarsal conjunctiva (Arlt line, *white arrows*) in a patient with subconjunctival fibrosis *(black arrow)* from previous trachoma. *(Courtesy of Vincent P. deLuise, MD.)*

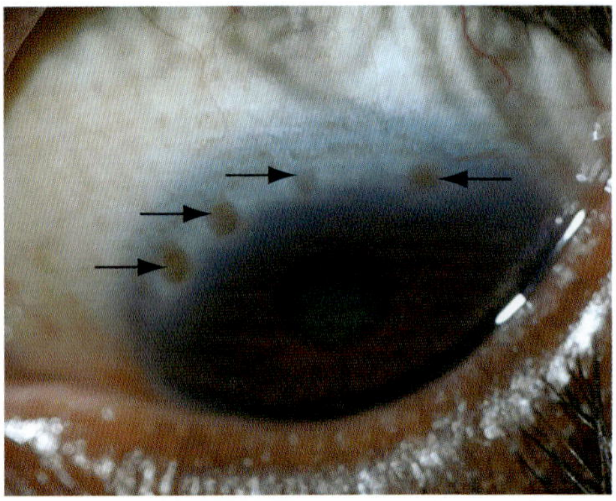

Figure 12-7 Trachoma exhibiting Herbert pits *(arrows)* of the superior limbus (round to oval, pigmented areas within pannus). *(Courtesy of Tom Lietman, MD.)*

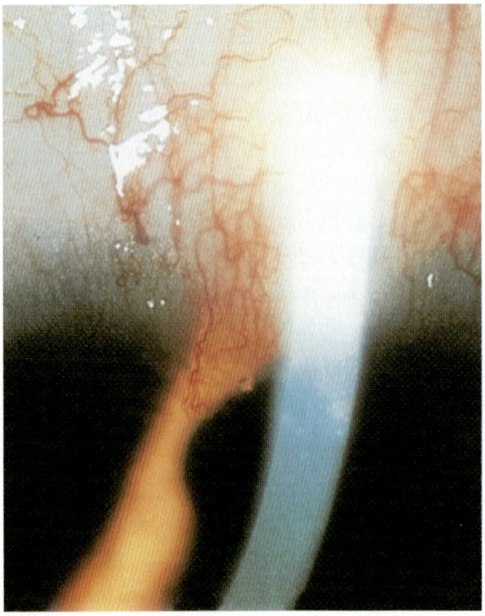

Figure 12-8 Superior micropannus in a patient with adult chlamydial conjunctivitis (trachoma).

Chronic trachoma can also result in tear-drainage obstruction, trichiasis, and entropion. The World Health Organization (WHO) has devised a simple grading system for trachoma severity based on the presence or absence of 5 key signs (see sidebar below). This grading system was developed for trained personnel, other than ophthalmologists, to assess the prevalence and severity of trachoma by means of findings from population-based surveys in endemic areas.

WORLD HEALTH ORGANIZATION: 5 KEY SIGNS FOR TRACHOMA SEVERITY GRADING

1. Follicular conjunctival inflammation
2. Diffuse papillary conjunctival hypertrophy
3. Tarsal conjunctival scarring
4. Aberrant lashes
5. Corneal opacification

Mohammadpour M, Abrishami M, Masoumi A. Trachoma: Past, present and future. *J Curr Ophthalmol.* 2016; 28(4):165–169.

Thylefors B, Dawson CR, Jones BR, West SK, Taylor HR. A simple system for the assessment of trachoma and its complications. *Bull World Health Organ.* 1987;65(4):477–483.

LABORATORY EVALUATION The primary mode of diagnosis of trachoma is on the basis of clinical manifestations in endemic areas. As an obligate intracellular pathogen, *C trachomatis* cannot be easily isolated by standard ophthalmic culture techniques and instead requires either direct observation of the intracellular bacterium or cell culture. Direct visualization is possible by Giemsa staining or direct fluorescent antibody staining. PCR probes are available for this purpose and are increasingly being used in place of other diagnostic methods.

MANAGEMENT The WHO, in conjunction with the International Trachoma Initiative, has implemented the SAFE strategy (surgery, antibiotics, facial cleanliness, and environmental control) for prevention and treatment of trachoma; as a result, the incidence of trachoma has decreased significantly in the Middle East and in North Africa.

Surgery is used to address the in-turned eye lashes of patients with trichiasis or entropion. Antibiotic treatment may include 1 of the following options:

- oral azithromycin 1000 mg, given as a single dose (preferred regimen)
- oral tetracycline, 1.5 g to 2.0 g, daily in divided doses for 3 weeks
- doxycycline 100 mg, twice daily for 2 weeks
- oral erythromycin (recommended for treatment of rare tetracycline-resistant cases)
- topical erythromycin or topical tetracycline 1%

The lack of facial cleanliness is strongly correlated with spread of trachoma; children with poor facial hygiene are more likely to acquire or transmit the disease. The environment must also be addressed; sanitation, water disposal, and water quality are essential for the success of any infectious disease eradication program.

Adult chlamydial conjunctivitis Adult chlamydial conjunctivitis is a sexually transmitted disease that is often associated with chlamydial urethritis or cervicitis. It is most prevalent in sexually active adolescents and young adults. Chlamydial infection is a systemic disease. The eye is usually infected by direct or indirect contact with infected genital secretions.

CLINICAL PRESENTATION Onset of conjunctivitis is typically 1 to 2 weeks after ocular inoculation and is not as acute as adenoviral keratoconjunctivitis. Patients may report having had mild symptoms for weeks to months. External signs of adult inclusion conjunctivitis include a follicular conjunctival response that is most prominent in the lower palpebral conjunctiva and fornix, mucopurulent discharge, and palpable preauricular adenopathy. Follicles in the bulbar conjunctiva and semilunar fold are frequently present, and this is a helpful and specific sign in patients not otherwise using topical medications associated with the findings. Unlike with neonatal forms, inflammatory conjunctival membranes do not develop in adult chlamydial keratoconjunctivitis.

Corneal involvement may involve fine or coarse epithelial infiltrates, occasionally associated with subepithelial infiltrates. Keratitis is more likely to be found in the superior cornea but also may occur centrally and resemble adenoviral keratitis. A micropannus, usually extending less than 3 mm from the superior cornea, may develop. The laboratory workup is as described in the previous section.

MANAGEMENT Left untreated, adult chlamydial conjunctivitis often resolves spontaneously in 6 to 18 months. The following oral antibiotic regimens are commonly used:

- azithromycin 1000 mg, given as a single dose
- doxycycline 100 mg, twice daily for 7 days
- tetracycline 250 mg, 4 times daily for 7 days
- erythromycin 500 mg, 4 times daily for 7 days

It is recommended that patients with laboratory-confirmed chlamydial conjunctivitis and their sexual contacts be evaluated for coinfection with other sexually transmitted diseases, such as syphilis or gonorrhea, before antibiotic treatment is started. Sexual partners should be treated concomitantly to avoid reinfection.

Centers for Disease Control and Prevention; Workowski KA, Berman SM. Sexually transmitted diseases treatment guidelines 2006. *MMWR Recomm Rep.* 2006;55(RR-11):1–94.

Neonatal chlamydial conjunctivitis Chlamydial conjunctivitis in neonates differs clinically from cases in adults in several ways and is more likely to respond to topical medications. The following features are characteristic of the neonatal form:

- no follicular response
- more mucopurulent discharge
- pseudomembranes may develop on the tarsal conjunctiva
- intracytoplasmic inclusions are seen more frequently in Giemsa-stained conjunctival specimens

Testing of Gram- and Giemsa-stained conjunctival scrapings is recommended in cases of neonatal conjunctivitis to identify *C trachomatis* and *N gonorrhoeae,* as well as other bacteria, as causative agents. Other *Chlamydia*-associated infections, such as pneumonitis and otitis media, may accompany inclusion conjunctivitis in neonates. Therefore, treatment with systemic erythromycin (12.5 mg/kg oral or IV 4 times daily for 14 days) is recommended, even though neonatal inclusion conjunctivitis usually responds to topical erythromycin or sulfacetamide.

Parinaud Oculoglandular Syndrome

Granulomatous conjunctivitis with regional lymphadenopathy is an uncommon condition also known as *Parinaud oculoglandular syndrome. Cat-scratch disease (CSD),* which precedes most cases of the syndrome, is estimated to affect 22,000 people annually in the United States, with conjunctivitis developing in approximately 10%. The primary causative agent is *Bartonella henselae.* Less frequent causes of Parinaud oculoglandular syndrome include *Afipia felis,* other *Bartonella* species, coccidioidomycosis, sporotrichosis, syphilis, tuberculosis, and tularemia.

CLINICAL PRESENTATION In CSD, unilateral granulomatous conjunctivitis develops approximately 3 to 10 days after inoculation, with 1 or more raised or flat gelatinous, hyperemic, granulomatous lesions on the superior or inferior tarsal conjunctiva, fornix, or bulbar conjunctiva. Either concurrently or 1 to 2 weeks later, the ipsilateral preauricular and submandibular lymph nodes, and occasionally the cervical nodes, become firm and tender. Approximately 10% to 40% of the nodes enlarge and become suppurative. Mild systemic symptoms of fever, malaise, headache, and anorexia develop in about 10% to 30% of patients, with severe, disseminated complications—including encephalopathy, encephalitis, thrombocytopenic purpura, osteolysis, hepatitis, and splenitis—occurring in approximately 2% of patients with CSD. Optic neuritis and neuroretinitis have also been reported infrequently.

PATHOGENESIS *B henselae* usually is transmitted by infected fleas to cats (especially kittens), its natural reservoir. Feline infection may be transient or may persist asymptomatically. Despite the name "cat-scratch" disease, scratches are not the only route of inoculation in humans; infection also may be transmitted by a bite or lick or by contact with the cat's fleas. Human-to-human transmission is not known to occur. Local infection causes a granulomatous reaction.

LABORATORY EVALUATION Serologic testing is the most cost-effective means of diagnosing typical CSD. Antibodies to *B henselae* can be detected by indirect fluorescent antibody testing or enzyme immunoassay. The latter is more sensitive and is available from specialty laboratories. A skin-test antigen for CSD is neither commercially available nor standardized. Atypical CSD is best approached by combining serologic testing with culture or PCR.

MANAGEMENT No ideal treatment for CSD has been determined, but some success has been noted with certain antibacterial treatment regimens, including azithromycin, erythromycin, and doxycycline. Rifampin is often used as an adjuvant. Responses to trimethoprim-sulfamethoxazole and fluoroquinolones have been reported but appear to be inconsistent.

Birnbaum AD, Tu EY. Parinaud's oculoglandular syndrome. In: Tasman W, Jaeger EA, eds. *Duane's Clinical Ophthalmology.* Vol 4. Lippincott Williams & Wilkins; 2011.

Infections of the Cornea and Sclera

Bacterial Keratitis

Bacterial infection of the eye is a common sight-threatening condition that may present with explosive onset and rapidly progressive stromal inflammation. Untreated, it often leads to progressive tissue destruction with corneal perforation or extension of infection to adjacent tissue. Bacterial keratitis is frequently associated with risk factors that disturb the corneal epithelial integrity.

In the United States, the most frequent risk factor for bacterial keratitis is contact lens (CL) wear, which has been identified in 19%–42% of patients with culture-proven microbial keratitis and accounts for up to one-third of emergency department visits for corneal infection. The risk of corneal infection is almost tenfold higher in those who wear contact lenses than in those who do not. The risk is higher still in patients who wear their contact lenses overnight, and it is positively correlated with the number of consecutive days that lenses are worn without removal. Results of a large epidemiologic study in Australia indicated an annual incidence of cosmetic contact lens–related microbial keratitis per 10,000 individuals of 1.2 for daily rigid gas-permeable CL wear, 1.9 for daily soft CL wear, and 19.5 for overnight soft CL wear. The use of disposable lenses for extended-wear and high–oxygen permeable silicone CL material did not appear to prevent microbial keratitis. Daily disposable soft CL use is felt by many clinicians to be the safest regimen. Poor CL hygiene is also a significant risk factor for microbial keratitis. Orthokeratology has been associated with an elevated incidence of corneal infection, similar to that of overnight contact lens wear.

The following are additional risk factors of bacterial keratitis:

- trauma
- contaminated ocular medications
- impaired local and systemic defense mechanisms
- disruption of the corneal surface

American Academy of Ophthalmology Refractive Management/Intervention Panel, Hoskins Center for Quality Eye Care. Preferred Practice Pattern Guidelines. Refractive Errors and Refractive Surgery. American Academy of Ophthalmology; 2017. www.aao.org/ppp

Stapleton F, Keay L, Edwards, K, et al. The incidence of contact lens–related microbial keratitis in Australia. *Ophthalmology.* 2008;115(10):1655–1662.

CLINICAL PRESENTATION In patients with bacterial corneal ulcers, there is rapid onset of pain accompanied by conjunctival injection, photophobia, and decreased vision. The rate of progression of these symptoms depends on the virulence of the infecting organism.

CLINICAL PEARL

Bacterial corneal ulcers typically present as a single infiltrate in the paracentral or midperipheral cornea with an epithelial defect and underlying superficial infiltrate (Fig 12-9). Some cases involve a more intense inflammatory response characterized by dense, suppurative stromal inflammation with indistinct edges and surrounding edema and stromal cells, even several millimeters away from the infiltrate (Fig 12-10).

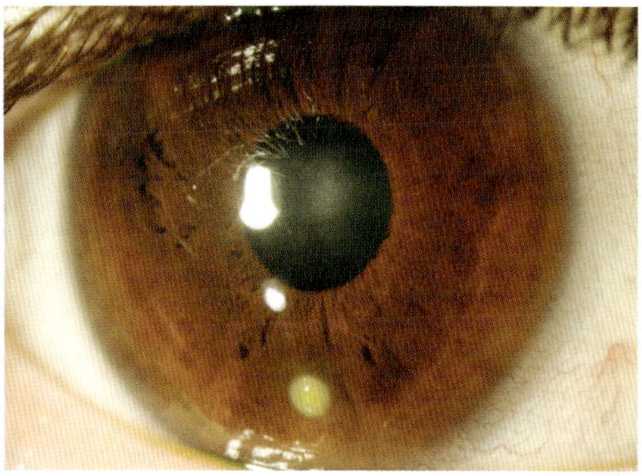

Figure 12-9 Bacterial keratitis with an epithelial defect and underlying superficial infiltrate. *(Courtesy of Shahzad I. Mian, MD.)*

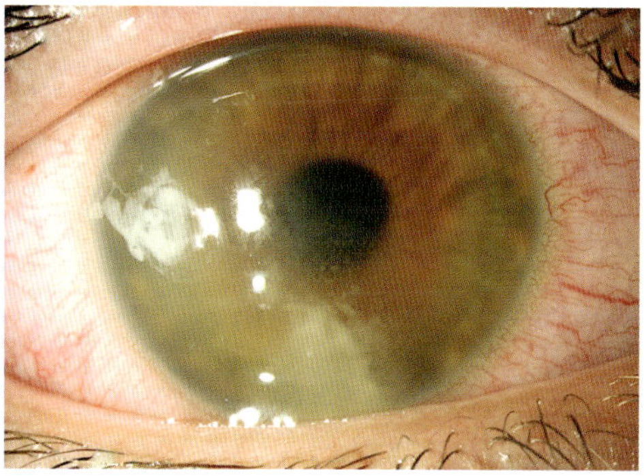

Figure 12-10 Bacterial keratitis with dense suppurative stromal inflammation and surrounding edema. *(Courtesy of Shahzad I. Mian, MD.)*

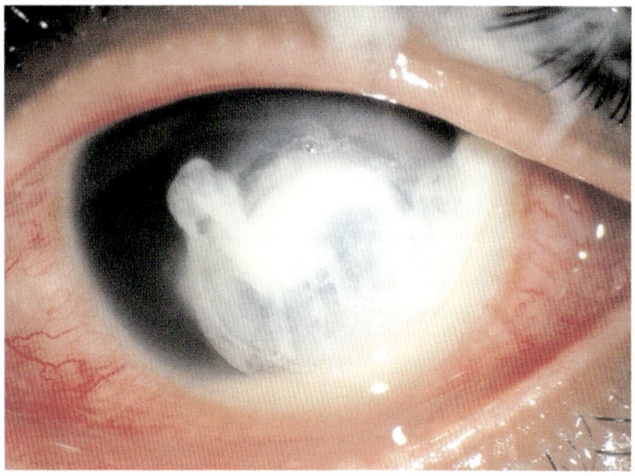

Figure 12-11 Suppurative ulcerative keratitis caused by *Pseudomonas aeruginosa.*

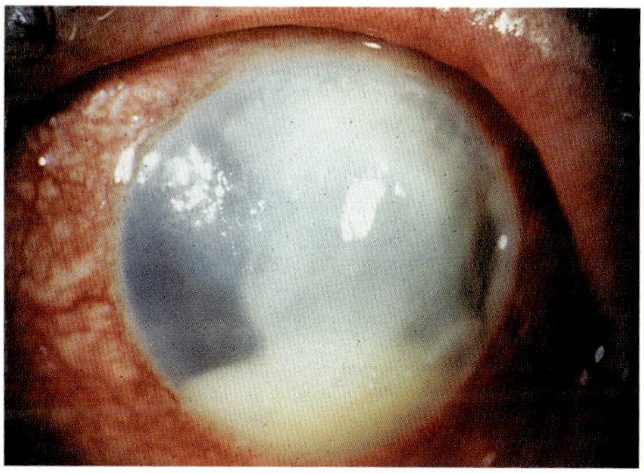

Figure 12-12 Bacterial keratitis with stromal infiltrate and hypopyon. *(Courtesy of Robert S. Feder, MD.)*

Pseudomonas aeruginosa typically causes stromal necrosis and adherent mucopurulent exudate (Fig 12-11). An endothelial inflammatory plaque, marked anterior chamber reaction, and hypopyon are also common in bacterial keratitis (Fig 12-12). The hypopyon can be subtle early on; it may be found nasally or temporally, if the patient has been lying down.

Patients with infections caused by slow-growing, fastidious organisms, such as mycobacteria or anaerobes, may have a nonsuppurative infiltrate and an intact epithelium. *Infectious crystalline keratopathy,* for example, presents as densely packed, white or crystalline, branching, snowflake-like aggregates with almost no host inflammatory response because the microorganisms are shielded by a biofilm. Risk factors of this condition include corticosteroid use, contact lens wear, and previous corneal surgery with or without retained sutures. Infectious crystalline keratopathy has been attributed to various bacterial and fungal agents, most commonly α-hemolytic *Streptococcus* species (Fig 12-13).

PATHOGENESIS Corneal pathogens adhere first to the corneal surface and then invade and proliferate in the corneal stroma. Certain risk factors tend to be selective for specific pathogens, based on the pathogen's mechanism of adherence. For example, *P aeruginosa* is more pathogenic in contact lens–related biofilms, in which binding to receptors on injured epithelial

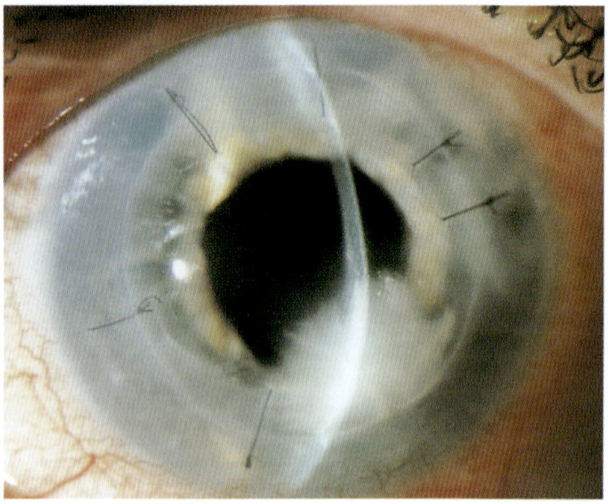

Figure 12-13 Infectious crystalline keratopathy in a corneal graft caused by α-hemolytic *Streptococcus* species.

cells is facilitated. After adhering, infiltration of the corneal stroma occurs, often mediated by bacteria proteases. The host responds with inflammation, comprising cytokine and chemokine expression, recruitment of inflammatory cells from the tears and limbal vessels, and secretion of matrix metalloproteinases, which result in characteristic corneal necrosis. Reduction of bacterial load and direct control of the inflammatory response are interventions aimed at decreasing keratolysis. See BCSC Section 1, *Update on General Medicine.*

LABORATORY EVALUATION For bacterial keratitis, the clinical appearance of the infection is not a reliable indicator of the causative pathogen. Instead, certain risk factors and geographic location may be helpful in ascertaining the disease agent. Causative organisms are listed in Table 12-8.

GUIDELINES FOR OBTAINING CULTURES AND SMEARS

According to guidelines from the American Academy of Ophthalmology (AAO), specimens should be obtained for smears or cultures in the following cases:

- the corneal infiltrate is central, large, or associated with significant stromal involvement or melting
- the infection is chronic or unresponsive to broad-spectrum antibiotic therapy
- there is a history of corneal surgeries
- atypical clinical features are present, suggestive of fungal, amebic, or mycobacterial keratitis.
- there are multiple sites of corneal infiltration
- perforation has increased the likelihood of endophthalmitis*

American Academy of Ophthalmology Cornea/External Disease Committee, Hoskins Center for Quality Eye Care. Preferred Practice Pattern Guidelines. *Bacterial Keratitis.* American Academy of Ophthalmology; 2018. www.aao.org/ppp

*Note: Anterior chamber tap for culture or intracameral antibiotic injection routinely performed in cases of endophthalmitis is generally not done in the presence of infectious corneal ulceration.

Table 12-8 Causes of Bacterial Keratitis

Common Organisms	Uncommon Organisms
Enterobacteriaceae (*Proteus* spp, *Enterobacter* spp, *Serratia* spp)	*Corynebacterium* spp
Pseudomonas aeruginosa (most common organism in soft contact lens wearers)	*Moraxella* spp
Staphylococcus aureus	*Mycobacterium* spp
Staphylococcus epidermidis	*Neisseria* spp
Streptococcus pneumoniae and other *Streptococcus* spp	*Nocardia* spp
	Non–spore-forming anaerobes, eg: *Actinomyces* spp, *Propionibacteria* spp

In addition to culturing corneal specimens, it may be helpful to culture samples obtained from contact lenses, contact lens cases and solutions, and any other potential sources of contamination, such as inflamed eyelids. The microbial yield in specimens collected for corneal cultures and smears is significantly higher before the initiation of antibiotic treatment, but specimens should still be cultured in cases of treatment failure. Some have suggested that antibiotics should be discontinued for 12 to 24 hours to increase the yield of the pathogen. Positive results of a smear do not obviate broad-spectrum treatment coverage but may guide coverage toward a different class of microorganism in the absence of positive culture findings. (See BCSC Section 4, *Ophthalmic Pathology and Intraocular Tumors,* for discussion of specimen collection, culturing, staining, and interpretation.) Culture results should always be interpreted in the context of the clinical condition of the patient. Negative results do not necessarily mean there is no infection. *Acanthamoeba* and fungal pathogens should be suspected if the history or appearance is suggestive, or if the clinical course has been atypical.

MANAGEMENT The primary goal of therapy is preservation of sight and of corneal integrity. Bacterial pathogens can cause irreversible corneal scarring over a period of hours because of their rapid proliferation, keratolytic enzyme activity, and stimulation of destructive host immune responses. To reduce bacterial load and minimize risk of visual loss, initiation of therapy is advised before a definitive diagnosis is obtained.

Initial therapy consists of empiric, broad-spectrum topical antibiotics. In routine corneal ulcers, topical fluoroquinolone monotherapy has excellent penetration at commercially available concentrations and provides outcomes equivalent to those of combination therapy. The recommended regimen for fluoroquinolones is every 30 to 60 minutes initially and then tapering in frequency according to the clinical response. In severe cases, administration of antibiotics every 5 minutes for 30 minutes as a loading dose may be considered. Second-generation fluoroquinolones (ciprofloxacin, ofloxacin) continue to have excellent *Pseudomonas* coverage but lack useful gram-positive activity. Third- and fourth-generation fluoroquinolones (eg, moxifloxacin, gatifloxacin, levofloxacin, and besifloxacin) have improved gram-positive and atypical mycobacterial coverage, compared with predecessors, but have limited activity against methicillin-resistant *Staphylococcus aureus* (MRSA). Alternatively, topical combination therapy with an agent active against gram-positive bacteria and another agent active against gram-negative bacteria can be given initially (Table 12-9).

Table 12-9 Initial Therapy for Bacterial Keratitis

Organism	Antibiotic	Topical Dose	Subconjunctival Dose
Gram-positive cocci	Cefazolin	50 mg/mL	100 mg in 0.5 mL
	Vancomycin 25–50 mg/mL[a]	25–50 mg/mL	25 mg in 0.5 mL
	Moxifloxacin, gatifloxacin, levofloxacin, besifloxacin	5–6 mg/mL	Not available
Gram-negative rods	Tobramycin	9–14 mg/mL	20 mg in 0.5 mL
	Ceftazidime	50 mg/mL	100 mg in 0.5 mL
	Ciprofloxacin, ofloxacin, moxifloxacin, gatifloxacin, levofloxacin, besifloxacin	3–6 mg/mL	Not available
No organism or multiple types of organisms	Fortified cefazolin	50 mg/mL	100 mg in 0.5 mL
	with		
	Fortified tobramycin	9–14 mg/mL	20 mg in 0.5 mL
	or		
	Fluoroquinolones	3–6 mg/mL	Not available
Gram-negative cocci	Ceftriaxone	50 mg/mL	100 mg in 0.5 mL
	Ceftazidime	50 mg/mL	100 mg in 0.5 mL
	Ciprofloxacin, ofloxacin, moxifloxacin, gatifloxacin, levofloxacin, besifloxacin	3–6 mg/mL	Not available
Mycobacteria	Clarithromycin	10 mg/mL 0.03%	
	Moxifloxacin, gatifloxacin, besifloxacin	5–6 mg/mL	Not available
	Amikacin	20–40 mg/mL	20 mg in 0.5 mL

[a] For resistant *Staphylococcus* spp.

Notes for Table 12-9: Preparation of topical antibiotics

Cefazolin 50 mg/mL

1. Add 9.2 mL of artificial tears to a vial of cefazolin in 1 g (powder for injection).
2. Dissolve. Take 5 mL of this solution and add it to 5 mL of artificial tears.
3. Refrigerate and shake well before instillation.

Vancomycin 50 mg/mL (Dilution can be extrapolated to a 15–25 mg/mL concentration by a compounding pharmacy.)

1. Add 10 mL of 0.9% sodium chloride for injection USP (no preservatives) or artificial tears to a 500-mg vial of vancomycin to produce a solution of 50 mg/mL.
2. Refrigerate and shake well before instillation.

Ceftazidime 50 mg/mL

1. Add 9.2 mL of artificial tears to a vial of ceftazidime 1 g (powder for injection).
2. Dissolve. Take 5 mL of this solution and add it to 5 mL of artificial tears.
3. Refrigerate and shake well before instillation.

Tobramycin 14 mg/mL

1. Withdraw 2 mL of tobramycin injectable from vial (40 mg/mL).
2. Add 2 mL to a tobramycin ophthalmic solution (5 mL) to give a 14 mg/mL solution.
3. Refrigerate and shake well before instillation.

In general, administration of a topical cycloglegic agent is recommended to reduce discomfort and prevent pupillary block related to inflammation. IOP should be monitored during therapy and may be reduced with topical medication if needed.

Fortified antibiotics (compounded at higher concentrations than the commercially available counterparts) may be administered for severe ulcers when increased drug concentration in the corneal stroma is desired. Fortified antibiotics generally are difficult to obtain and have greater toxicity. Fortified vancomycin may be considered for gram-positive coverage of large or vision-threatening ulcers, when MRSA is suspected, or after failure of the initial therapy. With effective treatment, most infectious keratitis cases will have negative culture results by 48 to 72 hours. Once the offending microbe is identified or there is clinical improvement, appropriate monotherapy may be considered (see Table 12-9) to reduce toxicity while maintaining coverage. Continued administration of fortified antibiotics beyond 7 days is not advisable because of increased toxicity. At times, bacterial keratitis will improve with antibiotic therapy even when in vitro data suggest resistance of the causative agent to that antibiotic. Therefore, the clinical response should guide the choice of medical therapy.

Several parameters are useful for monitoring improvement in the clinical response to antibiotic therapy:

- reepithelialization
- blunting of the perimeter of the stromal infiltrate
- decreased density of the stromal infiltrate (caution: stromal loss will also result in corneal clearing)
- cessation of corneal thinning
- reduction in stromal edema and endothelial inflammatory plaque
- reduction in anterior chamber inflammation

Systemic antibiotics—especially fluoroquinolones, which have excellent ocular penetration—and intensive topical antibiotics are indicated in cases with suspected scleral and/or intraocular extension of infection but generally are not used in routine cases of bacterial keratitis.

The role of corticosteroid therapy for bacterial keratitis remains controversial. Tissue destruction results from a combination of the direct effects of the bacteria and the host inflammatory response, including the release of proteolytic enzymes, which persist after corneal sterilization. Corticosteroids are effective at controlling inflammation but inhibit the host response to infection. The literature strongly suggests that corticosteroid therapy administered *prior to* appropriate antibiotic therapy worsens prognosis. In a randomized clinical trial in which topical corticosteroids were given 48 hours after initiation of topical antibiotics for bacterial keratitis, no effect on final visual outcome or complication rate was seen at 3 months. There were trends toward improved outcomes in patients with the poorest vision at baseline who received corticosteroids and for the entire corticosteroid group at 1 year. In this study, cases of keratitis caused by *Nocardia*, which is uncommon in the United States, had worse outcomes with corticosteroid treatment.

Although corticosteroid use is unsupported, it generally does not increase the risk of poor outcomes or complications in treated bacterial keratitis, and certain patients benefit from the addition of corticosteroids to antibiotic therapy.

The following are recommendations for conditions of bacterial keratitis in which corticosteroid therapy should not be given:

- in the absence of appropriate antibiotic therapy
- if the patient is unable to return for frequent follow-up or adhere to antibiotic therapy
- if any other virulent or difficult-to-eradicate organism is found or suspected

Corticosteroid 1% drops may be started every 6 hours beginning 48 hours after initiation of antibiotic therapy. If the patient experiences no adverse effects, the frequency of administration may be adjusted based on clinical response. If a patient on long-term topical steroid therapy presents with bacterial keratitis, the corticosteroids should be decreased, with an expectation of increased inflammation. If fungal or *Acanthamoeba* infection is suspected, corticosteroids should be stopped. Additional measures, including lubrication, bandage contact lenses, and patching, may be needed to promote reepithelialization and reduce keratolysis. Collagen crosslinking may be considered as adjunctive therapy for bacterial keratitis; however, there is not sufficient evidence to support its use in primary management of bacterial keratitis.

Surgical treatment of bacterial keratitis is indicated if the disease progresses despite therapy or is otherwise unresponsive to therapy—or if descemetocele formation or perforation occurs. Lamellar keratoplasty (LK) may be preferable to penetrating keratoplasty (PK) because LK is associated with lower risk of intraocular seeding of infection, formation of peripheral anterior synechiae, glaucoma, and cataract formation associated with entering the anterior chamber. Descemetocele and perforations smaller than 2 mm may be managed with tissue adhesive as a therapeutic modality (see Chapter 5). Amniotic membrane grafting is not recommended when the infection has not resolved completely, has not been clearly identified, or if a corneal perforation is present. Peripheral iridectomy should be performed during PK because extensive synechiae may develop from inflammatory membranes. Interrupted sutures are recommended, and the patient should be given appropriate topical antibiotics and cycloplegia. There is disagreement regarding topical corticosteroid use postkeratoplasty, particularly if the bacterial infection has not been controlled. See Chapter 16 in this volume for a more detailed discussion of LK and PK and BCSC Section 2, *Fundamentals and Principles of Ophthalmology,* for an in-depth discussion of ocular pharmacology.

American Academy of Ophthalmology Cornea/External Disease Panel, Hoskins Center for Quality Eye Care. Preferred Practice Pattern Guidelines. *Bacterial Keratitis.* American Academy of Ophthalmology; 2018. www.aao.org/ppp

Price MO, Tenkman LR, Schrier A, Fairchild KM, Trokel SL, Price FW Jr. Photoactivated riboflavin treatment of infectious keratitis using collagen cross-linking technology. *J Refract Surg.* 2012;28(10):706–713.

Schein OD, Glynn RJ, Poggio EC, Seddon JM, Kenyon KR. The relative risk of ulcerative keratitis among users of daily-wear and extended-wear soft contact lenses. A case-control study. Microbial Keratitis Study Group. *N Engl J Med.* 1989;321(12):773–778.

Srinivasan M, Mascarenhas J, Rajaraman R; Steroids for Corneal Ulcers Trial Group. Corticosteroids for bacterial keratitis: the Steroids for Corneal Ulcers Trial (SCUT). *Arch Ophthalmol.* 2012;130(2):143–150.

Srinivasan M, Mascarenhas J, Rajaraman R; Steroids for Corneal Ulcers Trial Group. The Steroids for Corneal Ulcers Trial (SCUT): Secondary 12-month clinical outcomes of a randomized controlled trial. *Am J Ophthalmol.* 2014;157(2):327–333.

Atypical mycobacteria

Although *Staphylococcus* is the most common causative agent in early onset keratitis following refractive surgery, atypical mycobacteria frequently are associated with laser in situ keratomileusis (LASIK)-related infections that occur 1 week or later postsurgically (Figs 12-14, 12-15). The most common atypical mycobacteria are *Mycobacterium fortuitum* and *M chelonae,* which are found in soil and water. These organisms should be suspected in delayed-onset post-LASIK infection, particularly with recalcitrant, nonsuppurative infiltrates. After LASIK, the surgical flap should be lifted to obtain specimens for culture. Positive results should be confirmed with acid-fast staining or culture on Löwenstein-Jensen medium. Medical treatment options include oral and topical clarithromycin, amikacin, linezolid, and fluoroquinolones with antimycobacterial activity, including moxifloxacin, besifloxacin, and gatifloxacin.

Chang MA, Jain S, Azar DT. Infections following laser in situ keratomileusis: an integration of the published literature. *Surv Ophthalmol.* 2004;49(3):269–280.

Hyon JY, Joo MJ, Hose S, Sinha D, Dick JD, O'Brien TP. Comparative efficacy of topical gatifloxacin with ciprofloxacin, amikacin, and clarithromycin in the treatment of experimental *Mycobacterium chelonae* keratitis. *Arch Ophthalmol.* 2004;122(8):1166–1169.

Fungal Keratitis

In the United States, fungal keratitis is less common than bacterial keratitis, accounting for less than 10% of corneal infections; filamentous fungal keratitis occurs more frequently in warm, humid regions.

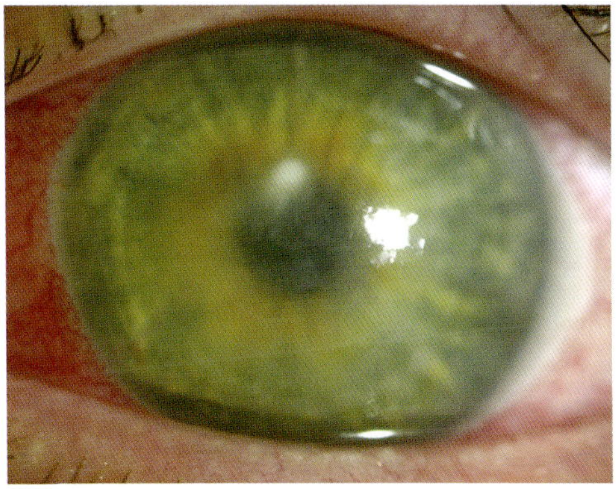

Figure 12-14 Atypical mycobacterial infection following laser in situ keratomileusis (LASIK). *(Courtesy of Elmer Y. Tu, MD.)*

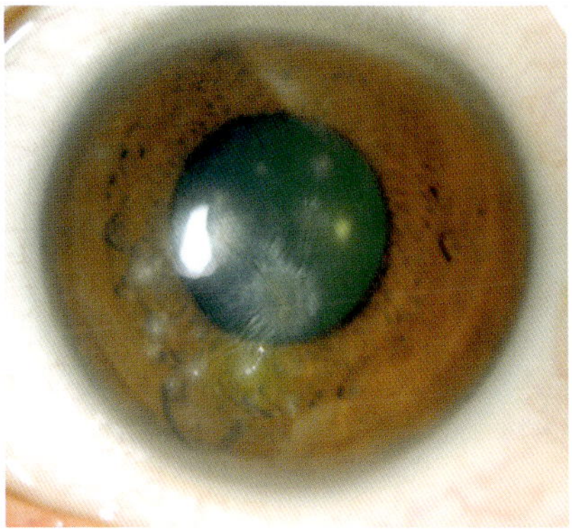

Figure 12-15 Atypical mycobacterial infection. *(Courtesy of Christopher J. Rapuano, MD.)*

Risk factors for fungal keratitis include the following:

- trauma to the cornea with plant or vegetable material (the leading risk factor)
- contact lens wear
- corticosteroid use (corticosteroids activate and increase the virulence of fungal organisms and dampen host resistance to infection.)
- chronic corneal erosions/ulceration from other causes
- chronic keratitis (eg, due to HSV, herpes zoster, or vernal/atopic keratoconjunctivitis)
- systemic immunosuppression (which predisposes individuals to fungal keratitis [eg, *Candida*])
- corneal surgery (eg, penetrating keratoplasty, endothelial keratoplasty)

Chang DC, Grant GB, O'Donnell K, et al; Fusarium Keratitis Investigation Team. Multistate outbreak of *Fusarium* keratitis associated with use of a contact lens solution. *JAMA*. 2006; 296(8):953–963.

CLINICAL PRESENTATION Patients with fungal keratitis tend to have fewer early signs and symptoms of an inflammatory response than do patients with bacterial keratitis and may have little or no conjunctival injection at presentation. However, the severity of pain in fungal keratitis can be disproportionately greater than the amount of corneal inflammation.

In the initial stage, filamentous fungal keratitis manifests as a gray-white, nonsuppurative infiltrate with irregular feathery or filamentous margins (Fig 12-16). Superficial lesions may elevate the surface of the cornea and have a dry, rough, or gritty texture detectable at time of diagnostic corneal scraping. Multifocal or satellite infiltrates may be present. In addition, a deep stromal infiltrate may develop in the presence of an intact epithelium. An endothelial plaque or hypopyon may also occur, particularly if the fungal infiltrate is deep or large, or if it has penetrated into the anterior chamber.

As fungal keratitis progresses, intense suppuration may develop, and the infiltrates may resemble those of bacterial keratitis. Rapidly progressive hypopyon and inflammatory membranes of the anterior chamber also may occur, potentially signaling extension of the fungal infection into the anterior chamber. Occasionally, fungus may invade the iris or posterior chamber, precipitating angle-closure glaucoma secondary to inflammatory pupillary block.

Candida species are the most common organisms causing yeast keratitis, which presents as superficial white, raised colonies. Infection is usually superficial, but deep

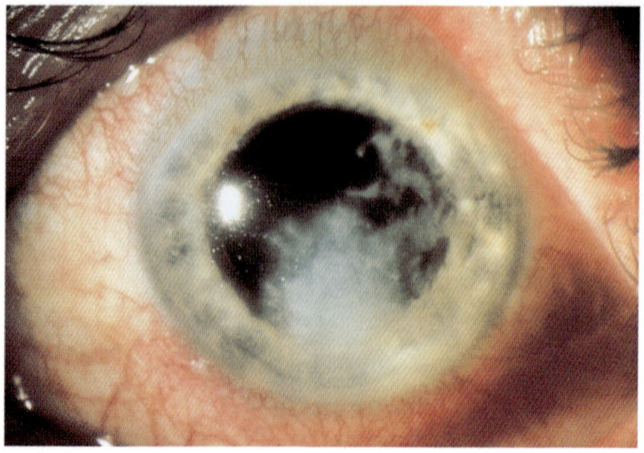

Figure 12-16 Fungal keratitis caused by *Fusarium solani* with characteristic dry-appearing, white stromal infiltrate with feathery edges.

invasion may occur, with suppuration resembling that of keratitis induced by gram-positive bacteria.

LABORATORY EVALUATION Results of smears stained with acridine orange, calcofluor white, or potassium hydroxide (KOH) can assist the clinician in making a rapid diagnosis. Blood agar, Sabouraud dextrose agar, and brain–heart infusion agar are the preferred media for fungal culture, and in vitro antifungal sensitivity testing can be helpful in optimizing medical treatment. Confocal microscopy is an effective tool for detecting branching filaments and individual septa, which are common findings of mold pathogens in the cornea. PCR may be applied for highly sensitive detection of fungal infections.

MANAGEMENT Natamycin 5% suspension is recommended for treatment of filamentous fungal keratitis, particularly those caused by *Fusarium* species. Topical amphotericin B 0.15% is highly efficacious in cases of yeast keratitis such as *Candida* species. Amphotericin B is also recommended for filamentous keratitis caused by *Aspergillus* species. Use of topical voriconazole 1% has increased, and efficacy has been demonstrated in cases of fungal keratitis unresponsive to other therapy; however, drug resistance has been reported, and a recent prospective, randomized clinical trial concluded that voriconazole is inferior to natamycin for empiric therapy, especially for *Fusarium solani*.

Systemic treatment may be considered for severe keratitis or keratitis with scleral or intracameral extension. Ketoconazole (200–600 mg/day), fluconazole (200–400 mg/day), or itraconazole (200 mg/day) may be used, but oral voriconazole (200–400 mg/day) and posaconazole (800 mg/day) have excellent intraocular penetration and broad coverage and have been rapidly supplanting these older drugs. Alternatively, intrastromal injection of aqueous-soluble amphotericin B (5–10 µg/0.1 mL) or voriconazole (50–100 µg/0.1 mL) as primary or secondary treatment of deep fungal keratitis, and intracameral injection of either agent for intraocular extension, are becoming more widely validated. Culture-proven or histologically proven fungal keratitis that does not respond to therapy warrants speciation of the pathogen and antifungal sensitivity testing. Corneal crosslinking has been investigated as an adjunct therapy for fungal keratitis, but it appears to have no effect in deep stromal disease and mixed results in superficial fungal infections.

When smear results are negative and fungal infection is suspected, repeat scrapings or corneal biopsy may be necessary. Mechanical debridement may be beneficial in cases of superficial fungal keratitis. In cases of fungal infiltration of the deep corneal stroma, topical antifungal therapy may be ineffective because penetration of these agents is reduced in the presence of an intact epithelium. Penetration of natamycin or amphotericin B can be enhanced by debridement of the corneal epithelium. Patients with progressive disease despite maximum topical and/or oral antifungal therapy may require therapeutic LK or PK to prevent scleral or intraocular extension of the fungal infection; however, the prognosis for salvaging the eye is poor.

Bunya VY, Hammersmith KM, Rapuano CJ, Ayres BD, Cohen EJ. Topical and oral voriconazole in the treatment of fungal keratitis. *Am J Ophthalmol.* 2007;143(1):151–153.

Ferrer C, Alio JL. Evaluation of molecular diagnosis in fungal keratitis. Ten years of experience. *J Ophthalmic Inflamm Infect.* 2011; 1(1):15–22.

Loh AR, Hong K, Lee S, Mannis M, Acharya NR. Practice patterns in the management of fungal corneal ulcers. *Cornea.* 2009;28(8):856–859.

Prajna NV, Krishnan T, Mascarenhas J; Mycotic Ulcer Treatment Trial Group. The mycotic ulcer treatment trial: a randomized trial comparing natamycin vs voriconazole. *JAMA Ophthalmol.* 2013;131(4):422–429.

Acanthamoeba *keratitis*

Since 2003, a growing number of *Acanthamoeba* cases have occurred in the United States, particularly on the East Coast and in the Midwest. Results of 2 case-control studies showed an association between *Acanthamoeba* keratitis and use of Complete Moisture Plus multipurpose solution (formerly Advanced Medical Optics) for cleaning soft contact lenses, resulting in the voluntary recall of the product in May 2007. Unfortunately, the outbreak persisted, prompting a second multistate case-control study in 2011, led by the Centers for Disease Control and Prevention.

Joslin CE, Tu EY, McMahon TT, Passaro DJ, Stayner LT, Sugar J. Epidemiological characteristics of a Chicago-area *Acanthamoeba* keratitis outbreak. *Am J Ophthalmol.* 2006;142(2): 212–217.

Joslin CE, Tu EY, Shoff ME, et al. The association of contact lens solution use and *Acanthamoeba* keratitis. *Am J Ophthalmol.* 2007;144(2):169–180.

CLINICAL PRESENTATION Patients with amebic keratitis usually experience the following:

- severe ocular pain that is greater than expected from clinical findings
- photophobia
- a protracted, progressive course

The disease is bilateral in 7%–11% of patients and often is unresponsive to topical antimicrobial agents. In the early stage, infection with *Acanthamoeba* is localized to the corneal epithelium or just posterior and may present as diffuse epitheliopathy with coarse punctate features, subepithelial opacities, or dendritic epithelial lesions. Epithelial pseudodendrites often are misdiagnosed as herpetic keratitis and treated with antiviral agents and/or corticosteroids. Stromal infection typically manifests in the central cornea; early cases have a gray-white, superficial, nonsuppurative infiltrate. As the disease progresses, a partial or complete central ring infiltrate is often encountered (Fig 12-17). When seen, inflamed corneal nerves, known as *radial perineuritis* or *radial keratoneuritis,* are nearly pathognomonic of amebic keratitis.

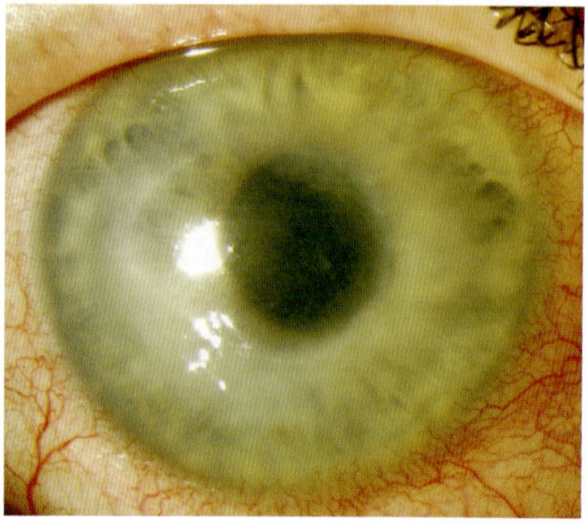

Figure 12-17 Ring infiltrate in *Acanthamoeba* keratitis. *(Courtesy of Shahzad I. Mian, MD.)*

Limbitis, scleritis (focal, nodular, or diffuse), or dacryoadenitis may be seen as well. Although intraocular extension may occur, consecutive encephalitis has not been reported.

Clinical features that favor a diagnosis of *Acanthamoeba* keratitis over HSV keratitis include the following:

- presence of epidemiologic risk factors, such as contact lens use or exposure to a hot tub or potentially contaminated freshwater
- disproportionately severe ocular pain (unlike the disproportionately mild pain secondary to trigeminal nerve involvement in HSV)
- a noncontiguous or multifocal pattern of granular epitheliopathy and subepithelial opacities (unlike the contiguous, dendritic pattern in HSV keratitis)
- failure of antiviral therapy to eradicate the infection

PATHOGENESIS *Acanthamoeba* is a genus of free-living ubiquitous protozoa found in freshwater and soil. Freezing, desiccation, and typical chlorine levels in municipal water supplies, swimming pools, and hot tubs are not sufficient to kill *Acanthamoeba*. Ocular exposure to well water and swimming in fresh water or ponds while wearing contact lenses increases risk of infection. *Acanthamoeba* may exist as motile trophozoites or dormant cysts. In Western countries, approximately 90% of reported cases of amebic keratitis have been associated with contact lens use, with the remainder linked to various other risk factors. Historically, episodic outbreaks of disease have been associated with water contamination, such as homemade saline contact lens solutions, groundwater affected by river flooding, or contaminated rooftop cisterns.

LABORATORY EVALUATION Diagnosis of *Acanthamoeba* keratitis is made by visualizing amebae in stained smears (eg, Giemsa, periodic acid–Schiff, calcofluor white, acridine orange) or by culturing organisms obtained from corneal scrapings on nonnutrient agar with overlay of *E coli* or *Enterobacter aerogenes*. Buffered charcoal–yeast agar also may be used as a substrate. In culture, characteristic trails form as the motile trophozoites travel across the surface of the plate. In vivo confocal microscopy can be performed to visualize *Acanthamoeba* cysts (Fig 12-18). Culture yield varies among laboratories, with findings of large studies indicating only 35% to 50% positivity for *Acanthamoeba* despite suggestive clinical presentation or

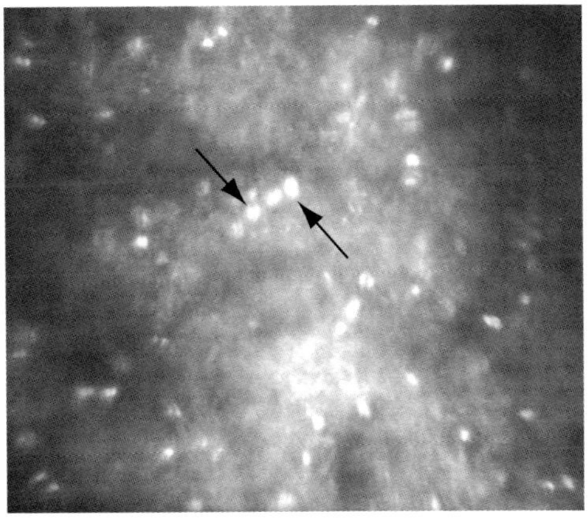

Figure 12-18 In vivo confocal microscopy image of *Acanthamoeba* cysts *(arrows)*. *(Courtesy of Elmer Y. Tu, MD.)*

confocal microscopy. Examination of contact lenses and related paraphernalia may be advisable. Lamellar corneal biopsy may be required to establish the diagnosis.

MANAGEMENT Early diagnosis of *Acanthamoeba* keratitis is the most important indicator of a good prognosis. However, diagnostic delay is common because of the nonspecific presentation of the disease and the specialized microbiological methods needed for diagnosis.

Cases identified early, which are defined as epithelial or anterior stromal, have an excellent visual prognosis and generally respond well to epithelial debridement, followed by a 3- to 4-month course of antiamebic therapy. Findings of deep stromal inflammation, a ring infiltrate, or extracorneal manifestations worsen the prognosis and often necessitate longer treatment (a year or more), other adjunctive therapy, or therapeutic keratoplasty.

Several antimicrobial agents have been recommended for medical treatment of *Acanthamoeba* keratitis based on their in vitro amebicidal effects as well as their clinical effectiveness. Topical agents include the following:

- *diamidines:* propamidine, hexamidine
- *biguanides:* polyhexamethylene biguanide (polyhexanide), chlorhexidine
- *aminoglycosides:* neomycin, paromomycin
- *imidazoles/triazoles:* voriconazole, miconazole, clotrimazole, ketoconazole, itraconazole

Only the biguanides have consistent in vitro and clinical efficacy against cysts and trophozoites; the other agents are effective primarily against trophozoites. Therefore, biguanides are the mainstay of pharmacologic treatment. Diamidines may be given early in the course of therapy, but resolution of the infection can be achieved with a biguanide alone. In a comparison of biguanides, chlorhexidine 0.02% and polyhexamethylene biguanide (PHMB) 0.02% performed similarly. Single-agent systemic treatment with voriconazole may be efficacious in recalcitrant cases.

CLINICAL PEARL

Corticosteroid exposure induces acanthamoebal excystment in vitro and may worsen clinical outcomes when used prior to effective anti-acanthamoebal therapy.

Much of the morbidity of *Acanthamoeba* keratitis, including scleritis, glaucoma, and cataract, can be attributed to the exuberant host response. The judicious use of topical and systemic immunosuppressants may be beneficial after the patient has received at least 2 weeks of anti-acanthamoebal therapy.

Traditionally, keratoplasty has been reserved for vision rehabilitation after completion of treatment or for cases that progress despite maximal medical therapy and are at risk of perforation. Recent results have indicated that LK and PK may reduce the rate of recurrent infection and improve visual outcomes when combined with adjunctive anti-acanthamoebal agents. However, medical treatment is preferred in the vast majority of cases. It is advisable to perform optical keratoplasty only after a full course of amebicidal therapy because recurrence is possible when medical therapy is ended prematurely. Corneal crosslinking is not currently recommended for the treatment of *Acanthamoeba* keratitis because of efficacy concerns.

Dart JK, Saw VP, Kilvington S. *Acanthamoeba* keratitis: diagnosis and treatment update 2009. *Am J Ophthalmol.* 2009;148(4):487–499.e2.
Robaei D, Carnt N, Minassian DC, Dart JK. The impact of topical corticosteroid use before diagnosis on the outcome of *Acanthamoeba* keratitis. *Ophthalmology.* 2014;121(7):1383–1388.
Robaei D, Carnt N, Minassian DC, Dart JK. Therapeutic and optical keratoplasty in the management of *Acanthamoeba* keratitis: risk factors, outcomes, and summary of the literature. *Ophthalmology.* 2015;122(1):17–24.
Tu EY. *Acanthamoeba* and other parasitic corneal infections. In: Mannis MJ, Holland EJ, eds. *Cornea.* Vol 1. 4th ed. Elsevier; 2017:976–985.
Tu EY, Joslin CE, Sugar J, Shoff ME, Booton GC. Prognostic factors affecting visual outcome in *Acanthamoeba* keratitis. *Ophthalmology.* 2008;115(11):1998–2003.

Corneal Stromal Inflammation Associated With Systemic Infection

Nonsuppurative stromal keratitis can be caused by the following:

- reactive arthritis
- congenital or acquired syphilis
- Lyme disease
- tuberculosis
- leprosy
- onchocerciasis

See BCSC Section 9, *Uveitis and Ocular Inflammation* for further discussion.

Microsporidiosis

CLINICAL PRESENTATION Based on the patient's immune status, 1 of 2 presentations of microsporidial infection may occur. Immunocompetent individuals may experience corneal stromal keratitis, whereas those who are immunocompromised (particularly those with AIDS) may have conjunctivitis and epithelial keratopathy (Fig 12-19). Immunocompromised

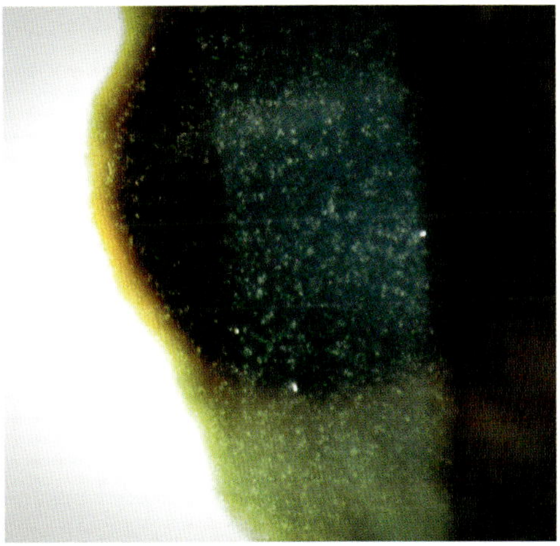

Figure 12-19 Microsporidial epitheliopathy. *(Courtesy of Woodford S. Van Meter, MD.)*

patients may also have disseminated microsporidiosis involving the sinuses, respiratory tract, or gastrointestinal tract.

Common symptoms include ocular irritation, photophobia, decreased vision, and bilateral conjunctival injection with little or no associated inflammation. Depending on the genus of the microsporidium, the condition may manifest as stromal keratitis or keratoconjunctivitis. In the keratoconjunctivitis variant, corneal findings include superficial nonstaining opacities described as "mucoid" in appearance, dense areas of fine punctate fluorescein staining, and a clear corneal stroma, with minimal or no iritis.

LABORATORY EVALUATION Microsporidosis-positive conjunctival biopsy specimens stained with Brown and Hopps solution and visualized with light microscopy exhibit small gram-positive spores in epithelial cells (Fig 12-20). Transmission electron microscopy (Fig 12-21), immunofluorescence antibody techniques, or elaborate tissue culture techniques may also be used for evaluation.

PATHOGENESIS Microsporidia are intracellular protozoa known to cause ocular infection. Initially recognized as an opportunistic pathogen in individuals with immunosuppression, this organism is increasingly being identified as the cause of infection in immunocompetent persons, especially in Southeast Asia. Deep stromal infection may present as chronic, progressive keratitis in immunocompetent patients.

MANAGEMENT Restoration of immune function can lead to resolution of microsporidial keratitis. Although there is no definitive treatment, topical fumagillin has been used successfully for microsporidial keratoconjunctivitis, with little toxic effect. Topical treatment with voriconazole 1% and oral itraconazole 200 mg 2 times per day may also be effective. In severe infection, granulomatous inflammation may lead to necrotic thinning and perforation necessitating PK. Medical therapy generally must be prolonged, and recurrence is common after treatment discontinuation. Topical fluoroquinolones (ciprofloxacin 0.3%,

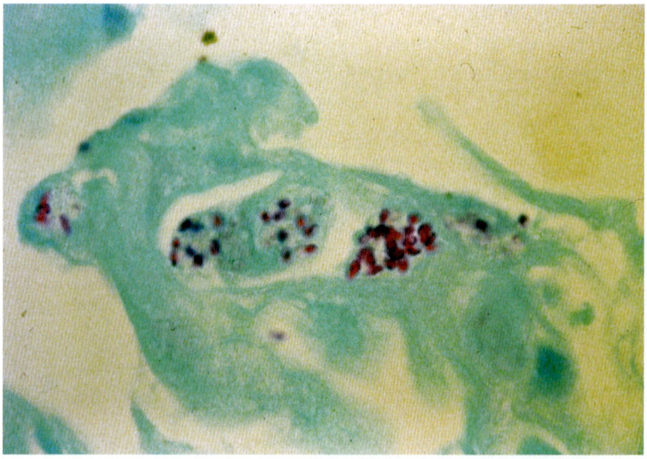

Figure 12-20 Intracellular spores of microsporidia viewed under light microscopy. *(Courtesy of Woodford S. Van Meter, MD.)*

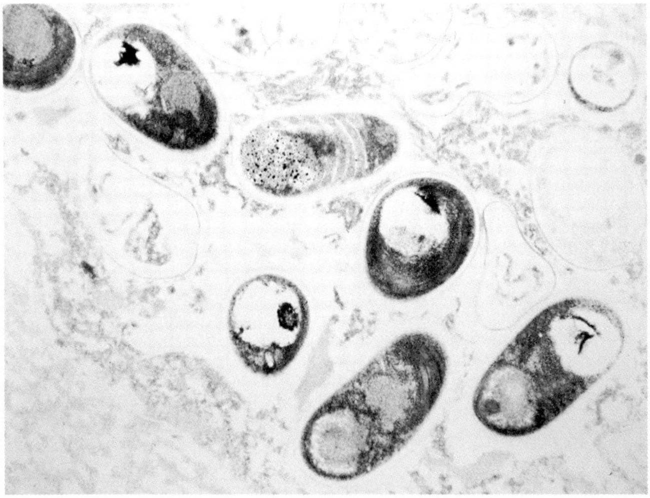

Figure 12-21 Visualization of microsporidia by electron microscopy. *(Courtesy of Woodford S. Van Meter, MD.)*

moxifloxacin 0.5%, gatifloxacin 0.5%, levofloxacin 0.5%, and norfloxacin 0.3%) as monotherapy or in combination with topical fumagillin or systemic albendazole have been effective for the treatment of microsporidial keratitis, with resolution in 99% of cases even on topical fluoroquinolone monotherapy.

Joseph J, Sridhar MS, Murthy S, Sharma S. Clinical and microbiological profile of microsporidial keratoconjunctivitis in southern India. *Ophthalmology.* 2006;113(4):531–537.

Loh RS, Chan CM, Ti SE, Lim L, Chan KS, Tan DT. Emerging prevalence of microsporidial keratitis in Singapore: epidemiology, clinical features, and management. *Ophthalmology.* 2009;116(12):2348–2353.

Loiasis

Infection with *Loa loa* (loiasis) and other filarial nematodes can result in conjunctivitis and dermatologic manifestations. The microfilarial stage of the parasite is transmitted from human to human by the bite of an infected female deerfly indigenous to West and Central Africa. A migrating worm burrows subcutaneously at about 1 cm/min but is most conspicuous when it is seen or felt wriggling under the periocular skin or bulbar conjunctiva (Fig 12-22). Extraction of the filarial worm cures the conjunctivitis; antiparasitic treatment then is administered for disseminated infestation. Diethylcarbamazine may be given 2 mg/kg 3 times a day for 3 weeks and repeated as necessary. Ivermectin 150 mg/kg may also be effective, but significant adverse effects have been reported in patients with prominent intravascular loiasis. Concurrent administration of corticosteroids and/or antihistamines may be necessary to minimize allergic reactions.

Microbial Scleritis

Bacterial and fungal infections of the sclera are rare. Most cases result from the extension of microbial keratitis involving the peripheral cornea. Trauma and exposure to contaminated

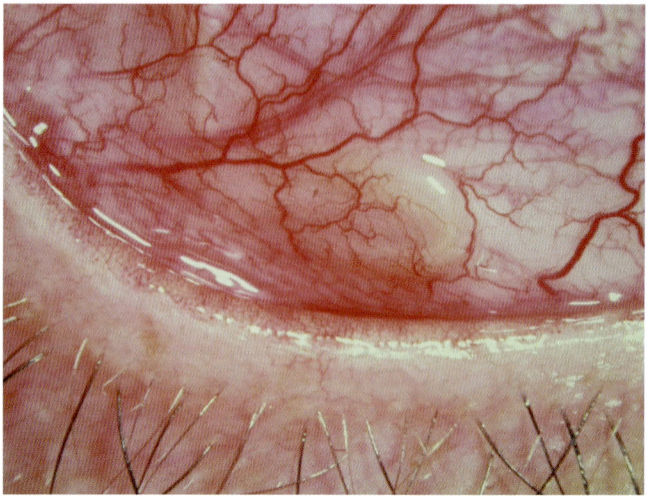

Figure 12-22 Subconjunctival loiasis. *(Courtesy of Woodford S. Van Meter, MD.)*

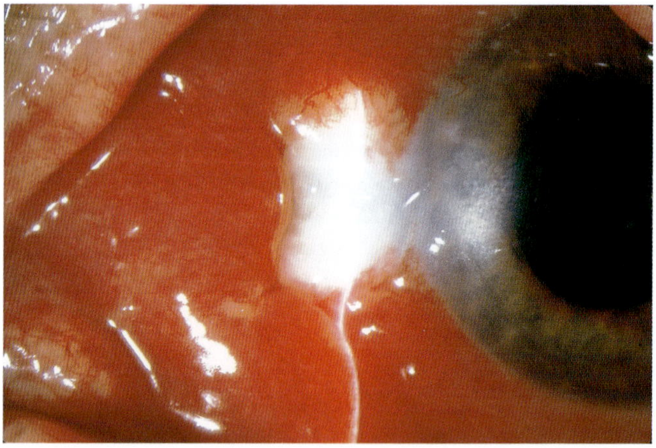

Figure 12-23 Bacterial scleritis occurring 2 weeks after pterygium surgery. *(Courtesy of Kirk R. Wilhelmus, MD.)*

foreign bodies (including scleral buckles) are possible risk factors. Bacterial scleritis may manifest in sclera damaged by previous pterygium surgery, especially when beta irradiation or mitomycin has been used (Fig 12-23). Bacteria and fungi can also invade tissue of the eye wall surrounding a scleral surgical wound, often leading to endophthalmitis. Scleral inflammation may accompany syphilis, tuberculosis, or leprosy, as well as infection with *Acanthamoeba* species, *Nocardia* species, or atypical mycobacteria. Tuberculous scleritis should be considered in chronic steroid-dependent scleritis or in surgically induced necrotizing scleritis. Diffuse or nodular scleritis is an occasional complication of ocular infection with varicella-zoster virus.

LABORATORY EVALUATION Suppurative scleritis can be assessed in the same manner as microbial keratitis. Antimicrobial therapy can be initiated after results of smears and cultures are obtained. If the overlying epithelium is intact, obtaining a scleral or episcleral biopsy specimen is recommended for culture, histologic examination, and molecular diagnostic testing. The workup of nonsuppurative scleritis is guided by the history and by findings from the examination.

MANAGEMENT Topical antimicrobial therapy is the same as for microbial keratitis. Because of the difficulty in controlling microbial scleritis, subconjunctival injections and intravenous antibiotics may also be used. Results of long-term oral therapy have been favorable.

CHAPTER 13

Diagnosis and Management of Immune-Related Disorders of the Cornea and External Eye

This chapter includes a related video. Go to www.aao.org/bcscvideo_section08 or scan the QR code in the text to access this content.

Indicates selected key points within the chapter.

Highlights

- Acute Stevens-Johnson syndrome/toxic epidermal necrolysis is a medical emergency associated with significant risk of morbidity and mortality.
- Covering the entire ocular surface with amniotic membrane, including the eyelid margins, early in the acute phase of severe Stevens-Johnson syndrome or toxic epidermal necrolysis can be very helpful.
- Signs of mucous membrane pemphigoid include subepithelial conjunctival fibrosis, forniceal shortening, and trichiasis. Early diagnosis and initiation of immunosuppressive therapy can arrest disease progression and prevent blindness.
- Scleritis and/or peripheral ulcerative keratitis with an underlying collagen-vascular disease is indicative of inadequate control of the systemic disease. Initiation of or change in immunosuppressive therapy may be required.

Definition

The Gell and Coombs classification divides hypersensitivity reactions into 4 types:

- type I: immediate hypersensitivity (anaphylaxis)
- type II: antibody-mediated cytotoxic reactions
- type III: immune complex–mediated reactions
- type IV: cell-mediated reactions (delayed hypersensitivity)

The modern classification divides the effector responses of adaptive immunity into 3 categories:

- antibody-mediated
- lymphocyte-mediated (delayed hypersensitivity, cytotoxic lymphocytes)
- combined antibody and cellular mechanisms

Despite this reclassification, the Gell and Coombs categories still appear in the literature and are mentioned in this chapter as well. See BCSC Section 9, *Uveitis and Ocular Inflammation.*

Immune-Mediated Diseases of the Eyelid

Contact Dermatoblepharitis

CLINICAL PRESENTATION Topical ophthalmic medications, cosmetics, and environmental substances can occasionally trigger a local allergic reaction. An immediate hypersensitivity immunoglobulin (Ig) E–mediated (type I) reaction typically occurs within minutes after exposure to an allergen. Ocular reactions are associated with itching, eyelid erythema and swelling, and conjunctival hyperemia and chemosis (Fig 13-1). In rare cases, signs of systemic anaphylaxis may develop in the patient.

Lymphocyte-mediated delayed hypersensitivity (type IV) reactions typically begin 24–72 hours following instillation of a topical agent but may not occur for weeks or months of continual use. Patients are often sensitized by previous exposure to the offending drug or preservative. An acute eczematous reaction develops with erythema, edema, and scaling of the eyelid (Fig 13-2). Sequelae of chronic contact blepharoconjunctivitis include hyperpigmentation, dermal scarring, and lower eyelid ectropion. A papillary conjunctivitis associated with mucoid or mucopurulent discharge may develop. Inferior punctate epithelial erosions may be noted.

CLINICAL PEARL

Contact blepharoconjunctivitis may be caused by medications and preservatives such as

- cycloplegics such as atropine and homatropine
- aminoglycosides such as neomycin, gentamicin, and tobramycin
- antiviral agents such as idoxuridine and trifluridine
- glaucoma medications such as α-adrenergic agents and β-blockers
- preservatives such as thimerosal, benzalkonium chloride, and EDTA

MANAGEMENT Treatment of hypersensitivity reactions requires the identification and discontinuation of the offending agent. The history usually provides the necessary clues, but sometimes a "challenge test" is necessary to confirm a suspicion. Such tests should never be done in patients with a known systemic allergy to a drug.

Immediate hypersensitivity reactions are initially managed by allergen avoidance or discontinuation of the causative agent. Adjunctive therapy may involve the use of cold compresses, artificial lubricants, topical antihistamines, and mast-cell stabilizers. Topical

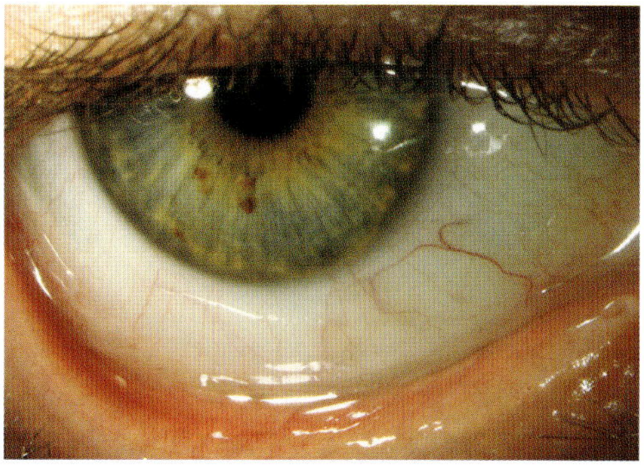

Figure 13-1 Acute anaphylactic reaction to a topical ophthalmic medication with chemosis and hyperemia of the palpebral conjunctiva. *(Courtesy of Arie L. Marcovich, MD, PhD.)*

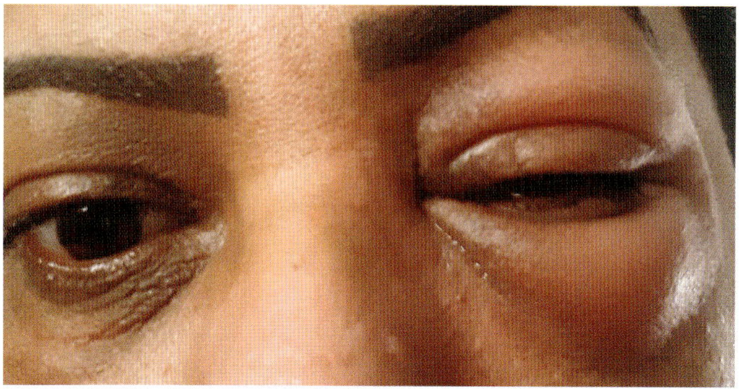

Figure 13-2 Delayed allergic contact conjunctivitis and dermatitis in the left eye secondary to use of a topical ophthalmic medication. *(Courtesy of Arie L. Marcovich, MD, PhD.)*

vasoconstrictors, either alone or in combination with antihistamines, may provide acute symptomatic relief, but long-term use is not recommended.

Delayed hypersensitivity reactions are also treated with allergen withdrawal. In severe cases, a several-day course of topical corticosteroids, tacrolimus ointment (0.03%), or pimecrolimus cream (1.0%; off-label use) applied to the eyelids and periocular skin may speed resolution of eyelid and conjunctival inflammation.

Atopic Dermatitis

CLINICAL PRESENTATION Atopic dermatitis is a chronic condition in genetically susceptible individuals that usually begins in infancy or childhood and may or may not involve the external eye. Patients report marked itching and eczematoid lesions on the eyelids and other sites (eg, joint flexures in adolescents and adults, face and extensor surfaces in infants and young children) (Fig 13-3). Affected patients usually have a personal or family history of atopic disorders, such as asthma, allergic rhinitis, nasal polyps, and aspirin hypersensitivity.

Ocular findings include periorbital darkening of the skin, exaggerated eyelid folds, meibomianitis, ectropion, and chronic papillary conjunctivitis. The appearance of the skin lesions varies depending on the age of the patient. Infants typically have an erythematous rash, children tend to have eczematous dermatitis with secondary lichenification from scratching, and adults have scaly patches with thickened and wrinkled dry skin.

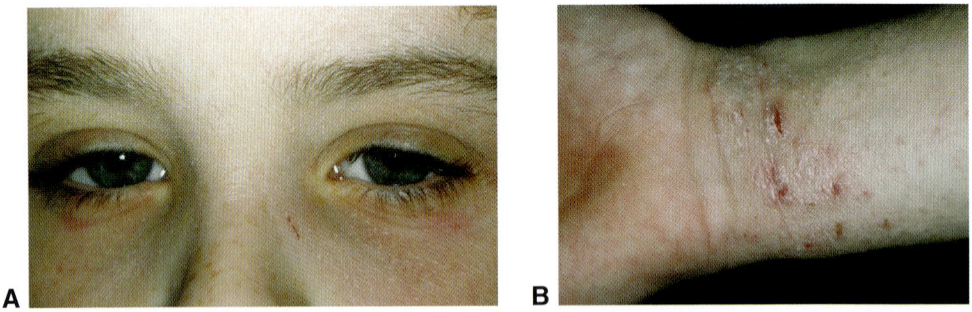

Figure 13-3 Atopic dermatitis in a child. **A,** Eyelid lesions. **B,** Eczematous dermatitis with secondary lichenification from scratching on joint flexures. *(Courtesy of Arie L. Marcovich, MD, PhD.)*

PATHOGENESIS The pathogenesis of atopic dermatitis involves a delayed hypersensitivity reaction and impaired cell-mediated immunity. In addition, there is an increase both in IgE hypersensitivity and in histamine release from mast cells and basophils.

MANAGEMENT It is important to identify and minimize allergens in the environment and in foods whenever possible. In general, it is advisable to consult with an allergist. Moisturizing lotions and petrolatum gels can be useful for skin hydration. Acute lesions can be controlled with a topical corticosteroid cream or ointment (clobetasone butyrate 0.05%), but long-term use of such medications is strongly discouraged to avoid skin thinning and ocular complications associated with corticosteroid use (eg, cataract, glaucoma). Topical tacrolimus ointment 0.03% and pimecrolimus cream 1.0% are also effective and have fewer adverse effects. Oral antipruritic agents such as antihistamines and mast-cell stabilizers can alleviate itching but may exacerbate dry eye symptoms secondary to anticholinergic activity. Dupilumab, an inhibitor of interleukins (ILs) 4 and 13, is an effective biologic treatment for atopic dermatitis. However, this treatment can induce mild to severe conjunctivitis and marked meibomian gland dysfunction that leads to the development of keratitis and signs and symptoms of evaporative dry eye disease. Treatment for these signs and symptoms consists of topical and oral corticosteroids, lubrication, eyelid hygiene, and warm compresses.

Delves PJ, Martin SJ, Burton DR, Roitt IM. *Roitt's Essential Immunology.* 13th ed. Wiley-Blackwell; 2017.

Langan SM, Irvine AD, Weidinger S. Atopic dermatitis. *Lancet.* 2020;396(10247):345–360.

Maudinet A, Law-Koune S, Duretz C, Lasek A, Modiano P, Tran THC. Ocular surface diseases induced by dupilumab in severe atopic dermatitis. *Ophthalmol Ther.* 2019;8(3):485–490.

Immune-Mediated Disorders of the Conjunctiva

Seasonal Allergic Conjunctivitis and Perennial Allergic Conjunctivitis

CLINICAL PRESENTATION Seasonal allergic conjunctivitis (SAC) can develop rapidly after airborne exposure to pollen, usually in spring and summer. Symptoms consist of itching (intense itching is a hallmark), eyelid swelling, conjunctival hyperemia, chemosis, and mucoid discharge. Attacks are usually short-lived and episodic. Affected individuals often have other atopic conditions, such as allergic rhinitis, asthma, and eczema (atopic dermatitis). Perennial allergic conjunctivitis (PAC) has a similar but milder presentation that can last year-round and is triggered by allergens like dust, occupational substances (eg, adhesives, metals, paints, latex), mites, molds, and animal dander.

PATHOGENESIS SAC and PAC are largely IgE-mediated hypersensitivity reactions. The allergen, which is typically airborne, enters the tear film and comes into contact with allergen-specific IgE bound to conjunctival mast cells. Degranulation of mast cells releases histamine and other inflammatory mediators that cause itching, vasodilation, and edema in the acute phase. Additional mediators signal recruitment of inflammatory cells, such as eosinophils in late-phase disease. In a presensitized individual, the activation and degranulation of mast cells can be triggered within minutes of allergen exposure.

LABORATORY EVALUATION The diagnosis of SAC is generally made through a careful patient history combined with the clinical signs and symptoms. Skin testing with a panel of allergens may be helpful in directing treatment.

MANAGEMENT Efforts are first directed at avoidance or elimination of the allergen. Thorough cleaning or replacing carpets, linens, and bedding in the patient's home can be effective in removing accumulated allergens, such as animal dander and dust mites. Having the patient shower and change clothing after exposure to allergens can also be helpful. It is important to identify contributing factors, including contact lenses and dry eye disease, because they can play an important role in facilitating allergen contact with the ocular surface. Glasses or goggles can serve as physical barriers. Treatment is based on the severity of patient symptoms and includes 1 or more of the following:

Supportive

- cold compresses
- artificial tears

Topical

- vasoconstrictors
- antihistamines and mast-cell stabilizers
- nonsteroidal anti-inflammatory drugs (NSAIDs)
- judicious use of corticosteroids

Systemic

- oral antihistamines
- desensitization injections

Artificial tears dilute and flush away allergens and other inflammatory mediators. Topical vasoconstrictors, alone or in combination with antihistamines, may provide acute symptom relief for redness. However, their use for more than 5–7 consecutive days may predispose the patient's eyes to a rebound effect of vascular dilation. Topical mast cell–stabilizing agents

Table 13-1 Topical Mast-Cell Stabilizers and Antihistamines for Allergic Conjunctivitis

Class	Drug
Mast cell stabilizers	Cromolyn 2% Lodoxamide 0.1% Nedocromil 2%
Antihistamines	Antazoline 0.5% Levocabastine 0.05% Pheniramine 0.3%
Mast cell stabilizers and antihistamines	Alcaftadine 0.25% Azelastine 0.05% Bepotastine 1.5% Epinastine 0.05% Ketotifen 0.035% Olopatadine 0.1% Pemirolast 0.1%

(Table 13-1) are useful in treating SAC. Oral antihistamines may provide symptom relief in some patients in the short term but may be associated with an increase in signs and symptoms of dry eye disease.

Desensitization injections (allergen-specific immunotherapy) can be beneficial if the offending allergen has been identified by skin testing. Certain topical NSAIDs have been approved by the US Food and Drug Administration for use in cases of ocular atopy, but their efficacy varies greatly. Reports of corneal perforations with the use of topical NSAIDs, especially the generic forms, suggest the need for careful monitoring. Topical corticosteroids are very effective in managing ocular allergy; however, they are typically reserved for cases unresponsive to other treatments and must be used with caution. If corticosteroids are prescribed, patients must be clearly informed of the associated risks and closely monitored for adverse effects. See BCSC Section 2, *Fundamentals and Principles of Ophthalmology,* for a discussion of topical antihistamines and mast-cell stabilizers.

American Academy of Ophthalmology Cornea/External Disease Committee, Hoskins Center for Quality Eye Care. Preferred Practice Pattern Guidelines. *Conjunctivitis.* American Academy of Ophthalmology; 2018. www.aao.org/ppp

Castillo M, Scott NW, Mustafa MZ, Mustafa MS, Azuara-Blanco A. Topical antihistamines and mast cell stabilisers for treating seasonal and perennial allergic conjunctivitis. *Cochrane Database Syst Rev.* 2015;6:CD009566. Epub 2015 Jun 1.

Mantelli F, Lambiase A, Bonini S, Bonini S. Clinical trials in allergic conjunctivitis: a systematic review. *Allergy.* 2011;66(7):919–924.

Mishra GP, Tamboli V, Jwala J, Mitra AK. Recent patents and emerging therapeutics in the treatment of allergic conjunctivitis. *Recent Pat Inflamm Allergy Drug Discov.* 2011;5(1): 26–36.

Ueta M, Kinoshita S. Ocular surface inflammation is regulated by innate immunity. *Prog Retin Eye Res.* 2012;31(6):551–575.

Vernal Keratoconjunctivitis

CLINICAL PRESENTATION Vernal keratoconjunctivitis (VKC) is a seasonally recurring, bilateral inflammation of the cornea and conjunctiva that occurs predominantly in children to young adults, with a 2:1 male predominance. Frequently, patients have a personal or family history of atopy that includes allergic rhinitis, asthma, or eczema. The disease may persist year-round in some patients. Symptoms consist of itching, photophobia, blurred vision, and copious mucoid discharge. There are 2 forms of VKC:

- *palpebral VKC,* which is associated with diffuse papillary hypertrophy that is usually more prominent on the tarsal conjunctiva of the upper eyelid. Bulbar hyperemia and chemosis are typically present. In more severe cases, giant papillae resembling cobblestones may develop on the upper tarsus (Fig 13-4; also see Fig 3-2).
- *limbal VKC,* which may develop alone or in association with palpebral VKC. The limbal conjunctiva has a thickened, gelatinous appearance, with opalescent spots called Horner-Trantas dots, which are aggregates of eosinophils and epithelial cells (Fig 13-5).

Corneal changes observed in VKC include punctate epithelial erosions in the superior and central cornea and pannus formation in the superior cornea. In severe cases, diffuse

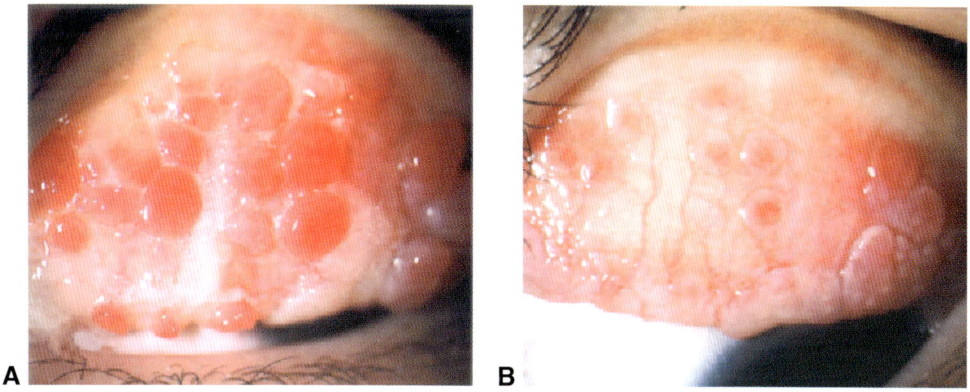

Figure 13-4 Palpebral vernal keratoconjunctivitis. **A,** Before treatment. **B,** After treatment with tacrolimus. *(Reproduced with permission from Ohashi Y, Ebihara N, Fujishima H, et al. A randomized, placebo-controlled clinical trial of tacrolimus ophthalmic suspension 0.1% in severe allergic conjunctivitis.* J Ocul Pharmacol Ther. *2010;26(2):165–174.)*

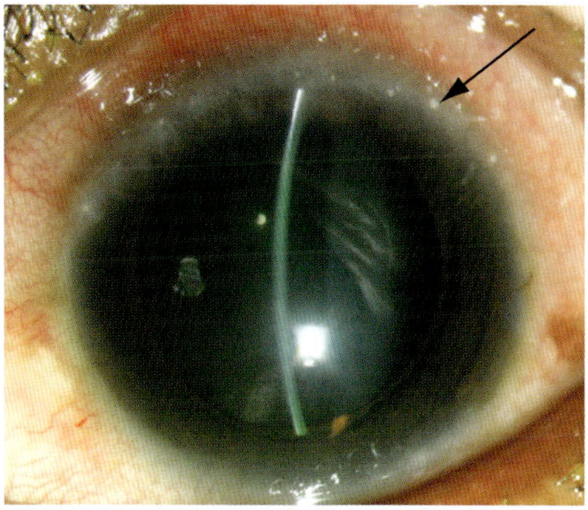

Figure 13-5 Limbal vernal keratoconjunctivitis. Note the Horner-Trantas dots *(arrow).* *(Courtesy of Arie L. Marcovich, MD, PhD.)*

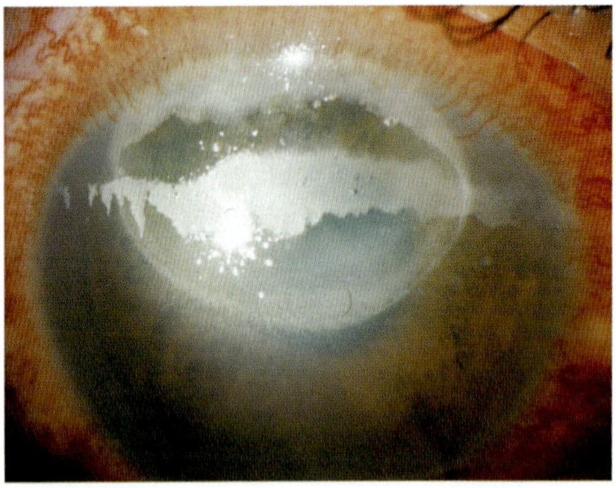

Figure 13-6 Shield ulcer in vernal keratoconjunctivitis. *(Courtesy of David Rootman MD.)*

peripheral corneal vascularization may develop. Corneal epithelial damage resulting from constant rubbing by superior tarsal giant papillae and cytotoxic agents secreted by eosinophils (major basic protein and eosinophil cationic protein) may lead to the formation of oval-shaped noninfectious ulcers, so-called shield ulcers, in the superior or central cornea (Fig 13-6). The secreted proteins form a dense plaque on the denuded stroma, preventing epithelialization. An association between VKC and keratoconus has been reported. Stem cell deficiency may also occur in severe cases.

PATHOGENESIS Both IgE and lymphocyte-mediated hypersensitivity reactions are involved. The conjunctival inflammatory infiltrate in VKC consists of eosinophils, lymphocytes, plasma cells, and monocytes.

MANAGEMENT Therapy is based on the severity of the patient's symptoms and the ocular surface disease. *Mild cases* are typically managed successfully with topical antihistamines. Environmental control may be helpful; home air-conditioning systems can filter and decrease exposure to the offending antigen. *Mild to moderate disease* may be responsive to topical mast-cell stabilizers; these drops are typically started in the month before symptoms usually begin in patients with seasonal exacerbations. *Year-round disease* may require long-term maintenance dosing.

Severe cases may require the use of topical corticosteroids. They are typically reserved for exacerbations that result in moderate to severe discomfort and/or decreased vision because of the possibility of corticosteroid-related complications from long-term administration. Fluorometholone may be preferred because it does not penetrate well into the anterior chamber. During those exacerbations, intermittent (pulse) therapy can be very effective. Topical corticosteroids can be used relatively frequently (eg, every 2 hours) for 5–7 days and then tapered for maintenance to 2 or 3 times daily during the allergy season. The use of corticosteroid ointment at bedtime may be effective and may also be less likely to be inappropriately used during the day, due to blurring of vision. Whenever corticosteroids are prescribed, it is critical to review the potential dangers of long-term topical corticosteroid use with the patient and family to emphasize the importance of close follow-up and monitoring for adverse effects.

Supratarsal injection of corticosteroid is an alternative to topical delivery in cooperative patients with severe VKC. The supratarsal subconjunctival space is located superior to the upper border of the superior tarsus and is most easily reached by everting the upper eyelid. After application of topical anesthesia, a supratarsal injection of 0.5–1.0 mL of either a relatively short-acting corticosteroid such as dexamethasone phosphate (4 mg/mL) or a longer-acting corticosteroid such as triamcinolone acetonide (40 mg/mL) can be performed. Monitoring of intraocular pressure (IOP) is mandatory, because corticosteroid-induced IOP spikes are possible. Close follow-up with an eye care provider is essential to monitor for cataract formation or permanent vision loss.

Steroid-sparing agents have been shown to be effective. Topical tacrolimus ointment 0.03% or 1.0% can be applied once to twice daily (off-label use), to treat refractory cases of VKC. Topical cyclosporine 0.05%–2.0% 2–4 times daily can also be used in an off-label fashion. Reported adverse effects of cyclosporine include punctate epithelial keratopathy and ocular surface irritation. Systemic anti-inflammatory therapy with oral prednisone given in a pulsed fashion can be helpful and is reserved for the most severe cases. Collaboration with an allergist is recommended.

Nonhealing shield ulcers can be treated by peeling or wiping of the corneal plaque followed by topical steroid and antibiotic drops (Video 13-1). A bandage contact lens may be applied. Use of amniotic membrane graft has been reported in severe cases.

VIDEO 13-1 Surgical treatment of shield ulcer.
Courtesy of Denise Wajnsztajn, MD; David Kohn, MD; Abraham Solomon, MD; and Joseph Frucht-Pery, MD.

Hazarika AK, Singh PK. Efficacy of topical application of 0.03% tacrolimus eye ointment in the management of allergic conjunctivitis. *J Nat Sci Biol Med.* 2015;6(Suppl 1):S10–S12.

Pucci N, Caputo R, di Grande L, et al. Tacrolimus vs. cyclosporine eyedrops in severe cyclosporine-resistant vernal keratoconjunctivitis: a randomized, comparative, double-blind, crossover study. *Pediatr Allergy Immunol.* 2015;26(3):256–261.

Sangwan VS, Jain V, Vemuganti GK, Murthy SI. Vernal keratoconjunctivitis with limbal stem cell deficiency. *Cornea.* 2011;30(5):491–496.

Singhal D, Sahay P, Maharana PK, Raj N, Sharma N, Titiyal JS. Vernal keratoconjunctivitis. *Surv Ophthalmol.* 2019;64(3):289–311.

Solomon A. Corneal complications of vernal keratoconjunctivitis. *Curr Opin Allergy Clin Immunol.* 2015;15(5):489–494.

Atopic Keratoconjunctivitis

CLINICAL PRESENTATION The ocular findings of atopic keratoconjunctivitis (AKC) are similar to those of VKC; Table 13-2 summarizes the differences. Specific findings in AKC include

- year-round disease, with minimal seasonal exacerbation
- older age, typically begins in late teens and peaks between the third and fifth decades of life
- eyelids that are typically scaly, indurated, and inflamed and frequently demonstrate keratinization

Table 13-2 Characteristics of Vernal and Atopic Keratoconjunctivitis

	Vernal Keratoconjunctivitis	Atopic Keratoconjunctivitis
Season	Spring and summer, but may exist year-round in severe cases	Year-round with acute exacerbations
Age	Children to young adults (2–22 years)	Adults (20–50 years)
Eyelids	Swelling of upper eyelids, ptosis	Scaly, indurated, and inflamed; keratinization of the margins can occur
Discharge	Copious, ropy, mucoid	Watery, clear
Conjunctival papillae	Giant papillae in upper tarsal conjunctiva	Small to medium-size papillae in the upper and lower tarsal conjunctiva
Limbal form	Limbal swelling with Horner-Trantas dots	No limbal form
Corneal involvement	Shield ulcer in severe cases; associated with keratoconus	Corneal vascularization and opacification can occur; associated with keratoconus, HSV
Cataract	Usually no cataract (unless corticosteroid-induced)	Posterior or anterior subcapsular cataract

- conjunctiva that has chemosis, often with subepithelial fibrosis and symblepharon formation (Fig 13-7)
- small or medium-sized papillae (as opposed to giant) that appear in the upper and lower palpebral conjunctiva
- eosinophils found in conjunctival cytology specimens that are less numerous and are less often degranulated
- vascularization and opacification of the cornea secondary to chronic epithelial disease, likely resulting from some degree of direct trauma from eyelid changes and/or limbal stem cell dysfunction (Fig 13-8)
- corneal findings that include
  - persistent epithelial defects
  - increased incidence of ectatic corneal diseases such as keratoconus and pellucid marginal degeneration, likely related to chronic eye rubbing
  - increased incidence of staphylococcal and herpes simplex infections
- development of posterior subcapsular and/or multifaceted or shield-shaped anterior subcapsular lens opacities

PATHOGENESIS Immunopathology of AKC combines IgE and lymphocyte-mediated reaction. One or more manifestations of AKC develop in approximately one-third of patients with atopic dermatitis. Atopic individuals demonstrate depressed systemic cell-mediated immunity. This altered immune status conveys a susceptibility to herpes simplex virus keratitis and colonization of the eyelids with *Staphylococcus aureus.*

MANAGEMENT AKC treatment involves allergen avoidance; cold compresses may also be of benefit. The use of pharmacotherapeutic agents similar to those used in the treatment of VKC is helpful. Just as in VKC, topical tacrolimus ointment 0.03% or 1.0% can be applied once to twice

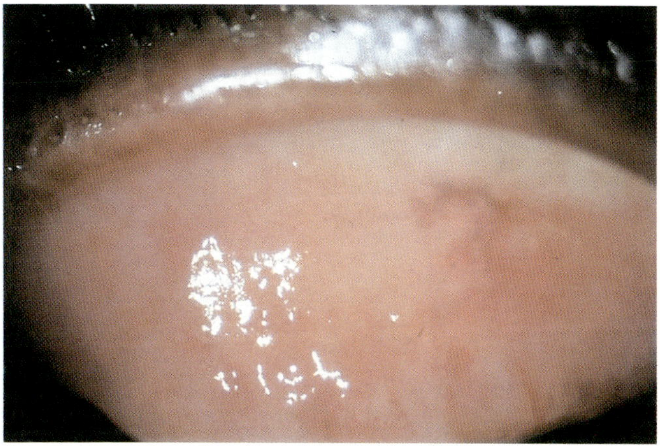

Figure 13-7 Atopic keratoconjunctivitis demonstrating small papillae, edema, and subepithelial fibrosis.

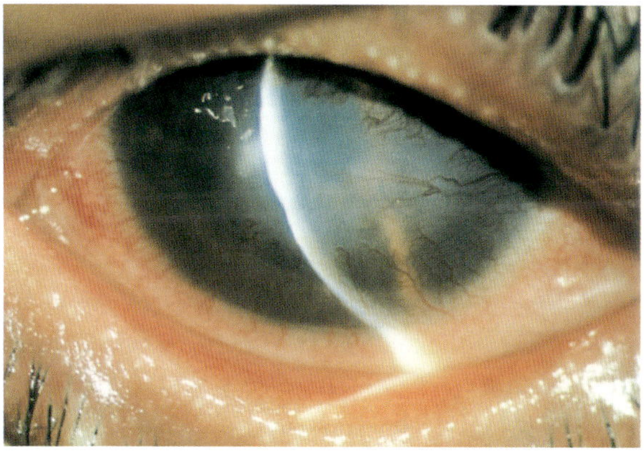

Figure 13-8 Severe corneal vascularization and scarring in an eye with atopic keratoconjunctivitis.

daily (off-label use) and topical cyclosporine 0.05%–2.0% 2–4 times daily can assist in limiting the topical corticosteroid required to control the inflammation. In addition, it is important to carefully monitor patients for infectious diseases that may warrant specific therapy, such as secondary staphylococcal infections and herpes simplex keratitis (see Chapters 11 and 12).

In severe cases, the indications for systemic therapy include chronic ocular surface inflammation unresponsive to topical treatment, ocular discomfort, progressive cicatrization, and peripheral ulcerative keratopathy. It is important to monitor the degree of systemic immunosuppression in coordination with an internist or rheumatologist. Systemic treatment of AKC may be beneficial in suppressing the IL-2 response, which promotes lymphocyte proliferation.

Brémond-Gignac D, Nischal KK, Mortemousque B, Gajdosova E, Granet DB, Chiambaretta F. Atopic keratoconjunctivitis in children: clinical features and diagnosis. *Ophthalmology.* 2016;123(2):435–437.

Chen JJ, Applebaum DS, Sun GS, Pflugfelder SC. Atopic keratoconjunctivitis: a review. *J Am Acad Dermatol.* 2014;70(3):569–575.

Erdinest N, Solomon A. Topical immunomodulators in the management of allergic eye disease. *Cur Opin Allergy Clin Immunol.* 2014;14(5):457–463.

García DP, Alperte JI, Cristóbal JA, et al. Topical tacrolimus ointment for treatment of intractable atopic keratoconjunctivitis: a case report and review of the literature. *Cornea.* 2011;30(4):462–465.

Ligneous Conjunctivitis

CLINICAL PRESENTATION Ligneous conjunctivitis is a rare, chronic autosomal recessive disorder characterized by the formation of firm woodlike yellowish fibrinous membranes on the conjunctival surface (Fig 13-9). Patients present with symptoms of ocular irritation and foreign-body sensation. The cardinal finding consists of yellowish, platelike masses that overlie 1 or more of the palpebral surfaces and are readily visible with eversion of the eyelid. Ligneous conjunctivitis is generally bilateral and can affect individuals of all ages.

PATHOGENESIS Ligneous conjunctivitis has been linked to severe type I plasminogen deficiency, with decreased fibrinolysis as the primary defect. More than 12% of patients have severe hypoplasminogenemia. The genetic defect in the plasminogen gene *(PLG)* is located at chromosome 6q26. The membranes are composed of fibrin, fibrin-bound tissue plasminogen activator (tPA), epithelial cells, and inflammatory cells that adhere to the conjunctival surface. Latent and activated forms of matrix metalloproteinase-9 (MMP-9) have also been identified.

MANAGEMENT Cultures can be taken at initial diagnosis to exclude a bacterial or viral pseudomembranous or membranous conjunctivitis. A complete surgical excision is typically combined with topical and systemic medical treatment. Amniotic membrane transplantation has been reported in some cases.

Topical treatment includes the following:

- plasminogen
- fresh frozen plasma
- heparin
- corticosteroids
- cyclosporine A 2%

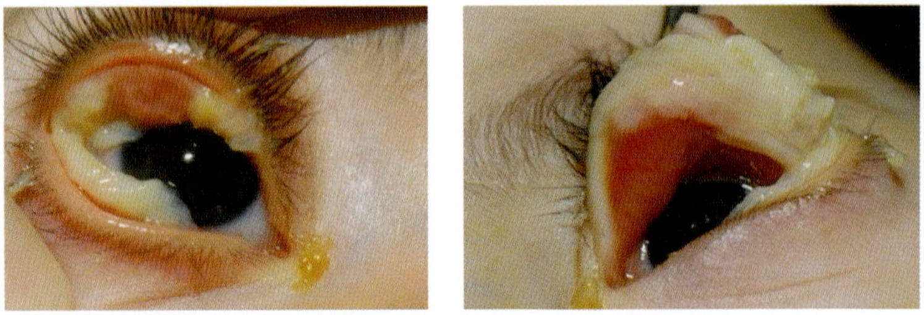

Figure 13-9 Firm yellowish lesions of the eyelids characteristic of ligneous conjunctivitis. *(Courtesy of John Dart, MD.)*

Intravenous treatment includes

- fresh frozen plasma
- lys-plasminogen

No single treatment has been shown to be consistently effective or superior. Recurrences are frequent and may require close follow-up and repeated excisions. Many cases of ligneous conjunctivitis eventually resolve spontaneously after several months to a few years.

Hiremath M, Elder J, Newall F, Mitchell S, Dyas R, Monagle P. Heparin in the long-term management of ligneous conjunctivitis: a case report and review of literature. *Blood Coagul Fibrinolysis.* 2011;22(7):606–609.

Ku JYF, Lichtinger A, Yeung SN, Kim P, Cserti-Gazdewich C, Slomovic AR. Topical fresh frozen plasma and heparin treatment of ligneous conjunctivitis in a Canadian hospital setting. *Can J Ophthalmol.* 2012;47(5):e27–e28.

Neff KD, Holland EJ, Schwartz GS. Ligneous conjunctivitis. In: Mannis MJ, Holland EJ, eds. *Cornea.* Vol 1. 4th ed. Elsevier; 2017:587–592.

Stevens-Johnson Syndrome, Stevens-Johnson Syndrome/Toxic Epidermal Necrolysis Overlap, and Toxic Epidermal Necrolysis

Stevens-Johnson syndrome (SJS), SJS/toxic epidermal necrolysis (SJS/TEN) overlap, and TEN are acute inflammatory, vesiculobullous reactions involving the skin and at least 2 mucous membranes. The conjunctiva and oropharynx are the tissues most frequently involved. In this chapter, the term SJS–TEN is used to refer collectively to SJS, SJS/TEN overlap, and TEN.

The current nomenclature is based on the amount of skin involvement:

- SJS: less than 10%
- SJS/TEN overlap: 10%–30%
- TEN: more than 30%

The reported incidence of SJS ranges from 1.2 to 6 per million patient-years, and the reported incidence of TEN ranges from 0.4 to 1.2 per million patient-years. The incidence increases with advancing age, and patients with HIV infection seem to be at higher risk. Reported mortality rates range from 1% to 5% in SJS and 25% to 35% in TEN.

Jain R, Sharma N, Basu S, et al. Stevens-Johnson syndrome: the role of an ophthalmologist. *Surv Ophthalmol.* 2016;61(4):369–399.

CLINICAL PRESENTATION Fever, arthralgia, malaise, and upper or lower respiratory tract symptoms are usually sudden in onset. Skin eruption follows within a few days, with a classic "target" lesion consisting of a red center surrounded by a pale ring and then a red ring. Maculopapular and bullous skin lesions are also common. The mucous membranes of the eyes, mouth, and genitalia may be affected by bullous lesions with membrane or pseudomembrane formation. New lesions may appear over 4–6 weeks, with approximately 2-week cycles for each crop of lesions.

The primary ocular finding is a mucopurulent conjunctivitis and episcleritis. Conjunctival and corneal epithelial sloughing and necrosis with severe inflammation and scarring may develop (Fig 13-10). Patients are at risk of infection because of loss of the

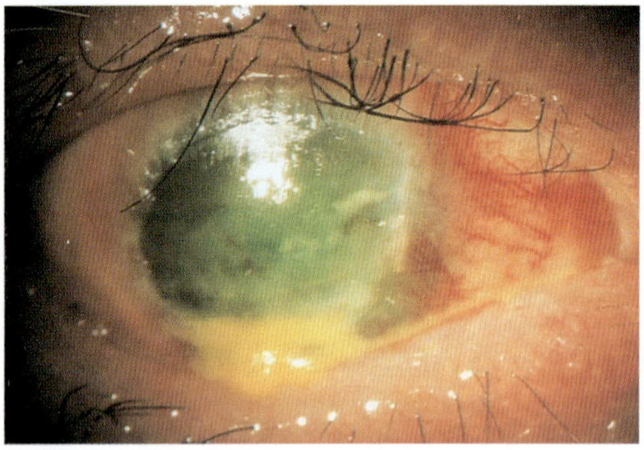

Figure 13-10 Stevens-Johnson syndrome with severe ocular surface disease and cicatricial entropion of the upper eyelid.

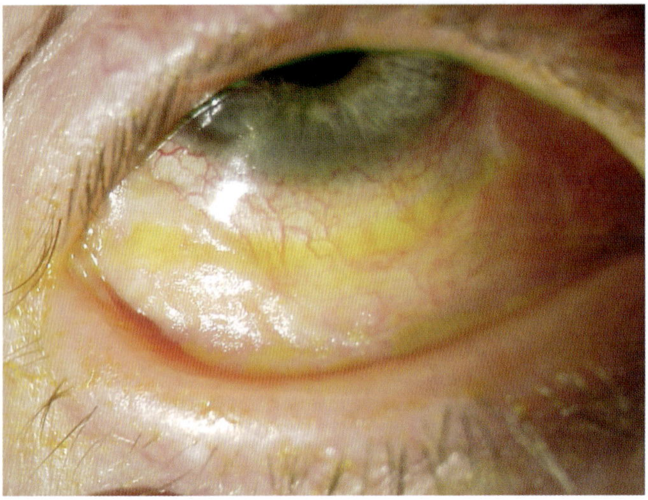

Figure 13-11 Stevens-Johnson syndrome demonstrating inferior eyelid symblepharon and ocular surface keratinization. *(Courtesy of Charles S. Bouchard, MD.)*

epithelial barrier. Ocular surface cicatrization results in long-term ocular complications such as formation of conjunctival symblepharon and forniceal shortening (Fig 13-11), eyelid margin keratinization, trichiasis, and tear deficiency. Eyelid margin keratinization and scarring are important risk factors for poor long-term outcomes in these patients.

Catt CJ, Hamilton GM, Fish J, Mireskandari K, Ali A. Ocular manifestations of Stevens-Johnson syndrome and toxic epidermal necrolysis in children. *Am J Ophthalmol.* 2016;166:68–75.

Gerull R, Nelle M, Schaible T. Toxic epidermal necrolysis and Stevens-Johnson syndrome: a review. *Crit Care Med.* 2011;39(6):1521–1532.

Sotozono C, Ueta M, Yokoi N. Severe dry eye with combined mechanisms is involved in the ocular sequelae of SJS/TEN at the chronic stage. *Invest Ophthalmol Vis Sci.* 2018;59(14):DES80–DES86.

PATHOGENESIS Approximately 80% of TEN cases and 50%–80% of SJS cases are thought to be drug induced, most frequently by the following medications:

- sulfonamides
- anticonvulsants

- NSAIDs
- allopurinol

The remaining SJS–TEN cases are attributed to infectious diseases such as

- *Mycoplasma pneumoniae*
- herpes simplex virus
- adenovirus
- streptococcal bacteria

A delayed-type hypersensitivity reaction usually occurs 4–28 days after exposure to the inciting agent.

Jun I, Rim JH, Kim MK, et al. Association of human antigen class I genes with cold medicine–related Stevens-Johnson syndrome with severe ocular complications in a Korean population. *Br J Ophthalmol.* 2019;103(4):573–576.

MANAGEMENT Acute SJS/TEN is a medical emergency associated with significant risk of morbidity and mortality. Management requires a team-based approach, similar to that used for thermal burn victims, and includes the intensive care provider, an anesthesiologist, a surgeon specializing in the treatment of burns, and the ophthalmologist. The offending agent must be immediately discontinued. Systemic therapy is mainly supportive and is aimed at managing dehydration and superinfection. Systemic treatment with immunosuppressive agents, immunomodulatory agents, or intravenous immunoglobulins remains controversial.

The mainstay of ocular therapy in the acute phase is lubrication with preservative-free artificial tears and ointments as well as vigilant surveillance for the early manifestations of ocular infection or epithelial defects, which are treated as follows:

- conjunctival hyperemia without epithelial defects: topical steroids and antibiotics
- conjunctival, corneal, or eyelid margin defects with or without membranes: amniotic membrane graft with topical steroids and antibiotics

CLINICAL PEARL

Significant long-term benefit has been demonstrated if early amniotic membrane grafting of the entire ocular surface, including the eyelid margins, is performed within the first 3 to 7 days. Various techniques can be used, and the procedure can be done in the operating room or at the bedside for patients who cannot be taken to the operating room immediately.

Management of *chronic* SJS/TEN is targeted at rehabilitation of visual function and treatment of secondary dry eye disease and the mechanical abnormalities of the eyelids and eyelashes, which can cause ocular surface trauma and inflammation.

Dry eye disease is a significant problem secondary to scarring of the ocular surface and damage to the meibomian and accessory lacrimal glands. Conjunctival scarring can also affect lacrimal gland function. Chronic aqueous deficiency contributes to the development of further ocular surface damage and epithelial defects and can lead to limbal stem cell deficiency. Eyelid sequelae such as entropion, trichiasis, and keratinization, which result from cicatrizing conjunctivitis, can cause chronic ocular surface irritation and inflammation. Treatment of dry eye includes lubrication with preservative-free drops and ointments, punctal occlusion, and eyelid hygiene. Topical and systemic corticosteroids have been reported to help reduce active inflammation but must be used with caution. Depending on the extent of the chronic disease, other treatment options include debridement of keratin from eyelid margins, use of scleral lenses, and mucous membrane grafting. See Chapter 3 for discussion of dry eye disease.

Vision rehabilitation in patients with chronic disease is challenging and can be high risk. Scleral contact lenses may improve patient comfort and vision and help some patients avoid surgery. Surgical treatments are risky and are generally avoided unless there are no other options. Living donor or cadaveric limbal stem cell transplantation and cultivated oral and nasal mucosal epithelial transplantation have been performed but are less successful in cases of extreme dry eye. Penetrating keratoplasty is associated with an extremely poor prognosis in patients with chronic disease and is generally reserved for eyes with progressive thinning or perforation. In severe cases, favorable results have been achieved with a keratoprosthesis, but success may be limited in cases of severe dry eye. Unfortunately, many patients with chronic SJS/TEN are young and will experience lifelong ocular morbidity. Rehabilitation is hindered not only by sequelae of the acute disease, but also by ongoing, chronic immunopathology of the ocular surface.

Basu S, Shanbhag SS, Gokani A, Kedar R, Bahuguna C, Sangwan VS. Chronic ocular sequelae of Stevens-Johnson syndrome in children: long-term impact of appropriate therapy on natural history of disease. *Am J Ophthalmol.* 2018;189:17–28.

Gregory, DG. New grading system and treatment guidelines for the acute ocular manifestations of Stevens-Johnson syndrome. *Ophthalmology.* 2016;123(8):1653–1658.

Jain R, Sharma N, Basu S, et al. Stevens-Johnson syndrome: the role of an ophthalmologist. *Surv Ophthalmol.* 2016;61(4):369–399.

Kohanim S, Palioura S, Saeed HN, et al. Stevens-Johnson syndrome/toxic epidermal necrolysis—a comprehensive review and guide to therapy. II. Ophthalmic disease. *Ocul Surf.* 2016;14(2):168–188.

Shanbhag SS, Chodosh J, Saeed HN. Sutureless amniotic membrane transplantation with cyanoacrylate glue for acute Stevens-Johnson syndrome/toxic epidermal necrolysis. *Ocul Surf.* 2019;17(3):560–564.

Shanbhag SS, Rashad R, Chodosh J, Saeed HN. Long-term effect of a treatment protocol for acute ocular involvement in Stevens-Johnson Syndrome/toxic epidermal necrolysis. *Am J Ophthalmol.* 2019;208:331–341.

Mucous Membrane Pemphigoid

CLINICAL PRESENTATION Mucous membrane pemphigoid (MMP), formerly called ocular cicatricial pemphigoid (OCP), is a chronic, cicatrizing conjunctivitis of autoimmune etiology. It is a vesiculobullous disease that may affect other mucous membranes, including those of the mouth, oropharynx, genitalia, and anus. Difficulty swallowing may be an important early symptom. Skin involvement can occur in some cases.

Patients with MMP are usually older than 60 years at the time of diagnosis. They often present with recurrent attacks of mild and nonspecific conjunctival inflammation with an occasional mucopurulent discharge. Patients with MMP may initially present with trichiasis. The need for repeated epilation may be indicative of MMP; it is important to examine such patients for fibrosis of the palpebral conjunctiva, which is an early sign of MMP, or symblephara and forniceal shortening, which are signs of more advanced disease.

The Foster staging system divides MMP severity into 4 stages:

- stage I: chronic conjunctivitis with subconjunctival fibrosis (Fig 13-12)
- stage II: fornix foreshortening (Fig 13-13)
- stage III: symblepharon formation (Fig 13-14)
- stage IV: ankyloblepharon, frozen globe (Fig 13-15)

It is important to diagnose MMP in its early stages. In many cases, the disease initially produces nonspecific symptoms with minimal overt physical findings, such as chronic red eye. Fine white linear opacities may appear on the tarsal conjunctiva (see Fig 13-12). Abnormal shortening of the inferior fornix warrants further evaluation. A subtle inferior symblepharon can be detected when the lower eyelid is pulled down while the patient looks up (see Fig 13-14). Oral mucosal lesions may be a clue that can lead to early diagnosis.

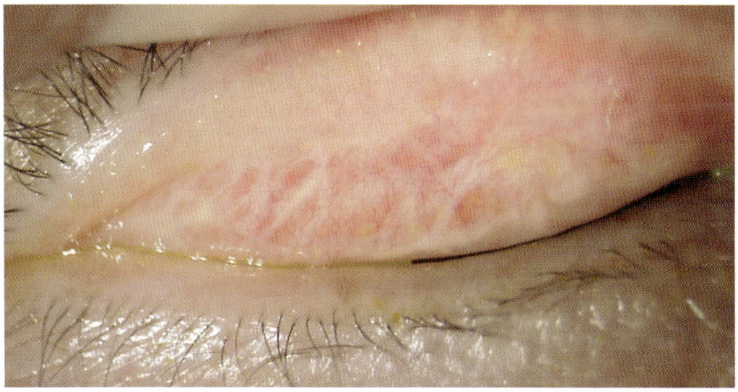

Figure 13-12 Ocular mucous membrane pemphigoid (MMP) showing subepithelial fibrosis of the tarsal conjunctiva of the upper eyelid. *(Courtesy of Charles S. Bouchard, MD.)*

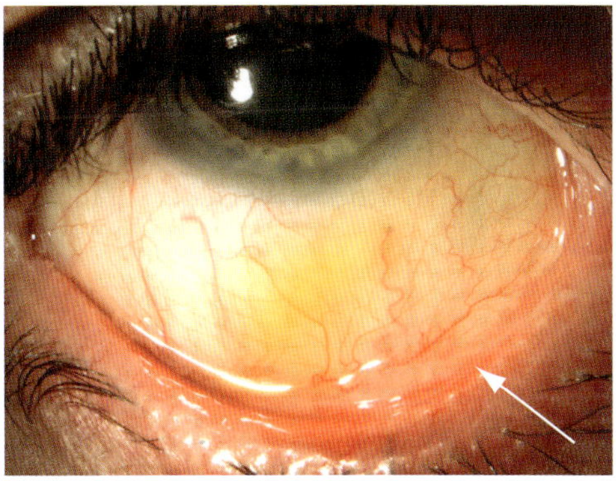

Figure 13-13 Shortening of the inferior fornix is present *(arrow)* in an eye with MMP stage II. *(Courtesy of Arie L. Marcovich, MD, PhD.)*

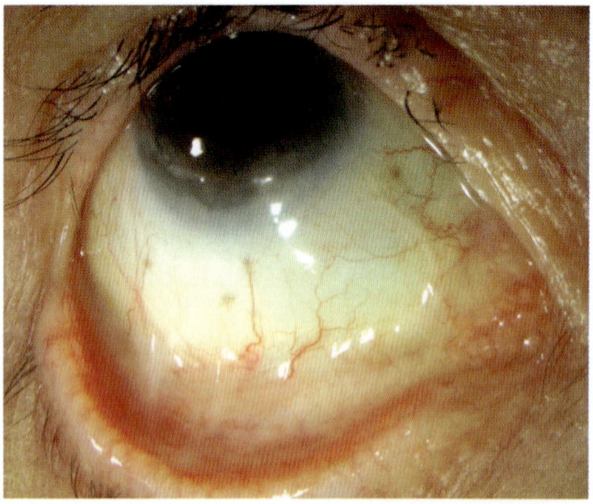

Figure 13-14 Inferior symblepharon is demonstrated in an eye with MMP stage III when the lower eyelid is pulled down with the patient in upgaze. *(Courtesy of Arie L. Marcovich, MD, PhD.)*

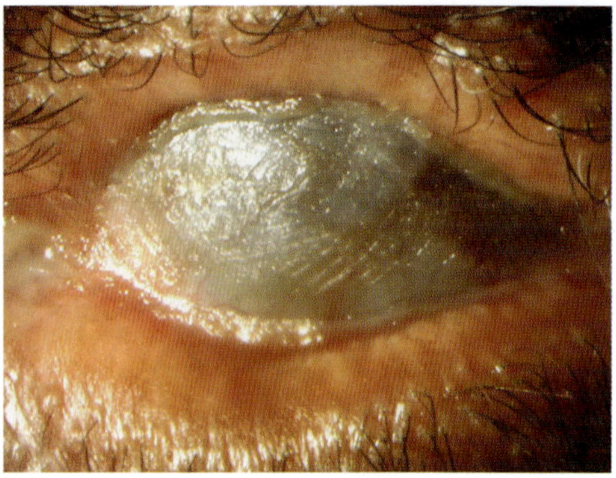

Figure 13-15 Eye with MMP stage IV shows a complete loss of the fornices, keratinization of the ocular surface, and ankyloblepharon. *(Courtesy of Arie L. Marcovich, MD, PhD.)*

Recurrent attacks of conjunctival inflammation can lead to destruction of goblet cells and eventually obstruction of the lacrimal gland orifices. The resultant aqueous and mucous tear deficiency leads to keratinization of the conjunctiva. Entropion and trichiasis may develop as scarring progresses, leading to corneal abrasions, vascularization (Fig 13-16), additional scarring, ulceration, and epidermalization of the ocular surface. Corneal abrasions in these patients are emergencies and must be treated immediately to minimize progression to ulceration, perforation, scarring, and ankyloblepharon formation (see Fig 13-15). Although the clinical course varies, progressive deterioration usually occurs in untreated cases. Remissions and exacerbations are common. Surgical intervention can incite further scarring but may be essential in managing entropion and trichiasis.

The differential diagnosis of cicatrizing conjunctivitis includes 4 major categories (Table 13-3). The diagnosis of unilateral MMP should be made with caution because other diseases, including many of those listed in Table 13-3, may masquerade as MMP. Also, linear IgA dermatosis, a rare dermatologic condition, can result in an ocular syndrome that is clinically identical to MMP and requires similar treatment.

Pseudopemphigoid, which has a clinical picture similar to that of MMP, has been associated with the long-term use of certain topical ophthalmic medications (eg, pilocarpine, epinephrine, timolol, idoxuridine). The main difference between pseudopemphigoid and true pemphigoid is that in the former, disease progression generally ceases once the offending agent is recognized and removed.

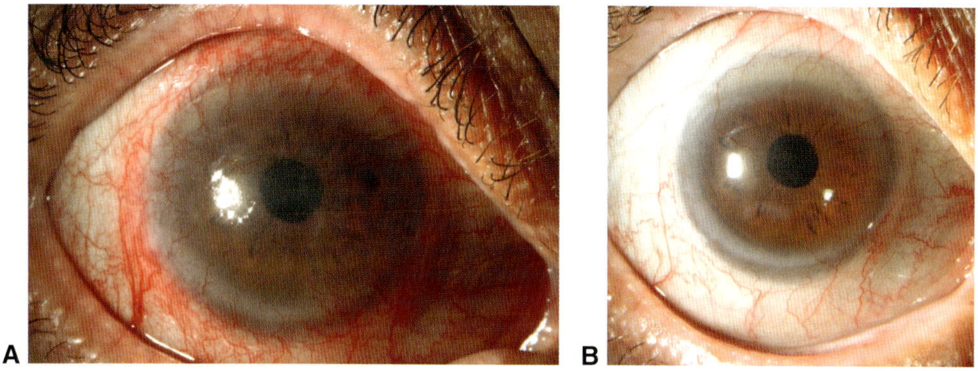

Figure 13-16 MMP stage III. **A,** Patient presents with corneal vascularization and severe inflammation. **B,** Same eye after 5 years of treatment with intravenous cyclophosphamide demonstrates regression of vascularization and inflammation. *(Courtesy of Arie L. Marcovich, MD, PhD.)*

Table 13-3 Differential Diagnosis of Cicatricial Conjunctivitis

Infectious	Allergic Reaction to Drug, Trauma, or Environment	Autoimmune	Miscellaneous
Adenovirus *Chlamydia trachomatis* Skin infections due to *Corynebacterium diphtheriae*	Atopic keratoconjunctivitis Stevens-Johnson syndrome	Lichen planus Lupus Mucous membrane pemphigoid Sarcoidosis Scleroderma	Chemical or thermal injury Medicamentosa Neoplasia (paraneoplastic) Ocular rosacea Radiation exposure Trauma

PATHOGENESIS The underlying cause of MMP is not completely clear. An impaired immune response leads to production of autoantibodies against adhesion molecules in the hemidesmosome–epithelial basement membrane complex. Activation of complement proteins and overexpression of proinflammatory cytokines leads to breakdown of the conjunctival membrane, fibroblast stimulation, collagen production, and fibrosis.

Williams GP, Radford C, Nightingale P, Dart JKG, Rauz S. Evaluation of early and late presentation of patients with ocular mucous membrane pemphigoid to two major tertiary referral hospitals in the United Kingdom. *Eye (Lond).* 2011;25(9):1207–1218.

LABORATORY EVALUATION Although MMP is a bilateral disease, 1 eye may be more severely involved than the other. A diagnosis of pemphigoid can be confirmed with direct immunofluorescence or immunoperoxidase staining of conjunctival biopsy specimens. The success rate of pathology labs in diagnosing MMP varies considerably; it is important to utilize a laboratory that specializes in dermatopathology.

Biopsy specimens are obtained from the junction between unaffected and actively affected areas of the conjunctiva or, if involvement is diffuse, from the inferior conjunctival fornix. Oral mucosal biopsies may be useful, especially in the presence of an active lesion. In pseudopemphigoid, conjunctival biopsies may or may not yield a positive result. Immunohistochemical staining techniques can demonstrate complement 3, IgG, IgM, and/or IgA

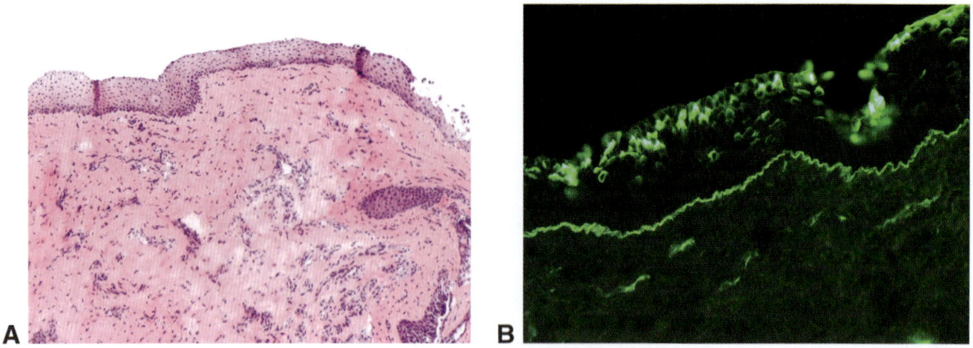

Figure 13-17 Conjunctival biopsy from a patient with MMP. **A,** Hematoxylin-eosin (×100) stain reveals fibrosis and few inflammatory cells. There is no pathognomonic appearance based on histopathology only. For a proper immunofluorescence evaluation, a sizable portion of unaffected basement membrane would be required. **B,** Direct immunofluorescence for IgA (×200) shows a linear staining of the basement membrane. In contrast to IgG, IgA is actively secreted by the epithelium and therefore always stains positive, but not in a linear pattern, as demonstrated at the top of the image. *(Courtesy of Robert M Verdijk, MD, PhD.)*

localized in the epithelial basement membrane of the conjunctiva in pemphigoid (Fig 13-17). Circulating anti–basement membrane antibody has been identified in some patients with pemphigoid. End-stage disease may produce negative results because of the destruction of basement membrane.

CLINICAL PEARL

The diagnosis and decision to treat MMP are made based on clinical findings even when biopsy results are negative; however, a positive biopsy can be important when weighing the risks of systemic immunosuppression. (See also BCSC Section 4, *Ophthalmic Pathology and Intraocular Tumors.*)

Radford CF, Rauz S, Williams GP, Saw VPJ, Dart JKG. Incidence, presenting features, and diagnosis of cicatrizing conjunctivitis in the United Kingdom. *Eye (Lond).* 2012;26(9):1199–1208.

MANAGEMENT The management of MMP requires a multidisciplinary approach. Collaboration with other medical specialists who have experience using systemic immunosuppressive treatment is recommended to maximize patient outcome. Classifying patients according to their risk for disease progression (low or high) is valuable when appropriate therapy is being determined. Because progression is often slow, careful clinical staging of the disease and photo documentation (with the patient in different positions of gaze) are generally recommended in evaluation of the disease course and response to therapy.

It is important to remember that MMP is a systemic disease requiring systemic therapy. Topical treatments (steroids, cyclosporine A, tacrolimus) may help alleviate symptoms but will not prevent disease progression. Oral corticosteroids can be helpful to reduce inflammation in the short run until agents used to achieve long-term immunosuppression take effect. Systemic treatment regimens depend on the severity of the disease and whether sight-threatening complications are present:

- *patients with mild disease:* methotrexate and mycophenolate mofetil
- *patients with sight-threatening disease:* cyclophosphamide with prednisone is a mainstay of therapy but is associated with greater risk of complications
- *patients who are unresponsive to or who experience complications with conventional treatments:* intravenous immunoglobulin, anti–TNF-α medications, and rituximab (Table 13-4)

It is critical for the ophthalmologist to partner with providers who are experienced in the administration and management of these treatments (ie, rheumatologists, hematologists, oncologists). Patients are treated for few months to several years until inflammation subsides (see Fig 13-16B). Blepharitis is treated with eyelid hygiene and daily oral doxycycline.

Any procedure or surgery (eyelid or intraocular) can cause the disease to flare, and the patient can be supported with adequate immunosuppression therapy as necessary. Surgical correction of eyelid deformities or treatment of trichiasis is important. In severe cases, hard palate and buccal mucosal grafting can be useful techniques in fornix reconstruction. Punctal occlusion, which may have already resulted from cicatrization, can be useful in the management of any associated dry eye condition. Because patients with cicatrizing conjunctivitis have a higher rate of spontaneous extrusion of silicone punctal plugs, permanent punctal occlusion with cautery is often required. Standard penetrating

Table 13-4 Systemic Immunomodulatory Drugs

Class	Drug	Mode of action
Alkylating agents	Cyclophosphamide	Forms crosslinks in DNA and RNA; inhibits DNA replication
	Chlorambucil	Forms crosslinks in DNA and RNA; inhibits DNA replication
Antimetabolites	Azathioprine	Purine analogue that inhibits DNA replication and RNA transcription
	Methotrexate	Folic acid analogue that inhibits DNA replication
	Mycophenolate mofetil	Inhibits inosine monophosphate dehydrogenase and DNA replication
Biologic immune modulators	Adalimumab	Monoclonal antibody against TNF-α
	Alemtuzumab (Campath-1H)	Monoclonal antibody against CD52 cells (T and B lymphocytes)
	Infliximab	Monoclonal antibody against TNF-α
	Rituximab	Monoclonal antibody against CD20 cells (mainly B lymphocytes)
	Tocilizumab	Monoclonal antibody against IL-6 receptor
Interleukin inhibitors	Dupilumab	Monoclonal antibody against IL-4 and IL-13 receptors
T-cell inhibitors	Cyclosporine A	Calcineurin inhibitor that downregulates transcription of IL-2
	Tacrolimus	Calcineurin inhibitor that downregulates transcription of IL-2

IL = interleukin; TNF = tumor necrosis factor.

keratoplasty in MMP patients with severe corneal disease carries a guarded prognosis. In patients who become blind due to MMP, keratoprosthesis surgery, performed as a last resort, has achieved greater success in the absence of severe dry eye.

Foster CS, Chang PY, Ahmed AR. Combination of rituximab and intravenous immunoglobulin for recalcitrant ocular cicatricial pemphigoid: a preliminary report. *Ophthalmology.* 2010; 117(5):861–869.

Friedman J, Marcovich AL, Kleinmann G, Schattner A. Low-dose pulsed intravenous cyclophosphamide for severe ocular cicatricial pemphigoid in elderly patients. *Cornea.* 2014;33(10):1066–1070.

Georgoudis P, Sabatino F, Szentmary N, et al. Ocular mucous membrane pemphigoid: current state of pathophysiology, diagnostics and treatment. *Ophthalmol Ther.* 2019;8(1):5–17.

Queisi MM, Zein M, Lamba N, Meese H, Foster CS. Update on ocular cicatricial pemphigoid and emerging treatments. *Surv Ophthalmol.* 2016;61(3):314–317.

Srikumaran D, Tzu JH, Akpek EK. Cicatrizing conjunctivitis. *Focal Points: Clinical Modules for Ophthalmologists.* American Academy of Ophthalmology; 2011, module 1.

Valenzuela FA, Perez VL. Mucous membrane pemphigoid. In: Mannis MJ, Holland EJ, eds. *Cornea.* Vol 1. 4th ed. Elsevier; 2017:549–557.

Ocular Graft-vs-Host Disease

Graft-vs-host disease (GVHD) is a relatively common complication of allogeneic bone marrow transplantation, which is performed most commonly for hematopoietic malignancies.

CLINICAL PRESENTATION The clinical features of ocular GVHD mirror those of other ocular inflammatory conditions associated with autoimmune and collagen-vascular diseases. GVHD has 2 main components:

- conjunctival inflammation, which can be severe and may be associated with subepithelial fibrosis, limbal stem cell deficiency, and secondary corneal scarring
- severe keratoconjunctivitis sicca from lacrimal gland infiltration, which occurs in 40%–60% of patients with chronic GVHD

PATHOGENESIS In this condition, the grafted cells can attack the patient's tissues, including the skin, gut, lungs, liver, and eyes. GVHD can be acute or chronic (developing more than 3 months after a bone marrow transplant); most ocular complications occur as a manifestation of chronic GVHD.

Inamoto Y, Chai X, Kurland BF, et al; Chronic GVHD Consortium. Validation of measurement scales in ocular graft-versus-host disease. *Ophthalmology.* 2012;119(3):487–493.

Lin X, Cavanagh HD. Ocular manifestations of graft-versus-host disease: 10 years' experience. *Clin Ophthalmol.* 2015;9:1209–1213.

Shikari H, Antin JH, Dana R. Ocular graft-versus-host disease: a review. *Surv Ophthalmol.* 2013;58(3):233–251.

MANAGEMENT Aggressive ocular lubrication and punctal occlusion are the mainstays of local therapy. Punctal fibrosis is common and must be monitored closely because it can lead to plug extrusion. Severe filamentary keratitis can be treated with a topical mucolytic agent such as acetylcysteine 10% or a bandage contact lens. Topical cyclosporine or

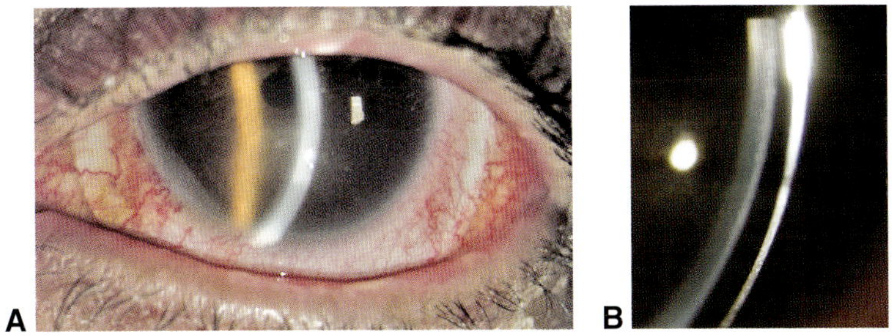

Figure 13-18 Graft-vs-host disease (GVHD). **A,** Patient with GVHD fitted with a therapeutic scleral contact lens. The inferior paracentral cornea demonstrates subepithelial scarring. **B,** High-magnification image shows the space between the contact lens and cornea. *(Courtesy of Charles S. Bouchard, MD.)*

tacrolimus may also be useful in controlling ocular GVHD. Autologous serum tears can help improve the ocular surface. Visual disturbances are typically due to surface irregularity; however, patients also have a high rate of posterior subcapsular cataract, which may contribute to decreased vision. Scleral contact lenses and therapeutic soft contact lenses (Fig 13-18) can be important management tools for patients with severe ocular surface disease. Keratoprosthesis may be a last-resort option for patients with end-stage ocular surface disease who are not candidates for other conventional corneal procedures. Severe GVHD may require systemic immunosuppressive therapy in consultation with the treating hematologist or oncologist.

Abud TB, Amparo F, Saboo US, et al. A clinical trial comparing the safety and efficacy of topical tacrolimus versus methylprednisolone in ocular graft-versus-host disease. *Ophthalmology*. 2016;123(7):1449–1457.

Avadhanam VS, Liu CS. A brief review of Boston type-1 and osteo-odonto keratoprostheses. *Br J Ophthalmol.* 2015;99(7):878–887.

DeLoss KS, Le HG, Gire A, Chiu GB, Jacobs DS, Carrasquillo KG. PROSE treatment for ocular chronic graft-versus-host disease as a clinical network expands. *Eye Contact Lens.* 2016;42(4):262–266.

Dietrich-Ntoukas T, Steven P. Okuläre graft-versus-host-disease [ocular graft-versus-host disease]. *Ophthalmologe.* 2015;112(12):1027–1040. German.

Tahmaz V, Gehlsen U, Sauerbier L, et al. Treatment of severe chronic ocular graft-versus-host disease using 100% autologous serum eye drops from a sealed manufacturing system: a retrospective cohort study. *Br J Ophthalmol.* 2017;101(3):322–326.

Conjunctivitis/Episcleritis Associated With Reactive Arthritis

Reactive arthritis (formerly called *Reiter syndrome*) is a systemic disorder characterized by the classic triad of ocular (conjunctivitis/episcleritis, iridocyclitis, or keratitis), urethral, and joint inflammation.

CLINICAL PRESENTATION The most common ocular finding in reactive arthritis is a bilateral papillary conjunctivitis with mucopurulent discharge, which has been reported in 30%–60% of patients. The conjunctivitis is self-limited, lasting for days to weeks. Some patients present more often with episcleritis rather than with conjunctivitis. Mild nongranulomatous anterior uveitis has been reported in 3%–12% of patients. Various forms of keratitis—including diffuse punctate epithelial erosions, superficial or deep focal infiltrates, or superficial or deep vascularization—can occur in rare cases. Reactive arthritis may be considered in any case of chronic, nonfollicular, mucopurulent conjunctivitis with negative culture results.

The joint inflammation is often highly asymmetric and involves a few joints (oligoarticular). These manifestations can appear simultaneously or separately, in any sequence. Less-common manifestations include keratoderma blennorrhagicum (a scaling skin eruption), balanitis (inflammation of the head of the penis), aphthous stomatitis, fever, lymphadenopathy, pneumonitis, pericarditis, and myocarditis. Attacks are self-limited, lasting from two to several months, but they may recur periodically over the course of several years.

PATHOGENESIS Reactive arthritis may occur after dysentery due to gram-negative bacteria (most frequently *Salmonella, Shigella,* and *Yersinia* species) or after nongonococcal urethritis caused by *Chlamydia trachomatis.* More than 75% of patients with reactive arthritis are HLA-B27–positive. See BCSC Section 9, *Uveitis and Ocular Inflammation,* for discussion of HLA-B27–related diseases and illustrations of nonocular manifestations of reactive arthritis.

MANAGEMENT Treatment is mainly palliative. Corneal infiltrates and vascularization often respond to topical corticosteroids. Systemic treatment of any related infection with oral antibiotics may be beneficial. Occasionally, the intraocular (uveitic) component of the disease can be very severe and require systemic immunosuppression (see BCSC Section 9, *Uveitis and Ocular Inflammation*).

Immune-Mediated Diseases of the Cornea

Thygeson Superficial Punctate Keratitis

CLINICAL PRESENTATION Thygeson superficial punctate keratitis (SPK) is characterized by recurrent episodes of tearing, foreign-body sensation, photophobia, and reduced vision. It affects children more commonly than older adults and is typically bilateral, although it may develop initially in 1 eye or may be markedly asymmetric in some cases. Symptoms may exceed the apparent signs. The hallmark finding noted during exacerbations is multiple (up to 40, but as few as 2–3) slightly elevated corneal epithelial infiltrates that demonstrate negative staining with fluorescein (Fig 13-19; also see Fig 3-6B). The epithelial lesions are small, round or oval, gray-white, granular opacities associated with minimal or no conjunctival reaction, in contrast to infiltrates seen in adenoviral keratoconjunctivitis. High-magnification imaging reveals each opacity to be a cluster of multiple smaller pinpoint opacities. A characteristic feature is the waxing and waning appearance of individual epithelial opacities, which change in location and number over time. The greatest density of these lesions is typically found in the central cornea. The raised punctate epithelial lesions often stain with rose bengal in addition to fluorescein. There is no conjunctival inflammatory reaction during exacerbations, but occasionally mild bulbar conjunctival hyperemia may be noted.

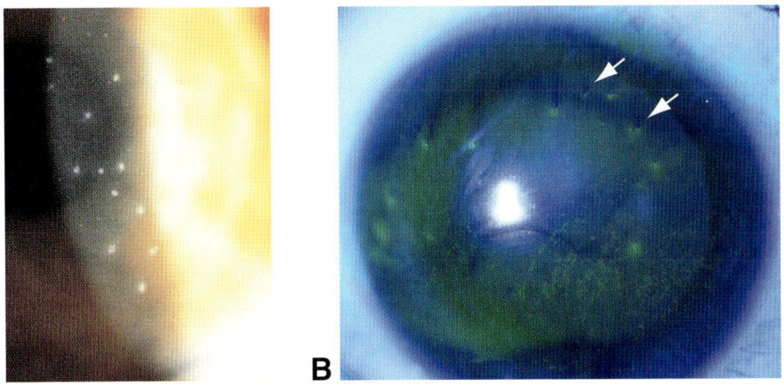

A B

Figure 13-19 Thygeson superficial punctate keratitis. **A,** Fine, superficial infiltrates with a granular appearance are typical. **B,** Characteristic negative staining is seen with fluorescein dye and cobalt blue illumination. *(Part B courtesy of Arie L. Marcovich, MD, PhD.)*

PATHOGENESIS The etiology of SPK is unknown. Although many of the clinical features resemble those of a viral infection of the corneal epithelium, attempts to confirm viral particles by electron microscopy or culture have been unsuccessful. No inflammatory cells are evident. The rapid response of the lesions to corticosteroid therapy suggests that SPK is largely immunogenically derived.

Chan TCY, Chau HHT, Bhat AK, Nischal KK, Jhanji V. Thygeson's superficial punctate keratitis. *J EuCornea.* 2019;3(3–5):5–8.

MANAGEMENT In general, it is preferable to treat the symptoms, rather than the clinical findings, of this condition. Supportive therapy with artificial tears is often adequate in mild cases. Treatment alternatives for symptomatic cases include topical corticosteroids and bandage contact lenses. Currently, antiviral therapy is not the standard of care, because the association with active viral infection has not been confirmed.

A mild topical corticosteroid (eg, fluorometholone 0.1%) may be effective, because the lesions are quite responsive to corticosteroids. Treatment will hasten infiltrate resolution, but the lesions frequently recur in the same or different locations on the cornea once the topical corticosteroids are stopped. Steroid use should be minimized due to the chronic nature of the disease, and it is important to monitor the patients for the risks associated with steroid use. Topical cyclosporine or tacrolimus ophthalmic preparations may also be effective in causing regression of the lesions.

Marquezan MC, Nascimento H, Vieira LA, et al. Effect of topical tacrolimus in the treatment of Thygeson's superficial punctate keratitis. *Am J Ophthalmol.* 2015;160(4):663–668.

Vieira AC, Schwab IR. Superficial punctate keratitis of Thygeson. In: Mannis MJ, Holland EJ, eds. *Cornea.* Vol 1. 4th ed. Elsevier; 2017:1030–1034.

Interstitial Keratitis Associated With Infectious Diseases

Interstitial keratitis (IK) is a nonsuppurative inflammation of the corneal stroma that features cellular infiltration and usually vascularization without primary involvement of the epithelium or endothelium. The geographic distribution (diffuse versus focal or multifocal) and depth of the stromal infiltration, in addition to associated systemic signs, are useful in determining the cause of IK.

CLINICAL PEARL

Congenital syphilis is the etiology in 80% of bilateral IK cases. Acquired syphilis and herpes simplex keratitis account for a high percentage of cases of unilateral IK. Herpes zoster keratitis is also an important cause of unilateral IK. These viral pathogens are discussed in Chapter 11.

Other microorganisms are the cause of IK in rare cases, including

- *Mycobacterium tuberculosis*
- *M leprae*
- *Borrelia burgdorferi* (Lyme disease)
- measles virus
- Epstein-Barr virus (infectious mononucleosis)
- *C trachomatis* (lymphogranuloma venereum)
- *Leishmania* species
- *Onchocerca volvulus* (onchocerciasis)

The exact mechanism of IK is not completely understood. Antigens of infectious microorganisms in the corneal stroma may elicit an immune response. IK does not necessarily indicate that active infection is present.

Syphilitic interstitial keratitis

Syphilitic eye disease is discussed further in Chapter 6 of this volume, in BCSC Section 6, *Pediatric Ophthalmology and Strabismus,* and in BCSC Section 9, *Uveitis and Ocular Inflammation.* Systemic aspects of syphilis are discussed in BCSC Section 1, *Update on General Medicine.*

CLINICAL PRESENTATION Manifestations of congenital syphilis that occur early in life (within the first 2 years) are infectious. However, IK is a later, immune-mediated manifestation of congenital syphilis. Affected children typically show no evidence of corneal disease in their first years; stromal keratitis lasting for several weeks develops late in the first or second decades of life. These patients may also have nonocular signs of congenital syphilis, including

- dental deformities: notched incisors and mulberry molars
- bone and cartilage abnormalities: saddle nose, palatal perforation, saber shins, and frontal bossing
- cranial nerve (CN) VIII (vestibulocochlear) deafness
- rhagades (circumoral radiating scars)
- cognitive impairment

Widely spaced, peg-shaped teeth; CN VIII deafness; and interstitial keratitis constitute the Hutchinson triad. Although congenital syphilitic keratitis is bilateral in 80% of cases, the eyes may not be affected simultaneously or to the same degree. Initial symptoms are pain, tearing, photophobia, and perilimbal injection. The inflammation may last for weeks if left untreated.

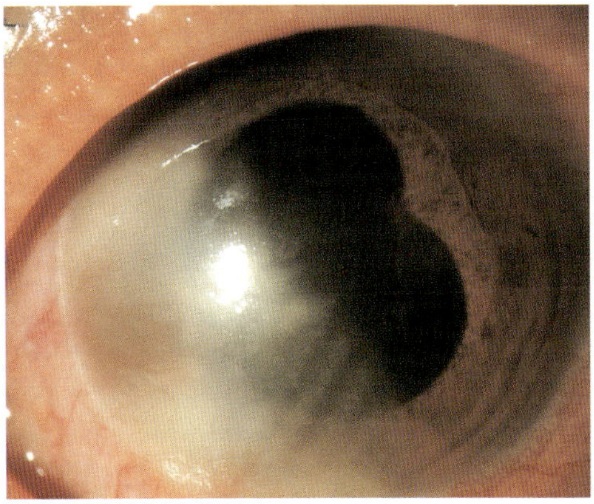

Figure 13-20 Active syphilitic interstitial keratitis with salmon patch.

Sectoral superior stromal inflammation and keratic precipitates are typically seen early in the disease course. As the disease progresses, deep stromal neovascularization develops. Eventually, the inflammation spreads centrally, and corneal opacification and edema may develop. In some cases, the deep corneal vascularization becomes so intense that the cornea appears pink—hence the term *salmon patch* (Fig 13-20). Sequelae of stromal keratitis include corneal scarring, thickening of Descemet membrane, corneal thinning, and ghost vessels in the deep layers of the stroma. Vision may be reduced because of irregular astigmatism and stromal opacification.

Stromal keratitis is less common in acquired syphilis; if it occurs, it is unilateral in 60% of cases. The ocular findings are similar to those seen in congenital syphilitic keratitis. In general, uveitis and retinitis are much more common manifestations of acquired syphilis than keratitis.

LABORATORY EVALUATION AND MANAGEMENT A diagnosis of congenital syphilis is confirmed by identification of *Treponema pallidum* by fluorescent antibody testing. The detection of specific IgM is currently the most sensitive serologic method. During the acute phase, ocular inflammation is treated with topical corticosteroids in order to limit stromal inflammation and late scarring. Cycloplegic drugs can be helpful as well. If untreated, the disease can "burn out" over time, but because chronic disease can lead to severe corneal opacification, early intervention is beneficial in preventing the late sequelae noted above. Patients with findings of IK should have a workup for syphilis. Patients with systemic syphilis or neuroretinal manifestations should be treated with penicillin or an appropriate alternative antibiotic in accordance with the protocol for either congenital or acquired syphilis. The necessity of lumbar puncture in syphilitic IK is uncertain, and any patient with suspected syphilis should be referred for immediate consultation with a specialist in infectious diseases.

Cogan Syndrome

Cogan syndrome is a rare autoimmune disorder of unknown etiology. However, the disease shares some clinicopathologic features with polyarteritis nodosa. The progressive ocular and audiovestibular symptoms that develop in affected patients can lead to blindness, deafness, and even death from systemic vasculitis.

CLINICAL PRESENTATION Cogan syndrome typically occurs in young adults and produces stromal keratitis, vertigo, and hearing loss. The history may reveal a recent upper respiratory tract infection, diarrhea, dental infection, or immunization. The earliest corneal findings are bilateral faint, white subepithelial infiltrates resembling those occurring in viral keratoconjunctivitis but located in the peripheral cornea. Multifocal nodular infiltrates may develop in the posterior cornea weeks to months later. A systemic vasculitis that presents as polyarteritis nodosa occurs in some patients.

LABORATORY EVALUATION When the cause of stromal keratitis is not apparent, a VDRL or rapid plasma reagin (RPR) test and FTA-ABS or microhemagglutination assay for *T pallidum* can be performed; VDRL and RPR tests may become nonreactive in cases of congenital syphilis, while FTA-ABS remains positive. Other infectious syndromes should also be considered. Antibodies to chlamydia have been reported in cases of Cogan syndrome. A hearing test should be performed when Cogan syndrome is being considered; the presence of autoantibodies against the inner ear and endothelial antigens has been reported. The erythrocyte sedimentation rate (ESR) and the C-reactive protein (CRP) level may be elevated. Also, case reports have noted that affected patients test positive for antineutrophil cytoplasmic antibody (ANCA), rheumatoid factor (RF), antinuclear antibody (ANA), and anticardiolipin antibodies. However, laboratory findings are not consistent in Cogan syndrome, and there is no definitive test. This syndrome thus remains a diagnosis of exclusion.

D'Aguanno V, Ralli M, de Vincentiis M, Greco A. Optimal management of Cogan's syndrome: a multidisciplinary approach. *J Multidiscip Healthc.* 2017;11:1–11.

Tirelli G, Tomietto P, Quatela E, et al. Sudden hearing loss and Crohn disease: when Cogan syndrome must be suspected. *Am J Otolaryngol.* 2015;36(4):590–597.

MANAGEMENT The acute keratitis of Cogan syndrome is treated with frequent topical corticosteroids. Oral corticosteroids are recommended for the vestibular and auditory symptoms because this treatment improves the long-term prognosis. Cytotoxic agents may also have a therapeutic role but are typically reserved for severe or unresponsive cases. Early recognition and treatment of Cogan syndrome are critical to prevent the rapid progression to vision loss, deafness, and death from systemic vasculitis. Early consultation with an otolaryngologist and rheumatologist is recommended.

Durtette C, Hachulla E, Resche-Rigon M, et al. Cogan syndrome: characteristics, outcome, and treatment in a French nationwide retrospective study and literature review. *Autoimmun Rev.* 2017;16(12):1219–1223.

Marginal Keratitis

The limbus plays an important role in immune-mediated corneal disorders. It has a population of antigen-presenting cells (APCs) that express MHC class II antigens and are capable of efficient mobilization and induction of T-cell responses. Immune-related corneal changes often occur in the periphery because this area is adjacent to the vascularized limbus. The proximity to blood vessels permits circulating immune cells, immune complexes, and complement factors to deposit in the cornea adjacent to the terminal capillary loops of the limbal vascular arcades, thereby producing a variety of immune phenomena that manifest in the periphery. Predisposing factors include

- blepharoconjunctivitis
- acne rosacea (see Chapter 3)
- contact lens wear

CLINICAL PRESENTATION Marginal keratitis is characterized by creamy white elliptical infiltrates, typically separated from the limbus by a relatively lucent zone of 1–2 mm (Fig 13-21). They most often occur near the point of intersection of the eyelid margin and the limbus, that is, at 10, 2, 4 and 8 o'clock (Fig 13-22). These infiltrates represent an inflammatory reaction to staphylococcal blepharitis. The presence of marginal keratitis does not always correlate with the degree of blepharitis; in fact, in some cases, the blepharitis is quite mild. In chronic disease, superficial blood vessels may cross the clear interval into the area of corneal infiltration. The epithelium overlying marginal infiltrates may be intact, show punctate epithelial erosions, or be absent. Stromal opacification, peripheral corneal thinning, and/or pannus may develop following resolution of the acute marginal keratitis. Although patients are often initially treated with topical antibiotics, the condition usually responds well to treatment with corticosteroids. Long-term control of the eyelid margin disease

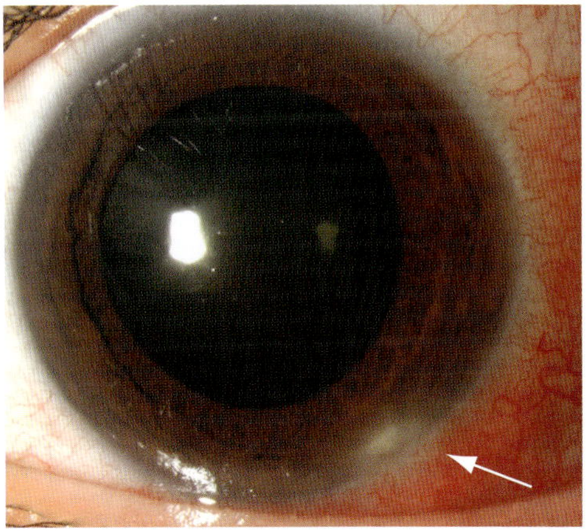

Figure 13-21 Marginal infiltrates are typically creamy white with little surrounding reaction. The epithelium is usually intact. *(Courtesy of Arie L. Marcovich, MD, PhD.)*

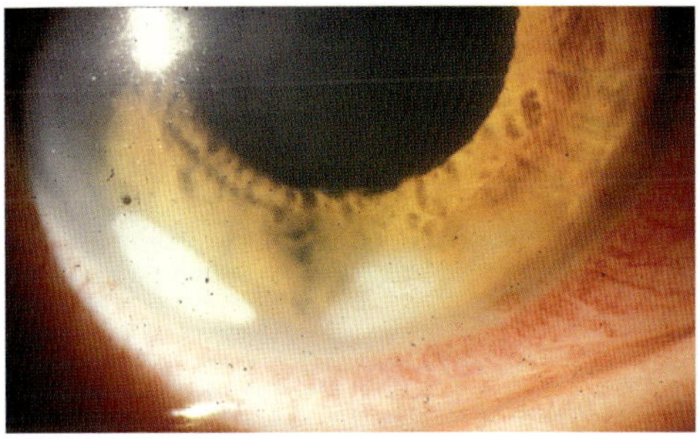

Figure 13-22 Marginal keratitis with a lucent area, which typically occurs between the infiltrate and the limbus. These are most commonly found where the limbus and eyelid intersect, at 10, 2, 4, and 8 o'clock. *(Courtesy of Robert S. Feder, MD.)*

reduces the likelihood of recurrence. The management of marginal keratitis is discussed in greater detail in Chapter 3.

Chung G, Iuorno JD. Phlyctenular keratoconjunctivitis and marginal staphylococcal keratitis. In: Mannis MJ, Holland EJ, eds. *Cornea*. Vol 1. 4th ed. Elsevier; 2017:1076–1081.

Peripheral Ulcerative Keratitis Associated With Systemic Immune-Mediated Diseases

CLINICAL PRESENTATION A history of autoimmune and rheumatologic disease is often (but not invariably) present in affected patients, although in some the ocular finding of peripheral corneal infiltration or frank stromal melting may be the first sign of the underlying systemic illness. Peripheral ulcerative keratitis (PUK) occurs most often in association with rheumatoid arthritis, but it is associated with other conditions as well (Table 13-5). The term *keratolysis* refers to the significant, often rapid, stromal melting seen in some cases. The onset of autoimmune PUK generally correlates with exacerbations of an underlying systemic disease. Left untreated or inadequately treated, a high number of patients with autoimmune PUK suffer severe disease-related morbidity and mortality.

Although autoimmune PUK can be bilateral and extensive, it is usually unilateral and limited to 1 sector of the peripheral cornea (Fig 13-23). The initial lesions appear in a zone within 2 mm of the limbus and are accompanied by varying degrees of vaso-occlusion

Table 13-5 Differential Diagnosis of Peripheral Ulcerative Keratitis

Ocular Conditions and Diseases	Systemic Conditions and Diseases
Microbial	Microbial
Viral (herpes simplex, herpes zoster)	Viral (herpes zoster, AIDS, hepatitis C)
Bacterial *(Staphylococcus, Streptococcus, Gonococcus, Moraxella, Haemophilus)*	Bacterial (tuberculosis, syphilis, gonorrhea, borreliosis, bacillary dysentery)
Acanthamoeba	Helminthiasis (macroparasitic infection, ie, worm infestation)
Fungal	α_1-Antitrypsin deficiency
Exposure keratopathy	Behçet disease
Mooren ulcer	Collagen-vascular disease
Rosacea	Polyarteritis nodosa
Terrien marginal degeneration (inflammatory type)	Progressive systemic sclerosis and scleroderma
Traumatic or postsurgical	Relapsing polychondritis
	Rheumatoid arthritis
	Sjögren syndrome
	Systemic lupus erythematosus
	Granulomatosis with polyangiitis (Wegener granulomatosis)
	Inflammatory bowel disease
	Malignancy
	Sarcoidosis

Modified with permission from Dana MR, Qian Y, Hamrah P. Twenty-five-year panorama of corneal immunology: emerging concepts in the immunopathogenesis of microbial keratitis, peripheral ulcerative keratitis, and corneal transplant rejection. *Cornea.* 2000;19(5):630.

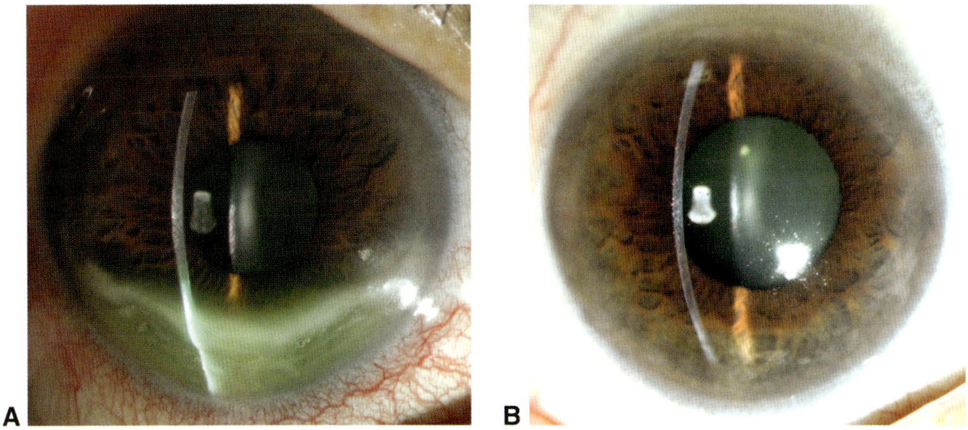

Figure 13-23 Peripheral ulcerative keratitis (PUK). **A,** PUK associated with rheumatoid arthritis that was treated with systemic corticosteroid and immunosuppressive treatment combined with a bandage contact lens and topical antibiotic. **B,** The same eye 4 years later with the patient continuing systemic immunosuppressive treatment. *(Courtesy of Arie L. Marcovich, MD, PhD.)*

of the adjacent limbal vascular network. In most cases, the epithelium is absent, and the underlying stroma thinned in the affected area; however, if the disease is detected early, epithelial loss may be patchy and stromal loss kept to a minimum. Ulceration may or may not be associated with a significant cellular infiltrate in the corneal stroma, and the adjacent conjunctiva can be minimally or severely inflamed. The sclera can also be involved in patients with systemic immune-mediated diseases (eg, necrotizing scleritis in patients with rheumatoid arthritis).

PATHOGENESIS Though not a standard diagnostic procedure, biopsy of conjunctival tissue adjacent to marginal corneal disease typically shows evidence of immune-mediated vaso-occlusive disease. In patients with systemic autoimmune disease, central or paracentral corneal melting that may progress to perforation can infrequently occur (Fig 13-24). The mechanism is not completely clear. Pathological studies have demonstrated T-lymphocyte infiltration.

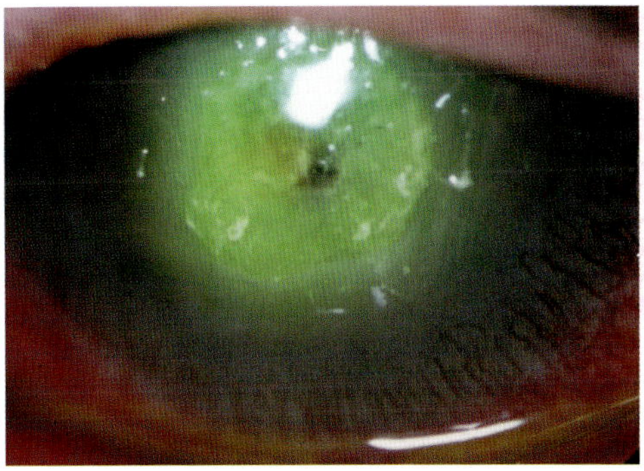

Figure 13-24 Central corneal melting with perforation associated with rheumatoid arthritis. *(Courtesy of Arie L. Marcovich, MD, PhD.)*

Foster CS. Ocular manifestations of the potentially lethal rheumatologic and vasculitic disorders. *J Fr Ophthalmol.* 2013;36(6):526–532.

Kalsow CM, Ching SSST, Plotnik RD. Cellular infiltrate in rheumatoid arthritis–associated paracentral corneal ulceration. *Ocul Immunol Inflamm.* 2017;25(6):878–883.

MANAGEMENT The goal of therapy is to provide local supportive measures to decrease stromal melting. This is achieved through treatment intended to promote epithelialization, improve ocular surface lubrication, and suppress immune-mediated inflammation both locally and systemically.

Maintaining enhanced lubrication of the ocular surface is very important, because keratoconjunctivitis sicca (KCS) is a manifestation of secondary Sjögren syndrome in many patients with rheumatoid arthritis. Some patients with rheumatoid arthritis with keratolysis do not have KCS. Melting may stop or slow appreciably when epithelial healing is achieved by means of enhanced tear function, patching, or a bandage contact lens.

Collagenase inhibitors (eg, topical sodium citrate 10%, acetylcysteine 20%, medroxyprogesterone 1%) and systemic collagenase and MMP-9 inhibitors (eg, doxycycline, minocycline) are of potential value. Topical cyclosporine has been shown to be effective in patients with central melting that is likely due to a T-cell–mediated process rather than occlusive vasculitis.

Systemic corticosteroids can help control the underlying disease and result in enhanced collagenase function. When considering topical corticosteroids, the clinician must weigh the benefits of treating inflammation against the risks of impaired healing, secondary infection, and potentiation of collagenase that may increase the chance of stromal melt.

Excision or recession of adjacent limbal conjunctiva, particularly in patients with rheumatoid arthritis, may be followed by rapid healing of the overlying epithelial defect and healing of the ulcer. This is presumably because the procedure eliminates the adjacent source of inflammatory cells and collagenolytic enzymes.

Systemic immunosuppression is required if healing with local measures alone is inadequate. Institution or escalation of systemic treatment, including immunosuppression therapy with immunomodulatory agents (eg, methotrexate, cyclophosphamide, cyclosporine) in addition to or in place of oral prednisone, may be helpful. Biologic agents such as infliximab have reportedly been used with some success in more severe cases. Patients with severe, rapid melting may require intravenous therapy with high-dose cyclophosphamide, with or without corticosteroid therapy.

Impending perforation is treated with temporizing measures such as cyanoacrylate glue (see Chapter 5, Video 5-7) and bandage contact lens placement until systemic therapy can control the underlying disease. Lamellar and penetrating grafts are susceptible to melting if the underlying systemic disease has not been controlled. Sometimes multiple tectonic grafts are required to preserve the globe while the systemic therapy is being adjusted. Once the underlying disease process has been controlled, keratoplasty for visual restoration can be performed (see Chapter 16). Although conjunctival flaps can be very helpful in controlling the stromal melting in many situations, they are probably best avoided in patients with immune-mediated disease, because bringing the conjunctival vasculature even closer to the area of corneal disease could potentially accelerate keratolysis. It is very important to partner with a rheumatologist in caring for patients with immune-mediated disease due to the significant risk of morbidity and death.

Bhat P, Birnbaum AD. Diagnosis and management of noninfectious corneal ulceration and melting. *Focal Points: Clinical Modules for Ophthalmologists.* American Academy of Ophthalmology; 2015, module 3.

Huerva V, Sanchez MC, Traveset A, Jurjo C, Ruiz A. Rituximab for peripheral ulcerative keratitis with Wegener granulomatosis. *Cornea.* 2010;29(6):708–710.

Kaçmaz RO, Kempen JH, Newcomb C, et al. Cyclosporine for ocular inflammatory diseases. *Ophthalmology.* 2010;117(3):576–584.

Pham M, Chow CC, Badawi D, Tu EY. Use of infliximab in the treatment of peripheral ulcerative keratitis in Crohn disease. *Am J Ophthalmol.* 2011;152(2):183–188.e2.

Mooren Ulcer

CLINICAL PRESENTATION Mooren ulcer is a chronic, painful, progressive ulceration of the peripheral cornea. Typically, the ulcer starts in the periphery of the cornea within the palpebral fissure and spreads circumferentially and then centrally, with undermining of the central edge (Fig 13-25). Ulceration toward the sclera is less common. The eye is inflamed, and pain can be intense, with photophobia and tearing. Perforation may occur with minor trauma or from secondary infection. Extensive vascularization and fibrosis of the cornea may occur. PUK due to known local (eg, rosacea) or systemic (eg, rheumatoid arthritis) diseases is not considered Mooren ulcer.

Two clinical types of Mooren ulcer have been described. Unilateral Mooren ulcer is a slowly progressive disease that typically occurs in an older patient population and has an equal sex distribution. The second type of Mooren ulcer, which is more common in Africa, is usually bilateral, progresses rapidly, and responds poorly to medical or surgical intervention (see Fig 13-25). Corneal ulceration frequently progresses to perforation (Fig 13-26). Many patients with this form of Mooren ulcer also have coexisting parasitemia. It is possible that in this subgroup of West African men, Mooren ulcer may be

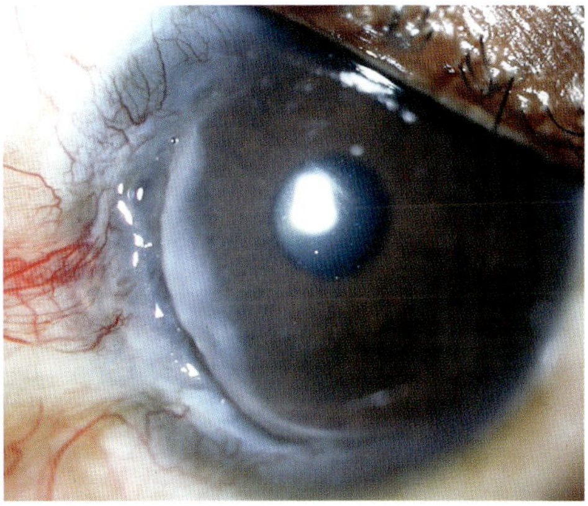

Figure 13-25 Mooren ulcer. Temporal cornea in the right eye demonstrates severe peripheral corneal ulceration. *(Courtesy of Arie L. Marcovich, MD, PhD.)*

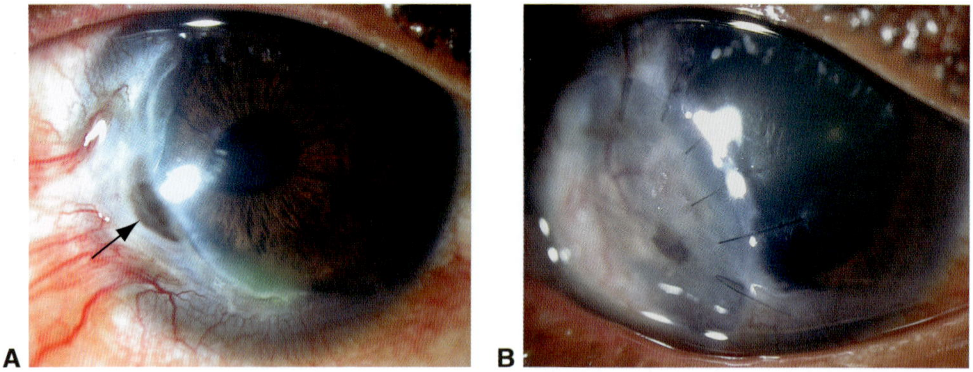

Figure 13-26 Mooren ulcer with severe exacerbation. **A,** Perforation and iris prolapse *(arrow)*. **B,** Anterior lamellar keratoplasty performed to seal the perforation. *(Courtesy of Arie L. Marcovich, MD, PhD.)*

triggered by antigen–antibody reaction to helminthic toxins or antigens deposited in the limbal cornea during the blood-borne phase of parasitic infection. Testing for hepatitis C should be considered in patients with Mooren ulcer–like findings, because there is increased prevalence of comorbid disease.

PATHOGENESIS Although the cause of Mooren ulcer is unknown, precipitating factors include accidental trauma, ocular surgery, hepatitis C, or exposure to parasitic infection. It has been suggested that inflammation associated with a previous injury or infection may alter the expression of corneal stromal antigens. These altered antigens stimulate humoral and cell-mediated immune mechanisms involved in the initiation and perpetuation of corneal destruction.

Kafkala C, Choi J, Zafirakis P, et al. Mooren ulcer: an immunopathologic study. *Cornea.* 2006;25(6):667–673.

MANAGEMENT The multitude of therapeutic strategies used against Mooren ulcer underscores the relative lack of effective treatment. Topical corticosteroids, contact lenses, acetylcysteine 10%, topical cyclosporine 2%, limbal conjunctival excision, and lamellar keratoplasty have all reportedly been used with variable success. Systemic immunosuppressive treatment of Mooren ulcer with agents such as oral corticosteroids, cyclophosphamide, methotrexate, cyclosporine, TNF-α inhibitors, and Campath-1H has been described (see Table 13-4). Hepatitis C–associated cases of Mooren ulcer–type PUK have responded to interferon therapy.

Alhassan MB, Rabiu M, Agbabiaka IO. Interventions for Mooren's ulcer. *Cochrane Database Syst Rev.* 2014;1:CD006131. Epub 2011 Jun 15.

Cordero-Coma M, Benito MF, Fuertes CL, Antolín SC, García Ruíz JM. Adalimumab for Mooren's ulcer. *Ophthalmology.* 2009;116(8):1589,1589.e1.

Garg P, Reddy JC, Sangwan VS. Mooren ulcer. In: Mannis MJ, Holland EJ, eds. *Cornea.* Vol 1. 4th ed. Elsevier; 2017:1082–1087.

van der Hoek J, Azuara-Blanco A, Greiner K, Forrester JV. Mooren's ulcer resolved with campath-1H. *Br J Ophthalmol.* 2003;87(7):924–925.

Immune-Mediated Diseases of the Episclera and Sclera

Episcleritis

CLINICAL PRESENTATION Episcleritis is typically a transient (usually days to weeks), self-limited disease of sudden onset affecting adults aged 20–50 years, with most cases occurring in women. The patient's chief complaint is usually ocular redness with irritation. If tenderness or dull pain is present, a diagnosis of scleritis should be considered. The disease occurs most often in the exposed interpalpebral area. It may recur in the same or different locations of the episclera. Approximately one-third of patients have bilateral disease.

Episcleritis is classified as simple (diffuse injection) or nodular. In simple episcleritis, inflammation is localized to a sector of the globe in 70% of cases and to the entire episclera in 30% of cases. In nodular episcleritis, a localized mobile nodule develops (Fig 13-27). Small peripheral corneal opacities can be observed adjacent to an area of episcleral inflammation in 10% of patients.

CLINICAL PEARL

Episcleral inflammation is superficial and will blanch with application of topical phenylephrine 2.5%. Episcleritis must be differentiated from the deeper inflammation seen in scleritis that is often associated with scleral edema discernible on slit-lamp examination. The inflamed episclera is characteristically bright red or salmon pink in natural light, unlike the violaceous darker hue seen in most forms of scleritis.

Sainz de la Maza M, Molina N, Gonzalez-Gonzalez LA, Doctor PP, Tauber J, Foster CS. Clinical characteristics of a large cohort of patients with scleritis and episcleritis. *Ophthalmology.* 2012;119(1):43–50.

PATHOGENESIS Episcleritis is a generally benign inflammation of the episcleral tissues. An underlying systemic cause is found in only a minority of patients.

MANAGEMENT A workup for underlying causes (eg, autoimmune connective tissue disease such as Sjögren syndrome or rheumatoid arthritis; other conditions such as gout, herpes zoster, syphilis, tuberculosis, Lyme disease, or rosacea) is indicated only in rare cases after multiple recurrences. Episcleritis generally clears without treatment, but topical or oral

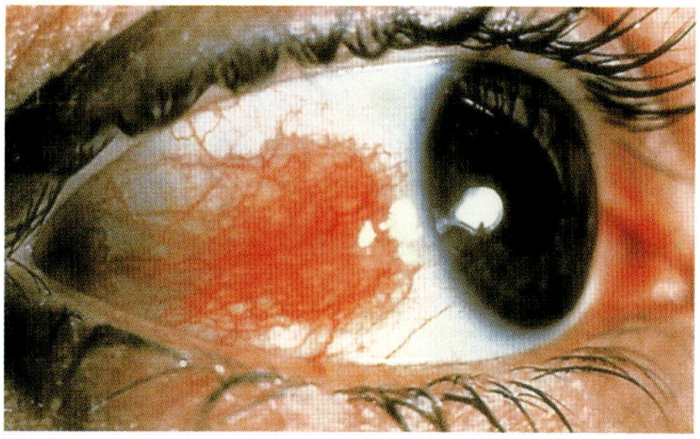

Figure 13-27 Nodular episcleritis.

NSAIDs may be prescribed for patients bothered by the pain. Most patients simply need reassurance that their condition is not sight threatening and can be treated with lubricants alone. Topical corticosteroid use should be kept to a minimum.

Scleritis

CLINICAL PRESENTATION Scleritis occurs most often in the fourth to sixth decades of life, is more common in women, and is exceedingly rare in children. About one-half of scleritis cases are bilateral at some time in their course. The onset of scleritis is usually gradual, extending over several days. Most patients with scleritis experience severe, boring ocular pain, which may worsen at night and occasionally awakens them from sleep. The pain may be referred to other regions of the head or face on the involved side, and the globe is often tender. The inflamed sclera has a violaceous hue that is best seen in natural light. Inflamed scleral vessels have a crisscross pattern, adhere to the sclera, and cannot be moved with a cotton-tipped applicator. Scleral edema, often with overlying episcleral edema, can be visualized with slit-lamp examination (Fig 13-28).

Scleritis can be classified clinically on the basis of the anatomical location (anterior versus posterior sclera) and the appearance of the scleral inflammation (Table 13-6). About one-third of patients with diffuse or nodular scleritis and two-thirds of patients with necrotizing scleritis have a detectable autoimmune connective tissue disease; the different forms of scleritis are discussed in the following subsections.

PATHOGENESIS An immune-mediated (typically immune-complex) vasculitis frequently leads to destruction of the sclera and subsequent visual morbidity. Scleritis can occur in association with various systemic infectious diseases, including syphilis, tuberculosis, herpes zoster, Lyme disease, "cat-scratch" disease, and leprosy. It is most frequently seen, however, in association with autoimmune or connective tissue diseases such as

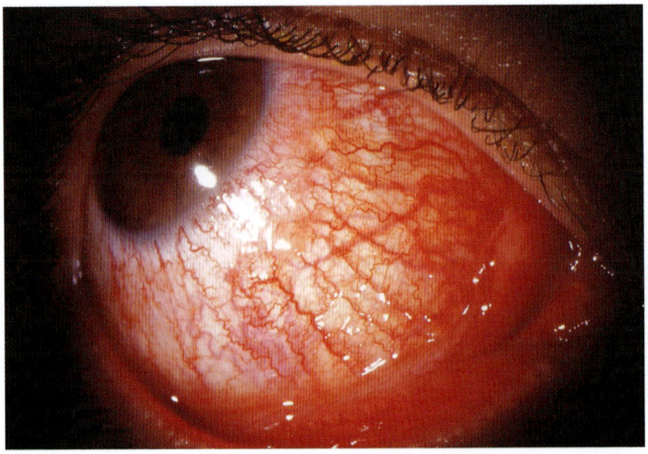

Figure 13-28 Diffuse anterior scleritis. *(Courtesy of Charles S. Bouchard, MD.)*

Table 13-6 Subtypes and Prevalence of Scleritis

Location	Subtype	Prevalence, %
Anterior sclera	Diffuse scleritis	75
	Nodular scleritis	14
	Necrotizing scleritis	5
	With inflammation	(4)
	Without inflammation (scleromalacia perforans)	(1)
Posterior sclera	Posterior scleritis	6

Data from Sainz de la Maza M, Molina N, Gonzalez-Gonzalez LA, et al. Clinical characteristics of a large cohort of patients with scleritis and episcleritis. *Ophthalmology.* 2012;119(1):43–50.

rheumatoid arthritis, systemic lupus erythematosus, and seronegative spondyloarthropathies (eg, ankylosing spondylitis) or secondary to vasculitides such as granulomatosis with polyangiitis (GPA, formerly Wegener granulomatosis), polyarteritis nodosa, and giant cell arteritis. Metabolic diseases such as gout may also, in rare instances, be associated with scleritis. More than 50% of patients with scleritis have an identifiable associated systemic disease.

See also BCSC Section 9, *Uveitis and Ocular Inflammation,* and BCSC Section 4, *Ophthalmic Pathology and Intraocular Tumors.*

Sainz de la Maza M, Biber JM, Schwam BL, Raizman MB. Scleritis. In: Mannis MJ, Holland EJ, eds. *Cornea.* Vol 1. 4th ed. Elsevier; 2017:1181–1194.

Diffuse versus nodular anterior scleritis

Diffuse anterior scleritis is characterized by a zone of scleral edema and redness. A portion of the anterior sclera (<50%) is involved in 60% of cases; the entire anterior sclera, in 40% (see Fig 13-28). In *nodular anterior scleritis,* the scleral nodule is a deep violaceous color, immobile, and separated from the overlying episcleral tissue, which is raised by the nodule (Fig 13-29).

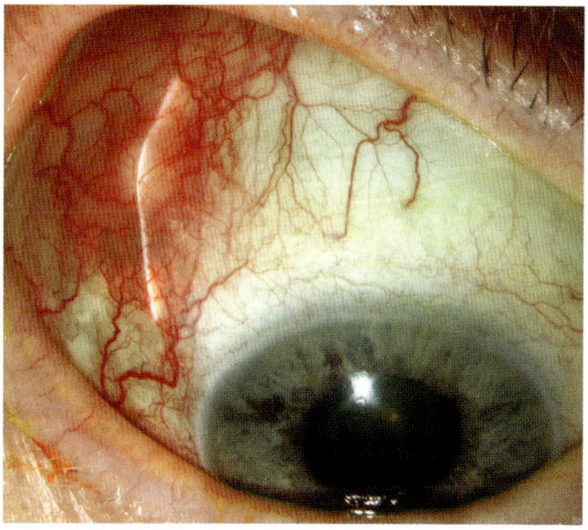

Figure 13-29 Nodular anterior scleritis. Note the scleral edema within the slit and scleral thinning and loss of normal vascularization inferiorly. *(Courtesy of Arie L. Marcovich, MD, PhD.)*

Necrotizing scleritis

Necrotizing scleritis is the most destructive form of scleritis. Ocular and systemic complications occur in 60% of affected patients, vision loss occurs in 40%, and if untreated, a significant percentage may die from complications of vasculitis.

Necrotizing scleritis with inflammation Patients with necrotizing scleritis with inflammation typically present with severe pain. Most commonly, a localized patch of inflammation is noted initially, with the edges of the lesion more inflamed than the center. In 25% of cases with more advanced disease, an avascular edematous patch of sclera is seen (Fig 13-30A). A conjunctival epithelial defect may be present (Fig 13-30B). Untreated, necrotizing scleritis may spread posteriorly and circumferentially until the entire anterior globe is involved. Severe tissue loss may result if treatment is not intensive and prompt. The sclera may develop a blue-gray appearance (due to thinning, which allows the underlying choroid to show) and reveal an altered deep episcleral blood vessel pattern with large anastomotic blood vessels that may circumscribe the involved area occurring after the inflammation subsides.

Necrotizing scleritis without inflammation Though undoubtedly due to inflammation, this form of scleritis, *scleromalacia perforans,* is said to be "without inflammation" because its clinical presentation is distinct from that of other forms of anterior scleritis, in which typical signs (redness, edema) and symptoms (pain) of inflammation are readily apparent.

Scleromalacia perforans typically occurs in patients with long-standing rheumatoid arthritis. Signs of inflammation are minimal, and affected individuals typically do not experience pain. As the disease progresses, the sclera becomes thinner and the underlying dark uveal tissue becomes visible (Fig 13-31). In many cases, the uvea is covered with only thin connective tissue and conjunctiva. Large abnormal blood vessels surround and cross the areas of scleral loss. A bulging staphyloma can develop if intraocular pressure is elevated (Fig 13-32); spontaneous perforation is rare, although these eyes may rupture with minimal trauma.

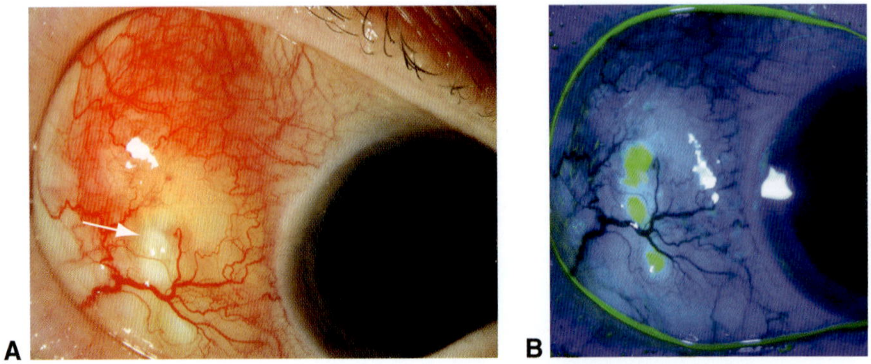

Figure 13-30 Necrotizing anterior scleritis with inflammation. **A,** Avascular edematous sclera *(arrow)* surrounded by inflammation. **B,** Conjunctival epithelial defects seen with fluorescein stain. *(Courtesy of Arie L. Marcovich, MD, PhD.)*

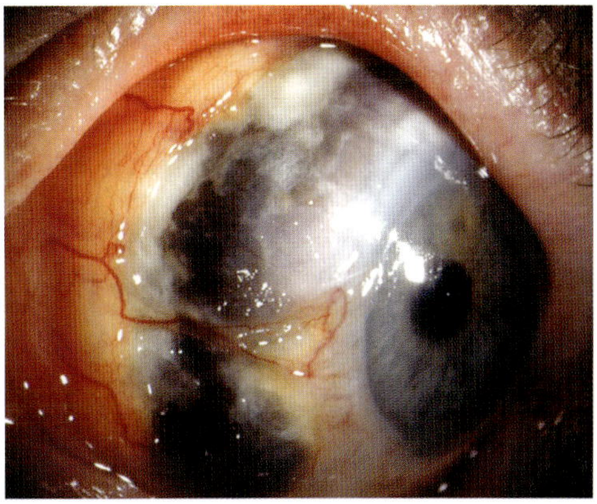

Figure 13-31 Necrotizing anterior scleritis without inflammation (scleromalacia perforans) in a patient with rheumatoid arthritis. *(Courtesy of Charles S. Bouchard, MD.)*

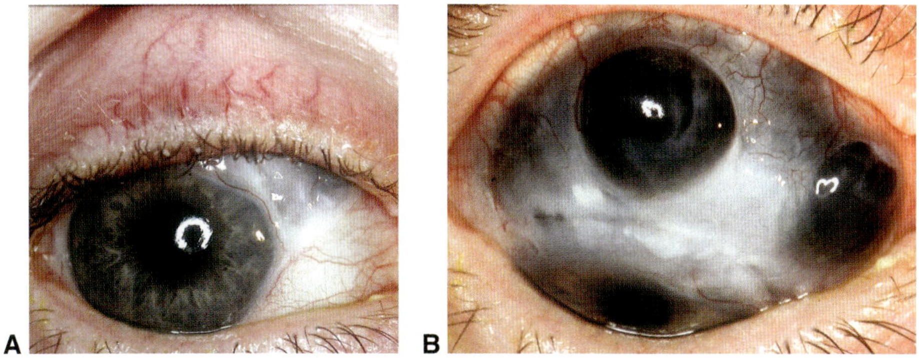

Figure 13-32 Necrotizing anterior scleritis without inflammation in a patient with rheumatoid arthritis with bulging staphylomas. **A,** Primary gaze. **B,** Down gaze. *(Courtesy of Arie L. Marcovich, MD, PhD.)*

Posterior scleritis

Posterior scleritis can occur in isolation or concomitantly with anterior scleritis. Posterior scleritis is sometimes considered an anterior variant of inflammatory pseudotumor. Patients present with pain, tenderness, proptosis, vision loss, and, occasionally, restricted motility. The pain may be referred to other parts of the head, and the diagnosis can be missed in the absence of associated anterior scleritis. Choroidal folds, exudative retinal detachment, papilledema, and angle-closure glaucoma secondary to choroidal thickening may develop. Retraction of the lower eyelid may occur in upgaze, presumably caused by infiltration of muscles in the region of the posterior scleritis. Demonstration of thickened posterior sclera with ultrasound (Fig 13-33), computed tomography, or magnetic resonance imaging may be helpful in establishing the diagnosis. Often, no related systemic disease can be found in patients with posterior scleritis.

Complications of scleritis

Complications of scleritis are frequent and include peripheral keratitis (occurring in 37% of cases), scleral thinning (33%), uveitis (30%), glaucoma (18%), and cataract (7%). In sclerokeratitis, the peripheral cornea becomes opacified by fibrosis and lipid deposition in conjunction with adjacent scleritis of varying intensity (Fig 13-34). With progression, the

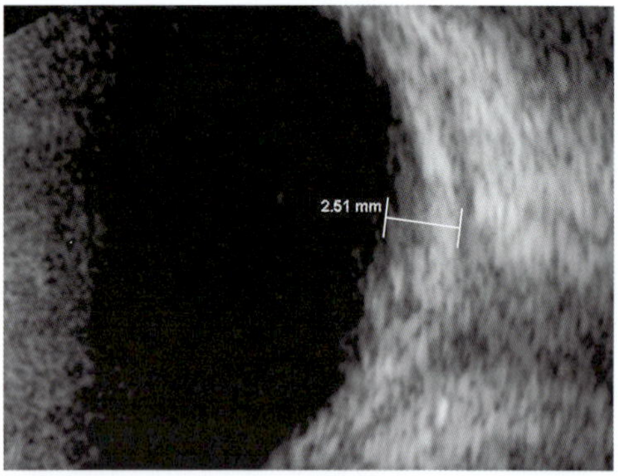

Figure 13-33 B-scan ultrasound image from a patient with posterior scleritis showing localized posterior scleral thickening (⊢⊣). *(Courtesy of James J. Reidy, MD.)*

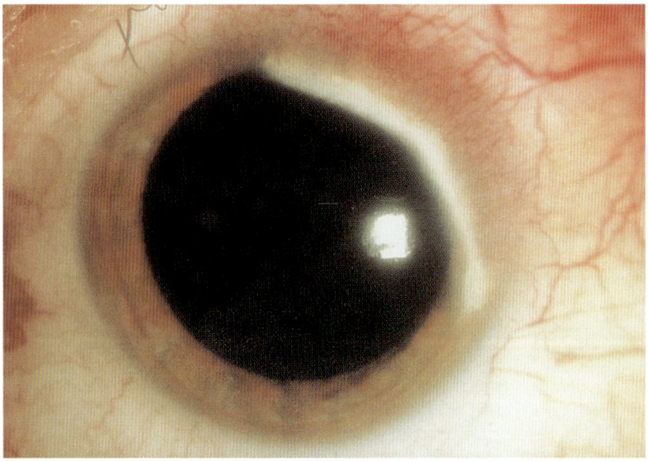

Figure 13-34 Sclerokeratitis.

central cornea becomes involved, resulting in opacification of a large segment of cornea. This type of keratitis commonly accompanies herpes zoster scleritis but may also occur in association with rheumatic diseases.

Anterior uveitis may occur as a spillover phenomenon in eyes with anterior scleritis. Some degree of posterior uveitis occurs in all patients with posterior scleritis and may also occur in those with anterior scleritis. Although one-third of patients with scleritis have evidence of scleral translucency and/or thinning, frank scleral defects are seen only in the most severe forms of necrotizing disease and in the late stages of scleromalacia perforans.

LABORATORY EVALUATION The differential diagnosis of scleritis is similar to that of PUK (see Table 13-5; see also BCSC Section 9, *Uveitis and Ocular Inflammation*, for associated diseases). The workup of scleritis therefore includes a complete physical examination, with attention to the joints, skin, and cardiovascular and respiratory systems. It is recommended that the ophthalmologist consult with a rheumatologist or other internist with experience in diagnosing and managing these conditions. Laboratory studies are guided by the history and findings of the physical examination. However, laboratory tests (see sidebar) are generally recommended as an initial screening. If infectious scleritis is suspected, scleral scraping or biopsy can be taken for microbiological analysis.

INITIAL LABORATORY WORKUP FOR SCLERITIS

- Chest x-ray
- Complete blood cell count (CBC) with differential
- Erythrocyte sedimentation rate (ESR) or C-reactive protein (CRP)
- Serum angiotensin-converting enzyme and lysozyme, as appropriate (ie, sarcoidosis screening)
- Serum autoantibody screening (antinuclear antibody [ANA], anti-DNA antibody, rheumatoid factor [RF], antineutrophil cytoplasmic antibody [ANCA])
- Serum uric acid test
- Syphilis serologic test
- Urinalysis

MANAGEMENT Although topical corticosteroids can be used to alleviate symptoms, the treatment of scleritis is systemic. A guideline for the treatment of patients with scleritis has been proposed by Sainz de la Maza, et al. It is important to clearly define treatment goals: treatment failure may be defined as progression of disease to a more severe form (eg, nodular to necrotizing) or failure to achieve a response to treatment after 2–3 weeks of therapy, in which case an alternate therapeutic strategy will need to be instituted. Idiopathic diffuse and nodular forms of scleritis, which have no ocular complications and little scleral inflammation, may be responsive to treatment with oral NSAIDs (eg, ibuprofen, indomethacin). If one NSAID is not effective, another may be substituted.

Systemic corticosteroid treatment may be used if the patient is unresponsive to NSAIDs or inflammation is more severe. To rule out tuberculosis exposure, a QuantiFERON-TB Gold test can be considered prior to initiating systemic immunosuppression with corticosteroids. NSAIDs and steroids should not be given simultaneously. Prednisone may be started at 1 mg/kg daily and then tapered within the first 2 weeks of treatment. Sustained remission may be obtained with NSAIDs. Acid-reducing medication can be given to patients prescribed NSAIDs or steroids to reduce the risk of gastritis and ulceration.

If corticosteroid treatment fails or the patient relapses after tapering the steroid, systemic immunosuppression therapy may be considered. (See Table 13-4 on immunomodulating drugs.) These cases often respond to antimetabolites (eg, methotrexate, azathioprine, mycophenolate mofetil). Patients with associated systemic disease, necrotizing scleritis, and/or progressive destructive ocular lesions may require treatment with

- immunosuppression therapy with antimetabolites:
  - T-cell inhibitors (eg, cyclosporin A, tacrolimus)
  - alkylating agents (eg, cyclophosphamide)
- biologic response modifiers:
  - anti-TNF-α medications (eg, infliximab)
  - anti-CD20 agents (eg, rituximab)
  - anti-CD52 agents (Campath-1H)

Antituberculosis and anti-*Pneumocystis* coverage may be necessary for at-risk patients. Patients receiving systemic treatment should be monitored closely by a physician specially trained in the administration of these medications and in the early detection and management of their complications. In addition, it is important to inform these patients that close follow-up with an ophthalmologist and partnering providers is necessary to monitor their disease status and treatment. In patients whose systemic evaluation is initially negative, it is important to repeat the workup annually.

Scleral reinforcement may at times be required to prevent spontaneous or impending perforation due to the destructive process of scleritis resulting in scleral thinning and ectasia. Ideally, any scleral surgery is performed only after systemic control of the inflammation or infection has been achieved. The thinned area of sclera may be covered with donor sclera or cornea, autologous periosteum, or fascia lata. Overlying conjunctiva should be carefully removed. The donor tissue patch is placed over the thinned area and is sutured to the adjacent healthier sclera with nylon or vicryl sutures. A core vitrectomy can be considered to facilitate flattening a bulging, staphylomatous area. It is recommended that the patch graft be covered either by advancing adjacent conjunctiva, using a conjunctival rotation flap, or by an amniotic membrane graft. This covering can be secured with sutures or fibrin glue.

Surgically induced scleritis (SIS) occurs in patients with rheumatoid arthritis following extracapsular cataract extraction through scleral approach. In patients with scleritis, a clear cornea approach to cataract surgery is recommended. If marked scleral thinning is present, maintaining lower IOP during cataract surgery can reduce the likelihood of scleral perforation.

Dick AD, Meyer P, James T, et al. Campath-1H therapy in refractory ocular inflammatory disease. *Br J Ophthalmol* 2000;84(1):107–109.

Levy-Clarke G, Jabs DA, Read RW, Rosenbaum JT, Vitale A, Van Gelder RN. Expert panel recommendations for the use of anti-tumor necrosis factor biologic agents in patients with ocular inflammatory disorders. *Ophthalmology.* 2014;121(3):785–796.e3.

Ragam A, Kolomeyer AM, Fang C, Xu Y, Chu DS. Treatment of chronic, noninfectious, nonnecrotizing scleritis with tumor necrosis factor alpha inhibitors. *Ocul Immunol Inflamm.* 2014;22(6):469–477.

Sainz de la Maza M, Molina N, Gonzalez-Gonzalez LA, Doctor PP, Tauber J, Foster CS. Scleritis therapy. *Ophthalmology.* 2012;119(1):51–58.

Singh J, Sallam A, Lightman S, Taylor S. Episcleritis and scleritis in rheumatic disease. *Curr Rheumatol Rev.* 2011;7(1):15–23.

Watson PG, Young RD. Scleral structure, organization and disease: a review. *Exp Eye Res.* 2004;78(3):609–623.

CHAPTER 14

Clinical Approach to Neoplastic Disorders of the Conjunctiva and Cornea

This chapter includes related videos. Go to www.aao.org/bcscvideo_section08 or scan the QR codes in the text to access this content.

This chapter includes a case study. Go to www.aao.org/bcsccasestudy_section08 or scan the QR code in the text to access this content.

Indicates selected key points within the chapter.

Highlights

- Topical interferon-α_{2b}, 5-fluorouracil, or mitomycin C can be used to treat ocular surface squamous neoplasia.
- Sebaceous carcinoma is initially misdiagnosed in more than 50% of cases, often masquerading as chalazia or chronic unilateral blepharoconjunctivitis.
- Primary acquired melanosis (PAM) with moderate to severe atypia has a high risk of progression to melanoma. Biopsy is therefore important for suspicious-appearing PAM lesions.
- Lymphoid hyperplasia is clinically indistinguishable from lymphoma; biopsy is required in order to differentiate these conditions.

Introduction

Ocular surface tumors of the conjunctiva and cornea are considered together because the lesions can affect both tissues concurrently. These lesions are classified by cell type: epithelium, melanocytes and nevus cells, vascular endothelium, mesenchymal cells, and lymphocytes. Many are analogous to lesions affecting the eyelid. Ocular surface tumors are associated with a spectrum of conditions, from benign to premalignant to malignant neoplasia, often with similar clinical appearance and presentation. Histopathological examination may be needed for definitive diagnosis. The most common ocular surface malignant tumors are malignant melanoma, squamous cell carcinoma, and lymphoma.

In the United States, approximately 1 person in 2500 (about 100,000 people per year) seeks ophthalmic care for a tumor of the eyelid or ocular surface. Benign neoplasms of the eyelid and ocular surface are at least 3 times more common than malignant lesions. Most of these tumors arise from the eyelid skin; see BCSC Section 4, *Ophthalmic Pathology and Intraocular Tumors,* and Section 7, *Oculofacial Plastic and Orbital Surgery.*

Shields CL, Chien JL, Surakiatchanukul T, Sioufi K, Lally SE, Shields JA. Conjunctival tumors: review of clinical features, risks, biomarkers, and outcomes—the 2017 J. Donald Gass lecture. *Asia-Pac J Ophthalmol (Phila).* 2017;6(2)109–120.

Shields JA, Shields CL. *Eyelid, Conjunctival, and Orbital Tumors: An Atlas and Textbook.* 3rd ed. Wolters Kluwer; 2016.

Approach to the Patient With a Neoplastic Ocular Surface Lesion

During the initial evaluation of a patient with a conjunctival or corneal neoplasm, it is important to obtain a detailed history, including sun exposure, prior skin cancer, and immunosuppression. The clinician should inquire about the duration and changes in the lesion appearance. The racial or ethnic background of the patient is relevant; conjunctival pigmentation may be normal in darker-skinned individuals but cause for concern in individuals with fair skin.

During the initial evaluation of the patient with a suspicious ocular surface lesion, a complete eye examination, including a dilated fundus examination, is warranted. It is important to examine the entire ocular surface, including the superior fornix, which requires eyelid eversion. Palpation for lymphadenopathy in the neck and preauricular region is an important part of the examination of patients with tumors, especially when malignancy is suspected, because malignant lesions (eg, conjunctival melanoma) can spread to regional lymph nodes. It is important to note the clinical characteristics of the lesion (see sidebar).

HOW TO DESCRIBE OCULAR SURFACE LESIONS

- Size, including clock hours, anterior/posterior extent, and shape
- Involvement of the bulbar conjunctiva, palpebral conjunctiva, fornix, limbus, and/or cornea
- Flat, elevated, invasive
- Pigmented or amelanotic
- Solid or cystic
- Fixed to underlying tissues or mobile
- Degree of vascularity, presence of feeder vessels
- Single or multifocal

It is important to document the appearance and extent of the lesion, using either photographs or a detailed diagram; this aids in surgical planning if the lesion is to be removed or in following the lesion if observation is recommended.

Management of Patients With Ocular Surface Tumors

The following sections describe the generally accepted approaches and principles in the management of patients with ocular surface tumors.

Observation

After completing the history and physical examination, an experienced clinician usually has an opinion about the nature of a conjunctival or corneal lesion. Many lesions are not suspicious for malignancy (eg, inclusion cysts); others will be indeterminate based on the history and results of the clinical examination. For these cases, observation may be a reasonable option. If the clinician decides to observe, regular (annual or even more frequent) ophthalmic examinations are essential. If growth or suspicious changes in the lesion are observed, surgery or topical chemotherapy is usually indicated. Tissue for histologic evaluation may be required for definitive diagnosis. Findings that raise concern for malignancy in such lesions include

- enlargement
- elevation
- extensive pigmentation, even if lesion is flat
- fixation to underlying tissues
- large feeder vessel

"Optical biopsy" using noninvasive imaging technologies such as optical coherence tomography (OCT; see Chapter 7, Fig 7-3, and BCSC Section 4, *Ophthalmic Pathology and Intraocular Tumors,* Chapter 5, Fig 5-18), confocal microscopy, or ultrasound biomicroscopy (UBM) may assist the clinician in deciding whether to continue observation or proceed with surgical excision, chemotherapy, or other treatment options.

Morkin MI, Wall SC, Karp CL. Ocular surface tumors. Focal Points: Clinical Modules for Ophthalmologists. American Academy of Ophthalmology; 2020, module 6.

Nanji AA, Mercado C, Galor A, Dubovy S, Karp CL. Updates in ocular surface tumor diagnostics. *Int Ophthalmol Clin.* 2017;57(3):47–62.

Singh S, Mittal R, Ghosh A, Tripathy D, Rath S. High-resolution anterior segment optical coherence tomography in intraepithelial versus invasive ocular surface squamous neoplasia. *Cornea.* 2018;37(10):1292–1298.

Surgery

Surgical resection has been the traditional approach to the treatment of ocular surface tumors. The advantages of surgical excision include providing tissue for definitive histopathological diagnosis, confirmation of clear margins, immediate results, fewer issues related to patient adherence to a therapeutic regimen, and, in some cases, cost efficiency due to fewer medications and office visits compared to alternative treatments. Potential disadvantages of surgical excision include incomplete treatment of microscopic, subclinical disease, as well as scarring and symblepharon. If more than two-thirds of the limbal epithelium is removed, stem cell deficiency and chronic epitheliopathy may result. Stem cell transplantation using tissue harvested from the fellow eye or an allograft may eventually be required.

Principles of surgical excision of ocular surface tumors include

- performing a complete excision with 2- to 4-mm clear margins
- using the "no-touch technique" to avoid touching the tumor during removal to prevent tumor seeding
- administering double freeze–thaw cryotherapy to surrounding conjunctival and limbal margins and applying absolute alcohol or cryotherapy to involved and surrounding corneal epithelium for squamous cell or melanocytic tumors

A conjunctival tumor should be evaluated by an ophthalmic pathologist because diagnoses in these cases can be challenging, especially for less-experienced clinicians. Once removed, the lesion can be placed on filter paper and the edges labeled with ink or suture to indicate the orientation of the lesion, which is helpful to the pathologist. The surgeon should take care to avoid damage to the specimen during removal, which could make histopathological assessment of the lesion more difficult. Immunostaining can help in distinguishing benign from malignant lesions. The clinical history is relevant to the pathologist's interpretation; thus, the label should include the age and race or ethnicity of the patient, the duration of the lesion, and whether the lesion has changed clinically.

See BCSC Section 4, *Ophthalmic Pathology and Intraocular Tumors,* for further discussion of specimen handling and histologic examination.

Shields JA, Shields CL, De Potter P. Surgical management of conjunctival tumors. The 1994 Lynn B. McMahan Lecture. *Arch Ophthalmol.* 1997;115(6):808–815.

Topical Chemotherapy

Topical chemotherapy may be used as an alternative to surgical excision for primary treatment of ocular surface tumors or as adjunctive therapy preceding or following surgical excision. Topical chemotherapy has the advantage of treating beyond areas of clinically visible involvement, but unlike surgical excision, it does not provide the opportunity for histologic diagnosis or the determination of clear margins.

Topical chemotherapeutic agents include interferon-α_{2b} (INF-α_{2b}), 5-fluorouracil (5-FU), and mitomycin C (MMC); their benefits and adverse effects are as follows:

- *INF-α_{2b}:* 1 million IU/ml solution
  - better tolerated than 5-FU and MMC, but may require longer treatment and greater expense
  - adverse effects are usually minimal, eg, mild conjunctival hyperemia, follicular conjunctivitis
  - subconjunctival or perilesional weekly injection of INF-α_{2b} 3 million units may be associated with flulike symptoms; use of an oral NSAID prior to injection may lessen these symptoms
- *5-FU:* 1% solution
  - adverse effects are usually mild: ocular pain, lid edema, hyperemia, keratitis, stem cell deficiency
  - lower cost than other options
  - does not require refrigeration

- *MMC:* 0.02% solution
  - less likely to be tolerated than INF-α_{2b} or 5-FU but is sometimes effective following INF-α_{2b} or 5-FU failure
  - ocular surface toxicity can be severe and include ocular pain, hyperemia, keratitis, corneal erosion, and limbal stem cell deficiency
  - placement of punctal plugs may help avoid punctal stenosis

Controlled studies have not yet determined optimal chemotherapy regimen for each tumor cell type. First-line therapy for ocular surface squamous neoplasia (OSSN) consists of 1 of the 3 topical agents listed in this section (Figs 14-1, 14-2). Melanocytic tumors are less likely to resolve with topical chemotherapy and may be more responsive to MMC than INF-α_{2b} or 5-FU.

Other Treatment Options

Immunomodulatory agents (eg, rituximab) and radiotherapy are effective treatments for ocular lymphoid tumors. Additional treatment options for ocular surface tumors are evolving and depend on the cell type; they include radiotherapy, radioimmunotherapy, targeted gene therapy, and checkpoint inhibitors.

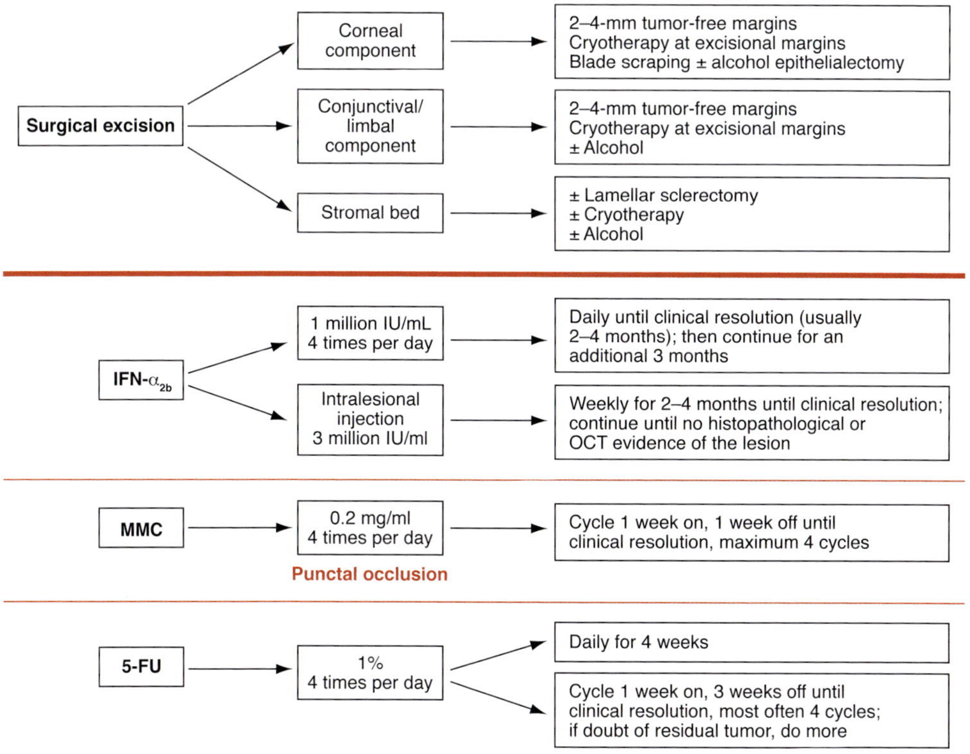

Figure 14-1 Treatment options for ocular surface squamous neoplasia (OSSN). 5-FU = 5-fluorouracil; IFN-α_{2b} = interferon-α_{2b}; MMC = mitomycin C.

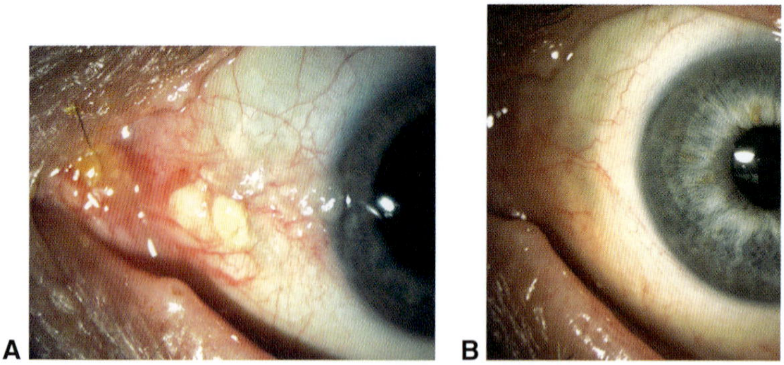

Figure 14-2 OSSN. **A,** OSSN prior to treatment. **B,** The same eye 7 weeks after topical treatment with INF-α_{2b} 1 million IU/mL 4 times daily. *(Courtesy of David D. Verdier, MD.)*

Treatment Follow-Up

Once a tumor has been managed, long-term (annual or more frequent) follow-up is essential because ocular surface tumors can recur. It is important to perform a complete examination of the ocular surface and palpation of regional lymph nodes at each visit. Patients with malignant epithelial or melanocytic ocular surface tumors should be referred to a dermatologist for a complete skin evaluation.

Tumors of Epithelial Origin

Epithelial tumors of the conjunctiva and cornea are listed in Table 14-1.

Warner MA, Stagner AM, Jakobiec FA. Epithelial tumors of the conjunctiva. In: Mannis MJ, Holland EJ, eds. *Cornea.* Vol 1. 4th ed. Elsevier; 2017:410–426.

Benign Epithelial Tumors

Conjunctival papilloma

Conjunctival papilloma has 2 forms, *sessile* and *pedunculated,* and they differ etiologically, histologically, and clinically. See BCSC Section 4, *Ophthalmic Pathology and Intraocular Tumors,* for discussion of the histologic findings.

CLINICAL PRESENTATION A pedunculated papilloma is a fleshy, exophytic growth with a fibrovascular core (Fig 14-3A). It often arises in the inferior fornix but can also present on the tarsal or bulbar conjunctiva or along the plica semilunaris. The lesion emanates from a stalk and has a multilobulated appearance with smooth, clear epithelium and numerous underlying small corkscrew blood vessels. Multiple lesions can occur, and the lesion may be extensive in patients with compromised immunity.

A sessile papilloma is typically found at the limbus and has a flat base (Fig 14-3B). With its glistening surface and numerous red dots, this form of papilloma resembles a strawberry. The lesion may spread onto the cornea. Signs of dysplasia include leukoplakia

Table 14-1 Tumors of Ocular Surface Epithelium

Benign	Preinvasive	Malignant
Papilloma Pseudoepitheliomatous hyperplasia Benign hereditary intraepithelial dyskeratosis	Conjunctival and corneal intraepithelial neoplasia	Squamous cell carcinoma Mucoepidermoid carcinoma

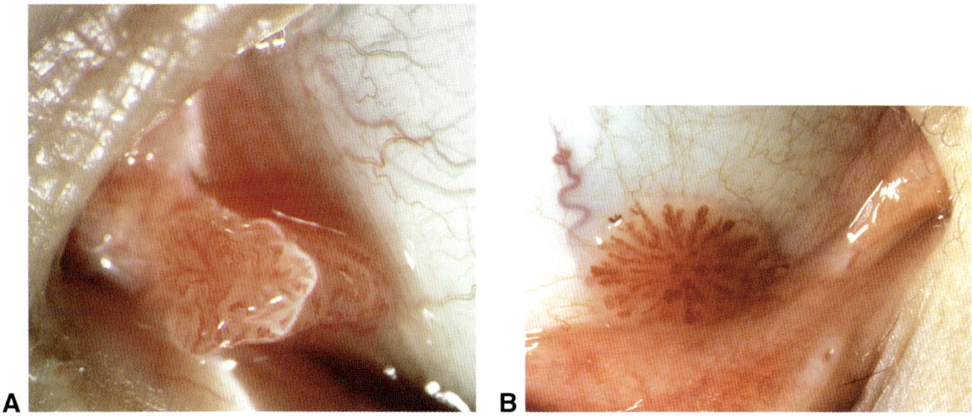

Figure 14-3 Conjunctival squamous papilloma. **A,** Pedunculated. **B,** Sessile. *(Reproduced with permission from Mannis MJ, Holland EJ, eds.* Cornea. *Vol 1. 4th ed. Elsevier; 2017:412.)*

(indicative of keratinization), symblepharon formation, inflammation, and invasion. A very rare variant is an inverted papilloma.

PATHOGENESIS *Human papillomavirus (HPV),* subtypes 6 and 11 (in children) or 16 (in adults), may initiate a neoplastic growth of epithelial cells with vascular proliferation that gives rise to a pedunculated conjunctival papilloma. A sessile lesion, though also usually benign, may represent a dysplastic or carcinomatous lesion, especially when caused by HPV subtypes 16, 18, or 33. HPV vaccination may be preventative.

MANAGEMENT A pedunculated papilloma that is small, cosmetically acceptable, and nonirritating may be observed; spontaneous resolution can occur over many months to years. Surgical excision with cryotherapy or cautery to the base of the lesion is curative in approximately 90% of cases. However, an incomplete excision can stimulate growth and lead to a worse cosmetic outcome. Surgical manipulation should be minimized to reduce the risk of dissemination of the virus to uninvolved healthy conjunctiva. Adjunctive treatment with topical INF-α_{2b} or oral cimetidine may be beneficial in cases of extensive or recalcitrant lesions.

A sessile limbal papilloma must be observed closely or excised. If the lesion enlarges or shows clinical features suggesting dysplastic or carcinomatous growth, excisional biopsy with adjunctive cryotherapy is indicated.

Kaliki S, Arepalli S, Shields CL, et al. Conjunctival papilloma: features and outcomes based on age at initial examination. *JAMA Ophthalmol.* 2013;131(5):585–593.

Theotoka D, Morkin MI, Galor A, Karp CL. Update on diagnosis and management of conjunctival papilloma. *Eye Vis (Lond).* 2019;6:18.

Ocular Surface Squamous Neoplasia

Ocular surface squamous neoplasia (*OSSN;* Case Study 14-1) is an inclusive term that comprises a wide spectrum of conjunctival and corneal squamous tumors that may have similar clinical findings but require biopsy for differentiation. The traditional categorization of OSSN lesions as conjunctival or corneal intraepithelial neoplasia or squamous cell carcinoma is made on the basis of histologic criteria. See also BCSC Section 4, *Ophthalmic Pathology and Intraocular Tumors.*

CASE STUDY 14-1 Ocular surface lesion.
Courtesy of David D. Verdier, MD.

Risk factors associated with OSSN include ultraviolet light exposure, prior skin cancer, older age, male sex, smoking, HPV, and HIV. Systemic immunosuppression seems to potentiate squamous neoplasia. Rapid growth of a lesion may occur in a person with AIDS. In a young adult, OSSN may prompt consideration of a serologic test for HIV infection.

Kamal S, Kaliki S, Mishra DK, Batra J, Naik MN. Ocular surface squamous neoplasia in 200 patients: a case-control study of immunosuppression resulting from human immunodeficiency virus versus immunocompetency. *Ophthalmology.* 2015;122(8): 1688–1694.

Sayed-Ahmed IO, Palioura S, Galor A, Karp CL. Diagnosis and medical management of ocular surface squamous neoplasia. *Expert Rev Ophthalmol.* 2017;12(1):11–19.

Shields CL, Ramasubramanian A, Mellen PL, Shields JA. Conjunctival squamous cell carcinoma arising in immunosuppressed patients (organ transplant, human immunodeficiency virus infection). *Ophthalmology.* 2011;118(11):2133–2137.e1.

Noninvasive OSSN: conjunctival or corneal intraepithelial neoplasia

Conjunctival or corneal intraepithelial neoplasia (CIN), or *dysplasia,* is analogous to actinic keratosis of the skin. In CIN, the dysplastic process does not involve the underlying basement membrane. CIN is considered a premalignant condition that is at risk of transforming into squamous cell carcinoma. Related terms include *squamous dysplasia,* which is used when atypical cells invade only part of the epithelium, and *squamous carcinoma in situ,* used when cellular atypia involves the entire thickness of the epithelial layer.

CLINICAL PRESENTATION The 3 principal clinical variants of conjunctival disease (Fig 14-4) are as follows:

1. *papilliform,* in which a sessile papilloma harbors dysplastic cells
2. *gelatinous,* which occurs as a result of acanthosis and dysplasia
3. *leukoplakic,* which is caused by hyperkeratosis, parakeratosis, and dyskeratosis

A B C
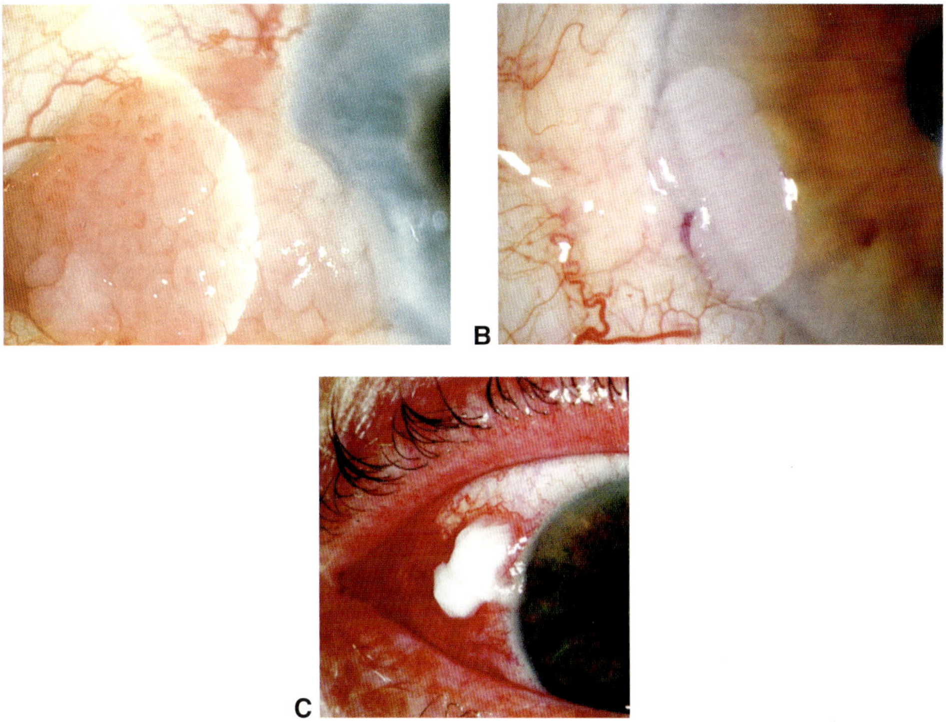

Figure 14-4 Conjunctival intraepithelial neoplasia. **A,** Papilliform. **B,** Gelatinous. **C,** Leukoplakic. *(Part A courtesy of James Chodosh, MD, MPH; parts B and C courtesy of James J. Reidy, MD.)*

CIN lesions are slow-growing tumors that are nearly always centered at the limbus but are able to spread to other areas of the ocular surface. Mild inflammation and various degrees of abnormal vascularization may accompany CIN lesions; large feeder blood vessels indicate an increased probability of invasion beneath the epithelial basement membrane.

Corneal involvement may present as a translucent, sometimes granular, mildly elevated gray epithelial sheet that is based at the limbus and extends onto the cornea. The edges of corneal lesions have characteristic fimbriated margins and pseudopodia-like extensions (Fig 14-5). Topical rose bengal, lissamine green, and toluidine blue staining can help define the extent of the lesion. In some cases, the conjunctival or limbal component is not clinically apparent. Occasionally, free islands of corneal involvement are present.

Invasive OSSN: squamous cell carcinoma

In squamous cell carcinoma (SCC), involvement extends beyond the basement membrane into stroma, with metastatic potential. SCC is more common and aggressive in patients with compromised immunity and in those with xeroderma pigmentosum.

CLINICAL PRESENTATION A plaquelike, gelatinous, or papilliform growth occurs in limbal and bulbar conjunctiva, usually in the interpalpebral fissure zone. A broad base is often present along the limbus. The lesion typically grows outward and has sharp borders; it may appear leukoplakic (Fig 14-6). Although histologic invasion of the epithelial basement membrane is present, growth usually remains superficial, with neoplastic cells

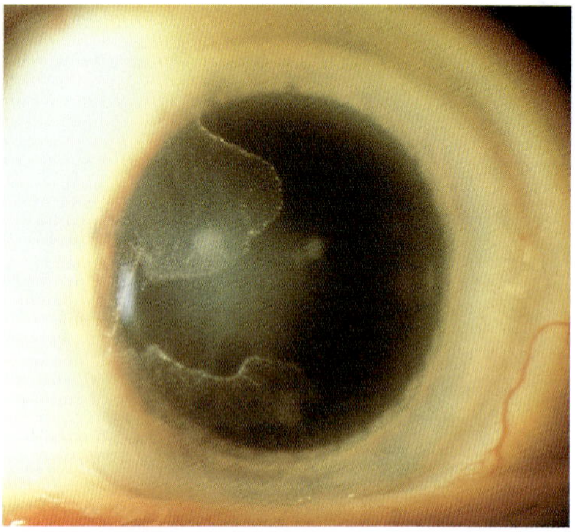

Figure 14-5 Corneal intraepithelial neoplasia. A fimbriated central edge is typical. *(Courtesy of James Chodosh, MD, MPH.)*

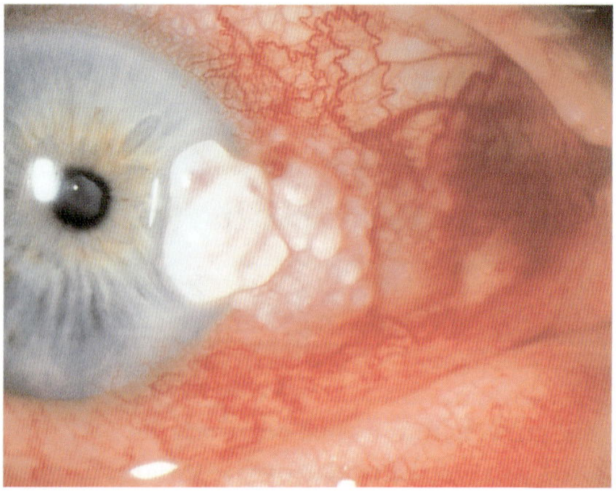

Figure 14-6 Limbal squamous cell carcinoma (SCC). The leukoplakia shown here is not uncommon in SCC.

infrequently penetrating the sclera or Bowman layer. Pigmentation can occur in individuals with darker skin. Engorged conjunctival vessels suggest malignancy. Note that the clinical appearance of CIN and invasive SCC may be similar (compare Figs 14-4C and 14-6).

Variants of squamous cell carcinoma *Mucoepidermoid carcinoma* is an aggressive variant of SCC that is more likely to invade the globe or orbit. It occurs more commonly in the salivary glands and occurs in the conjunctiva only in rare cases. In addition to neoplastic epithelial cells, malignant goblet cells can be visualized histopathologically with mucin stains. Treatment consists of surgical excision with wide margins; adjuvant therapy may include cryotherapy and radiotherapy.

Spindle cell carcinoma, another variant, is a rare, highly malignant SCC of the bulbar or limbal conjunctiva in which the anaplastic cells appear spindle shaped, like fibroblasts.

Shields JA, Shields CL. Premalignant and malignant lesions of the conjunctival epithelium. In: *Eyelid, Conjunctival, and Orbital Tumors: An Atlas and Textbook.* 3rd ed. Wolters Kluwer; 2016:283–306.

Management of OSSN

Surgical and topical chemotherapeutic treatment options for OSSN are summarized in Figure 14-1.

All OSSN lesions should be regarded as possible carcinoma with metastatic potential because it may be difficult to distinguish dysplasia from invasive SCC clinically. OSSN lesions that appear stable and have a more benign appearance can be observed with meticulous follow-up exams, including drawings, photographs, and imaging with optical coherence tomography (OCT). OCT imaging can assist the clinician in determining whether the tumor is confined to the epithelium (CIN) or penetrates basement membrane (SCC). Classic OCT findings of OSSN are a hyperreflective, thickened epithelial layer with an abrupt transition from normal to abnormal epithelium (Fig 14-7).

Lesions that are growing or appear suspicious for malignancy should be treated with surgical excision and/or topical chemotherapy. Success rates for treatment with topical INF-α_{2b}, MMC, or 5-FU are similar at more than 85%, comparable to success rates seen with wide-margin surgical excision followed by cryotherapy.

SCC can grow into the iris, trabecular meshwork, or the orbit, providing a portal to systemic circulation and metastasis. Orbital invasion may require orbital exenteration. Radiation therapy may be indicated as adjunctive treatment in select cases.

Surgical treatment The standard surgical treatment of a suspicious OSSN conjunctival/corneal lesion is complete removal of the tumor, including a 2- to 4-mm margin of uninvolved tissue surrounding the lesion, when possible. See sidebar and Video 14-1.

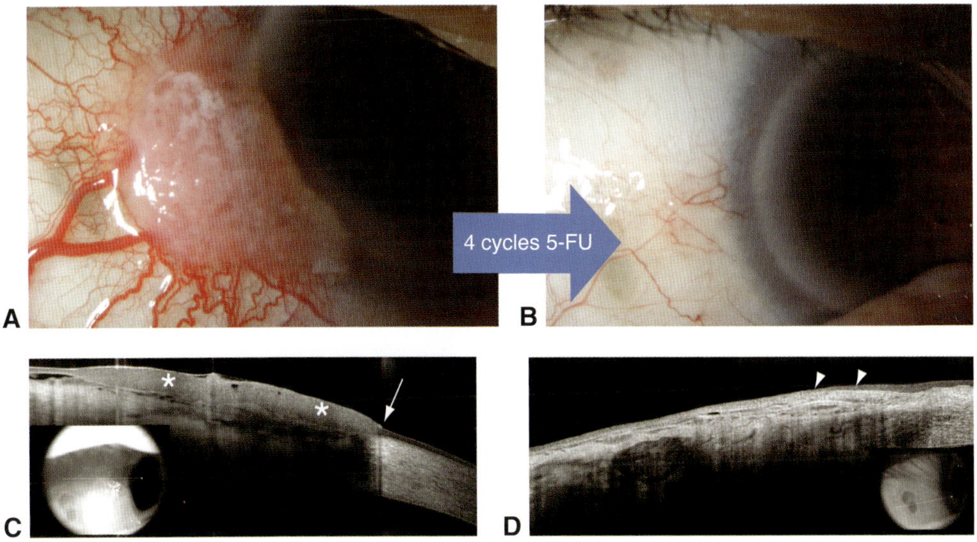

Figure 14-7 OCT images of OSSN. Clinical and OCT images of OSSN before (**A** and **C**) and after (**B** and **D**) 4 cycles of topical 5-FU 1% 4 times daily for 1 week, with 3 weeks off between each cycle. **C,** Note the thickened hyperreflective epithelium *(asterisks)* with abrupt transition *(arrow)* from normal to abnormal tissue, characteristic of OSSN. **D,** Resolution following 5-FU treatment; note the thin normal epithelium *(arrowheads)*. *Insets* shows location of scan. *(Courtesy of Carol L. Karp, MD.)*

STEPS IN SURGICAL TREATMENT OF OSSN

1. *Corneal epitheliectomy:* Apply absolute alcohol with a surgical sponge to the involved epithelial surface for 60 seconds, followed by gentle epithelial scrolling/debridement with a blade or blunt spatula. Avoid violating Bowman membrane, which is a natural barrier to tumor extension into the corneal stroma. (Alternative treatment: Double freeze–thaw cryotherapy to involved corneal epithelium and 2-mm of surrounding epithelium.)
2. *Conjunctival resection:* Perform a wide resection of the involved conjunctiva using the "no-touch" technique to prevent seeding of tumor. Some lesions may require lamellar sclerectomy for complete removal.
3. *Double freeze–thaw cryotherapy to surrounding conjunctival border:* Lift the edge and apply a cryoprobe to the exposed conjunctival underside until full blanching occurs; thaw for approximately 10 seconds; then refreeze. Move 3 mm from previously treated adjacent spot and repeat to encompass the entire border. Treat the limbal border with direct application of cryoprobe to the limbal surface.
4. *Scleral bed:* Treat with absolute alcohol; alternatively, can treat with double freeze–thaw cryotherapy, but it is more likely to cause increased inflammation and damage to the ciliary body.
5. *Wound closure:* Consider primary conjunctival closure or a conjunctival autograft if the conjunctival defect is small. Ocular surface reconstruction with glued or sutured amniotic membrane transplantation allows for wider tumor margins and reduced risk of postoperative scarring.

VIDEO 14-1 No-touch technique for conjunctival squamous cell carcinoma removal.
Courtesy of Brian P. Marr, MD, and Spencer Langevin, MD.

Topical chemotherapy Of the 3 agents, INF-α_{2b} is often the first choice because it has fewer adverse effects than 5-FU or MMC. INF-α_{2b} 1 million IU/mL is typically given 4 times daily until clinical resolution, on average 4 months. It is not unusual for tumors to appear unresponsive during the first few months of treatment and then show abrupt regression. Once clinical resolution occurs, treatment is continued for several additional months; ultra-high-resolution OCT has demonstrated that residual tumor may be present for up to 3 months following clinical resolution. Subconjunctival/perilesional injection of INF-α_{2b} (3 million IU/0.5 mL) can be given weekly in addition to, or as an alternative to, topical eyedrops, especially if patient adherence to the treatment regimen is an issue. Subconjunctival INF-α_{2b} is associated with flulike symptoms in 10% of patients, which can be managed with oral NSAIDs administered prior to the injection.

5-FU is cheaper and just as effective as INF-α_{2b} and does not require refrigeration. 5-FU 1% may be administered topically 4 times daily for 1 week, followed by a 3-week structured treatment interruption (drug holiday), until clinical resolution. This typically requires 4 cycles, but if there is any doubt of residual tumor, treatment can be continued for several additional cycles. Alternatively, 5-FU may be given 4 times daily for 1 month, with a structured treatment interruption of at least several months if repeat treatment is needed.

MMC can be used for a shorter duration than the other 2 agents, typically for weeks rather than months, but it may result in more severe adverse effects. MMC 0.2mg/ml is typically administered 4 times daily for 1 week, followed by a 1-week structured treatment interruption, for a maximum of 3 or 4 treatment cycles. If residual tumor persists, alternative treatment should be considered to avoid potential MMC toxicity. The ocular pain and surface toxicity associated with topical chemotherapy can be reduced with fluorometholone eyedrops once or twice per day.

Morkin MI, Karp CL. Medical and surgical management of ocular surface squamous neoplasia. In: Mannis MJ, Holland EJ, eds. *Cornea*. Vol 1. 5th ed. Elsevier; 2022:497–506.

Nanji AA, Moon CS, Galor A, Sein J, Oellers P, Karp CL. Surgical versus medical treatment of ocular surface squamous neoplasia: a comparison of recurrences and complications. *Ophthalmology.* 2014;121(5):994–1000.

Thomas BJ, Galor A, Nanji AA, et al. Ultra high-resolution anterior segment optical coherence tomography in the diagnosis and management of ocular surface squamous neoplasia. *Ocul Surf.* 2014;12(1):46–58.

Venkateswaran N, Mercado C, Galor A, Karp CL. Comparison of topical 5-fluorouracil and interferon alpha-2b as primary treatment modalities for ocular surface squamous neoplasia. *Am J Ophthalmol.* 2019;199:216–222.

Glandular Tumors of the Conjunctiva

Oncocytoma

A slow-growing cystadenoma, an oncocytoma is a benign tumor arising from ductal and acinar cells of main and accessory lacrimal glands. Oncocytoma most commonly occurs in older persons and may present as a reddish-brown nodule on the surface of the caruncle.

Sebaceous Carcinoma

Sebaceous carcinoma accounts for approximately 1% of all eyelid tumors and 5% of eyelid malignancies. It usually occurs in individuals older than 50 years but may be seen in younger persons after radiation therapy. These tumors may masquerade as chalazia or as chronic unilateral blepharoconjunctivitis (Fig 14-8). Consequently, more than 50% of cases are initially misdiagnosed. Epithelial invasion of the conjunctiva occurs in almost 50% of cases and extends onto the cornea in more than 25% of cases. Map biopsies (consisting of 3–4 mm diameter tissue samples harvested from multiple areas of concern) of palpebral and bulbar conjunctiva can be considered to identify areas of possible multicentric involvement and clinically inapparent pagetoid spread. Primary tumor involvement is treated with wide margin excision and cryotherapy, or exenteration if disease is extensive. Adjunctive use of topical MMC may offer some benefit. See BCSC Section 7, *Oculofacial Plastic and Orbital Surgery.*

Shields JA, Saktanasate J, Lally SE, Carrasco JR, Shields CL. Sebaceous carcinoma of the ocular region: the 2014 Professor Winifred Mao lecture. *Asia Pac J Ophthalmol (Phila).* 2015;4(4):221–227.

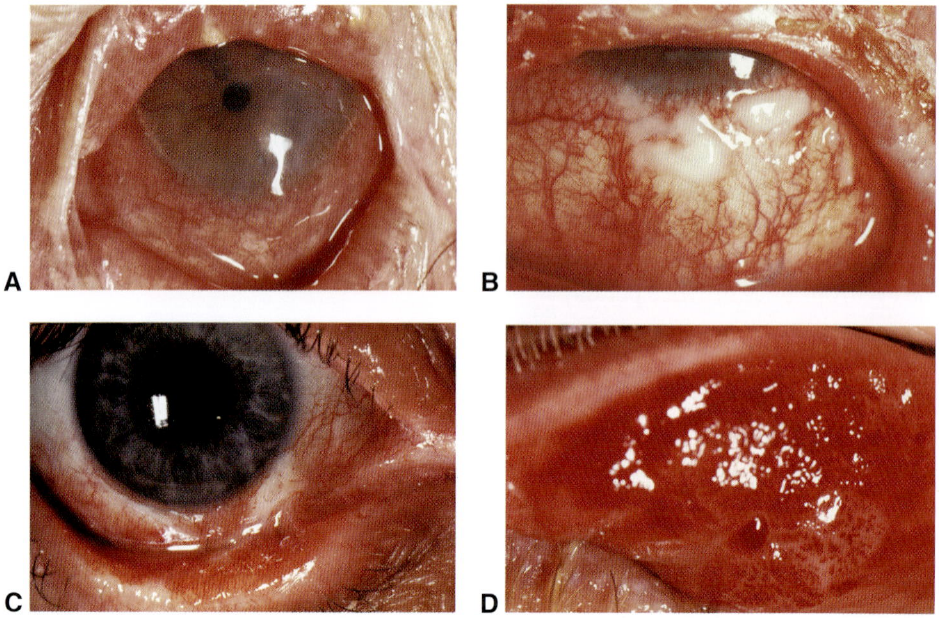

Figure 14-8 Various presentations of sebaceous carcinoma. **A,** Unilateral blepharoconjunctivitis with injection, pannus, thickened eyelid margin, and eyelash loss. **B,** White nodules composed of neoplastic sebaceous cells may be present near the limbus. **C,** Neoplastic symblepharon is present nasally. **D,** Upper palpebral conjunctival thickening. Papillary fronds may be present. *(Reproduced with permission from Mannis MJ, Holland EJ, eds.* Cornea. *Vol 1. 4th ed. Elsevier; 2017:422.)*

Tumors of Neuroectodermal Origin

Ocular surface tumors that arise from melanocytes, nevus cells, and other neuroectodermal cells are listed in Table 14-2. Some pigmented lesions of the globe are considered normal. For example, a *pigment spot of the sclera* is a collection of melanocytes associated with an intrascleral nerve loop or perforating anterior ciliary vessel. The term *melanosis* refers to excessive pigmentation without an elevated mass that may be congenital (epithelial or subepithelial) or acquired (primary or secondary). Conjunctival pigmentation can also occur because of long-term exposure to topical epinephrine compounds, oral minocycline, systemic or topical preparations containing silver, or mascara. See Video 14-2 for guidelines to managing conjunctival pigmented lesions.

VIDEO 14-2 Conjunctival pigmented lesions: planning your approach.
Courtesy of Carol L. Shields, MD.

Aggarwal S, Cameron JD, Karp CL. Melanocytic neoplasms of the conjunctiva. In: Mannis MJ, Holland EJ, eds. *Cornea*. Vol 1. 5th ed. Elsevier; 2022:507–515.

Shields JA, Shields CL. Conjunctival melanocytic lesions. In: *Eyelid, Conjunctival, and Orbital Tumors: An Atlas and Textbook.* 3rd ed. Wolters Kluwer; 2016:307–348.

Table 14-2 Tumors and Related Conditions of Neuroectodermal Cells of the Ocular Surface

Cell of Origin	Benign	Preinvasive/Malignant
Epithelial melanocytes	Freckle Complexion-associated melanosis	Primary acquired melanosis Melanoma
Subepithelial melanocytes	Ocular melanocytosis Melanocytoma	Melanoma
Nevus cells	Intraepithelial (junctional) nevus Compound nevus Subepithelial nevus	Melanoma
Neural and other cells	Neurofibroma	Leiomyosarcoma

Benign Pigmented Lesions

Ocular melanocytosis

Ocular melanocytosis represents a focal proliferation of subepithelial melanocytes. Congenital melanosis of the episclera occurs in approximately 1 in every 2500 individuals and is more common in Black, Hispanic, and Asian populations.

CLINICAL PRESENTATION Patches of episcleral pigmentation appear slate gray through the normal conjunctiva (Fig 14-9) and are immobile and usually unilateral. Affected patients may have a diffuse nevus of the uveal tract, evident as increased pigmentation of the iris and choroid. In approximately 50% of patients with ocular melanocytosis, ipsilateral dermal melanocytosis and a proliferation of dermal melanocytes is present in the periocular skin of the first and second dermatomes of cranial nerve V. The combined ocular and cutaneous pigmentations are referred to as *oculodermal melanocytosis* or *nevus of Ota*

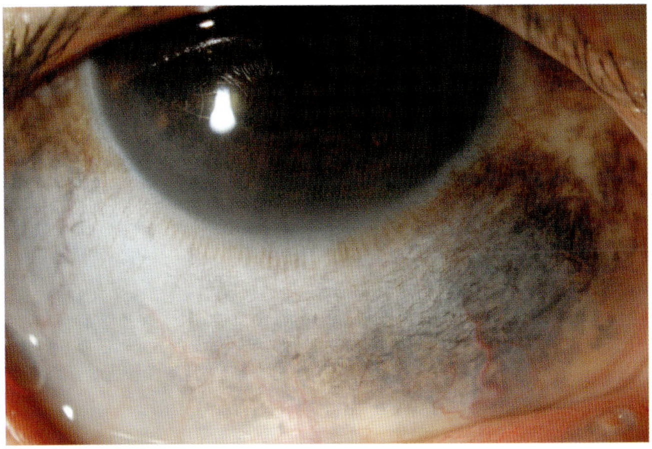

Figure 14-9 Episcleral pigmentation in a patient with congenital ocular melanocytosis. *(Courtesy of Kathryn Colby, MD, PhD.)*

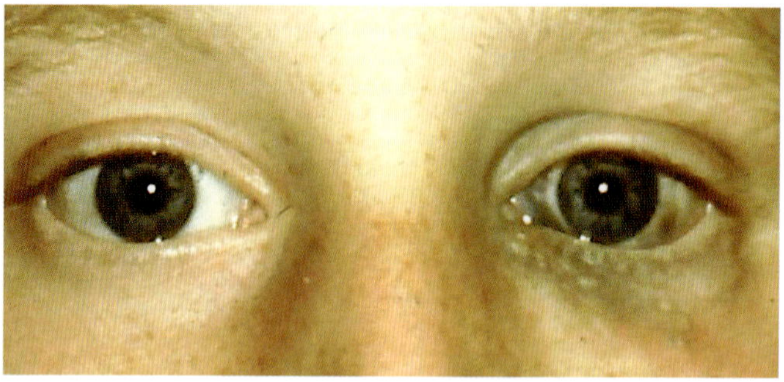

Figure 14-10 Nevus of Ota. *(Courtesy of Kenneth V. Cahill, MD.)*

(Fig 14-10). Approximately 5% of cases are bilateral. See Table 14-3 and BCSC Section 7, *Oculofacial Plastic and Orbital Surgery.*

In 10% of patients with ocular melanocytosis, secondary glaucoma occurs in the affected eye. Malignant transformation is possible but rare and seems to occur only in patients with fair complexions. Malignant melanoma can develop in the skin, conjunctiva, uvea, or orbit. The lifetime risk of uveal melanoma in a patient with ocular melanocytosis is about 1 in 400, significantly greater than the approximate 6-per-million risk of the general population. Twice-yearly ophthalmic examinations that include funduscopy is recommended in these patients.

Shields CL, Kaliki S, Livesey M, et al. Association of ocular and oculodermal melanocytosis with the rate of uveal melanoma metastasis: analysis of 7872 consecutive eyes. *JAMA Ophthalmol.* 2013;131(8):993–1003.

Nevus

Nevocellular nevi of the conjunctiva consist of nests or more diffuse infiltrations of benign melanocytes. They arise during the first or second decade of life.

CLINICAL PRESENTATION A nevus near the limbus is usually almost flat. Nevi appearing elsewhere on the bulbar conjunctiva, plica semilunaris, caruncle, or eyelid margin tend to be elevated. Intralesional cysts are present in 50% or more of conjunctival nevi, but seldom if ever in conjunctival melanoma (see BCSC Section 4, *Ophthalmic Pathology and Intraocular Tumors,* Chapter 5, Fig 5-19). Pigmentation of conjunctival nevi is variable. They may be light tan to brown or, in 15% of cases, amelanotic (Fig 14-11). Mild enlargement associated with hormonal influences can occur at puberty or pregnancy, creating a clinical impression of conjunctival melanoma. When inflamed, an amelanotic, vascularized nevus may resemble an angioma, or it may be misdiagnosed as chronic conjunctivitis. See Table 14-3.

Shields CL, Fasiuddin AF, Mashayekhi A, Shields JA. Conjunctival nevi: clinical features and natural course in 410 consecutive patients. *Arch Ophthalmol.* 2004;122(2):167–175.

HISTOPATHOLOGY Conjunctival nevi are classified as junctional (confined to the epithelial–stromal junction); subepithelial, or stromal (confined to the stroma); or compound (combines

Table 14-3 Clinical Comparison of Conjunctival Pigmented Lesions

Lesion	Onset	Characteristics	Location	Malignant Potential
Ocular and oculodermal melanocytosis	Congenital	Usually unilateral; flat, slate gray	Episclera	<1%, uveal melanoma
Nevus	First or second decade of life	Discrete, light tan to brown or amelanotic; may be flat or elevated 50% contain epithelial inclusion cysts	Conjunctival epithelium and/or stroma	5%
Complexion-associated melanosis (CAM)	Adulthood	Bilateral, flat, patchy, brown Occurs mainly in adults with darker skin	Conjunctival epithelium	None to low
Primary acquired melanosis (PAM)	Middle age	Unilateral, flat, patchy or diffuse, tan to brown Occurs most often in adults with fairer skin	Conjunctival epithelium	30% risk with moderate to severe cellular atypia
Malignant melanoma	Middle to late adulthood	Brown or amelanotic, often nodular, often vascular	Conjunctival stroma	Overall mortality rate 25%

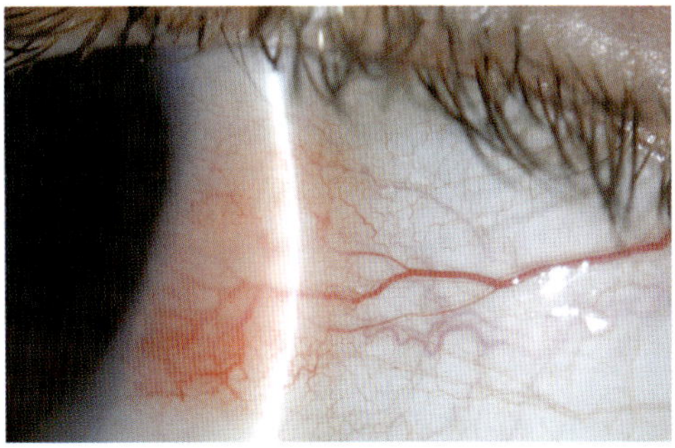

Figure 14-11 Amelanotic conjunctival nevus. *(Courtesy of Kathryn Colby, MD, PhD.)*

junctional and stromal components). Pure intraepithelial nevi are rare except in children. On histologic examination, nevi can occasionally be very difficult to differentiate from melanoma. Junctional nevi may be difficult to distinguish from primary acquired melanosis. Small epithelial inclusion cysts occur within approximately half of all conjunctival nevi, particularly the compound or subepithelial varieties. Secretion of mucin by goblet cells in the inclusion cysts can cause a nevus to enlarge, giving a false impression of malignant change. Cellular proliferation may induce secondary lymphocytic inflammation.

MANAGEMENT Only a small percentage of conjunctival nevi become malignant; therefore, nevi should not be considered precancerous. They can be followed every 6–12 months

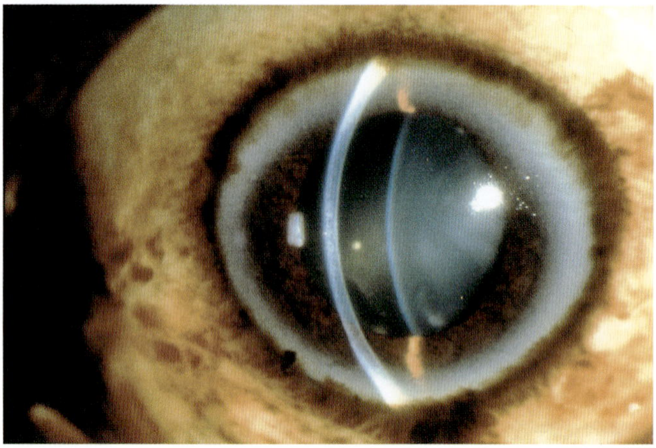

Figure 14-12 Complexion-associated melanosis in a patient with corneal arcus. *(Courtesy of James Chodosh, MD, MPH.)*

with an examination that includes serial photography or detailed slit-lamp drawings incorporating dimensional measurements. Patients should be instructed to periodically inspect the lesion, looking for changes in size, coloration, elevation, or vascularization. Lesions showing suspicious change or growth warrant an excisional biopsy. A biopsy can also be considered for pigmented lesions on the palpebral conjunctiva or cornea or in the fornix, because nevi are rare in these locations.

Complexion-associated melanosis

Complexion-associated melanosis (CAM; also called racial melanosis) is more commonly seen in individuals with darker complexions, but it occurs in persons of all races (approximately 95% of Black individuals, 35% of Asian individuals, 30% of Hispanic individuals, and 5% of White individuals). CAM appears as flat, light to dark-brown conjunctival patches with irregular margins that are most apparent at the limbus and less prominent as it extends into the fornix (Fig 14-12). The pigmentation can also involve the caruncle and palpebral conjunctiva as well as extend into the cornea with streaks or whorls (striate melanokeratosis). Histologic findings consist of hyperpigmentation of the conjunctival basal epithelial cells without atypia or hyperplasia. CAM is bilateral, fairly symmetric, and benign, with little risk of progression to melanoma. It is important to differentiate CAM from primary acquired melanosis (see Table 14-3), which seldom occurs in individuals with darker skin, is usually unilateral or highly asymmetric, and can transform to melanoma.

Preinvasive Pigmented Lesions

Primary acquired melanosis

CLINICAL PRESENTATION Primary acquired melanosis (PAM) is an acquired noncystic, flat, patchy or diffuse, tan to brown pigmentation of the conjunctival epithelium. PAM is usually unilateral or asymmetric if bilateral and is most often seen in individuals with fair skin

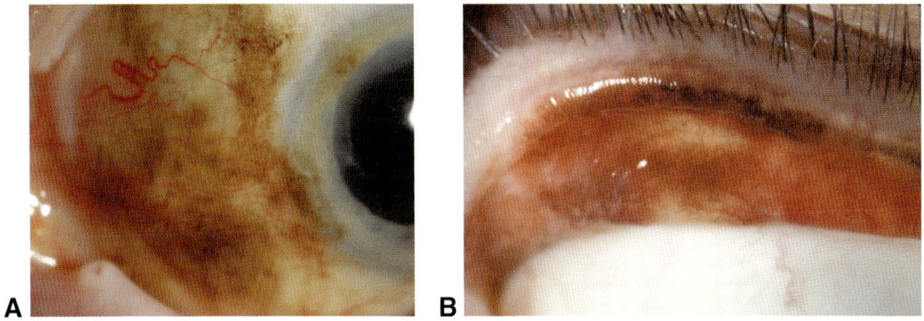

Figure 14-13 Primary acquired melanosis (PAM). **A,** Diffuse PAM of the bulbar conjunctiva. **B,** PAM of the palpebral conjunctiva. *(Courtesy of Kathryn Colby, MD, PhD.)*

(Fig 14-13). Secondary acquired melanosis has a similar appearance but is associated with systemic disease (eg, Addison disease), previous radiation, or pregnancy, or is secondary to another conjunctival lesion (eg, squamous papilloma or carcinoma). See Table 14-3.

Changes in the size of PAM may be associated with inflammation or may be the result of hormonal influences. Complete examination of the ocular surface (including double eversion of the upper eyelid) is essential in any patient with conjunctival pigmentation.

MANAGEMENT Most cases of PAM are benign, but a substantial minority of cases may progress to melanoma. It is difficult to predict which lesions may progress, but a worse prognosis is associated with

- larger size
- caruncular, forniceal, or palpebral location
- progressive enlargement
- a nodular component
- thickening
- feeder vessels

Two clock-hours or less of conjunctival involvement is associated with a lower risk of malignant transformation; involvement of more than 2 clock-hours is an indication to remove the lesion for histologic diagnosis. Lesions should be completely excised with the no-touch technique, if feasible, without jeopardizing the health of adjacent ocular structures. If disease is diffuse, map biopsies can help direct whether to proceed with excision and/or adjuvant therapy including cryotherapy, topical MMC, and alcohol-assisted keratectomy.

The most important finding in predicting progression to melanoma is the presence of cellular atypia, which can be determined only by excisional biopsy for histologic examination and immunohistochemistry. PAM without atypia has little malignant potential. These patients may be followed with examination every 6–12 months. PAM with mild atypia has a minimal risk of malignant transformation but should be followed more closely. PAM with moderate to severe atypia carries a 30% risk of progression to melanoma. Every effort should be made to eliminate all conjunctival pigment in patients with moderate to severe atypia. If the pigmentation is diffuse and not amenable to complete excision, adjuvant topical chemotherapy with MMC may be useful to treat the entire ocular surface. Secondary acquired melanosis has no significant risk of progression to melanoma. See BCSC Section 4, *Ophthalmic Pathology and Intraocular Tumors.*

Folberg R, McLean IW, Zimmerman LE. Conjunctival melanosis and melanoma. *Ophthalmology.* 1984;91(6):673–678.

Shields JA, Shields CL, Mashayekhi A, et al. Primary acquired melanosis of the conjunctiva: risks for progression to melanoma in 311 eyes. The 2006 Lorenz E. Zimmerman lecture. *Ophthalmology.* 2008;115(3):511–519.e2.

Malignant Pigmented Lesions

Melanoma

With a prevalence of approximately 1 per 2 million in the population with European ancestry, conjunctival melanomas make up 2% of ocular malignancies. Conjunctival melanomas are rare in Black and Asian populations.

Conjunctival melanomas may arise from PAM (70%) or nevi (5%) or they may arise de novo (25%). In rare cases, an underlying ciliary body melanoma can extend through the sclera and mimic a conjunctival melanoma. Malignant melanoma of the conjunctiva has a better prognosis than cutaneous melanoma, but the overall mortality rate is 25%.

Video 14-3 details the differential diagnosis, prognosis, and treatment guidelines for conjunctival melanoma.

VIDEO 14-3 Conjunctival melanoma: what you should know.
Courtesy of Fairooz P. Manjandavida, MD; Sandor Ferenczy, CRA; Tessa Tintle, BS; Sara E. Lally, MD; Carol L. Shields, MD; and Jerry A. Shields, MD.

CLINICAL PRESENTATION Although conjunctival melanomas can arise in palpebral conjunctiva, they are most commonly found in the bulbar conjunctiva or at the limbus (Fig 14-14A). The degree of pigmentation is variable; approximately 25% of conjunctival melanomas are amelanotic. Recurrent melanomas are often amelanotic, even if the primary tumor was pigmented (Fig 14-14B). Because heavy vascularization is common, these tumors may bleed easily. They grow in a nodular fashion and can invade the globe or orbit. Poor prognostic indicators include

- location in the palpebral conjunctiva, caruncle, or fornix (Fig 14-14C)
- invasion into deeper tissues
- thickness >1.8 mm (Fig 14-14D)
- involvement of the eyelid margin
- pagetoid or full-thickness intraepithelial spread
- lymphatic invasion
- mixed cell type

Conjunctival melanomas may metastasize to regional lymph nodes, the brain, lungs, liver, and bone.

MANAGEMENT Ocular surface lesions suspicious for melanoma should be treated expeditiously with complete wide-margin (2- to 4-mm) surgical excision and double freeze–thaw

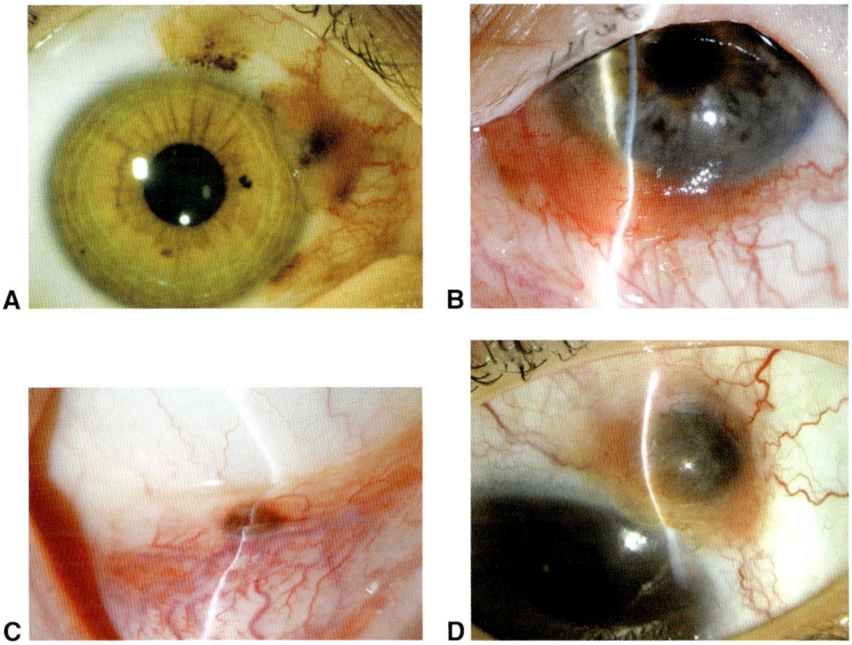

Figure 14-14 Malignant melanoma. **A,** Multifocal, partially pigmented malignant melanoma of the limbal conjunctiva. **B,** Recurrent amelanotic conjunctival melanoma; the primary tumor was pigmented. **C,** Small conjunctival melanoma in the inferior fornix. **D,** Conjunctival melanoma with thickness >1.8 mm. *(Parts A–C courtesy of Kathryn Colby, MD, PhD; part D courtesy of Arie L. Marcovich, MD, PhD.)*

cryotherapy to conjunctival margins, avoiding direct manipulation of the tumor (see Video 14-3). Some surgeons advocate for sentinel lymph node biopsy, but it has not been widely adopted. Adjunctive treatments that may improve local control include radiotherapy and topical chemotherapy with MMC. Orbital exenteration is occasionally performed in cases of advanced disease when the tumor cannot be completely excised by local excision or enucleation, provided metastatic disease has been excluded. It may also be appropriate as palliative treatment for advanced, aggressive tumors that cannot be controlled locally. Metastatic conjunctival melanoma may respond to treatment with immune checkpoint inhibitors such as nivolumab (a PD-1 inhibitor) and ipilimumab (a CTLA-4 inhibitor). Identification of melanoma biomarkers may assist in determining prognosis and selection of targeted therapy.

Conjunctival melanoma has a high rate of recurrence (>50%). Patients with a history of conjunctival melanoma require lifelong, close ophthalmic follow-up and should be counseled to contact their physician immediately if they notice any changes in the involved eye. Metastasis at 15 years exceeds 35%. Factors associated with a poorer prognosis include

- melanomas arising de novo (ie, not from preexisting nevi or PAM)
- tumors that do not involve the limbus
- residual involvement at the surgical margin

Cohen VML, O'Day RF. Management issues in conjunctival tumours: conjunctival melanoma and primary acquired melanosis. *Ophthalmol Ther.* 2019;8(4):501–510.

Cohen VML, Tsimpida M, Hungerford JL, Jan H, Cerio R, Moir G. Prospective study of sentinel lymph node biopsy for conjunctival melanoma. *Br J Ophthalmol.* 2013; 97(12):1525–1529.

Sagiv O, Thakar SD, Kandl TJ, et al. Immunotherapy with programmed cell death 1 inhibitors for 5 patients with conjunctival melanoma. *JAMA Ophthalmol.* 2018;136(11):1236–1241.

Shields CL, Markowitz JS, Belinsky I, et al. Conjunctival melanoma: outcomes based on tumor origin in 382 consecutive cases. *Ophthalmology.* 2011;118(2):389–395.e1.

Shields JA, Shields CL. Conjunctival melanocytic lesions. In: *Eyelid, Conjunctival, and Orbital Tumors: An Atlas and Textbook.* 3rd ed. Wolters Kluwer. 2016:307–348.

Neurogenic and Smooth-Muscle Tumors

Subconjunctival peripheral nerve sheath tumors such as *neurofibromas, schwannomas,* and *neuromas* have been reported, especially in cases of multiple endocrine neoplasia (MEN). A neurofibroma of the conjunctiva or eyelid is almost always a manifestation of neurofibromatosis, an autosomal dominant phakomatosis (see BCSC Section 6, *Pediatric Ophthalmology and Strabismus*). A *neurilemoma* is a very rare tumor of the conjunctiva that originates from Schwann cells of a peripheral nerve sheath. A *leiomyosarcoma* is a very rare limbal lesion with the potential for orbital invasion.

Vascular and Mesenchymal Tumors

Vascular lesions of the eyelid margin or conjunctiva generally are benign hamartomas or secondary reactions to infection or other stimuli (Table 14-4).

Benign Tumors

Vascular lesions

Hemangioma A capillary hemangioma is an unencapsulated hamartomatous growth of proliferating capillary endothelium. It usually presents within the first 6 weeks of life and may enlarge during the first year, after which it typically regresses spontaneously. The palpebral conjunctiva is frequently involved with a capillary hemangioma of the eyelid. The presence of diffuse hemangiomatosis of the palpebral conjunctiva or conjunctival fornix is suggestive of an orbital capillary hemangioma. Treatment options include observation, systemic or topical propranolol, and intralesional or systemic corticosteroids.

Table 14-4 Vascular Tumors of the Eyelid and Conjunctiva[a]

Hamartomatous	Reactive	Malignant
Capillary hemangioma	Glomus tumor	Angiosarcoma
Cavernous hemangioma	Intravascular papillary endothelial hyperplasia	Kaposi sarcoma
Nevus flammeus	Pyogenic granuloma	

[a] Tumors are not listed in any order, and lesions in 1 column do not correspond to those in parallel columns.

Malformations Vascular malformations include a spectrum of benign lesions that contain anomalous capillary venous, arterial, or lymphatic vessel elements. They can fluctuate in size but typically remain static.

Cavernous hemangiomas are the most common primary orbital tumor of adults. They contain dilated congested veins typically encapsulated with a thick fibrosed wall. Because of this encapsulation, they are more amenable to surgical excision. Isolated cavernous hemangiomas of the bulbar conjunctiva are rare and are more likely to represent extension from adjacent structures.

Nevus flammeus, a congenital lesion described as a port-wine birthmark, may occur alone or as part of Sturge-Weber syndrome and may be associated with vascular hamartomas, secondary glaucoma, and/or leptomeningeal angiomatosis. Some cases result from a mutation in the gene coding for the vascular endothelial protein receptor for angiopoietin 1, which controls the assembly of perivascular smooth muscle.

Ataxia-telangiectasia (also called Louis-Bar syndrome) is primarily associated with epibulbar telangiectasis, cerebellar abnormalities, and immune alterations. In this autosomal recessive disease, the epibulbar and interpalpebral telangiectasia of the arteries lacks an associated lymphatic component. The epibulbar vascular lesions seen in ataxia-telangiectasia can grow with the patient and the eyeball, but episodes of hemorrhage or swelling do not occur. See BCSC Section 6, *Pediatric Ophthalmology and Strabismus,* for additional discussion of ataxia-telangiectasia.

Lymphangiectasia appears in the eye as irregularly dilated lymphatic channels in the bulbar conjunctiva. It may be a developmental anomaly, or it can occur following trauma or inflammation. Anomalous communication with a venule can lead to spontaneous filling of the lymphatic vessels with blood.

Lymphatic malformation (previously called lymphangioma) is the term applied when the collection of anomalous lymphatic channels has a formed rather than an amorphous appearance. Involvement can be solitary or multifocal. Often, there is a deeper orbital component that can result in pain, proptosis, motility problems, and vision loss. Like a capillary hemangioma, a lymphatic malformation is usually present at birth and may enlarge slowly. Intralesional hemorrhage can produce a "chocolate cyst."

Jakobiec FA, Werdich XQ, Chodosh J, Freitag SK. An analysis of conjunctival and periocular venous malformations: clinicopathologic and immunohistochemical features with a comparison of racemose and cirsoid lesions. *Surv Ophthalmol.* 2014;59(2):236–244.

Nassiri N, Rootman J, Rootman DB, Goldberg RA. Orbital lymphaticovenous malformations: current and future treatments. *Surv Ophthalmol.* 2015;60(5):383–405.

Inflammatory vascular tumors

Vascular proliferation is often present in inflammatory conjunctival lesions. *Pyogenic granuloma,* a common type of reactive hemangioma, is misnamed because it is not suppurative and does not contain giant cells. The lesion may occur over a chalazion or when minor trauma or surgery stimulates exuberant healing tissue with fibroblasts (granulation tissue) and proliferating capillaries that grow in a radiating pattern. This rapidly growing lesion is red, pedunculated, and smooth (Fig 14-15); it bleeds easily and stains with fluorescein dye.

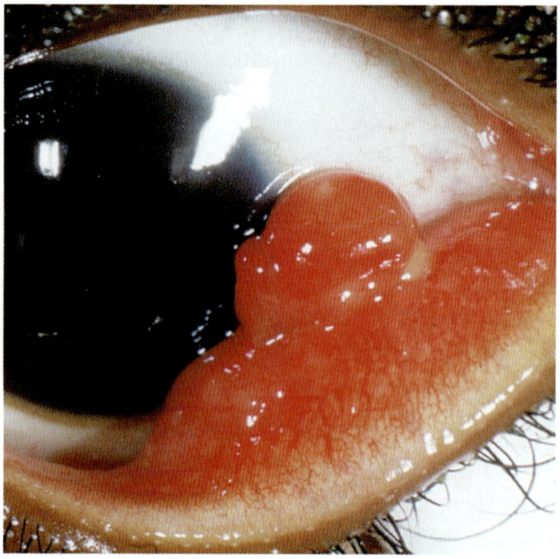

Figure 14-15 Pyogenic granuloma (in association with a chronically inflamed chalazion). *(Reproduced with permission from Mannis MJ, Holland EJ, eds.* Cornea. *Vol 1. 4th ed. Elsevier; 2017:326.)*

Topical or intralesional corticosteroids may be curative. Excision with cauterization to the base and generous postoperative topical corticosteroids may minimize recurrences.

Subconjunctival granulomas may form around parasitic and mycotic infectious foci. They have also occurred with connective tissue diseases such as rheumatoid arthritis. Sarcoid nodules appear as tan-yellow elevations that can resemble follicles. *Juvenile xanthogranuloma* is a histiocytic disorder that can present as a conjunctival mass. A *fibrous histiocytoma,* composed of fibroblasts and histiocytes with lipid vacuoles, arises, in rare cases, on the conjunctiva or limbus. *Nodular fasciitis* is a very rare benign tumor of fibrovascular tissue in the eyelid or under the conjunctiva; it may originate at the insertion site of a rectus muscle.

Malignant Tumors

Kaposi sarcoma

Kaposi sarcoma, a malignant neoplasm of vascular endothelium, involves the skin and mucous membranes. Internal organs are occasionally involved as well. Kaposi sarcoma–associated herpesvirus (human herpesvirus 8) is known to cause this disease. In young patients, Kaposi sarcoma occurs most often in patients with AIDS. Organ-transplant recipients and other highly immunosuppressed patients are at higher risk of developing Kaposi sarcoma.

CLINICAL PRESENTATION On the eyelid skin, Kaposi sarcoma presents as a purplish nodule. Orbital involvement may produce eyelid and conjunctival edema. In the conjunctiva, Kaposi sarcoma presents as a reddish, highly vascular subconjunctival lesion that may simulate a subconjunctival hemorrhage. The lesions are most often found in the inferior fornix and may be nodular or diffuse (Fig 14-16). Nodular lesions may be relatively less responsive to therapy than diffuse lesions.

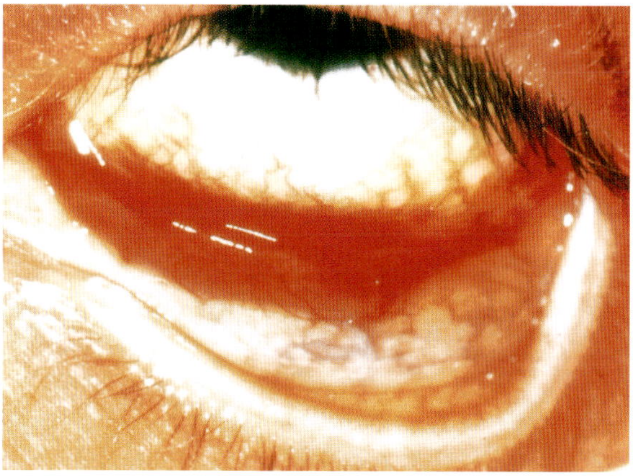

Figure 14-16 Kaposi sarcoma of the conjunctiva. *(Reproduced with permission from Holland GN, Pepose JS, Pettit TH, Gottlieb MS, Yee RD, Foos RY. Acquired immune deficiency syndrome. Ocular manifestations.* Ophthalmology. *1983;90(8):859–873. Photograph courtesy of Gary N. Holland, MD.)*

MANAGEMENT Treatment may not be curative. In addition to optimization of HAART (highly active antiretroviral therapy), options for controlling symptoms include surgical debulking, cryotherapy, and radiotherapy. Local or systemic chemotherapy may be required. Intralesional INF-α_{2a} (rather than INF-α_{2b}) has been reported to be effective.

Other malignant tumors

Malignant mesenchymal lesions that infrequently involve the conjunctiva include malignant fibrous histiocytoma, liposarcoma, leiomyosarcoma, and rhabdomyosarcoma.

Lymphocytic Tumors

Lymphoid tumors of the conjunctiva may be benign, malignant, or indeterminate. Many of these lesions have overlapping clinical and pathologic features. Approximately 20% of patients with a conjunctival lymphoid tumor have detectable extraocular lymphoma.

Lymphoid Hyperplasia

Formerly called *reactive lymphoid hyperplasia,* this benign-appearing accumulation of lymphocytes and other leukocytes may represent a low-grade B-cell lymphoma.

CLINICAL PRESENTATION Lymphoid hyperplasia presents as a minimally elevated, salmon-colored subepithelial tumor that usually has a smooth surface but may have a pebbly appearance corresponding to follicle formation (Fig 14-17). The lesion is often moderately or highly vascularized. Lymphoid hyperplasia is clinically indistinguishable from conjunctival lymphoma and requires biopsy to differentiate. Lymphoid hyperplasia may have a similar appearance to primary localized amyloidosis (discussed in Chapter 10). Most patients with lymphoid hyperplasia are older than 40 years, although it occurs in children in rare instances.

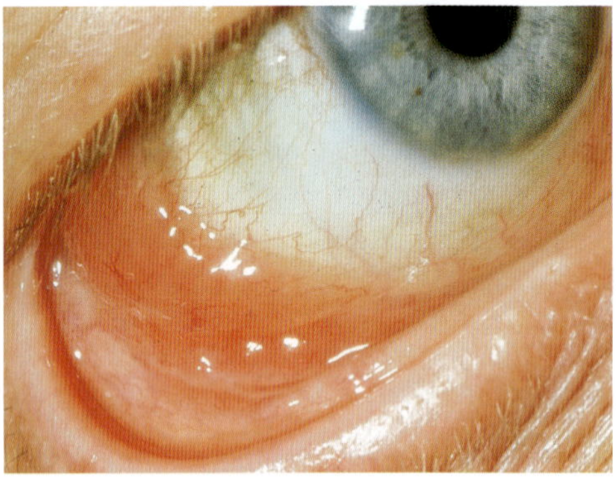

Figure 14-17 Conjunctival lymphoid hyperplasia.

MANAGEMENT Lymphoid hyperplasia may resolve spontaneously, but these lesions can be treated with local excision, topical corticosteroids, or radiation. Biopsy specimens require special handling to complete many of the histochemical and immunologic studies. Fresh tissue is required for immunohistochemistry, flow cytometry, and gene rearrangement studies. Because systemic lymphoma could potentially develop in a patient with an apparently benign polyclonal lymphoid lesion, general medical consultation is advisable.

Lymphoma

Conjunctival lymphoma usually occurs in immunosuppressed individuals or in persons older than 50 years. Some conjunctival lymphomas are limited to the conjunctiva; others occur in conjunction with systemic malignant lymphoma. Patients with Sjögren syndrome are at increased risk of developing lymphoma (see Chapter 3).

Histopathology is required to differentiate conjunctival lymphoma from benign lymphoid hyperplasia. Conjunctival lymphoma predominately occurs as a B-cell non-Hodgkin lymphoma with 1 of the following 4 subtypes, which are major predictors for outcome:

- *extranodal marginal zone lymphoma* (68%): 5-year survival rate 97% (Note: previously known as mucosa-associated lymphoid tissue [MALT] lymphoma)
- *follicular lymphoma* (16%): 5-year survival rate 82%
- *diffuse large B-cell lymphoma* (5%): 5-year survival rate 55%
- *mantle cell lymphoma* (7%): 5-year survival rate 9%

Conjunctival Hodgkin lymphoma and T-cell lymphoma are less common.

Kirkegaard MM, Rasmussen PK, Coupland SE, et al. Conjunctival lymphoma—an international multicenter retrospective study. *JAMA Ophthalmol.* 2016;134(4):406–414.

CLINICAL PRESENTATION Conjunctival lymphoma has essentially the same clinical appearance as benign lymphoid hyperplasia. It appears as a mobile, salmon-pink mass on the conjunctiva (Fig 14-18). It is typically unilateral; 20% of patients have bilateral lesions. Conjunctival lymphoma can also masquerade as a chronic follicular conjunctivitis (Fig 14-19). An epibulbar mass fixed to the underlying sclera may be a sign of extrascleral extension of uveal lymphoid neoplasia.

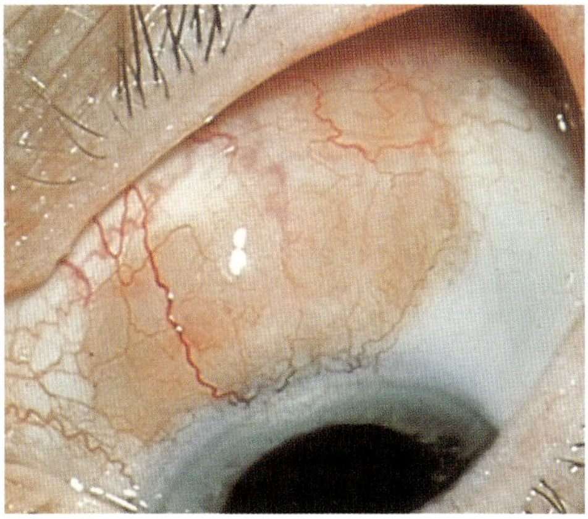

Figure 14-18 Conjunctival lymphoma.

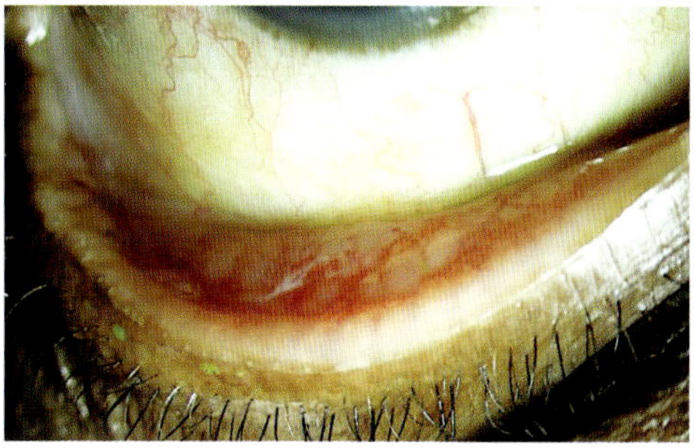

Figure 14-19 Follicular conjunctival lymphoma. *(Courtesy of Natalie C. Chueng, MD.)*

MANAGEMENT Patients with conjunctival lymphoma should be referred to an oncologist for systemic evaluation because underlying systemic lymphoma may be present or may eventually develop in up to 31% of these patients. Unless a tumor is small enough to be removed completely, incisional biopsy is indicated for histologic diagnosis. Local low-dose or ultra-low-dose external-beam radiation therapy is often curative for lesions confined to the conjunctiva; intralesional INF-α_{2b} or rituximab may also be effective. Intravenous rituximab is increasingly being administered for both local and systemic disease. Systemic chemotherapy is required for the treatment of systemic lymphoma.

Blasi MA, Tiberti AC, Valente P, et al. Intralesional interferon-α for conjunctival mucosa-associated lymphoid tissue lymphoma: long-term results. *Ophthalmology.* 2012;119(3): 494–500.

Pinnix CC, Dabaja BS, Milgrom SA, et al. Ultra-low-dose radiotherapy for definitive management of ocular adnexal B-cell lymphoma. *Head Neck.* 2017;39(6):1095–1100.

Raderer M, Kiesewetter B, Ferreri AJ. Clinicopathologic characteristics and treatment of marginal zone lymphoma of mucosa-associated lymphoid tissue (MALT lymphoma). *CA Cancer J Clin.* 2016;66(2):153–171.

Shields CL, Shields JA, Carvalho C, Rundle P, Smith AF. Conjunctival lymphoid tumors: clinical analysis of 117 cases and relationship to systemic lymphoma. *Ophthalmology.* 2001;108(5):979–984.

Tanenbaum RE, Galor A, Dubovy SR, Karp CL. Classification, diagnosis, and management of conjunctival lymphoma. *Eye Vis (Lond).* 2019;6:22.

Metastatic Tumors

Metastatic tumors to the conjunctiva are much less common than those to the uveal tract and orbit, but such tumors have arisen from cancer of the breast, lung, kidney, and elsewhere, including cutaneous melanoma. Metastatic lesions to the uveal tract, orbit, or paranasal sinuses can extend into the conjunctiva. Metastases or leukemic infiltrates to the limbus or cornea also occur.

CHAPTER 15

Clinical Aspects of Toxic and Traumatic Injuries of the Anterior Segment

This chapter includes related videos. Go to www.aao.org/bcscvideo_section08 or scan the QR codes in the text to access this content.

Indicates selected key points within the chapter.

Highlights

- Chemical solutions, especially strong alkaline substances, should be irrigated from the eye as soon as possible.
- Surgical repair of iridodialysis should be attempted as soon as possible to minimize corectopia from permanent contracture of the radial iris fibers.
- Blood in the anterior chamber, elevated intraocular pressure, and corneal endothelial damage increase the risk of corneal blood staining.
- Prolapsed uveal tissue following penetrating ocular injuries is usually reposited rather than resected, unless it is grossly necrotic or contaminated.
- Children at risk of amblyopia should undergo patching of the uninjured eye as soon as possible.

Chemical Injuries

Chemical injuries to the external eye can range in severity from mild irritation to complete destruction of the ocular surface and adnexa (eyelids), resulting in corneal opacification, loss of vision, and even loss of the eye. Chemical injuries may occur in the home or workplace. Some of the most severe ocular chemical injuries are caused by strong alkalis or acids used in assault. Table 15-1 lists some common caustic chemicals that can cause ocular injury.

Whenever possible, the offending chemical agent should be identified. The severity of a chemical injury depends on the pH (acid or alkali), volume, concentration, duration of contact, and inherent toxicity of the chemical. Frequently, the container of the toxic agent offers instructions for treatment or a phone number to call for detailed assistance (Video 15-1).

Table 15-1 Common Alkalis and Acids That Cause Eye Injuries

Substance	Compound	pH[a]	Use
Alkali	Ammonia	11.60	General-purpose cleaner, fertilizer, refrigerant
	Potassium hydroxide	10.98	Caustic potash
	Sodium hydroxide: lye, caustic soda	10.98	Drain cleaner, agent in air bag reaction
	Calcium hydroxide: lime	11.27	Plaster, mortar, cement, whitewash
	Magnesium hydroxide	10.40	Fireworks
Acid	Sulfuric acid	2.75	Car battery
	Hydrofluoric acid	3.27	Glass polisher, mineral refiner
	Acetic acid	3.91	Vinegar, glacial acetic acid
	Hydrochloric acid	3.01	Control of pH in swimming pools, pickling (removal of impurities) of steel

[a] pH in 1.0 M aqueous.

VIDEO 15-1 Chemical injuries.
Courtesy of James Chodosh, MD, MPH.

Alkali Burns

The most severe chemical injuries occur after contact with alkaline (high-pH) solutions because they cause saponification of fatty acids in cell membranes and ultimately cellular disruption. Once the surface epithelium is damaged, alkaline solutions readily penetrate the corneal stroma, where they rapidly destroy the proteoglycan ground substance and collagen fibers of the stromal matrix. Strong alkaline substances may also penetrate through the endothelium into the anterior chamber, causing severe tissue damage and intense inflammation. The vision prognosis is often determined by the extent of ocular surface injury and the effect of skin burns on eyelid function.

Classification and grading schemes for chemical injuries help characterize the severity of the injury. The Hughes classification scheme (modified by Thoft) divides chemical injuries of the cornea into 4 categories (Table 15-2) on the basis of clinical findings. The scheme shown in Table 15-3 establishes the grade of injury based on clinical signs, symptoms, and expected outcomes.

The poorest vision prognosis occurs in patients with extensive limbal epithelial damage. The limbus contains corneal epithelial stem cells (see Chapters 1 and 4); damage to this region can cause disruption in the cells repopulating the corneal epithelium. Blanching occurs when the vascular supply to this critical area is disrupted by death of vascular endothelial cells in the conjunctiva. The resultant limbal and anterior segment ischemia is a poor prognostic feature (Figs 15-1 through 15-4). If the conjunctiva recovers, vascularization may occur (Fig 15-5). Severe trauma leads to repopulation of the corneal surface epithelium with

Table 15-2 Prognostic Features of Chemical Injury of the Eye

Grade of Injury	Clinical Findings	Prognosis
Grade I	Corneal epithelial defect No corneal haze No loss of limbal stem cells	Excellent
Grade II (see Fig 15-1)	Cornea mildly hazy Focal limbal ischemia	Generally good; may have focal vascularization of cornea in area of limbal stem cell loss
Grade III (see Fig 15-2)	Severe corneal haze limits view of anterior segment structures Extensive limbal ischemia with loss of most limbal stem cells	Guarded; cornea must be repopulated with conjunctiva; surgery needed for vision rehabilitation
Grade IV (see Fig 15-3)	Complete loss of corneal and proximal conjunctival epithelium Cornea opaque Complete limbal ischemia and loss of all limbal stem cells	Extremely poor; melting likely; globe salvage may not be possible

Modified from Colby KA. Chemical injuries of the cornea. *Focal Points: Clinical Modules for Ophthalmologists.* American Academy of Ophthalmology; 2010, module 1.

undifferentiated conjunctival cells, which leads to reduced epithelial adhesion, recurrent breakdown, and chronic inflammation. Intraocular chemical penetration may result in cataract formation and secondary glaucoma; the latter is thought to result from damage to the trabecular meshwork, which can affect outflow facility.

Patients with severe alkali burns are fortunate if the conjunctival and corneal surface vascularize and stabilize. Patients with alkali burns may not be candidates for penetrating keratoplasty because the loss of surface goblet cells impairs graft survival. Limbal stem cell transplantation with subsequent keratoplasty or keratoprosthesis may be options. In the most severe cases, phthisis may occur. The absence of vascularization may lead to stromal melting, threatening globe integrity, which may lead to enucleation.

Bagley DM, Casterton PL, Dressler WE, et al. Proposed new classification scheme for chemical injury to the human eye. *Regul Toxicol Pharmacol.* 2006;45(2):206–213.

Colby KA. Chemical injuries of the cornea. *Focal Points: Clinical Modules for Ophthalmologists.* American Academy of Ophthalmology; 2010, module 1.

Acid Burns

Acid solutions with low pH tend to cause less-severe tissue damage than do alkaline solutions because acids denature and precipitate proteins in the tissues they contact, forming a barrier to penetration. Mild acid burns can cause an epithelial defect (Fig 15-6). Acid burns can severely damage the ocular surface, but in contrast to alkali burns, there is a lower chance of corneal melting or penetration of the solution into the anterior chamber. The exception to diminished penetration is a hydrofluoric acid burn, which can cause significant anterior segment destruction.

Table 15-3 Classification Scheme for Chemical Injury to the Human Eye Based on Clinical Findings

	Class 0						
	a	b	c	Class I	Class II	Class III	Class IV
Criteria to Be Used in Grading Clinical Cases							
Symptoms	Possible pain, excess tearing		Pain, excess tearing, foreign-body sensation; possible glare, photophobia, blurred vision	Symptoms include pain and loss of visual acuity (ranging from blurred vision and glare on the low end through complete loss of vision on the high end)			
Limbal blood vessel ischemia (circumference affected, %)	No ischemia; no injection present	No ischemia; injection may be present	No ischemia; injection present	<25%	25%–50%	50%–75%	70%–100%
Corneal epithelium	Appears normal		Punctate damage (expected to clear within 24 hours)	<33% loss in a geographic or punctate pattern	>33% to completely destroyed	Destroyed	
Corneal stroma	Details of iris clearly visible				Opacity causes blurriness of iris details	Pupil is discernible despite opacity	Unable to discern pupil; complete opacity
Depth of corneal injury	Corneal epithelium				<⅓, including epithelium and anterior stroma	>⅓, including epithelium and stroma	Entire cornea damaged

Corneal endothelial cell loss (% of total)	None		0%–10%	10%–60%	>40%	100%
Expected outcome	No consequence		Recovery of full vision	Recovery, but possibly with some degree of vision impairment	Loss of sight in the eye possible without extensive medical intervention	Loss of globe possible without extensive medical intervention
Prevention: Possible Approaches						
First aid labels	None	Wash/irrigate eye for 2–5 minutes; see an ophthalmologist if symptoms persist for 24 hours[a]	Wash/irrigate eye for 15–30 minutes; see an ophthalmologist immediately thereafter			
Packaging			Childproof closure		Safety packaging	

[a] For alkali-containing materials, irrigate for 15–30 minutes and see an ophthalmologist.

Modified with permission from Bagley DM, Casterton PL, Dressler WE, et al. Proposed new classification scheme for chemical injury to the human eye. *Regul Toxicol Pharmacol.* 2006;45(2):206–213.

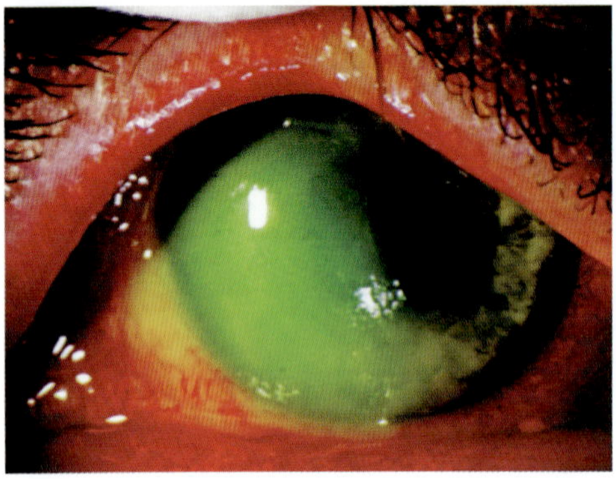

Figure 15-1 Grade II alkali burn, with inferior scleral ischemia (see Table 15-2). *(Courtesy of James J. Reidy, MD.)*

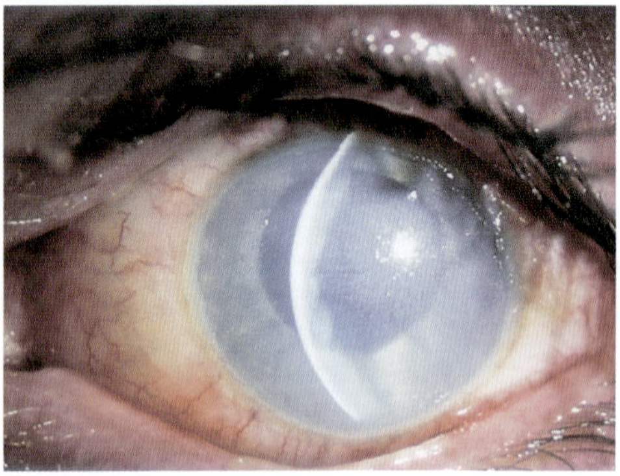

Figure 15-2 Grade III alkali burn with corneal edema and haze (see Table 15-2).

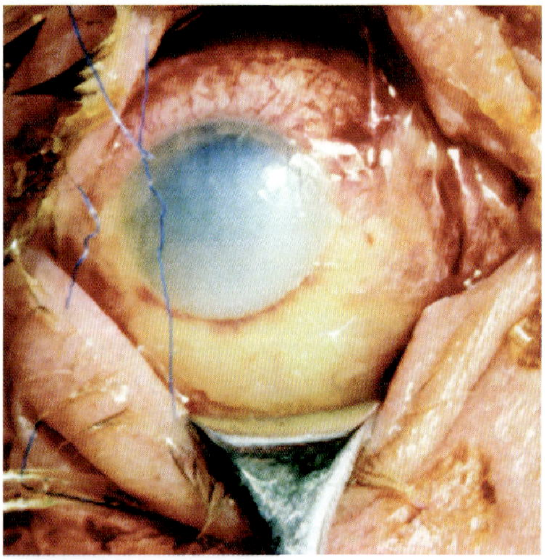

Figure 15-3 Grade IV alkali burn with corneal epithelial loss and stromal necrosis (see Table 15-2). The blue polypropylene sutures are holding the amniotic membrane in place over the cornea and eyelid margin. *(Courtesy of James J. Reidy, MD.)*

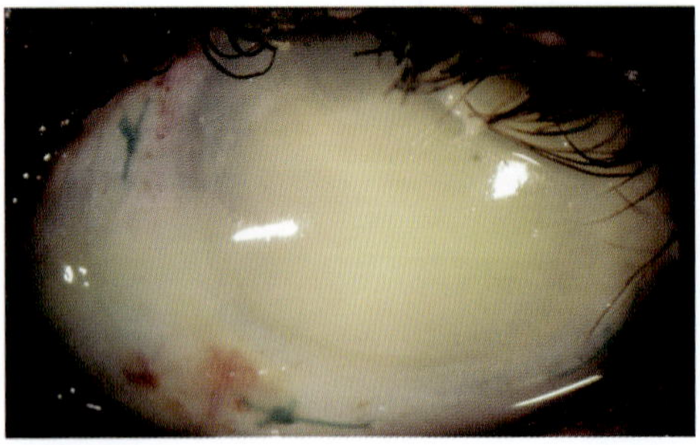

Figure 15-4 Severe alkali burn with opaque cornea and total limbal blanching. Sutures have secured an amniotic tissue graft over the cornea. *(Courtesy of Woodford S. Van Meter, MD.)*

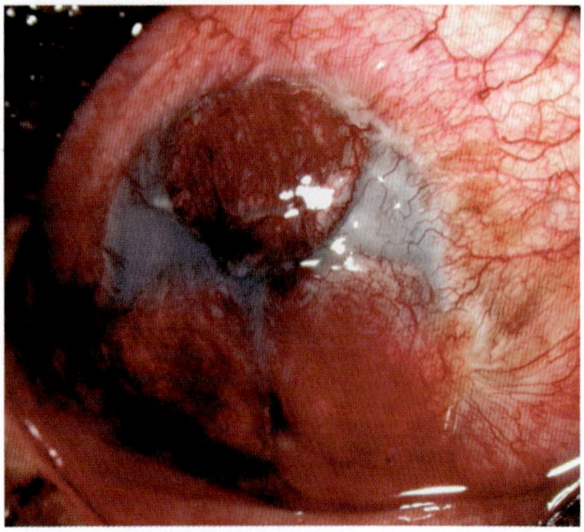

Figure 15-5 Intense corneal neovascularization following severe alkali burn. *(Courtesy of Woodford S. Van Meter, MD.)*

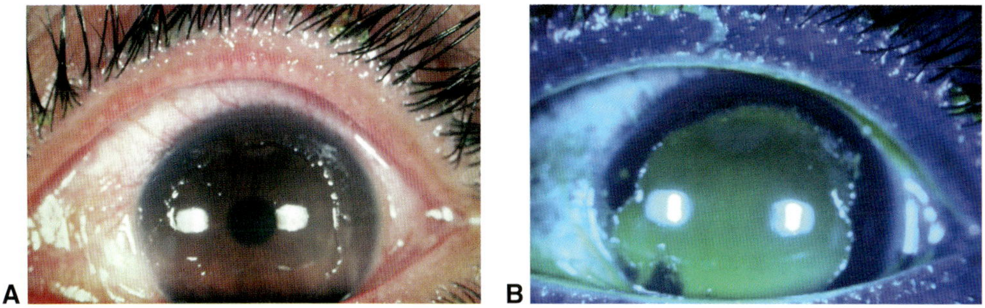

Figure 15-6 Epithelial defect from acid burn. **A,** Mild acid burn with central corneal epithelial defect. **B,** Fluorescein staining highlights the epithelial defect. *(Courtesy of Woodford S. Van Meter, MD.)*

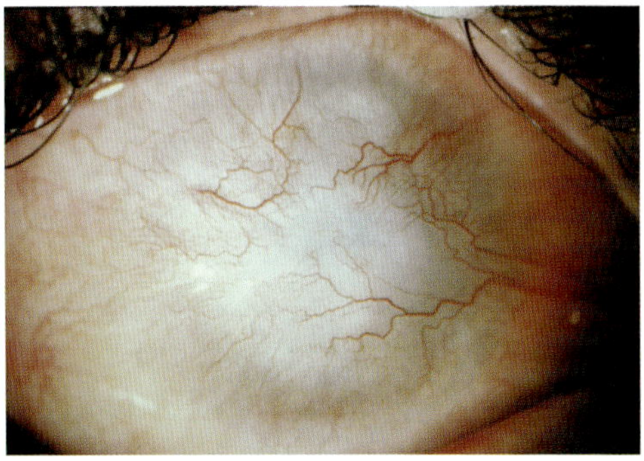

Figure 15-7 Corneal keratinization and opacification following a severe acid burn. *(Courtesy of Woodford S. Van Meter, MD.)*

Acid burns do not directly cause loss of the proteoglycan ground substance in the cornea, but they can incite severe inflammation and damage to the corneal matrix and result in corneal opacification (Fig 15-7) or symblepharon formation (Fig 15-8).

Management

Immediate, copious irrigation of the ocular surface with water or balanced saline solution is the most important step in the management of chemical injuries. If these liquids are not available, the clinician may use any other pure, nontoxic solution to rinse the ocular surface and dilute the offending agent. Buffer solutions may also be considered after initial irrigation. Alkali burns are true emergencies, and irrigation should be initiated at the site of the chemical injury and continued until an ophthalmologist evaluates the patient.

Irrigation The eyelid can be opened with a retractor or eyelid speculum, followed by instillation of topical anesthetic. Irrigation may be accomplished using handheld intravenous tubing; an irrigating eyelid speculum; or a Morgan lens, a special scleral contact lens that connects to intravenous tubing. Irrigation should continue until the pH of the conjunctival sac normalizes (pH 7.0–7.3). The conjunctival pH can be checked with a urinary pH strip. If this strip is not available, it is better to overtreat with prolonged periods of irrigation than to assume that the pH has normalized and discontinue treatment too early.

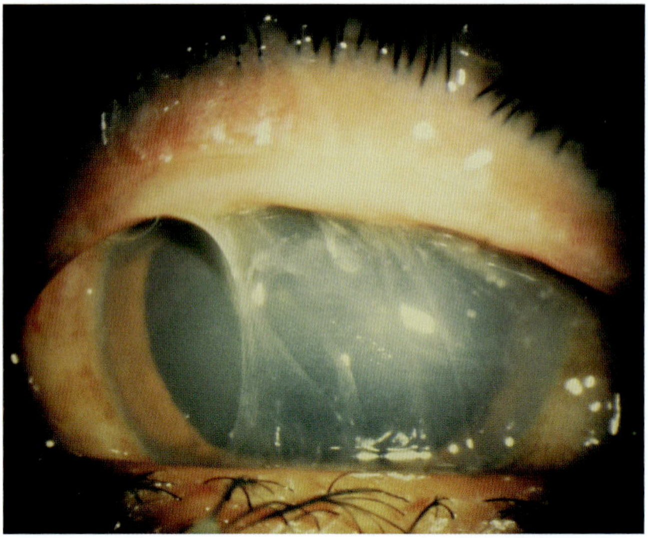

Figure 15-8 Symblepharon formation after a moderately severe acid burn. *(Courtesy of Woodford S. Van Meter, MD.)*

Removal of particulates Particulate chemicals are removed from the ocular surface with cotton-tipped applicators and/or forceps, as prolonged exposure to toxic particles can exacerbate chemical damage to the ocular surface. The upper eyelid is everted in order to search for material in the upper fornix (Fig 15-9), and the fornices are swept with an applicator to ensure that no particulate matter remains in the eye. Debridement of the necrotic corneal epithelium minimizes the release of inflammatory mediators from damaged epithelial cells and to promote reepithelialization.

Medications Use of topical cycloplegics is recommended and may be continued for patients experiencing discomfort or significant anterior chamber reaction. In the early stage of a chemical injury, intraocular pressure (IOP) may increase; IOP can be controlled by use of oral carbonic anhydrase inhibitors in order to avoid toxicity from topical glaucoma medications. However, if the corneal epithelium is healing normally, topical therapies may be used as well. See BCSC Section 10, *Glaucoma,* for a detailed discussion of medications used to control IOP.

Management in the intermediate period (ie, over the next week or more) aims to decrease inflammation, monitor IOP, limit matrix degradation, and promote reepithelialization of the cornea. An intense polymorphonucleocyte (PMN) infiltration of the corneal stroma can occur following acute alkali burns. PMNs deliver proteolytic enzymes that, in the absence of an intact epithelium, dissolve corneal stromal collagen and ground substance. Corticosteroids are excellent inhibitors of PMN function, and intensive treatment with a topical corticosteroid is recommended for up to 10–14 days following a chemical injury. Thereafter, the frequency of the corticosteroid drops is markedly reduced to prevent inhibition of wound healing and exacerbation of stromal melting. Corticosteroids retard epithelial wound healing and increase the risk of secondary infection by inhibiting

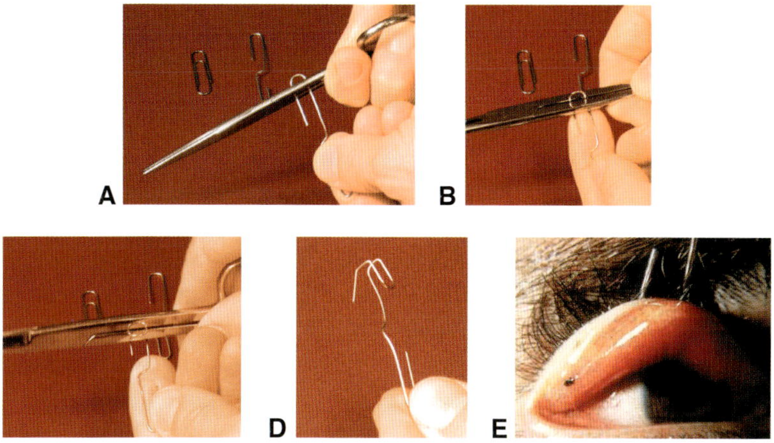

Figure 15-9 Fashioning an eyelid retractor from a paper clip. **A,** Bend the paper clip open. **B,** Grasp distal end of clip, leaving at least 1 cm for blade of retractor. **C,** Create the bend, ensuring bend leaves retractor thick enough to fit lid; bend sharp end of clip away from blunt end. **D,** Use retractor in same fashion as a Desmarres retractor. **E,** Use of the retractor for double eversion reveals a foreign body on the upper eyelid. *(Courtesy of John E. Sutphin, MD.)*

normal ocular surface immune defense mechanisms, so the associated risks in the chronic phase may exceed the benefits.

Oral tetracyclines and topical sodium citrate 10% can chelate extracellular calcium, which can inhibit PMN degranulation. In theory, this process can help inhibit PMN-induced collagenolysis. Topical medroxyprogesterone 1% may also be effective in suppressing collagen breakdown. Measures that promote wound healing and inhibit collagenolytic activity prevent stromal ulceration.

Systemic administration of ascorbic acid to rabbits with acute corneal alkaline injuries has been shown to restore the level of aqueous humor ascorbate to normal and significantly reduce the incidence of ulceration. High-dose ascorbic acid is believed to promote collagen synthesis in an alkali-burned eye, given that ascorbic acid is required as a cofactor for collagen synthesis. Some studies recommend that patients take 1–2 g of vitamin C per day. Because this therapy is potentially toxic to the kidneys, ascorbic acid generally is not administered to patients with compromised renal function.

Frequent use of nonpreserved topical lubricants helps facilitate epithelial healing in the intermediate and chronic stages of chemical injury.

Brodovsky SC, McCarty CA, Snibson G, et al. Management of alkali burns: an 11-year retrospective review. *Ophthalmology.* 2000;107(10):1829–1835.

Bandage contact lenses and surgical procedures A bandage contact lens or amniotic membrane graft or ring may help protect ocular surface epithelium once migration onto the peripheral cornea has begun. Acute conjunctival swelling and inflammation or late symblepharon formation may prevent retention of the contact lens. Amniotic membrane may be helpful in suppressing inflammation, promoting reepithelialization, and preventing symblepharon formation; this option can be considered 1–2 weeks after injury. A temporary or permanent tarsorrhaphy facilitates reepithelialization due to increased corneal coverage. Avascular sclera usually does not epithelialize until revascularization occurs. If scleral melting occurs, a rotational graft of tarsoconjunctival tissue from the adjacent eyelid can be performed to promote revascularization.

Autologous conjunctival or limbal stem cell transplantation using tissue from the patient's uninjured eye may facilitate healing of the corneal epithelial defect. Limbal stem cell transplantation may be performed after chemical injury when there are no signs of corneal epithelialization. However, the prognosis of limbal grafts is better when the eye is not inflamed; therefore, it is preferable to wait until the acute inflammation has subsided. A technique known as *simple limbal epithelial transplantation (SLET)* combines limbal stem cell transplantation with the use of amniotic membrane (see Chapter 5). If there is damage to the conjunctiva of both eyes, then either amniotic membrane alone or oral mucosal grafts may be necessary.

Cornea transplant prognosis in the long term is improved if the ocular surface inflammation has resolved either over time (months to years) or after limbal stem cell grafting (ocular surface reconstruction). Even when there is no active ocular surface inflammation, stromal vascularization in the host bed is associated with a much higher risk of rejection following keratoplasty. Keratoprosthesis is another surgical option, but again, the prognosis is best when the inflammation is under control.

Chan CC, Biber JM, Holland EJ. The modified Cincinnati procedure: combined conjunctival limbal autografts and keratolimbal allografts for severe unilateral ocular surface failure. *Cornea.* 2012;31(11):1264–1272.

Tejwani S, Kolari RS, Sangwan VS, Rao GN. Role of amniotic membrane graft for ocular chemical and thermal injuries. *Cornea.* 2007;26(1):21–26.

Vazirani J, Basu S, Sangwan V. Successful simple limbal epithelial transplantation (SLET) in lime injury–induced limbal stem cell deficiency with ocular surface granuloma. *BMJ Case Rep.* 2013;bcr2013009405.

Thermal and Radiation Injuries

Thermal Burns

Heat

Heat is a primary cause of inflammation and stromal protease expression and, if severe, can lead to collagen destruction. Rapid-reflex eyelid closure, Bell phenomenon, and reflex movement away from the source of intense heat usually limit damage to the globe from flames. Burns from molten metal that stays in contact with the eye are more likely to cause corneal injuries that result in permanent scarring.

Curling irons, cigarettes, and hot liquids splashing into the eye, especially during cooking, are common household causes of corneal burns (Fig 15-10). These burns are usually limited to the epithelium and generally require only a brief period of antibiotic and cycloplegic therapy; the patient should be followed closely for infection and traumatic anterior uveitis. Corneal wound burns related to cataract surgery are an iatrogenic cause of thermal

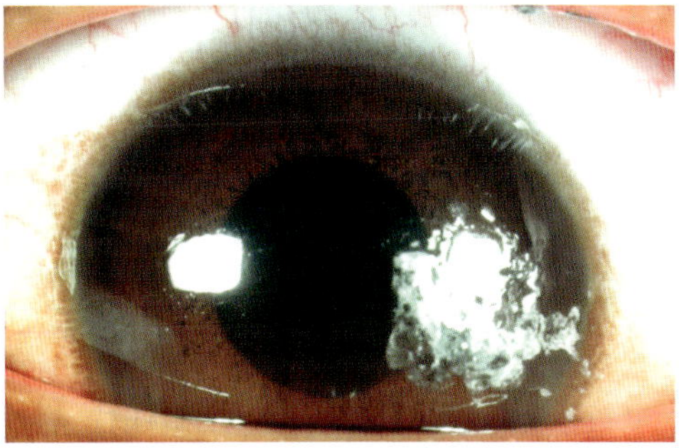

Figure 15-10 Cigarette burn on the cornea. *(Courtesy of Woodford S. Van Meter, MD.)*

injury that may lead to irregular astigmatism or difficulty obtaining a watertight wound after phacoemulsification.

The primary objectives of therapy for burns caused by heat are to

- relieve discomfort
- prevent secondary corneal inflammation, ulceration, and perforation from infection or from exposure caused by eyelid damage
- minimize eyelid scarring and resultant malfunction

A cycloplegic agent can help relieve discomfort from ciliary spasm or iridocyclitis. Use of prophylactic antibiotics (topical and/or systemic) can help prevent infection of burned eyelids and/or reduce the chances of infectious corneal ulceration. Limited debridement of devitalized tissues and granulation tissue, combined with full-thickness skin grafts and tarsorrhaphy, helps minimize eyelid scarring and ectropion. Burned ocular tissue can be temporarily protected by covering the eye with a lubricant and a piece of sterile plastic wrap. Amniotic membrane grafts can also be considered. Topical corticosteroids help suppress associated inflammation, but they can also inhibit corneal wound healing and increase the risk of infection. For this reason, they must be used with caution and, in general, for short periods.

Cold

Transient corneal stromal edema induced by cold has been reported in a variety of settings, including prolonged exposure to cold when skiing or mountain climbing. Cold temperatures adversely affect the pump function of the endothelial cells, rendering it less effective. Individuals with Raynaud disease and those with cranial nerve V dysfunction may be especially susceptible.

Ultraviolet Radiation

The corneal epithelium is susceptible to injury from natural and mechanically produced ultraviolet (UV) radiation. Common causes of UV-radiation injury to the eye are arc welding and unprotected exposure to sunlamps or tanning beds. Prolonged outdoor exposure to reflected sunlight, or *snow blindness,* occurs in skiers and mountain climbers at high elevations, where there is less atmospheric diffraction of UV radiation.

Patients with ocular UV-radiation injuries present with eyelid edema, conjunctival hyperemia, and diffuse punctate keratitis. Treatment options consist of

- patching to minimize discomfort from eyelid movement
- placement of a bandage contact lens
- placement of an amniotic membrane ring or graft
- topical antibiotic ointment or eyedrop therapy
- topical cycloplegia
- oral analgesics

Complete epithelial healing usually occurs within 24–72 hours. Appropriate protection with UV-blocking glasses can help protect the patient from such injuries. Medical use of UV light such as PUVA (psoralen and ultraviolet A) and corneal crosslinking in thin corneas can result in iatrogenic endothelial injury. (See Chapter 9, Appendix 9.2, Corneal Crosslinking for Corneal Ectasia.)

Ionizing Radiation

Exposure to ionizing radiation may occur with UV light, x-rays, gamma rays, medical imaging equipment, nuclear explosions, and radioisotopes. The level of exposure is related to the amount of energy in the ionizing radiation, the type of rays emitted, the duration of exposure, and the patient's proximity to the ionizing source. Tissue destruction may result from direct killing of cells, cellular DNA changes that produce lethal or other mutations, or radiation damage to blood vessels with secondary ischemic necrosis.

Ionizing radiation can damage the conjunctiva, cornea, and occasionally the lacrimal glands. Conjunctival edema occurs acutely, often followed by scarring, shrinkage, loss of tear production, and alterations in conjunctival blood vessels with telangiectasia. Necrosis of the conjunctiva and underlying sclera can occur if radioactive material (or a radiomimetic agent such as mitomycin C) is embedded in the conjunctiva. Punctate corneal epithelial erosions are noted acutely. Explosions involving ionizing radiation may lead to perforation of ocular tissues with immediate radiation necrosis.

The first step in management of acute radiation injury is the removal of all foreign bodies. Poor wound healing is a hallmark of ionizing radiation injuries. Late complications are related to decreased tear production, loss of corneal sensation, sloughing of corneal epithelial cells, and failure of the cornea to heal. Secondary microbial keratitis, vascularization, and ocular surface disease can result from dry eyes and compromised epithelial cells. In mild cases, ocular surface stabilization may occur with the use of artificial tears or a bandage contact lens.

In more severe cases the following options can be considered:

- tarsorrhaphy
- conjunctival flap from the affected eye
- autologous conjunctival flap from the fellow eye
- amniotic membrane transplant
- limbal stem cell transplant
- mucous membrane graft

The vision prognosis following penetrating keratoplasty or limbal stem cell transplantation in these patients is guarded because of the severely compromised ocular surface.

Injuries Caused by Animal and Plant Substances

Insect and Arachnid Injuries

Bee and wasp stings to the cornea and/or conjunctiva cause conjunctival hyperemia and chemosis acutely, sometimes associated with severe pain, corneal edema, stromal infiltration, and subsequent decreased vision. The significant variation in the acute response results from differences in the quantity of the venom injected and whether the reaction is primarily toxic or immunologic. In rare instances, other sequelae have been documented, including hyphema, lenticular opacities, anterior uveitis, secondary glaucoma, and heterochromia. Initial therapy with topical cycloplegics, topical (and occasionally systemic) corticosteroids, and topical antibiotics is beneficial. Removal of externalized stingers may be attempted. After the acute episode, retained stingers may remain inert in the cornea for years. Caterpillar and tarantula hairs *(urticating hairs)* may also become embedded in the cornea and conjunctiva. These hairs are very fine and usually cannot be removed manually. Because of their structure, these urticating hairs tend to migrate more deeply into ocular tissues and elicit a localized granulomatous inflammatory response *(ophthalmia nodosum)* (Fig 15-11). In these cases, the patient will have an extreme foreign-body sensation until the hairs migrate below the corneal surface. Inflammatory sequelae usually respond to topical corticosteroids.

Mangat SS, Newman B. Tarantula hair keratitis. *N Z Med J.* 2012;125(1364):107–110.

Shrum KR, Robertson DM, Baratz KH, Casperson TJ, Rostvold JA. Keratitis and retinitis secondary to tarantula hair. *Arch Ophthalmol.* 1999;117(8):1096–1097.

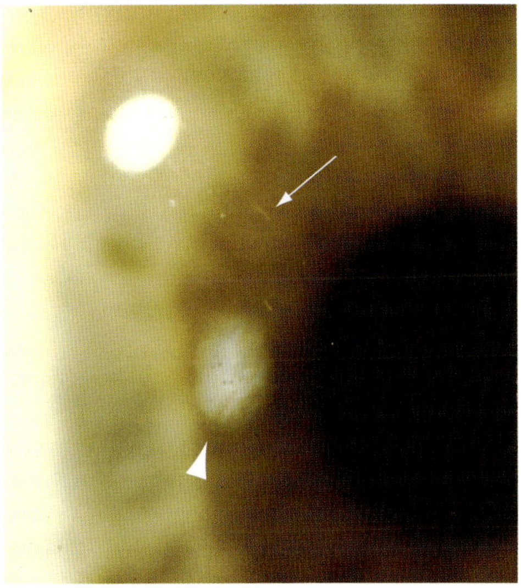

Figure 15-11 Tarantula hair keratitis. Note the stromal infiltrate *(arrowhead)* and tarantula hairs in the anterior stroma *(arrow)*. *(Courtesy of Steven P. Dunn, MD.)*

Plant Injuries

Milky sap (latex) from a variety of trees can cause toxic reactions manifested by acute keratoconjunctivitis, epithelial defects, and stromal infiltration. The pencil tree and the manchineel tree, widely found in tropical regions, are known offenders.

Calcium oxalate crystals released from crunching the leaves of houseplants in the genus *Dieffenbachia* can shoot into the cornea and cause keratoconjunctivitis. The crystals cause a foreign-body sensation and are difficult to see on slit-lamp examination. The diagnosis of *Dieffenbachia* keratitis is generally made based on the patient history. Corneal foreign bodies from coconut shell, sunflower stalk, and ornamental cactus have also been reported.

Initial management of injuries caused by all such plant materials includes

- irrigation and removal of foreign bodies when possible
- administration of topical cycloplegics
- prophylactic antibiotic coverage, as indicated by the clinical situation
- avoidance of corticosteroids

Corticosteroids are best avoided because they suppress immunity to microbes and may promote fungal infection, which poses a risk in all trauma cases involving vegetable matter. Surgical removal of vegetative foreign bodies should be attempted in order to mitigate the inflammatory response or associated secondary infection. If a patient with a severe injury from plant sources fails to improve after supportive therapy, the possibility of bacterial or fungal infection should be considered and an appropriate workup (including culture and/or biopsy) performed. For additional discussion of microbial keratitis, see Chapter 12.

Blunt Trauma

Subconjunctival Hemorrhage

A subconjunctival hemorrhage, blood beneath the conjunctiva, is heralded by an alarming bright red appearance against the adjacent white sclera (Fig 15-12). Patients with

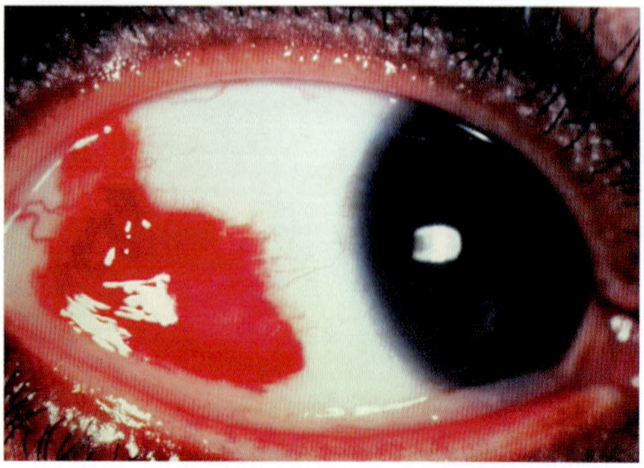

Figure 15-12 Subconjunctival hemorrhage shows prominently against white sclera. *(Courtesy of Woodford S. Van Meter, MD.)*

subconjunctival hemorrhage typically have no history of antecedent trauma. When associated with trauma, damage to deeper structures of the eye that risk globe integrity must be ruled out, particularly when there is extensive and raised hemorrhage. Subconjunctival hemorrhage is usually not associated with an underlying systemic disease and rarely has an identifiable cause. Occasionally, a history of vomiting, coughing, constipation, or other activities involving repeated Valsalva maneuver can be elicited. Patient medications should be reviewed for those associated with reduced clotting or inhibition of platelet function.

Typically, no therapy is necessary for the hemorrhage; it usually resolves in 7–12 days, and the patient simply requires reassurance that the condition is not serious. If the hemorrhage elevates the limbal conjunctiva significantly, dellen may occur. Patients should be warned that the hemorrhage can spread around the circumference of the globe before it resolves and that it may change in color from red to yellow during its dissolution.

Repeated episodes of spontaneous subconjunctival hemorrhage may indicate a possible bleeding diathesis, and a careful systemic medical evaluation may be warranted. Recurrent subconjunctival hemorrhages can be seen in association with uncontrolled hypertension; diabetes; systemic blood disorders; lymphangioma; amyloidosis; use of nonsteroidal anti-inflammatory drugs (NSAIDs); and use of antiplatelet (aspirin, clopidogrel), anticoagulant (heparin or warfarin), and thrombolytic (streptokinase) drugs.

Corneal Involvement

Blunt trauma to the cornea can result in abrasions, edema, tears in Descemet membrane (Fig 15-13; also see Chapter 6, Fig 6-11), and corneoscleral lacerations, usually located at the limbus or at the insertion of the extraocular muscles. Traumatic posterior annular keratopathy or corneal endothelial rings have also been described; these rings are whitish

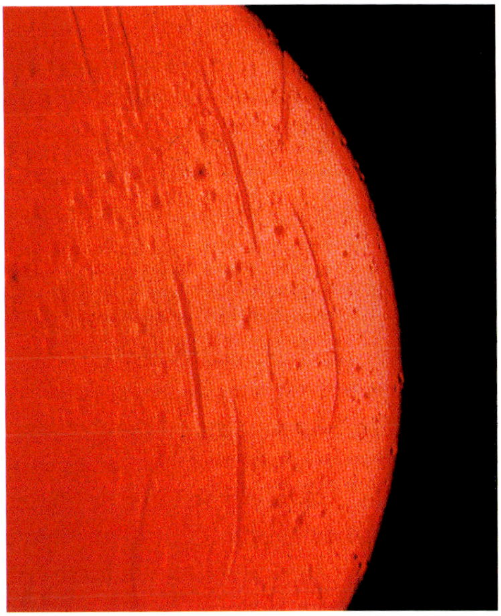

Figure 15-13 Tears in Descemet membrane due to blunt trauma from forceps delivery. *(Courtesy of Woodford S. Van Meter, MD.)*

gray and occur directly posterior to the traumatic impact. The endothelial rings appear within several hours of a contusive injury and usually disappear within a few days.

Corneal abrasion

Disruption of the corneal epithelium is usually associated with immediate pain, foreign-body sensation, tearing, and discomfort with blinking. A slit-lamp examination is essential in determining (1) the presence and extent of the erosion and (2) whether stromal loss is present. Fluorescein staining of the cornea can be helpful in determining the presence of an epithelial defect (see Chapter 2). A corneal abrasion has sharply defined edges and little to no associated inflammation (when seen acutely), in contrast to a corneal ulcer, which is characterized by opacification and breakdown of the stromal matrix with possible thinning. It is also important to rule out a foreign body as the cause of the abrasion. Associated traumatic stromal keratitis can cause symptoms of photophobia and reduced vision even after the abrasion has healed. Occasionally, a patient may not recall a definite history of trauma but still presents with signs and symptoms suggestive of a corneal abrasion. A patient with a corneal abrasion from a fingernail, piece of paper, or tree branch is more likely to develop recurrent erosions (see Chapter 4 for a discussion of recurrent corneal erosions). Herpes simplex virus keratitis should also be included in the differential diagnosis. A corneal abrasion associated with significant stromal edema may not stain as brightly with flourescein as expected.

MANAGEMENT Treatment for abrasion includes pressure patching, which can relieve pain from an abrasion by immobilizing the upper eyelid to prevent rubbing against the corneal defect. Patching is not necessary for most abrasions, and some patients may find patches and obstructed vision disturbing. It is important to ensure that the eye stays closed under the patch. Topical antibiotic ointment is commonly applied prior to patching.

Another alternative is a bandage contact lens, which provides pain relief, facilitates reepithelialization, and allows the patient to see. Antibiotic eyedrops rather than ointment are typically used with a bandage lens until the epithelium heals. Cycloplegics can help with associated ciliary spasm. It is important to choose an agent with an effect that does not exceed the expected duration of ciliary spasm. Topical NSAIDs may be used for pain relief in selected patients during the first 24–48 hours; however, these agents can potentially cause local toxicity and ulceration and delay wound healing. Oral analgesics within the first 24–48 hours can be helpful for many patients. Traumatic stromal keratitis responds well to a short course of topical corticosteroids.

Patients with abrasions caused by organic material require close follow-up to monitor for fungal infection. Abrasions caused by a fingernail or by vegetable matter such as paper, leaves, or thorns heal more slowly than abrasions caused by inorganic materials such as steel, glass, or plastic. A patch may increase the risk of infection in these cases. Topical corticosteroids are not appropriate in this situation.

Patients with contact lens–associated epithelial defects should not receive a patch or have a therapeutic contact lens applied due to the risk of promoting or worsening a corneal infection. These patients should be treated with topical antibiotic eyedrops or ointment and a topical cycloplegic agent selected for the appropriate duration of effect. Topical anesthetic drops (eg, tetracaine, proparacaine) should not be prescribed for patients with corneal abrasion because the use of such agents substantially increases the risk of complications, such as delayed epithelial healing and infection.

Traumatic Anterior Uveitis

The inflammation present in traumatic anterior uveitis is often associated with decreased vision and perilimbal conjunctival hyperemia. Photophobia, tearing, and ocular pain may occur within 24 hours of injury. The anterior chamber reaction can be surprisingly minimal, given the symptoms of pain and photophobia.

MANAGEMENT Treatment consists of a topical cycloplegic agent to relieve patient discomfort, as well as topical corticosteroid eyedrops if significant inflammation is present. Once the anterior uveitis has diminished, cycloplegia may be discontinued, and topical corticosteroids should be tapered slowly to prevent rebound anterior uveitis. See BCSC Section 9, *Uveitis and Ocular Inflammation,* for a more detailed discussion of uveitis.

Traumatic Mydriasis and Miosis

Traumatic mydriasis results from iris sphincter tears that can permanently dilate or otherwise alter the shape of the pupil (Fig 15-14). The iris tears may result in a hyphema. The pupil changes are generally permanent; patients are encouraged to use sunglasses for resultant photophobia. The clinician can consider surgical correction using an artificial iris if the defect is large or iris suture if it is smaller. Iris diaphragm contact lenses are also available.

Miosis tends to be associated with anterior chamber inflammation. Topical corticosteroid eyedrops to reduce inflammation and cycloplegia to prevent formation of posterior synechiae are helpful in controlling symptoms.

Arbisser LB, Miller KM. *Artificial Iris Implantation* [2019 American Academy of Ophthalmology Annual Meeting Video]. American Academy of Ophthalmology; 2019. Accessed November 13, 2021. www.aao.org/interview/artificial-iris-implantation

Masket, SM. *Using the HumanOptics Custom Artificial Iris.* Video Journal of Cataract & Refractive Surgery. American Academy of Ophthalmology; 2017. Accessed November 13, 2021. www.aao.org/clinical-video/using-humanoptics-custom-artificial-iris

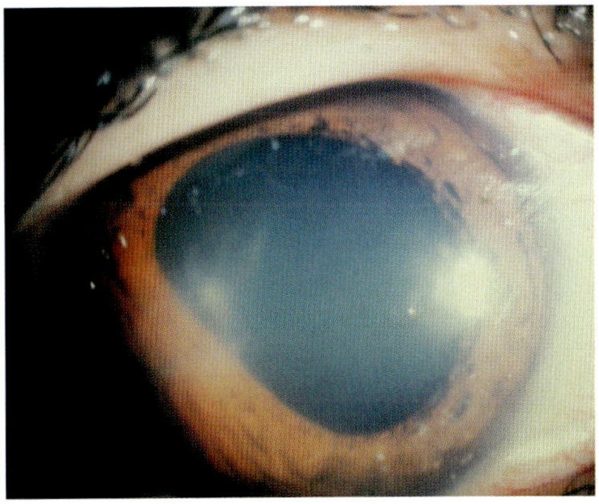

Figure 15-14 Traumatic mydriasis caused by tears in the iris sphincter muscle, resulting from blunt trauma. *(Courtesy of Woodford S. Van Meter, MD.)*

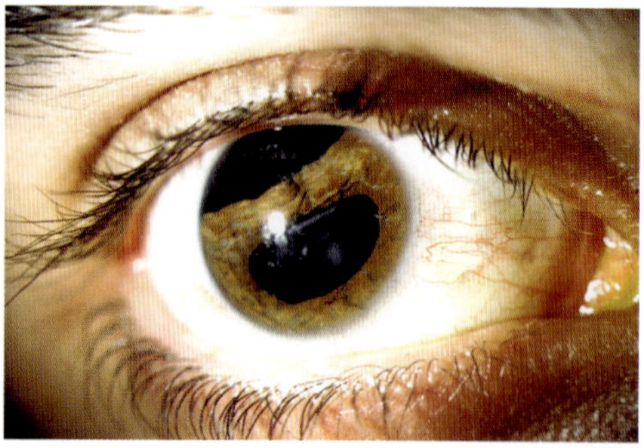

Figure 15-15 Severe iridodialysis resulting from blunt trauma. *(Courtesy of David Rootman, MD.)*

Iridodialysis and Cyclodialysis

Iridodialysis

Blunt trauma may cause iridodialysis, or traumatic separation of the iris root from the ciliary body (Fig 15-15). Anterior segment hemorrhage often ensues, and the iridodialysis may not be recognized until the hyphema has cleared. A small iridodialysis requires no treatment. A large iridodialysis may cause polycoria and monocular diplopia, requiring surgical repair (Figs 15-16, 15-17). If possible, the iridodialysis should be repaired within a few weeks of the injury, because prolonged contracture of the radial iris fibers may prevent a round pupil after normal iris anatomy is reestablished.

Cyclodialysis

Traumatic cyclodialysis is characterized by separation of the ciliary body from its attachment to the scleral spur, resulting in a cleft. A hyphema may result from the tearing of the tissue. On gonioscopic examination, this cleft appears as a gap at the posterior edge of the scleral spur from posterior displacement of the ciliary body band. Sclera may be visible through the gap. Ultrasound biomicroscopy can be useful in identifying the location and extent of the cyclodialysis (Fig 15-18). A cyclodialysis cleft can cause increased uveoscleral outflow, leading to chronic hypotony and macular edema. If treatment with topical cycloplegics does not suffice, closure may be attempted using laser therapy, diathermy, cryotherapy, or direct suturing. If repair is necessary, it should be performed after resolution of the hyphema.

Traumatic Hyphema

Traumatic hyphema usually occurs in young men; this demographic experiences more ocular trauma than any other. Trauma causes posterior displacement of the lens–iris interface with equatorial scleral expansion. The increase in equatorial diameter stretches the major iris arterial circle, arterial branches of the ciliary body, and/or recurrent choroidal arteries and veins. The hyphema results from injury to the vessels of the peripheral iris, iris sphincter, or anterior ciliary body (Fig 15-19). The extent of the bleeding may vary from a few circulating red blood cells observed on slit-lamp examination (microscopic hyphema; Fig 15-20) to a clot in the anterior chamber (layered hyphema; Fig 15-21) or to bleeding

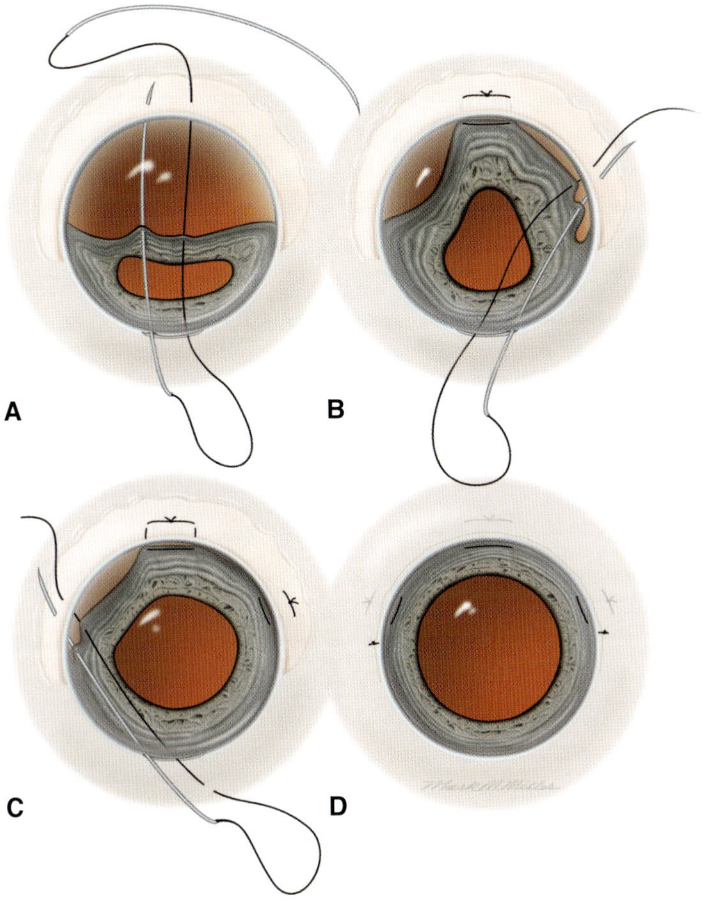

Figure 15-16 Repair of iridodialysis. **A,** A fornix-based conjunctival flap is made at the site of iridodialysis or iris disinsertion. A paracentesis is fashioned 180° from the center of the iris defect. A double-armed, 10-0 polypropylene suture on a CIF needle is passed through paracentesis and peripheral edge of the iris and out through the angle. The second needle is passed, similarly engaging the edge of the iris and exiting through the angle. **B,** The mattress suture is tied on the surface of the globe or alternatively under a partial-thickness scleral flap. The procedure is repeated to repair another section of the defect. **C,** The final portion of the defect is repaired. **D,** The knots can be buried in the sclera and the conjunctival flap is closed. *(Figure developed by Natalie Afshari, MD, and illustrated by Mark Miller.)*

so severe that it fills the anterior chamber completely. The prognosis for traumatic hyphema is generally good and is independent of the size of the hyphema, provided that no additional complications are present. Even *total,* or *eight-ball, hyphemas* (Fig 15-22) can resolve without sequelae. Traumatic hyphema is frequently associated with corneal abrasion, anterior uveitis, and mydriasis, as well as with injuries to the angle structures, lens, posterior segment, and orbit.

Spontaneous hyphema (ie, a hyphema that occurs without any history of trauma) is much less common and should alert the clinician to the possibility of rubeosis iridis

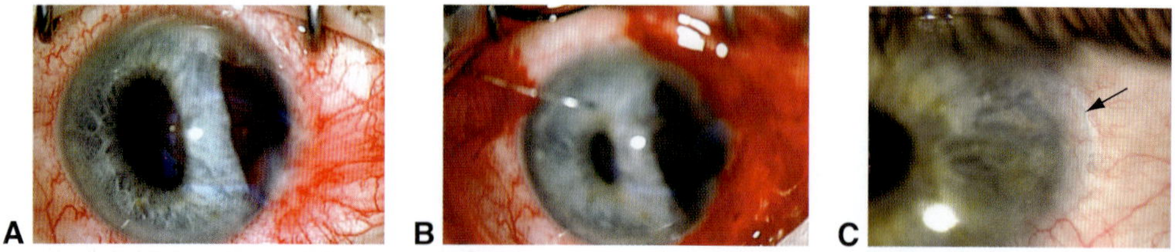

Figure 15-17 Repair of iridodialysis with polypropylene sutures. **A,** Traumatic iridodialysis. **B,** A needle is passed across the anterior chamber through the limbus opposite the dialysis for reattachment. **C,** Normal pupil following suturing of the iridodialysis. The *arrow* points to the polypropylene suture. *(Courtesy of Woodford S. Van Meter, MD.)*

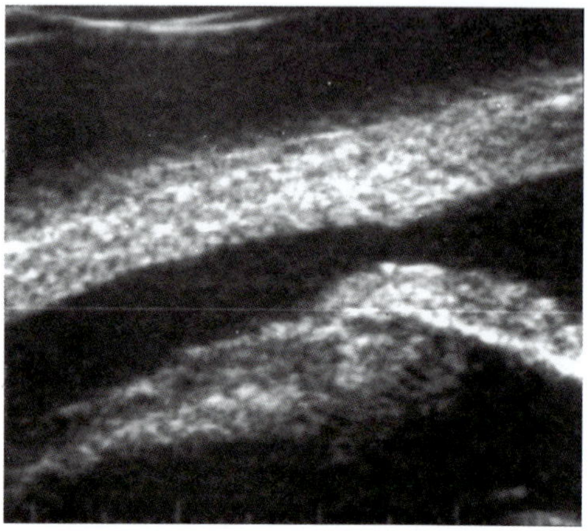

Figure 15-18 Ultrasound biomicroscopy of cyclodialysis. Note that the iris root and ciliary body are pulled away from the sclera. *(Courtesy of David Rootman, MD.)*

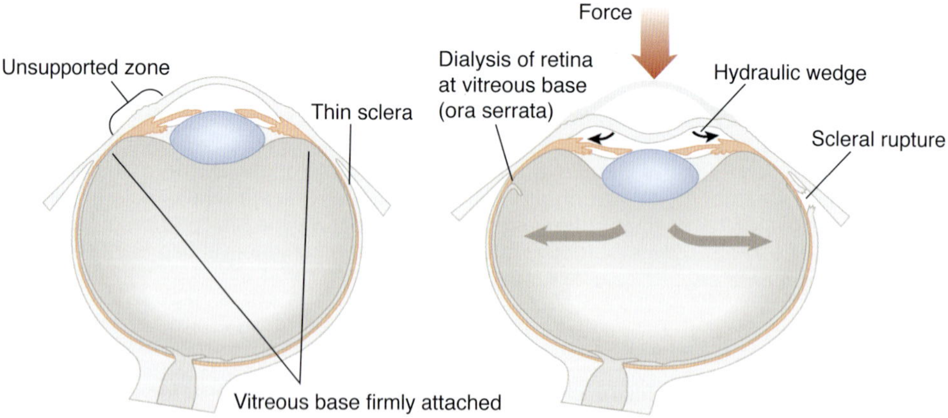

Figure 15-19 Mechanism of hyphema and blunt force injury to the eye. Blunt force applied to the eye displaces the aqueous volume peripherally, causing an increase in hydraulic pressure at the lens, iris root, and trabecular meshwork. If this "wedge of pressure" exceeds the tensile strength of ocular structures, the vessels in the peripheral iris and the anterior ciliary body may rupture, leading to hyphema. The force may cause scleral ruptures, typically at the limbus and posterior to the rectus muscle insertions, where the sclera is thinner and unsupported by the orbital bones. Severe trauma leads to lens subluxation, retinal dialysis, optic nerve avulsion, and/or vitreous hemorrhage. *(Illustration by Cyndie C.H. Wooley.)*

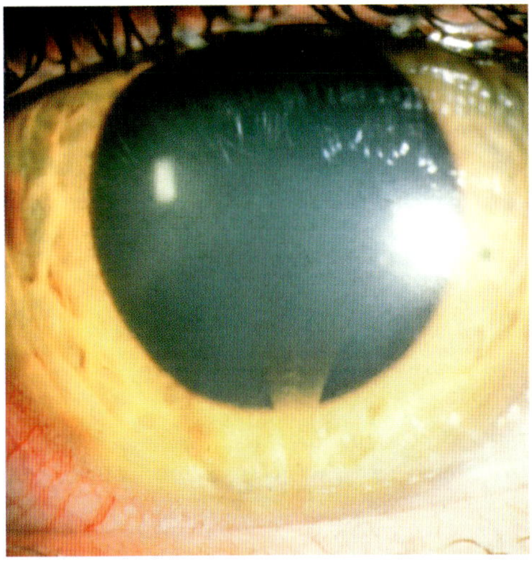

Figure 15-20 Microscopic hyphema with blood on the endothelial surface following blunt trauma. *(Courtesy of Woodford S. Van Meter, MD.)*

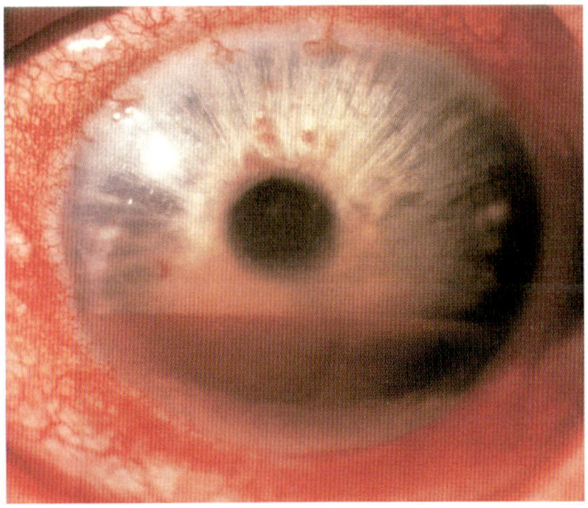

Figure 15-21 Layered hyphema from blunt trauma.

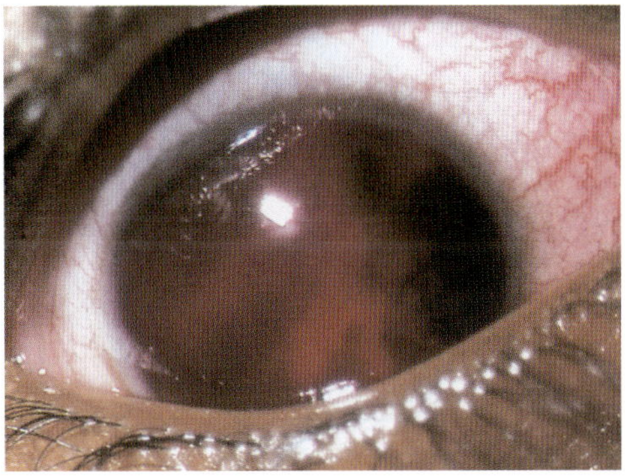

Figure 15-22 Total, or "eight-ball," hyphema.

(typically related to central retinal vein obstruction and/or diabetic retinopathy), clotting abnormalities, herpetic disease, or iris chafing from a sulcus placed intraocular lens (IOL). Juvenile xanthogranuloma, retinoblastoma, iris vascular hamartomas, and leukemia are associated with spontaneous hyphema in children.

Rebleeding

The greatest concern after a traumatic hyphema is rebleeding, which occurs in less than 5% of cases. Rebleeding is usually seen between 3 and 7 days after injury as a result of clot lysis and retraction. A complication associated with rebleeding is elevated IOP (in 50% of patients), which can potentially lead to glaucoma and optic atrophy.

The combination of blood in the anterior chamber, corneal endothelial damage, and elevated IOP can result in corneal blood staining (Fig 15-23A). Red blood cells within the anterior chamber release hemoglobin that penetrates the posterior corneal stroma, where

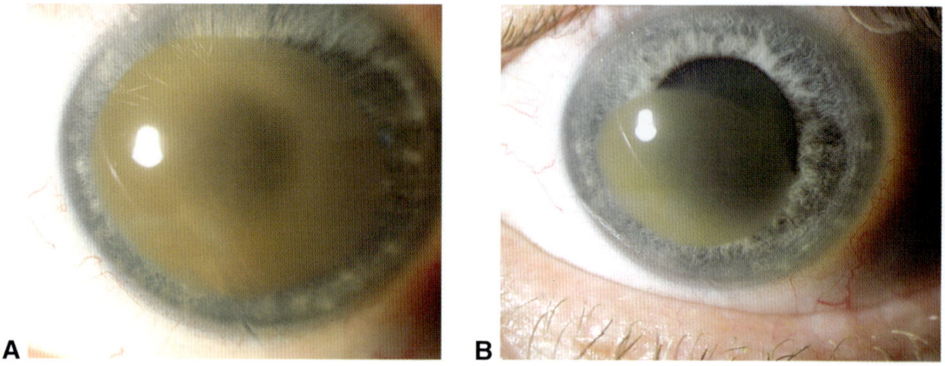

Figure 15-23 Corneal blood staining. **A,** Dense corneal blood staining after a traumatic hyphema. **B,** Clearing of corneal blood staining starts in the periphery. *(Courtesy of Robert W. Weisenthal, MD.)*

it is absorbed by keratocytes. Within the keratocytes, breakdown of the hemoglobin into hemosiderin can result in the death of the keratocytes. Close observation at the slit lamp may reveal early blood staining as yellow granular changes and reduced fibrillar definition in the posterior corneal stroma. Blood staining can lead to a reduction in corneal transparency that may be permanent. On histologic examination, red blood cells and their breakdown products can be seen within the corneal stroma. Corneal blood staining often clears slowly, starting in the periphery (Fig 15-23B), which poses a problem in children at risk of amblyopia.

Medical management

The treatment plan for traumatic hyphema aims to minimize the possibility of rebleeding, control inflammation, and control IOP. The essentials of patient care include

- a protective shield over the injured eye
- restriction of physical activity
- limiting Valsalva-related activities
- elevation of the head of the bed
- use of long-acting topical cycloplegic agents, initially to
  - improve patient comfort
  - control inflammation
  - eliminate iris movement
  - facilitate posterior segment evaluation
- use of topical corticosteroids, beneficial for
  - controlling anterior chamber inflammation
  - preventing synechiae formation
  - helping prevent rebleeding
- aggressive management of IOP with topical, oral, and even intravenous medication as needed
- oral corticosteroids (use is controversial, but may help control severe inflammation and/or prevent rebleeding)
- close outpatient observation (initially daily); admission to the hospital may be required

Aggressive treatment of elevated IOP is important to reduce the risk of corneal blood staining and optic atrophy. Topical antihypertensive agents (β-blockers and α-agonists) are the mainstay of therapy, although intravenous or oral hyperosmotic agents may occasionally be required. If medical management fails to control IOP, surgical evacuation of the blood may be required in order to reduce the risk of permanent corneal blood staining.

Antifibrinolytic agents (eg, aminocaproic acid or tranexamic acid) were previously thought to reduce the incidence of rebleeding, but studies have shown no statistical improvement in vision outcome. Because these agents can have significant adverse effects such as nausea, vomiting, postural hypotension, muscle cramps, nasal stuffiness, headache, rash, pruritus, dyspnea, toxic confusional states, and arrhythmias, they are seldom used today in the treatment of hyphema.

Gharaibeh A, Savage HI, Scherer RW, Goldberg MF, Lindsley K. Medical interventions for traumatic hyphema. *Cochrane Database Syst Rev.* 2019;19(1):CD005431.

Sickle cell complications

When a traumatic hyphema develops in an African American patient, a sickle cell workup should be performed to investigate the possibility of sickle cell hemoglobinopathy. Patients with sickle cell disease and carriers of the sickle cell trait are predisposed to sickling of red blood cells in the anterior chamber. Because sickle cells have restricted outflow through the trabecular meshwork, they may raise IOP dramatically. In addition, the optic nerve seems to be at greater risk of damage in patients with sickle cell disease, even those with modest IOP elevation, presumably as a result of a decrease in blood flow to the optic nerve.

The clinician must make every effort to control elevated IOP in these patients. Carbonic anhydrase inhibitors and osmotic agents reduce aqueous pH and lead to hemoconcentration, both of which may exacerbate sickling of red blood cells. The use of carbonic anhydrase inhibitors is avoided in sickle cell patients for this reason. Surgical intervention is recommended if average IOP remains 25 mm Hg or higher after the first 24 hours or if there are repeated, transient elevations, with IOP higher than 30 mm Hg for 2–4 days, despite medical intervention.

Bansal S, Gunasekeran DV, Ang B, et al. Controversies in the pathophysiology and management of hyphema. *Surv Ophthalmol.* 2015;61(3):297–308.
Campagna JA. Traumatic hyphema: current strategies. *Focal Points: Clinical Modules for Ophthalmologists.* American Academy of Ophthalmology; 2007, module 10.

Surgical intervention

Surgery should be performed at the first sign of corneal blood staining. Some studies suggest that surgery is indicated when IOP is higher than 25 mm Hg on average for 5 days with a total hyphema or when IOP is higher than 60 mm Hg for 2 days. Patients with preexisting optic nerve damage or sickle cell hemoglobinopathies may require earlier intervention. Indications for surgical intervention are summarized in Table 15-4.

The simplest way to surgically treat a persistent anterior chamber clot is to irrigate the anterior chamber with balanced salt solution through a limbal paracentesis. The goal is to remove circulating red blood cells that may obstruct the trabecular meshwork; removal of the entire clot is neither necessary nor wise because of the risk of a secondary hemorrhage.

Table 15-4 Indications for Surgical Intervention in Traumatic Hyphema

To prevent optic atrophy
IOP averages >60 mm Hg for 2 days
IOP averages >35 mm Hg for 7 days
To prevent corneal blood staining
IOP averages >25 mm Hg for 5 days
Evidence of early corneal blood staining
To prevent peripheral anterior synechiae
Total hyphema that persists for 5 days
Any hyphema failing to resolve to a volume of <50% within 8 days
In hyphema patients with sickle cell hemoglobinopathies
IOP averages >25 mm Hg for 24 hours
IOP has repeated transient elevations to >30 mm Hg for 2–4 days, despite medical intervention

IOP = intraocular pressure.

Adapted from Deutsch TA, Goldberg MF. Traumatic hyphema: medical and surgical management. *Focal Points: Clinical Modules for Ophthalmologists.* American Academy of Ophthalmology; 1984, module 5.

The irrigation procedure can be repeated. If irrigation is not successful, the irrigation/aspiration handpiece, used in cataract surgery, may be effective. The use of a cutting instrument or intraocular diathermy may be necessary in severe cases. Iris damage, lens injury, endothelial cell trauma, and additional bleeding are potentially serious complications of surgical intervention.

Penetrating and Perforating Ocular Trauma

It is important to understand the difference between a penetrating wound and a perforating wound for accurate communication and documentation. In a *penetrating wound,* a foreign body passes into an anatomical structure; in a *perforating wound,* a foreign body passes through such a structure. In a penetrating corneal injury, an object enters but does not pass all the way through the cornea, as in the case of a metallic foreign body that enters the corneal stroma but lodges anterior to Descemet membrane. In a perforating corneal injury, an object passes through the cornea and lodges in the anterior chamber. A perforating corneal foreign-body injury can also be called a *penetrating ocular injury* if the foreign body passes through the cornea but does not exit through the globe. In a *perforating ocular injury,* the foreign body enters and exits the globe.

Conjunctival Laceration

When managing conjunctival lacerations associated with trauma, the physician must be certain that the deeper structures of the eye have not been damaged and that no foreign body is present. After a topical anesthetic has been applied, the clinician can explore the conjunctival laceration with sterile forceps or cotton-tipped applicators, at the slit lamp. If it is still unclear whether the globe has been penetrated, exploration in the operating room can be considered. If it is obvious that globe integrity has been violated, exploration at the slit lamp should be limited and the patient prepared for surgical repair. In general, small linear conjunctival lacerations do not need to be sutured. However, stellate conjunctival lacerations, lacerations with bare sclera exposed, or lacerations with lost or retracted conjunctival tissue will heal faster if sutured closed.

Conjunctival Foreign Bodies

Foreign bodies on the conjunctival surface are best recognized during slit-lamp evaluation. Foreign bodies can lodge in the cul-de-sac, or they may be located on the palpebral conjunctival surface of the upper eyelid (Fig 15-24). If a patient is experiencing foreign-body sensation, topical fluorescein can be instilled to check for the fine, vertical, linear corneal abrasions characteristic of retained foreign bodies on the eyelid margin or superior tarsal plate (Fig 15-25). Foreign matter embedded in tissue can be removed with a sterile, disposable hypodermic needle. Glass particles, cactus spines, and insect hairs are often difficult to see, but a careful search of the cul-de-sac with high magnification aids in identification and removal. These foreign bodies may be removed with fine-tipped jeweler's forceps or a blunt spatula. If a foreign body is suspected but not seen, the cul-de-sac can be irrigated and wiped with a cotton-tipped applicator moistened with topical anesthetic. Double eversion of the eyelid with a Desmarres retractor or a bent paper clip may be necessary to allow the examiner to effectively search the entire arc of the superior cul-de-sac (Video 15-2; also see Fig 15-9).

VIDEO 15-2 Conjunctival foreign-body removal.
Courtesy of Joseph D. Iuorno, MD.

If no foreign body is found after a thorough examination, the next step is copious irrigation to cleanse the conjunctival fornices. Gunpowder or carbon fragments, such as

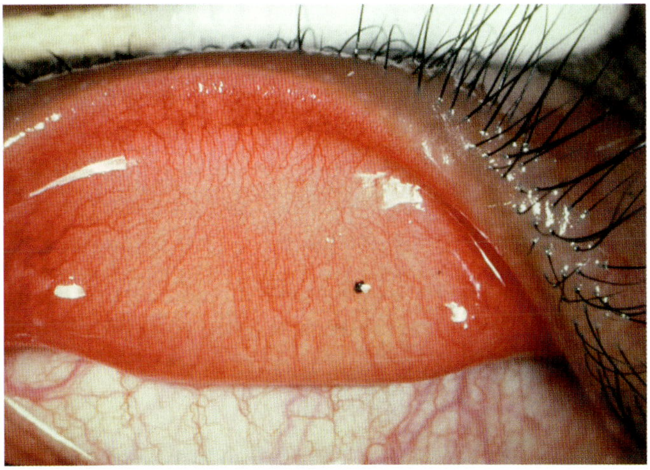

Figure 15-24 Rust foreign body embedded on the superior tarsal plate. *(Courtesy of Woodford S. Van Meter, MD.)*

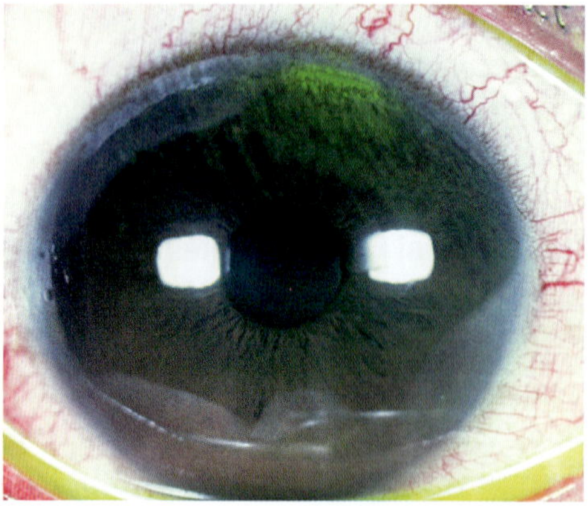

Figure 15-25 Vertical linear abrasions in the superior cornea are suggestive of a foreign body embedded in the superior tarsal conjunctiva. *(Courtesy of Woodford S. Van Meter, MD.)*

those that may be embedded in the conjunctiva by a blast injury, should be removed if possible. Because deeper fragments may be well tolerated, there is no need for extensive "digging" in an effort to achieve complete removal.

Corneal Foreign Bodies

Small foreign bodies can become embedded in the corneal epithelial surface. Larger foreign bodies can cause a corneal abrasion and then leave the eye. Because of the density of corneal pain fibers in the normal eye, an abrasion and a foreign body feel the same to the patient.

Corneal foreign bodies are identified most effectively by slit-lamp examination. Before removing a corneal foreign body, it is important to assess the depth of corneal penetration. Occult intraocular foreign bodies must be ruled out when there is a history of exposure to high-speed metallic foreign bodies, typically from grinding tools and metal-on-metal hammering. Identifying the composition of a corneal foreign body by either history or examination is important.

Vegetable or organic matter Leaves, thorns, bark, and dirt present an increased risk of fungal keratitis, so corticosteroid eyedrops are contraindicated in patients with these types of foreign bodies. Contaminated foreign material from a hospital, medical, or dental setting may pose a higher risk of bacterial infection.

Glass foreign bodies All exposed glass fragments should be removed. Fragments deeply embedded in the cornea are often inert and can be left in place (Fig 15-26). Careful gonioscopic evaluation of the anterior chamber is essential to ensure that the iris and the angle are free of any retained glass particles. Glass particles in the anterior chamber indicate a perforating corneal injury.

Iron foreign bodies Iron foreign bodies embedded in the cornea for more than a few hours can result in an orange-brown "rust ring" (Fig 15-27). Corneal iron foreign bodies

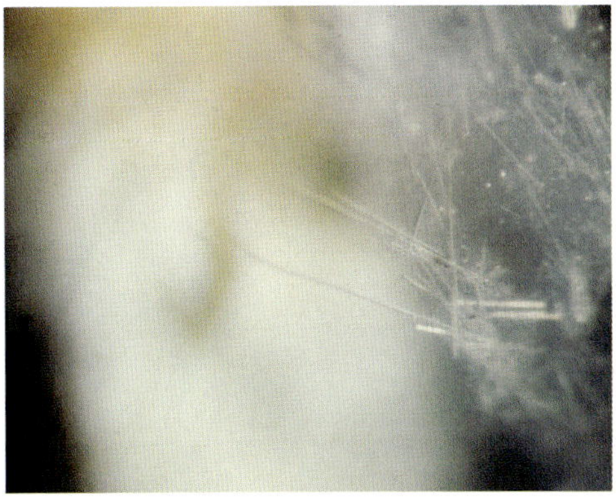

Figure 15-26 Glass or fiberglass foreign bodies (as seen in this photograph) may be well tolerated in the corneal stroma. *(Courtesy of Woodford S. Van Meter, MD.)*

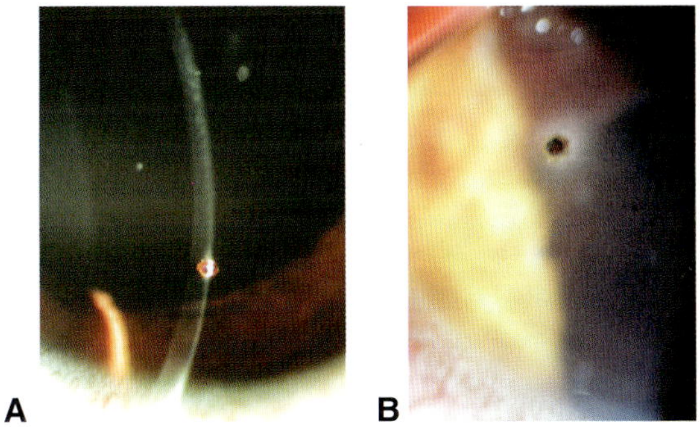

Figure 15-27 Iron foreign body in the cornea. **A,** Orange-brown "rust ring" around an iron foreign body present for 24–48 hours. **B,** White infiltrate around an iron foreign body present for 3–5 days. *(Courtesy of Woodford S. Van Meter, MD.)*

and rust rings can usually be removed at the slit lamp with a disposable (25- or 26-gauge) hypodermic needle, following application of a topical anesthetic. A battery-powered dental burr with a sterile tip may also be utilized; however, the rotating burr can cause excessive tissue disruption and increased scar formation. A foreign body that enters the corneal stroma deep to Bowman layer always results in some degree of scar formation. When such scars occur in the visual axis, they may result in glare and decreased vision from irregular astigmatism. Minimal disruption of Bowman layer during foreign-body removal will help minimize scarring and obstruction of the visual axis; this may mean retaining small amounts of the metallic foreign body.

MANAGEMENT Therapy following the removal of a corneal foreign body includes the use of topical antibiotics, cycloplegia, and occasionally the application of a firm pressure patch or bandage contact lens to help the healing process. If a pressure patch or bandage contact lens is used, the risk of infection due to the foreign body is increased, and the patient should be closely monitored until this risk has passed.

For the treatment of blast injuries, which may cause both penetrating and perforating corneal foreign bodies (Fig 15-28), the clinician should meticulously remove all possible

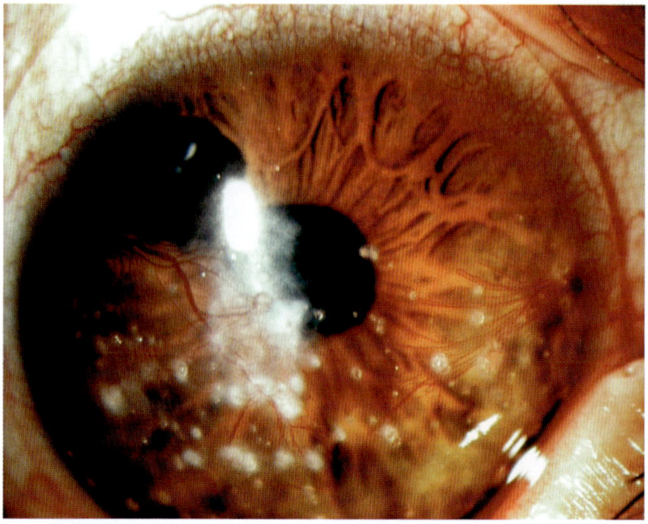

Figure 15-28 Multiple foreign bodies in the cornea following a blast injury. *(Courtesy of Woodford S. Van Meter, MD.)*

foreign bodies on or near the surface of the cornea to prevent subsequent erosion of the superficial foreign bodies and accompanying discomfort.

Scott R. The injured eye. *Philos Trans R Soc Lond B Biol Sci.* 2011;366(1562):251–260.

Evaluation and Management of Perforating Ocular Trauma

Evaluation

History

If a patient presents with both ocular and systemic trauma, diagnosis and treatment of any life-threatening injury takes precedence over evaluation and management of the ophthalmic injury. Once the patient is medically stable, the ophthalmologist should elicit a complete history, including past ocular history. The diagnosis of a traumatic ocular injury may be obvious from casual examination of the eye. However, a thorough history of the nature of the injury is crucial and should include questions regarding any association with

- metal-on-metal strike
- high-velocity projectile
- high-energy globe impact
- involvement of a sharp object
- lack of eye protection

Examination

Evaluation of a patient with a traumatic ocular injury includes a complete general and ophthalmic examination. As soon as possible, the examiner should determine and record

Table 15-5 Signs of Penetrating or Perforating Ocular Trauma

Suggestive	Diagnostic
Deep eyelid laceration	Exposed uvea, vitreous, retina
Conjunctival chemosis	Positive Seidel test result
Conjunctival laceration/hemorrhage	Visualization of intraocular foreign body
Focal iris–corneal adhesion	Intraocular foreign body seen on x-ray or ultrasonography
Shallow anterior chamber	
Iris defect	
Hypotony	
Lens capsule defect	
Acute lens opacity	
Retinal tear/hemorrhage	

visual acuity, which is the most reliable predictor of final vision outcome in traumatized eyes. Pupillary examination is then performed to detect the presence of an afferent pupillary defect (including a reverse Marcus Gunn response) or abnormality in pupil size or contour. The pupil may be peaked toward an area of corneal or scleral perforation. The examiner then looks for key signs that are suggestive or diagnostic of a penetrating or perforating ocular injury (Table 15-5).

If a significant perforating injury is suspected, it is important to avoid forced duction testing, gonioscopy, tonometry, and scleral depression. It is also important to instruct the patient to avoid straining, forced eye closure, or touching the eye, and a metal shield should be secured over the eye. Ancillary tests that may be useful in this setting are summarized in Table 15-6. All cases should be managed with safeguards appropriate for patients known to have blood-borne infections.

Nonsurgical Management

Some perforating injuries are so minimal that they seal spontaneously before ophthalmic examination, with no intraocular damage, iris prolapse, or adherence. These cases may require only systemic and/or topical antibiotic therapy along with close observation. Small, nongaping wounds may be treated as corneal abrasions with patching or a bandage contact lens until the epithelial defect has resolved and the patient is comfortable.

If a corneal wound is leaking (ie, the Seidel test result is positive; see Chapter 2, Fig 2-7) but the anterior chamber remains formed, the clinician can attempt to repair the leak with the following interventions, either alone or in combination:

- pharmacologic aqueous suppression (topical or systemic)
- patching
- therapeutic contact lens
- tissue adhesive

Generally, if these measures fail to seal the wound within 2 days, suture closure is recommended. If the corneal wound is leaking in the presence of a very shallow or flat anterior chamber, urgent surgical repair is required.

Table 15-6 Ancillary Tests in the Evaluation of Penetrating Ocular Trauma

Useful in many cases (to assess extent of injury and provide needed information for preoperative assessment of patient)
CT scan
Plain-film x-ray (generally not as useful as CT scan)
CBC, differential, platelet level
Complete metabolic panel
Useful in selected cases
MRI (especially in cases of suspected organic foreign objects in the eye or orbit; this should ***never*** be used if a metallic foreign object is suspected)
Prothrombin time, partial thromboplastin time, bleeding time
Consider tests for HIV status, hepatitis, sickle cell
Consider tests for drug and/or ethanol levels

CBC = complete blood count; CT = computed tomography; MRI = magnetic resonance imaging.

When a foreign body is present, management of the corneal perforation can be challenging. Descemet membrane is a strong structural barrier to perforation of the cornea; foreign bodies may penetrate through the stroma and lodge anterior to Descemet membrane. It may be difficult to determine whether removal of a deep foreign body will dislodge a self-sealed wound, so judicious decision making is mandatory. If multiple, very small foreign bodies are seen in the deep stroma (as may occur after an explosion) with no resultant inflammation or sign of infection, the patient may be monitored closely, given that removal of the very last particle may be unnecessary. If anterior chamber extension is present or suspected, the foreign body can be removed in the operating room. Overly aggressive attempts to remove deeply embedded foreign bodies at the slit lamp may cause leakage of aqueous humor and collapse of the anterior chamber and could dislodge the foreign body into the anterior chamber.

Surgical Management

Preoperative management

If surgical repair is required, the timing of the operation is crucial. Although studies have not documented any disadvantage in delaying the repair of an open globe for up to 24 hours, intervention ideally should occur as soon as possible. Prompt closure of the wound to restore the integrity of the globe helps minimize the risk of additional damage to intraocular contents, inflammation, microbial proliferation, and endophthalmitis.

Before proceeding to the operating room, it is important that the clinician

- apply a protective shield
- avoid excessive manipulation
- instruct the patient not to eat or drink
- prescribe appropriate medications for sedation and pain control once surgical consent has been signed
- initiate intravenous antibiotics and antiemetics, if necessary
- provide tetanus prophylaxis
- seek anesthesia consultation

Injuries associated with soil contamination and/or retained intraocular foreign bodies increase the risk of *Bacillus* endophthalmitis. Because this organism can destroy the eye within 24 hours, intravenous and/or intravitreal therapy with an antibiotic effective against *Bacillus* species may be necessary; fluoroquinolones (eg, levofloxacin, moxifloxacin, or gatifloxacin), clindamycin, or vancomycin can be considered. Surgical repair should be undertaken with minimal delay in cases at risk for contamination with this organism.

Anesthesia

General anesthesia is almost always preferred for repair of an open globe because retrobulbar or peribulbar anesthetic injection increases posterior orbital pressure, which may cause or exacerbate the extrusion of intraocular contents. Local or topical anesthesia may be considered in rare instances, such as in a patient with a small laceration who is at medical risk from general anesthesia. After the surgical repair is complete, a periocular anesthetic injection may be used to control postoperative pain.

Surgical repair considerations

Management of a typical full-thickness corneoscleral laceration with uveal prolapse generally requires surgical repair in the operating room (Fig 15-29). Repair of a corneoscleral laceration takes precedence over non–life-threatening surgical problems elsewhere on the body. Repair of an adnexal injury follows repair of the globe itself because eyelid surgery can put pressure on an open globe, and certain eyelid lacerations may actually improve exposure of the globe during surgery. The primary goal of the repair is to restore the integrity of the globe. The secondary goal at the time of the primary repair or during subsequent procedures is to restore vision. The surgeon is encouraged not to overpromise or be overly optimistic regarding the outcome in this setting. Because subsequent surgeries may be required, this procedure might be described as eye-saving rather than sight-saving surgery.

Primary enucleation is recommended only for an injury so devastating that restoration of the anatomy is impossible, or when it would be important to spare the patient another procedure. Prior to operating in such a case, it is helpful to add "and possible enucleation" to the consent form. Delay in enucleation following attempted repair with subsequent loss of light perception allows the patient time to acknowledge both loss of

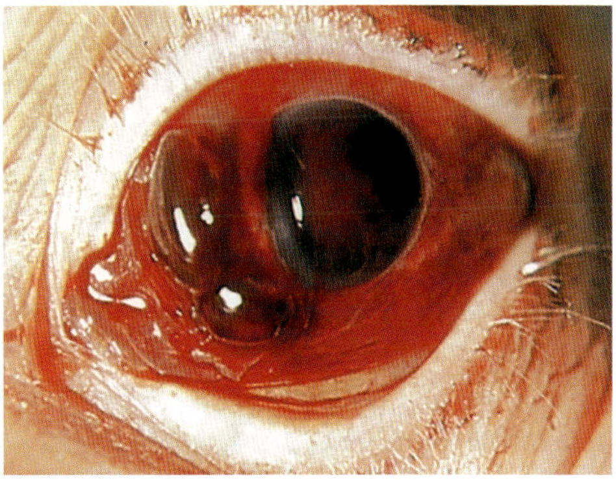

Figure 15-29 Scleral laceration with prolapse of uveal tissue secondary to blunt trauma.

vision and accompanying disfigurement, as well as to thoughtfully consider the benefits of enucleation in a nonemergent setting.

Agrawal R, Rao G, Naigaonkar R, Ou X, Desai S. Prognostic factors for vision outcome after surgical repair of open globe injuries. *Indian J Ophthalmol.* 2011;59(6):465–470.

Castiblanco CP, Adelman RA. Sympathetic ophthalmia. *Graefe's Arch Clin Exp Ophthalmol.* 2009;247(3):289–302.

Galor A, Davis JL, Flynn HW Jr, et al. Sympathetic ophthalmia: incidence of ocular complications and vision loss in the sympathizing eye. *Am J Ophthalmol.* 2009;148(5): 704–710.e2.

Repair of a corneoscleral laceration

If vitreous or lens fragments have prolapsed through the corneal wound, the surgeon cuts these fragments flush with the surface of the globe (Fig 15-30), taking care not to exert traction on the vitreous or zonular fibers. If uvea or retina (seen as translucent, tan tissue with extremely fine vessels) protrudes, the surgeon reposits it using a cannula or spatula in a gentle sweeping motion through a separate limbal incision, while keeping the anterior chamber formed with viscoelastic. If epithelium has obviously migrated onto a uveal surface or into the wound, the surgeon can attempt to peel the epithelial layer off. Only in cases of frankly necrotic macerated tissue should uveal tissue be excised.

The limbus is an important landmark for suturing a corneoscleral laceration. The limbus is sutured before the rest of the wound with 9-0 or 10-0 nylon suture, followed by closure of the remaining corneal components of the laceration with 10-0 nylon suture. The wound is divided in half with each successive suture until watertight closure is achieved. It may be necessary to reposit iris tissue repeatedly after each suture is placed in order to avoid entrapment of iris in the wound. A side port incision is of great utility during surgical repair for sweeping the iris from the wound and reforming the anterior chamber, thus reducing the manipulation of the traumatic wound. Despite these efforts, uvea may remain apposed to the posterior corneal surface. Superficial sutures may be helpful at this stage of closure to avoid incorporating the uvea into the wound closure. Once watertight, the uvea can be separated from the cornea with viscoelastic injection, followed by replacement of the superficial sutures with near–full-thickness sutures. It is best to bury suture knots to provide postoperative comfort. Viscoelastic is removed, if possible, prior to a final test of wound integrity and to reduce the risk of a postoperative IOP spike. Testing wound integrity when the eye is filled with air or viscoelastic does not guarantee a watertight closure.

It may be impossible to achieve a watertight closure because of unusual laceration configuration or loss of tissue. In such cases, X-shaped or purse-string sutures or other customized techniques may suffice. Cyanoacrylate glue or even primary lamellar keratoplasty may be required when watertight closure cannot be achieved. A bandage contact lens over the glue is necessary for comfort. A conjunctival flap or amniotic tissue graft should not be used to treat a wound leak.

Specific suturing techniques may be helpful in restoring a more normal corneal contour, when the anatomy of the wound allows. Longer, more widely spaced sutures create flattening in the area of the suture and are therefore placed in the peripheral cornea to re-create the aspheric curvature of the cornea (flatter in the periphery and steeper centrally).

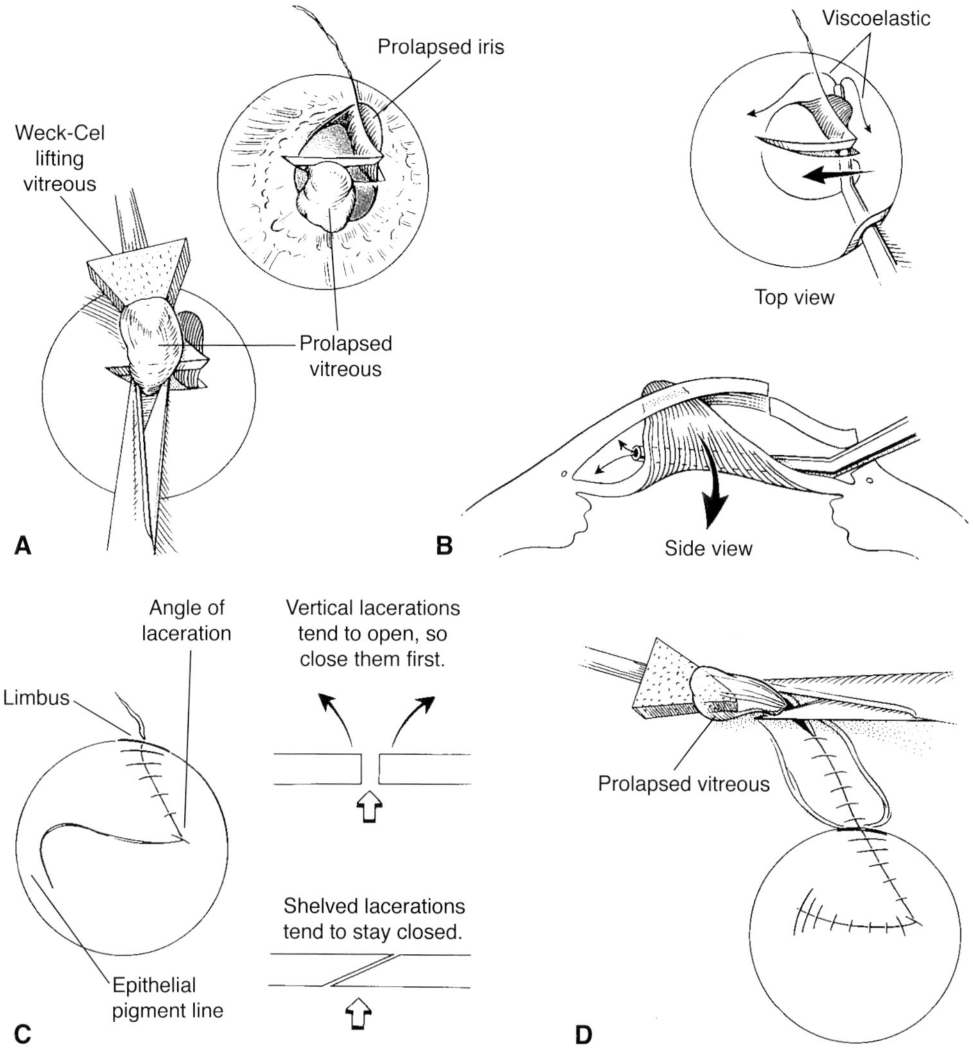

Figure 15-30 Restoring anatomical relationships in corneoscleral laceration repair. **A,** Prolapsed vitreous or lens fragments are excised. **B,** Iris is reposited by means of viscoelastic and a cannula inserted through a separate paracentesis. **C,** Landmarks such as limbus, laceration angles, or epithelial pigment lines are closed. Vertical lacerations are closed first to create a watertight globe more quickly, followed by shelved lacerations. **D,** The scleral part of the wound is exposed, prolapsed vitreous is severed, and the wound is closed from the limbus, working posteriorly. *(Reproduced from Hamill MB. Repair of the traumatized anterior segment.* Focal Points: Clinical Modules for Ophthalmologists. *American Academy of Ophthalmology; 1992, module 1. Illustrations by Christine Gralapp.)*

Shorter, more closely spaced sutures are then used centrally, when possible, in order to close the wound without excessive central flattening (Figs 15-31, 15-32). When the sutures are being tied, it is important to have sufficient tension to create a watertight closure without inducing corneal striae, astigmatism, or maceration of the inflamed stromal tissue. That said, establishing wound integrity takes priority over concerns about induced astigmatism.

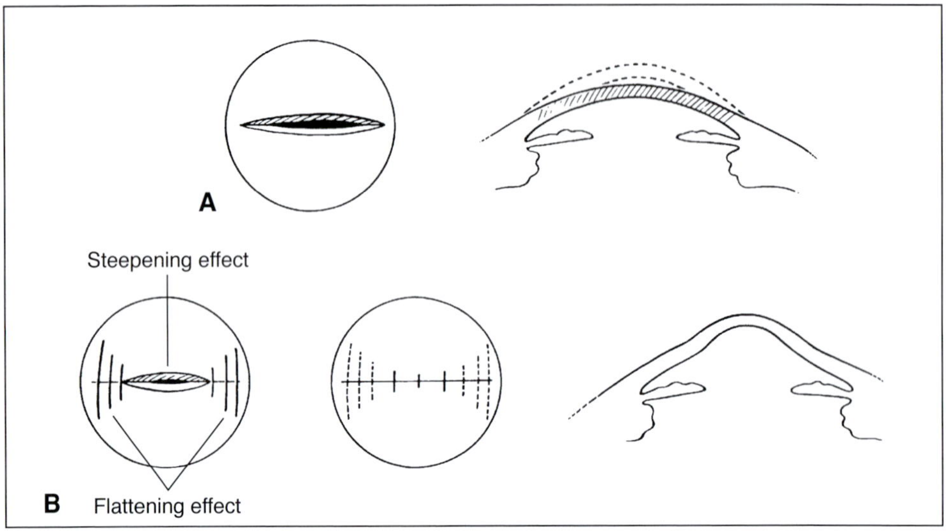

Figure 15-31 Restoring functional architecture in corneal wound closure. **A,** Laceration has a flattening effect on the cornea. **B,** Long, compressive sutures are placed in the periphery to flatten the peripheral cornea and steepen the central cornea. Subsequently, short, minimally compressive sutures are placed in the steepened central cornea to preserve sphericity despite the flattening effect of the sutures. *(Reproduced from Hamill MB. Repair of the traumatized anterior segment.* Focal Points: Clinical Modules for Ophthalmologists. *American Academy of Ophthalmology; 1992, module 1.)*

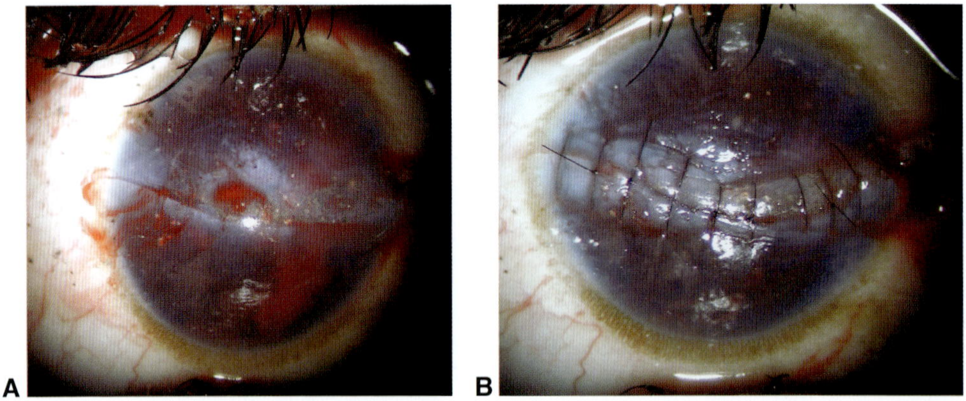

Figure 15-32 Repair of corneoscleral laceration. **A,** Corneoscleral laceration from improvised explosive device, Craig Joint Theater hospital, Bagram Air Base, Afghanistan. **B,** Repair with short central sutures and longer peripheral sutures, all uvea reposited. *(Courtesy of Charles D. Reilly, MD.)*

The scleral component of the laceration is evaluated with a gentle peritomy and conjunctival separation in order to expose the wound. Prolapsed vitreous is excised, and prolapsed nonnecrotic uvea and retina are reposited (Fig 15-33). The scleral wound is closed with 9-0 nylon or 8-0 nylon or silk sutures. Often, resection of Tenon capsule and management of prolapsed tissue must be repeated incrementally after each suture is placed.

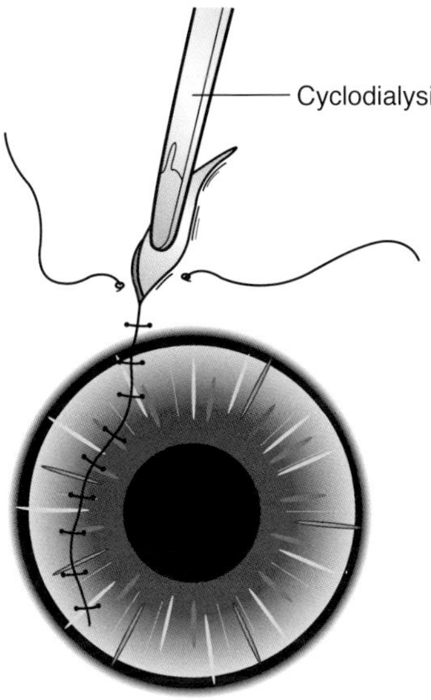

Figure 15-33 The zippering technique of scleral wound closure. Prolapsed uveal tissue is depressed while the scleral wound is progressively closed, moving in an anterior-to-posterior direction. *(Redrawn from Hersh PS, Shingleton BJ, Kenyon KR. Management of corneoscleral lacerations. In: Hersh PS, Shingleton BJ, Kenyon KR, eds.* Eye Trauma. *Mosby Year Book; 1991.)*

If the laceration might extend under an extraocular muscle, the muscle may be carefully removed at its insertion after preplacing a suture and then reinserting it following repair. Closure of the laceration should continue posteriorly only to the point at which it becomes technically difficult or requires undue pressure on the globe to complete. Very posterior lacerations may be tamponaded effectively by orbital tissue and are best left alone.

The decision of whether to perform additional intraocular surgery during the primary repair is made once the globe is watertight. The surgeon must decide whether intraocular surgery is needed and, if so, whether it should be attempted immediately or postponed. Factors to consider include the expertise of the surgeon, the quality of the facility and nursing personnel, the availability of technical equipment and instruments, the adequacy of the view of anterior segment structures, and issues of informed consent. If there are concerns regarding any of these factors, the surgeon should restore globe integrity and postpone the secondary procedures until a later date. For example, an anterior segment surgeon might not attempt a lens extraction with limited visualization. When attempting removal of opacified lens material, it is helpful to know whether the posterior capsule has been violated. Ultrasound biomicroscopy can be beneficial in this setting. Removal of a ruptured lens may be performed from a posterior approach with vitrectomy during a second procedure. See BCSC Section 11, *Lens and Cataract,* for further discussion of the issues of cataract surgery and IOL placement following trauma to the eye.

If a foreign body is visible in the anterior segment and can be grasped, it is reasonable to remove it, either through the wound or through a separate limbal incision. Metal fragments are difficult to remove through their entrance wounds because the rough metal edges usually require a larger wound for extraction than would appear necessary (Fig 15-34). A retained intraocular metallic foreign body can cause ocular siderosis (Fig 15-35). Yellow

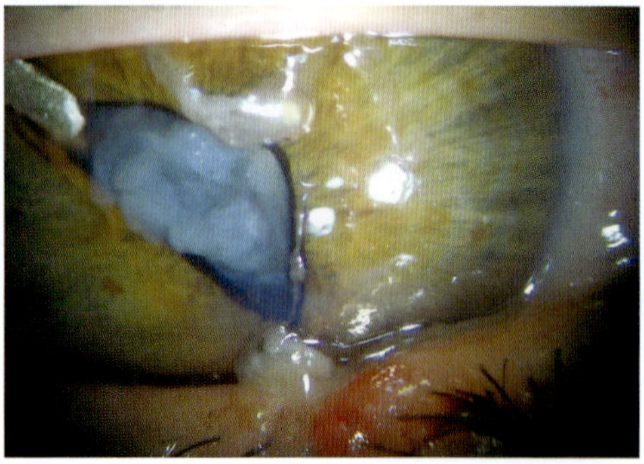

Figure 15-34 Penetrating metallic foreign body from rocket-propelled grenade, Craig Joint Theater hospital, Bagram Air Base, Afghanistan. Note iris incarceration at entrance wound at the limbus, anterior capsule laceration, and cortical fluffing of lens material within the pupil and metallic foreign body lodged in the angle superiorly. *(Courtesy of Charles D. Reilly, MD.)*

discoloration of the endothelium and deep stroma is visible. Removal of the foreign body can ameliorate the discoloration (Video 15-3). If left untreated, ocular siderosis can cause permanent damage to the retinal pigment epithelium and inner retinal layers and ultimately induce optic nerve atrophy.

VIDEO 15-3 Removal of metallic foreign body causing siderosis from angle.
Courtesy of Joseph D. Iuorno, MD.

Closure of iris lacerations may decrease the formation of anterior or posterior synechiae while reducing glare and polyopia from severe corectopia; however, it may be difficult to achieve during the primary procedure. Iridodialysis may cause monocular diplopia and an eccentric pupil if left untreated. If corneal opacity prevents safe repair of internal ocular injury, repairs can be performed secondarily. The McCannel technique and the Siepser knot are popular approaches for repair of an iris defect (Video 15-4; Fig 15-36).

VIDEO 15-4 Modified Siepser knot.
Courtesy of Michael E. Snyder, MD.

Prophylactic intraoperative antibiotics to cover both gram-positive and gram-negative organisms may be given by subconjunctival injection at the conclusion of the repair. Intravitreal antibiotics such as vancomycin 1 mg and ceftazidime 2.25 mg can be considered for contaminated wounds involving the vitreous.

Postoperative management

Postoperatively, therapy is directed at preventing infection, suppressing inflammation, controlling IOP, and relieving pain. Patients may be given intravenous antibiotics (eg, a cephalosporin and an aminoglycoside) for 48 hours or an oral antibiotic with good vitreous penetration, such as moxifloxacin 400 mg per day for 3–5 days. Topical antibiotics

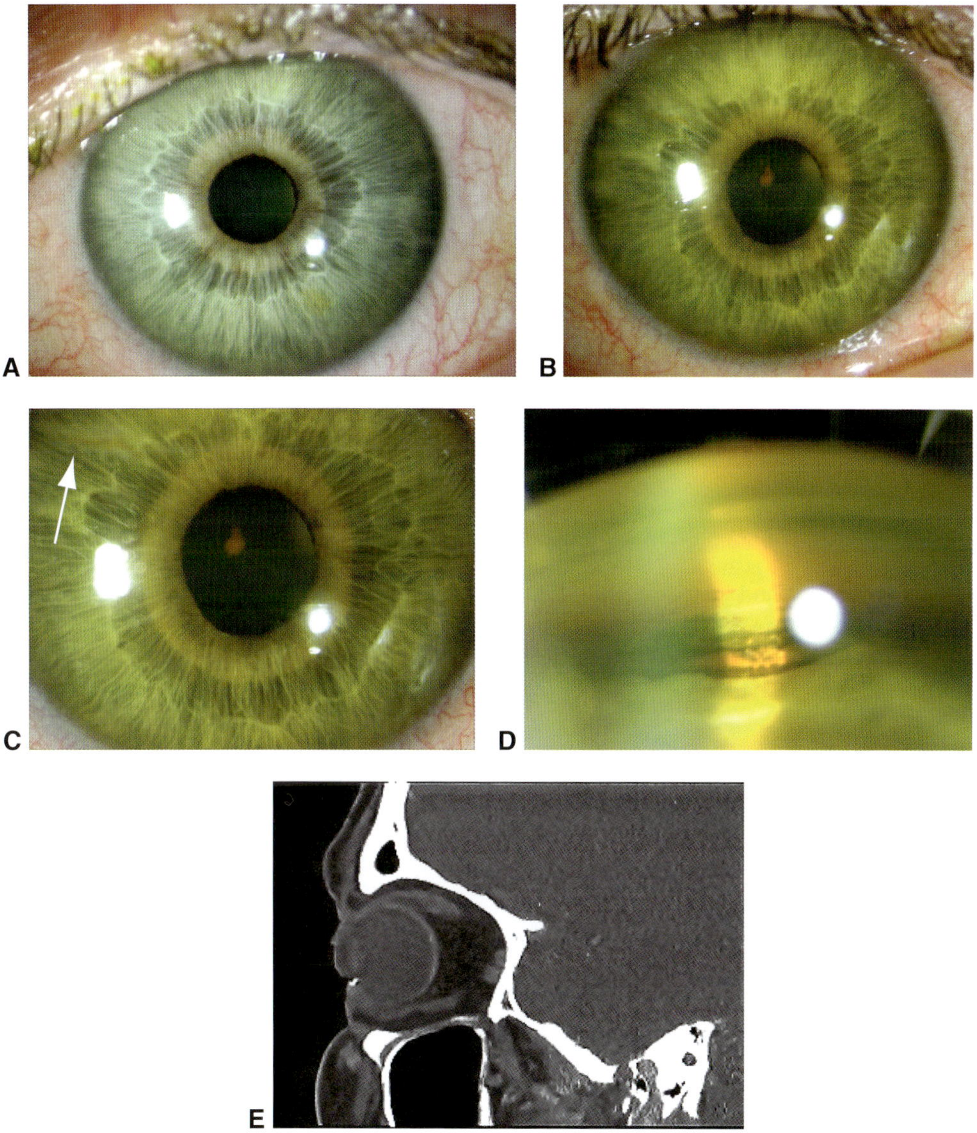

Figure 15-35 Retained intraocular foreign body. **A,** Normal fellow eye with blue iris. **B,** Siderosis causes yellow discoloration of iris and endothelium. **C,** Note entry wound *(arrow)* and pigment on the crystalline lens, likely representing the ricochet site of the projectile. **D,** Gonioscopy reveals foreign body in inferior angle. **E,** Visualization of angle with computed tomography imaging. *(Courtesy of Joseph D. Iuorno, MD.)*

are generally instilled 4 times a day for 7 days or until epithelial closure of the ocular surface is complete. Topical corticosteroids may be given 4–8 times a day, depending on the amount of inflammation or the risk of infection. Corticosteroid eyedrops and cycloplegics are slowly tapered as the inflammation subsides. A fibrinous response in the anterior chamber may respond well to a short course of systemic prednisone. IOP should

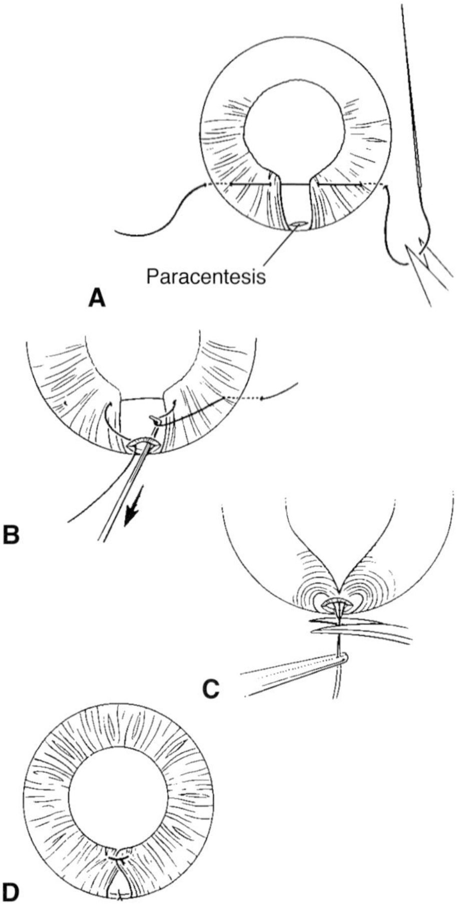

Figure 15-36 The McCannel technique for repairing iris lacerations. With large lacerations, multiple sutures may be used. **A,** A limbal paracentesis is made over the iris discontinuity. A long curved (CIF) needle with 10-0 polypropylene is then passed through the peripheral cornea, the edges of the iris, and exiting the peripheral cornea opposite, and the needle and suture are cut. **B,** A Sinskey hook is introduced through the paracentesis and around the suture peripherally, and both ends of the suture are drawn out through the paracentesis. **C,** The suture is securely tied. **D,** After the suture is secure, it is cut, and the iris is repositioned in the anterior chamber. *(Reproduced from Hamill MB. Repair of the traumatized anterior segment.* Focal Points: Clinical Modules for Ophthalmologists. *American Academy of Ophthalmology; 1992, module 1. Illustrations by Christine Gralapp.)*

be monitored, and elevated IOP should be controlled to minimize the risk of optic nerve damage. Postoperative hypotony is associated with

- wound leak
- cyclodialysis cleft
- ciliary body shutdown due to inflammation
- choroidal effusion
- intraocular hemorrhage

Corneal sutures that do not loosen spontaneously are generally left in place for at least 3 months, depending on wound healing and patient age, and then removed incrementally over the next few months. In children, sutures can be removed as early as 6–8 weeks. In general, wounds near the limbus heal faster than wounds in the paracentral cornea. Fibrosis and vascularization are indicators that enough healing has occurred to render suture removal safe. Loose sutures can be identified by applying fluorescein at each postoperative visit and looking for erosion through the epithelium. Eroded sutures do not provide structural support. They cause pain and increase the risk of infection and inflammation.

Injured eyes are at increased risk of choroidal effusion or retinal detachment, so frequent examination of the posterior segment is essential. If media opacity precludes an adequate fundus examination, evaluation for an afferent pupillary defect and B-scan ultrasonography are useful tools for monitoring retinal status.

Refraction and vision correction with contact lenses or glasses can proceed when the ocular surface and media clear. Partial or complete suture removal can be performed once adequately healed in order to facilitate improvement in vision. Because of the risk of amblyopia in a child or loss of fusion in an adult, vision correction should not be unnecessarily delayed. The uninvolved eye of a child at risk of amblyopia should be patched as soon as the first postoperative day.

Once the wound has healed and if the visual axis is clear, a rigid gas-permeable contact lens can create a new refractive surface and may help improve vision. Keratoplasty may be considered for cases of reduced vision function due to corneal opacity, marked irregular astigmatism, or endothelial failure (see Chapter 16).

For more information on wound repair, see BCSC Section 4, *Ophthalmic Pathology and Intraocular Tumors.*

Macsai MS, Rohr A. Surgical management and rehabilitation of anterior segment trauma. In: Mannis MJ, Holland EJ, eds. *Cornea.* Vol 2. 4th ed. Elsevier; 2017:1588–1600.

CHAPTER 16

Clinical Approach to Corneal Transplantation

This chapter includes related videos. Go to www.aao.org/bcscvideo_section08 or scan the QR codes in the text to access this content.

Indicates selected key points within the chapter.

Highlights

- Advantages of selectively replacing pathologic corneal tissue have led to a shift in surgeon preference from penetrating keratoplasty to lamellar keratoplasty.
- Deep anterior lamellar keratoplasty (DALK) preserves the host corneal endothelium, eliminating the risk of endothelial rejection and providing additional structural support in the case of trauma. However, DALK does not reduce postoperative astigmatism or prevent stromal rejection.
- Endothelial keratoplasty is the procedure of choice for treating endothelial cell dysfunction. Advantages include preservation of structural integrity, faster recovery of vision, more predictable refractive outcomes, and reduced risk of endothelial rejection compared with penetrating keratoplasty.
- In cases of endothelial rejection with edema, the use of systemic corticosteroids is recommended either orally or intravenously, in addition to topical treatment.

Corneal Transplantation

Corneal transplantation refers to surgical replacement of the host cornea with full-thickness (penetrating keratoplasty) or partial-thickness (lamellar keratoplasty) donor corneal tissue. If the donor is another person, the tissue is called an *allograft* and the procedure is referred to as *allogeneic transplantation*. If the donor tissue is from the same eye or fellow eye, it is called an *autograft* and the procedure is referred to as *autologous transplantation*. Innovations in keratoplasty (see sidebar) have produced a veritable alphabet soup of nomenclature to describe the various procedures (Table 16-1).

Table 16-1 Contemporary Keratoplasty Procedures

Abbreviation	Procedure
ALK (ALTK)	Anterior lamellar (therapeutic) keratoplasty
DALK	Deep anterior lamellar keratoplasty
dDALK	Descemetic deep anterior lamellar keratoplasty
pdDALK	Pre-Descemetic deep anterior lamellar keratoplasty
DMEK	Descemet membrane endothelial keratoplasty
DSEK (DSAEK)	Descemet stripping (automated) endothelial keratoplasty
DSO/DWEK	Descemet stripping only/Descemet without endothelial keratoplasty
EK	Endothelial keratoplasty
FLAK	Femtosecond laser–assisted keratoplasty
PKP/PK	Penetrating keratoplasty

Modified from American Academy of Ophthalmology Cornea/External Disease Panel. Preferred Practice Pattern Guidelines. *Corneal Edema and Opacification.* American Academy of Ophthalmology; 2018. www.aao.org/ppp

MILESTONES IN THE HISTORY OF CORNEAL TRANSPLANTATION

- 1905: First successful penetrating keratoplasty performed, using human tissue from a live donor
- 1911: Anterior lamellar keratoplasty performed, with preserved donor cornea from a human cadaver
- 1944: First eye bank established to provide a source of donated human eye tissue for keratoplasty
- 1954: Posterior lamellar keratoplasty performed
- 1963: Osteo-odonto-keratoprosthesis performed
- 1992: Boston keratoprosthesis type I (Kpro) approved by the US Food and Drug Administration
- 1998–2006: Renaissance of lamellar keratoplasty advances, including
  - 1998: Posterior lamellar keratoplasty reintroduced and refined
  - 2000: Deep lamellar endothelial keratoplasty performed
  - 2002: Deep anterior lamellar keratoplasty (DALK) big-bubble technique performed
  - 2004: Descemet stripping endothelial keratoplasty (DSEK) performed
  - 2005: Descemet stripping automated endothelial keratoplasty (DSAEK) performed
  - 2006: Descemet membrane endothelial keratoplasty (DMEK) performed
- 2012: Descemet stripping only (DSO) performed
- 2017: DSO with topical Rho kinase inhibitor supplementation
- 2018: Injected cultured endothelial cells with Rho kinase inhibitor supplementation

Arenas E, Esquenazi S, Anwar M, Terry M. Lamellar corneal transplantation. *Surv Ophthalmol.* 2012;57(6):510–529.

Melles GRJ. Posterior lamellar keratoplasty. DLEK to DSEK to DMEK. *Cornea.* 2006;25(8):879–881.

Corneal Transplant Procedures and Trends

Indications for corneal transplantation procedures performed in the United States in 2019 are listed in Table 16-2.

There has been a dramatic and continuing shift in surgeon preference from penetrating keratoplasty (PK; also abbreviated as PKP) to lamellar keratoplasty (LK or LKP) over the past 20 years. In 2000, 99.3% of US corneal transplant procedures were PKs. In 2012, endothelial keratoplasty (EK) surpassed PK. Among EK procedures, the proportion of Descemet membrane endothelial keratoplasty (DMEK) surgeries steadily increased from 3% in 2012 to 43% in 2019, with Descemet stripping endothelial keratoplasty (DSEK) making up the remaining 57%. By 2019, the mix of US keratoplasty procedures had evolved as follows:

- 62.4% EK, comprising
  - 57% DSEK
  - 43% DMEK
- 35.4% PK
- 1.5% anterior lamellar keratoplasty (ALK), comprising deep anterior lamellar keratoplasty (DALK) and anterior or midstromal ALK
- 0.5% keratoprosthesis (KPro)
- 0.1% keratolimbal allograft (KLA)

Internationally, DALK is becoming more common, perhaps because tissue suitable for DALK is more readily available than for PK. Other advantages of DALK include a vision outcome similar to that for PK without the risk of endothelial rejection or increased risk of intraoperative suprachoroidal hemorrhage and postoperative or traumatic ruptured globe. The slower acceptance of DALK in the United States may be explained by the increased surgical time and skill required, the lower reimbursement, and the easy access to tissue suitable for PK.

Eye Bank Association of America (EBAA). *2019 Eye Banking Statistical Report*. EBAA; 2020.

Park CY, Lee JK, Gore PK, Lim CY, Chuck RS. Keratoplasty in the United States: a 10-year review from 2005 through 2014. *Ophthalmology*. 2015;122(12):2432–2442.

Keratoplasty and Eye Banking

Tissue Processing and Preservation

Eye banks in the United States typically preserve tissue in either Optisol GS (Bausch + Lomb) or Life 4°C (NuMedis). Each type of media contains chondroitin sulfate, dextran, gentamycin, and streptomycin; Life 4°C also contains insulin. Tissue is stored at 2–8° C and can remain viable for up to 2 weeks.

Eye banks in Europe typically incubate donor corneal tissue in organ culture storage at 37°C. Organ culture allows tissue to be stored for up to 35 days but requires a culture at the end of the storage period to confirm sterility before the tissue is used. The organ culture system is more complex, costly, and labor-intensive than intermediate storage at 4°C, but the longer storage time is advantageous in places where the supply of donor corneas is limited.

Table 16-2 Domestic Indications for Transplant in US Eye Banks, 2019

Surgical Diagnosis	PK		ALK		EK		Total
Endothelial Cell Failure							
Post–cataract surgery edema	866	19.4%	—	—	3595	80.6%	4461
Endothelial dystrophies	765	4.4%	—	—	16,652	95.6%	17,417
Other causes of endothelial dysfunction	1263	22.4%	—	—	4366	77.6%	5629
Subtotal	**2894**	**10.5%**	**0**	**0%**	**24,613**	**89.5%**	**27,507**
	16.6% of PK				80.3% of EK		56.4% of grafts
Stromal or Full-Thickness (Nonendothelial) Disease							
Ectasias/thinning	2433	88.9%	304	11.1%	—	—	2737
Noninfectious ulcerative keratitis or perforations	1199	96.7%	41	3.3%	—	—	1240
Degenerations or dystrophies	744	91.7%	67	8.3%	—	—	811
Microbial keratitis	419	97.2%	12	2.8%	—	—	431
Mechanical or chemical trauma	433	94.5%	25	5.5%	—	—	458
Congenital opacities	265	95.7%	12	4.3%	—	—	277
Refractive issue	32	94.1%	2	5.9%	—	—	34
Pterygium	4	100.0%	0	0.0%	—	—	4
Other causes of corneal dysfunction or distortion	1683	92.3%	141	7.7%	—	—	1824
Subtotal	**7212**	**92.3%**	**604**	**7.7%**	**0**	**0%**	**7816**
	41.4% of PK		81.1% of ALK				16.0% of grafts
Regraft							
Repeat corneal transplant	3220	51.4%	27	0.4%	3020	48.2%	6267
	18.5% of PK		3.6% of ALK		9.9% of EK		12.8% of grafts
Unknown/Unspecified							
Unknown, unreported, or unspecified	4083	56.6%	114	1.6%	3017	41.8%	7214
	23.5% of PK		15.3% of ALK		9.8% of EK		14.8% of grafts
	PK		**ALK**		**EK**		**Total**
Total for each procedure	**17,409**	**35.7%**	**745**	**1.5%**	**30,650**	**62.8%**	**48,804**

ALK = anterior lamellar keratoplasty; EK = endothelial keratoplasty; PK = penetrating keratoplasty.

Modified with permission from the Eye Bank Association of America (EBAA). *2019 Eye Banking Statistical Report.* EBAA; 2020.

The process of tissue recovery and preparation includes a detailed donor history, a slit-lamp evaluation, and an endothelial cell count at the eye bank before release for transplantation. The optimal time from death to recovery is less than 12 hours, or up to 24 hours if the donor body is refrigerated or ice is placed over the eyes. Most eye banks prepare precut tissue for Descemet stripping automated endothelial keratoplasty (DSAEK) and prestripped tissue for DMEK, placing an "S" stamp on the anterior side to aid orientation. The option of preloaded tissue, particularly for DMEK, is increasingly being utilized.

Eye Bank Association of America (EBAA). *Eye Bank Association of America Medical Standards, June 2020.* EBAA; 2020.

Drury DC, Ramos S. Eye banking: structure and function. In Mannis MJ, Holland EJ, eds. *Cornea.* Vol 1. 5th ed. Elsevier; 2022:246–249.

Glasser DB, DeMatteo J. Medical standards for eye banking. In: Mannis MJ, Holland EJ, eds. *Cornea.* Vol 1. 5th ed. Elsevier; 2022:250–258.

Donor-Cornea Selection

Eye bank personnel screen the donor's medical record and obtain blood samples to rule out potentially transmissible diseases. Medical criteria that render a potential donor unsuitable for tissue recovery are listed in Table 16-3. Diseases that can be transmitted from donor corneas are listed in Table 16-4. Responsibility for determining whether a donor cornea is suitable for transplantation ultimately rests with the transplant surgeon.

Donor tissue from a person younger than 2 years is typically not used for PK because it is extremely steep and difficult to handle, which poses challenges in creating a watertight closure and achieving a predictable refractive outcome. Corneas from donors who have undergone cataract surgery are acceptable if they exceed the minimum acceptable cell count outlined in the eye bank's policy (typically 2000 cells/mm^2). Corneas with low endothelial cell counts and clear stroma may be suitable for anterior lamellar procedures. Conversely, corneas with anterior stromal opacities but acceptable cell counts may be used for EK. Tissue from a donor under age 50 is often avoided for DMEK because it is more difficult to unscroll.

Results from 2 landmark studies of eye bank–supplied corneal tissue, the Cornea Donor Study (CDS) and the Cornea Preservation Time Study (CPTS), provide guidance for selection of donor tissue. The CDS evaluated the effect of donor age on graft survival in patients with PK. Donors were grouped into 2 cohorts according to age: 10–64 years and 65–75 years. At 5-year follow-up, the study showed no difference in the rate of graft survival between the 2 groups. However, at 10-year follow-up, the rate of graft survival was slightly lower in patients who received tissue from donors older than age 70. The CPTS provides guidelines for the use of DSEK tissue preserved in Optisol GS or Life 4°C, finding comparable graft success rates for tissue stored up to 11 days after death and even up to 14 days in some circumstances.

Rosenwasser GO, Szczotka-Flynn LB, Ayala AR, et al. Effect of cornea preservation time on success of Descemet stripping automated endothelial keratoplasty: a randomized trial. *JAMA Ophthalmol.* 2017;135(12):1401–1409.

Writing Committee for the Corneal Donor Study Research Group; Mannis MJ, Holland EJ, Gal RL, et al. The effect of donor age on penetrating keratoplasty for endothelial disease. *Ophthalmology.* 2013;120(12):2419–2427.

Table 16-3 Medical Criteria Contraindicating Donor-Cornea Use

Death of unknown cause with likelihood of other exclusion criteria
Congenital rubella
Reye syndrome within the past 3 months
Active viral encephalitis of unknown origin or progressive encephalopathy (eg, subacute sclerosing panencephalitis, progressive multifocal leukoencephalopathy)
Active bacterial or viral encephalitis
Active bacterial or fungal endocarditis
Suspected rabies virus infection or history of being bitten, within the past 6 months, by an animal suspected to be infected with rabies virus
Down syndrome (exclusion criterion for PK or ALK)
Intrinsic eye diseases
- Retinoblastoma
- Malignant tumor of the anterior ocular segment or known adenocarcinoma in the eye (primary or metastatic origin)
- Active ocular or intraocular inflammation: conjunctivitis, keratitis, scleritis, uveitis, vitritis, choroiditis, or retinitis
- Congenital or acquired disorders of the eye that would preclude a successful outcome for the intended use (eg, a central donor corneal scar for an intended PK, keratoconus, or keratoglobus)

Active leukemias
Active disseminated lymphomas
High-risk behavior or incarceration in prison
Prior refractive corneal surgery, such as radial keratotomy, PRK, LASIK, and lamellar inserts, with the exception that previous laser refractive surgery may not disqualify a donor's tissue for use in EK
Positive test for anti-HIV-1 and anti-HIV-2 (or combination test) and nonreactive for HBsAg and anti-HCV antibody
Parkinson disease, amyotrophic lateral sclerosis, multiple sclerosis, Alzheimer disease
CJD, variant CJD, or family member with CJD
History of Ebola virus disease
History of melanoma with known metastatic disease

Donors for PK

Prior intraocular or anterior segment surgery
- Refractive corneal procedures (radial keratotomy, lamellar inserts)
- Laser photoablation surgery

Pterygium or other disorders involving the optical center of the cornea

Donors for ALK

Criteria are the same as those listed for PK, except that tissue with local eye disease affecting the corneal endothelium or previous ocular surgery that does not compromise the corneal stroma can be used.

Donors for EK

Criteria are the same as those listed for PK, except that tissue with noninfectious anterior pathology that does not affect the posterior stroma and endothelium is acceptable.

ALK = anterior lamellar keratoplasty; CJD = Creutzfeldt-Jakob disease; EK; endothelial keratoplasty; HBsAg = hepatitis B surface antigen; HCV = hepatitis C virus; LASIK = laser in situ keratomileusis; PK = penetrating keratoplasty; PRK = photorefractive keratectomy.

Data from the Eye Bank Association of America (EBAA). *EBAA Medical Standards, June 2021.* EBAA; 2021.

Table 16-4 Disease Transmission From Corneal Transplantation

Proven disease transmission from corneal transplantation
Rabies
Hepatitis B
Creutzfeldt-Jakob disease (previously diagnosed)
Retinoblastoma
Bacterial or fungal keratitis
Bacterial or fungal endophthalmitis
Potential disease transmission from corneal transplantation[a]
Hepatitis C virus infection
Herpes simplex virus infection
HIV (types 1 and 2) infection
West Nile virus
Zika virus
Prion diseases

[a] Other diseases that contraindicate donor-cornea use and that could be transmitted via corneal transplantation are listed in Table 16-3.

Data from the Eye Bank Association of America (EBAA). *EBAA Medical Standards, June 2021.* EBAA; 2021.

Transplantation for the Treatment of Corneal Disease

Ophthalmologists have many options for surgically treating the wide spectrum of corneal disease. The procedure of choice depends primarily on the depth and extent of corneal pathology (Table 16-5). Discussion of the surgical technique for these procedures is beyond the scope of this book; however, many excellent resources are listed in the references provided throughout this chapter (also see the videos in this chapter).

Table 16-5 Layer-Based Approach to the Surgical Management of Corneal Opacities and Edema

Layer of Pathology	Representative Disease	ED	SK	PTK	ALK	EK	PK	DSO
Epithelium	Redundant, irregular epithelium	•						
Subepithelial layer	Epithelial (anterior) basement membrane dystrophy	•						
	Salzmann nodular degeneration	•	•					
Bowman layer	Band keratopathy	•	•	•				
	Reis-Bücklers dystrophy		•	•	•			
Anterior–midstroma	Granular corneal dystrophy		•	•	•		•	
Midposterior stroma	Scarring				•		•	
Endothelium						•	•	•

ALK = anterior lamellar keratoplasty; DSO = Descemet stripping only; ED = epithelial debridement; EK = endothelial keratoplasty; PK = penetrating keratoplasty; PTK = phototherapeutic keratectomy; SK = superficial keratectomy.

From American Academy of Ophthalmology Cornea/External Disease Panel. Preferred Practice Pattern Guidelines. *Corneal Edema and Opacification.* American Academy of Ophthalmology; 2018. www.aao.org/ppp

Hausheer JR, ed. *Basic Techniques of Ophthalmic Surgery.* 3rd ed. American Academy of Ophthalmology; 2019.

Mannis MJ, Holland EJ, eds. *Cornea.* Vol 2. 5th ed. Elsevier; 2022.

Preoperative Evaluation and Preparation of the Transplant Patient

A complete ophthalmic evaluation, including a history (see sidebar) and examination, is necessary before considering corneal transplantation. It is important to obtain a detailed social history to help determine whether the patient or caretakers can adhere to the potentially complex postoperative treatment regimen.

FACTORS OBTAINED IN HISTORY THAT IMPACT KERATOPLASTY OUTCOME

History can reveal important considerations, including

- conditions that could affect vision prognosis and decision to operate, namely
  - amblyopia
  - macular degeneration
  - glaucoma or other optic neuropathy
  - macular edema
- risk factors for rejection such as
  - young age
  - prior rejection
  - multiple prior grafts
  - stromal vascularization
  - large diameter graft required
- prior herpes simplex or herpes zoster ocular involvement, which may result in
  - reduced corneal sensation
  - likelihood of recurrent disease
- prior trabeculectomy or tube shunt surgery, which
  - reduces endothelial cell survival
  - increases the risk of graft failure
  - makes EK (especially DMEK) technically more difficult
- Prior vitrectomy, which makes DMEK technically much more difficult

Examination begins with an assessment of vision and of vision potential. Overrefraction with a rigid contact lens can aid in determining the cause of decreased vision. Improvement in visual acuity with the contact lens indicates the impact of superficial irregular astigmatism on vision (see Chapters 2 and 8 for further discussion of contact lens use). If improved, the patient can be offered treatment with a rigid scleral or corneal contact lens rather than surgery. In patients with a clouded cornea, simple clinical tests, such as checking color vision,

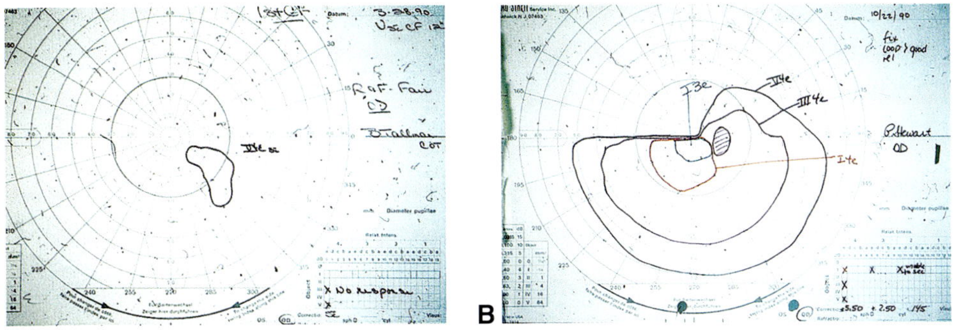

Figure 16-1 Opacities such as corneal edema and cataract can dramatically reduce the visual field. **A,** Goldmann visual field OD in a 78-year-old glaucoma patient with decompensated Fuchs endothelial corneal dystrophy and cataract. **B,** Visual field OD in the same patient 7 months after combined keratoplasty and cataract extraction with intraocular lens (IOL) insertion. *(Courtesy of Robert S. Feder, MD.)*

light projection, entoptic phenomenon, and afferent pupillary defect (ie, reverse Marcus-Gunn pupil), may reveal additional conditions contributing to visual disability. Visual fields in patients with corneal and lens opacities are often dramatically constricted (Fig 16-1). Prior to considering PK, DALK, ALK, or another corneal procedure, it is important to check for reduced corneal sensation.

Preexisting external eye conditions that may compromise corneal transplant healing and maintenance should be identified and controlled or corrected, if possible, prior to surgery. Conditions that compromise the ocular surface include dry eye disease, corneal hypoesthesia, acne rosacea, blepharitis, lagophthalmos, trichiasis, and abnormalities of eyelid position, and likely will require continued care even after surgery.

A careful slit-lamp examination is a critical step in the evaluation process. In some patients, extensive guttae alone may cause enough reduction in vision or symptoms of glare to warrant surgery. Subtle stromal edema can be seen at the slit lamp and can be measured with ultrasonic pachymetry, Scheimpflug imaging, or anterior segment optical coherence tomography (OCT). (See Chapter 2 for discussion of these tests.) Typically, corneal edema is worse in the morning and improves throughout the day. Diurnal fluctuation can be either documented by testing in the early morning and in the afternoon or simulated by having patients close their eyes for 30 minutes followed by repeat pachymetry and a slit-lamp examination. The presence of peripheral anterior synechiae, large iris defects, or cataract may impact the surgical approach. The presence of active keratitis or uveitis at the time of surgery is associated with a higher incidence of postoperative complications, such as graft rejection or failure, glaucoma, and cystoid macular edema. Ideally, there should be no ocular inflammation for several months prior to surgery.

It is important to measure intraocular pressure (IOP). If possible, hypotony or elevated IOP should be normalized prior to considering intraocular surgery. Poorly controlled glaucoma reduces endothelial cell survival and increases the risk of graft failure. Postoperative corticosteroid use may affect IOP.

Additional testing such as OCT imaging may help detect retinal problems such as macular edema (cystoid or diabetic), epiretinal membrane, or age-related macular degeneration. If the media are completely opaque, B-scan ultrasonography can help rule out a retinal detachment or mass lesion.

American Academy of Ophthalmology Cornea/External Disease Panel. Preferred Practice Pattern Guidelines. *Corneal Edema and Opacification.* American Academy of Ophthalmology; 2018. www.aao.org/ppp

Hannush SB, Riveroll-Hannush L. Preoperative considerations and decision-making in keratoplasty. In: Mannis MJ, Holland EJ. eds. *Cornea.* Vol 2. 5th ed. Elsevier; 2022:1155–1161.

Watanabe S, Oie Y, Fujimoto H, et al. Relationship between corneal guttae and quality of vision in patients with mild Fuchs endothelial corneal dystrophy. *Ophthalmology.* 2015;122(10):2103–2109.

Penetrating Keratoplasty

The most common indications for PK are

- keratoconus (although DALK is often a better option)
- combined stromal and endothelial pathology (Video 16-1)
- graft failure (EK is preferred for endothelial graft failure)
- corneal opacity with concomitant intraocular lens (IOL) exchange, implantation or manipulation and/or anterior segment reconstruction (Video 16-2)

VIDEO 16-1 Penetrating keratoplasty (PK) for stromal scarring and endothelial dysfunction in congenital hereditary endothelial dystrophy.
Courtesy of Robert W. Weisenthal, MD.

VIDEO 16-2 PK with scleral-sutured intraocular lens (IOL) using an open-sky approach.
Courtesy of Robert W. Weisenthal, MD.

Therapeutic PK may be performed to restore the structural integrity of the eye or to resolve an infectious or inflammatory keratitis that is refractory to conventional medical therapy.

To educate the patient about the risks and benefits of corneal transplant surgery, the surgeon must understand potential intraoperative and postoperative complications, as well as postoperative management; these are summarized in Table 16-6 and discussed in the following subsections.

Chan CC, Perez MA, Verdier DD. Penetrating keratoplasty: the fundamentals. In: Mannis MJ, Holland EJ, eds. *Cornea.* Vol 2. 5th ed. Elsevier; 2022:1162–1173.

Verdier DD, Rosenberg ED, Donnenfeld ED. Therapeutic keratoplasty. In: Mannis MJ, Holland EJ, eds. *Cornea.* Vol 2. 5th ed. Elsevier; 2022:1431–1444.

Table 16-6 **Comparison of Procedures for Penetrating and Selective Lamellar Keratoplasty**

	Penetrating Keratoplasty (PK)	Anterior Lamellar/Deep Anterior Lamellar Keratoplasty (ALK/DALK)	Descemet Stripping/Membrane Endothelial Keratoplasty (DSEK/DMEK)
Indications	Combined stromal and endothelial pathology Diseased cornea precludes adequate view for performing endothelial keratoplasty (EK) or combined anterior segment reconstruction or intraocular lens (IOL) positioning or exchange Stromal pathology (ALK usually preferred) Endothelial pathology (EK usually preferred) Infection extending to deep corneal stroma or endothelium, or EK interface infection	Stromal pathology not involving endothelium (unless very focal endothelial involvement, eg, descemetocele or localized scar) Combined epithelial and/or anterior basement membrane and stromal pathology	Corneal pathology primarily attributed to endothelial disease
Intraoperative complications	Expulsive or choroidal hemorrhage Excessive posterior pressure with extrusion of lens and/or vitreous Damage to iris or lens Damage to donor endothelium Excessive bleeding from iris or wound edge Scleral perforation with fixation sutures Irregular trephination Poor graft centration Iris or vitreous incarceration in the wound Retinal tear or detachment	Corneal perforation; may require transition to PK Irregular dissection of host stromal tissue Poor microkeratome dissection for donor tissue Double (pseudo-) anterior chamber or Descemet membrane detachment Placement of air bubble to tamponade Descemet membrane can cause formation of an anterior subcapsular cataract	Poor microkeratome dissection of donor tissue (DSEK) or inability to harvest Descemet membrane with endothelium (DMEK) Inability to strip host Descemet tissue Excessive manipulation of donor tissue, leading to cell loss and possible graft failure Improper orientation or loss of donor tissue Tearing of donor tissue Anterior chamber hemorrhage or fibrin formation compromising graft unfolding and placement Vitreous or blood in the interface Choroidal hemorrhage (lower risk than PK)

(Continued)

Table 16-6 *(continued)*

	Penetrating Keratoplasty (PK)	Anterior Lamellar/Deep Anterior Lamellar Keratoplasty (ALK/DALK)	Descemet Stripping/Membrane Endothelial Keratoplasty (DSEK/DMEK)
Postoperative complications	Wound leak/misalignment Flat chamber Persistent epithelial defect Suture-related problems Neovascularization Elevated intraocular pressure/glaucoma Graft rejection Graft failure Infectious keratitis Endophthalmitis Cystoid macular edema Recurrent primary disease Ruptured globe	Persistent epithelial defect Suture-related problems Neovascularization Retained interface debris Opacification and/or vascularization of the interface Visually significant wrinkling of the interface or Descemet membrane Graft rejection (stromal or epithelial) Graft failure Inflammatory necrosis of the graft Infectious keratitis Epithelial ingrowth Recurrent primary disease	Dislocated or decentered lenticule Pupillary block glaucoma Primary graft failure (usually iatrogenic) Interface opacification Interface infection Graft rejection (lower risk than PK) Graft failure Epithelial ingrowth Glaucoma Cystoid macular edema
Advantages	Full-thickness tissue eliminates interface-related visual problems. Ability to treat epithelial, stromal, and endothelial disease and allow anterior segment reconstruction in a single procedure if necessary	Selective removal of pathological tissue Reduced risk of penetration of anterior chamber Less chance of graft rejection without donor endothelium, allowing more flexibility in dose and duration of postoperative steroid prophylaxis Lower risk of ruptured globe compared to PK Preservation of globe integrity due to stronger wound than in PK Less risk of intraoperative choroidal hemorrhage Minimal requirements for donor tissue Less risk for patients who do not adhere to treatment or rub their eyes	Selective removal of pathological tissue Rapid vision rehabilitation Reduction in suture-related problems Less induced astigmatism, less refractive shift than with PK or ALK/DALK Greater accuracy in selection of IOL for combined transplant/lens procedures Reduced incidence of graft rejection (DMEK < DSEK < ALK/DALK < PK) Preservation of ocular surface and corneal sensation Smaller incision with preservation of globe integrity

	Penetrating Keratoplasty (PK)	Anterior Lamellar/Deep Anterior Lamellar Keratoplasty (ALK/DALK)	Descemet Stripping/Membrane Endothelial Keratoplasty (DSEK/DMEK)
Disadvantages	Irregular and/or high corneal astigmatism and refractive error Difficulty controlling anterior corneal curvature, potentially leading to anisometropia Ocular surface disease or neurotrophic cornea leads to prolonged healing or persistent epithelial defect.	Irregular and/or high corneal astigmatism and refractive error Difficulty determining anterior corneal curvature, potentially leading to anisometropia Ocular surface disease or neurotrophic cornea leads to prolonged healing or persistent epithelial defect. Stromal opacification/interface debris Irregular interface Procedure more technically demanding and time-consuming	Increased risk of primary graft failure, especially during surgical learning curve Significant stromal haze, subepithelial fibrosis, or epithelial irregularity may require second procedure.

Intraoperative Complications

Complications that can occur during surgery are listed in Table 16-6.

Chen MC, Mannis MJ. Intraoperative complications of penetrating keratoplasty. In: Mannis MJ, Holland EJ, eds. *Cornea.* Vol 2. 5th ed. Elsevier; 2022:1174–1179.

Postoperative Care and Complications

The long-term success of a PK procedure depends on appropriate postoperative management and conscientious patient adherence. Routine postsurgical care includes short-term use of topical antibiotics and a prolonged, perhaps indefinite, course of topical corticosteroids (prednisolone, difluprednate ophthalmic emulsion 0.05%, or fluorometholone 0.25% or 0.1%). Frequent office visits are necessary to facilitate rapid vision rehabilitation and early recognition of the many complications that can occur after PK. The following subsections review some common postsurgical complications.

Penetrating keratoplasty: postoperative management. In: Mannis MJ, Holland EJ, eds. *Cornea.* Vol 2. 5th ed. Elsevier; 2022:1187–1241.

Primary donor failure (primary endothelial failure)

When a graft is edematous from the first postoperative day and remains so without inflammatory signs, the reason may be a deficiency of donor endothelium (Fig 16-2). Most surgeons allow at least 4 weeks and up to 2 months for spontaneous resolution of edema before considering regrafting. The cause of the donor failure is not always clear and may be related to intraoperative handling of the tissue.

Wound misalignment or leak

The wound is always checked carefully for aqueous leakage at the end of surgery. A Seidel test can be helpful postoperatively in assessing wound integrity, particularly in patients with low IOP and a normal or shallow anterior chamber. Small wound leaks or suture track leaks without iris incarceration often close spontaneously. Patching, therapeutic contact lenses,

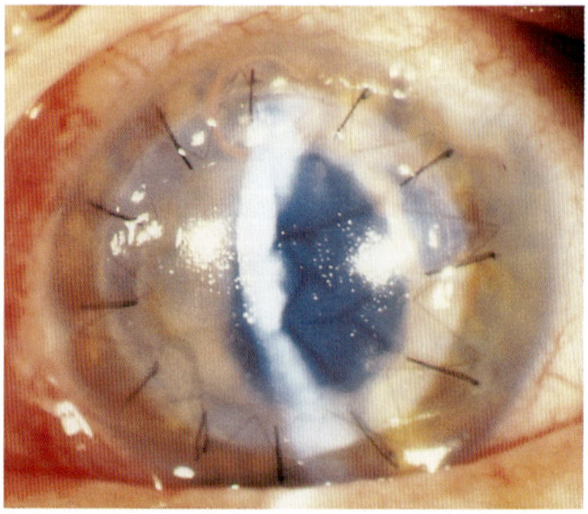

Figure 16-2 Slit-lamp photograph showing primary donor failure after penetrating keratoplasty (PK).

and use of aqueous suppressants may facilitate a watertight seal. Resuturing is advised for leaks associated with a shallow anterior chamber and low IOP lasting longer than 3 days.

Flat chamber or iris incarceration in the wound

If the IOP is low and there is a flat chamber or iris incarceration in the wound, it is best to reposit the iris, re-form the anterior chamber, and suture the wound in the operating room. If the problem is not addressed promptly and appropriately, anterior synechiae may form, increasing the risk of graft rejection, glaucoma, or graft failure. Normal or high IOP with a shallow or flat anterior chamber may signify pupillary block or malignant glaucoma (aqueous misdirection). Initially, dilation of the pupil may help break the pupillary block; if this is not successful, other measures are required. See BCSC Section 10, *Glaucoma,* for discussion of pupillary block and malignant glaucoma.

Endophthalmitis

Postoperative endophthalmitis may result from intraoperative contamination, contamination of the donor corneal button, or persistent wound leak with invasion of microorganisms. The incidence of endophthalmitis is considerably higher in PK patients than in cataract surgery patients, particularly if the vitreous is invaded or if the donor died of infection. Immunosuppressed patients with moderate to severe eyelid inflammation are also at greater risk for infection. Early recognition and aggressive intervention can save the eye and possibly preserve vision in some cases. Donor rim culture may identify any potential contaminants. A rim culture positive for fungus is associated with endophthalmitis in 3% of recipients and in the case of a positive bacterial rim culture, the risk is 1%. See also BCSC Section 9, *Uveitis and Ocular Inflammation.*

Borkar DS, Wibbelsman TD, Buch PM, et al. Endophthalmitis rates and clinical outcomes following penetrating and endothelial keratoplasty. *Am J Ophthalmol.* 2019;205:82–90.

Chen JY, Jones MN, Srinivasan S, Neal TJ, Armitage WJ, Kaye SB; NHSBT Ocular Tissue Advisory Group and Contributing Ophthalmologists (OTAG Audit Study 18). Endophthalmitis after penetrating keratoplasty. *Ophthalmology.* 2015;122(1):25–30.

Persistent epithelial defect

Large epithelial defects are common after PK, but they generally heal within 7–14 days. After this time, irreversible scarring and ulceration may occur. Patients who have reduced corneal sensation or decreased blink rate before surgery are at greater risk. It is important to appropriately manage ocular surface disease that contributes to the nonhealing epithelial defect (eg, dry eye, exposure, acne rosacea, blepharitis, or abnormal eyelid position). Lubrication, punctal occlusion with plugs or cautery, patching, or therapeutic bandage soft lenses represents the first line of treatment. Amniotic membrane graft and temporary or permanent lateral tarsorrhaphy may be helpful in difficult cases. (See the sections on neurotrophic keratopathy and persistent epithelial defects in Chapter 4 and tarsorrhaphy in Chapter 5.) If these measures are not successful, the diagnosis of herpetic keratitis should be considered even if this was not the underlying reason for the graft. Oral antivirals can be used as a therapeutic trial.

Elevated intraocular pressure

Routine measurement of IOP and evaluation of the optic nerve head for cupping is an important part of postoperative care. High IOP may occur at any time after PK. Often, the first clinical sign is the loss of folds in Descemet membrane. IOP elevation early in the postoperative period can be due to pupillary block, aqueous misdirection, hemorrhage or pigment blocking the trabecular meshwork, or an overly tight running suture. Elevated IOP starting within 1 month postoperatively may be due to a corticosteroid response. The onset of high IOP can occur many months or even years after uncomplicated use of topical corticosteroid. If glaucoma develops, aggressive treatment with appropriate topical medications, laser surgery, or other surgical intervention is indicated. Though uncommon, epithelial downgrowth or fibrous ingrowth can also cause postoperative pressure elevation. (See BCSC Section 10, *Glaucoma.*)

Recurrence of primary disease

Bacterial, fungal, viral, or amebic keratitis can recur in a graft in the early postoperative period. Herpetic keratitis can recur at any time (Fig 16-3). In recurrent infections, medical treatment directed at the causative agent is the initial form of therapy (see Chapters 11 and 12). With regard to topical corticosteroid use, management of infection must be balanced against the risk of rejection. Typically, the frequency or potency is significantly reduced in an effort to control the infection. In the case of herpes simplex, fungal, or amebic disease, topical corticosteroids are likely to potentiate the infection. Epithelial–stromal dystrophies such as granular or lattice dystrophy can recur in the superficial cornea up to a year or more after the initial procedure (Fig 16-4; also see Chapter 8). Dystrophic recurrence in the superficial stroma can be treated with phototherapeutic keratectomy (PTK); see Chapter 5.

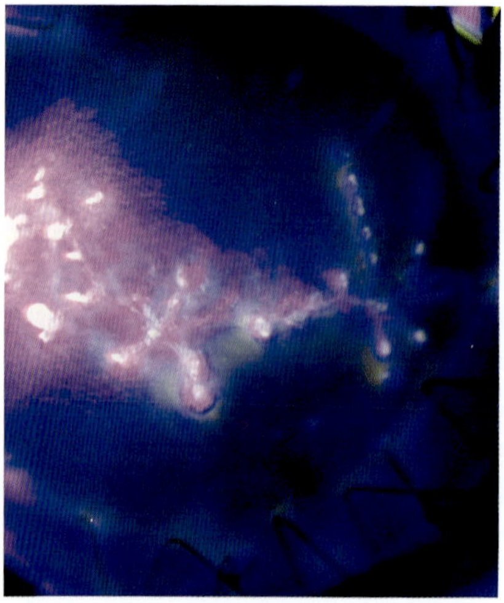

Figure 16-3 Slit-lamp photograph shows recurrence of herpes simplex keratitis in a graft. *(Courtesy of Robert W. Weisenthal, MD.)*

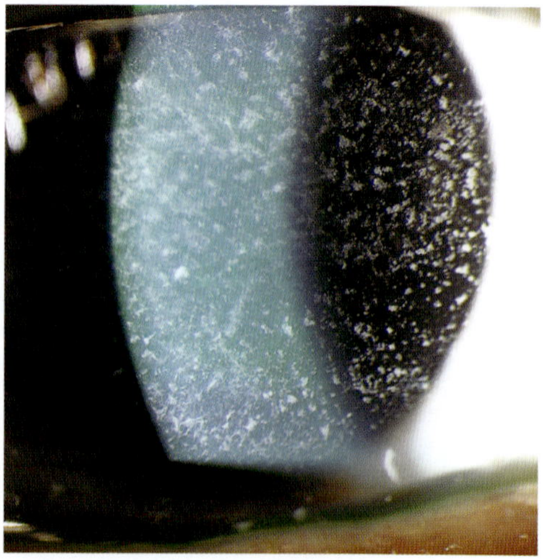

Figure 16-4 Slit-lamp photograph shows recurrence of granular corneal dystrophy after corneal transplantation. *(Courtesy of Robert W. Weisenthal, MD.)*

Suture-related problems

Postoperative problems related to sutures that may necessitate removal include

- excessive tightness, producing an irregular astigmatism or elevated IOP
- loosening (usually as a result of wound contraction, suture breakage, resolution of wound edema, or suture cheese-wiring; Fig 16-5)
- broken interrupted or continuous suture
- infectious abscesses (usually localized around loose, broken, or exposed sutures; Fig 16-6)
- noninfectious (toxic) suture infiltrates, often multiple and in areas of pannus, or extension of sutures beyond the limbus
- giant papillary conjunctivitis from exposed knots
- vascularization along suture tracks

Loose or broken sutures do not contribute to wound stability and should be removed as soon as possible. Loose sutures stain with fluorescein because they usually have broken through the corneal epithelium. For this reason, the application of topical fluorescein and inspection of the suture integrity is an important part of routine postoperative examination. Decolorizing nylon sutures are a signal that the sutures may soon break. Retained intrastromal suture fragments may be left in place. Vascularization along the suture indicates that the wound is adequately healed in that area and that sutures may safely be removed. Vascularized sutures are also prone to loosening and may increase the likelihood of graft rejection. After the sutures are removed, the refractive error or astigmatism may shift dramatically, so it is important that the surgeon see the patient in 3–4 weeks to ensure wound stability and to recheck refraction. The shift may occur even when sutures are removed years after surgery. Suture removal within the first few weeks of surgery may need to be replaced to avoid wound leak or marked astigmatism.

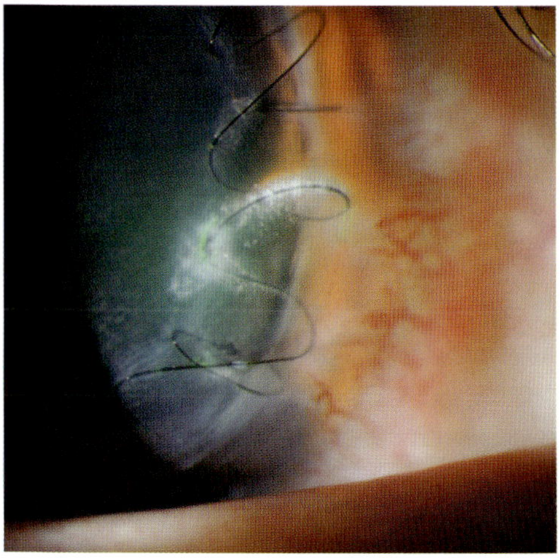

Figure 16-5 Slit-lamp photograph of an eroded continuous suture after PK. *(Courtesy of Robert W. Weisenthal, MD)*

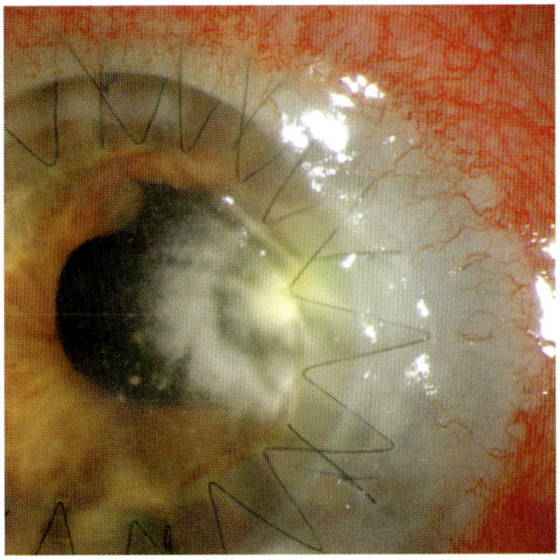

Figure 16-6 Slit-lamp photograph of a suture abscess in a corneal graft. *(Courtesy of Stephen E. Orlin, MD.)*

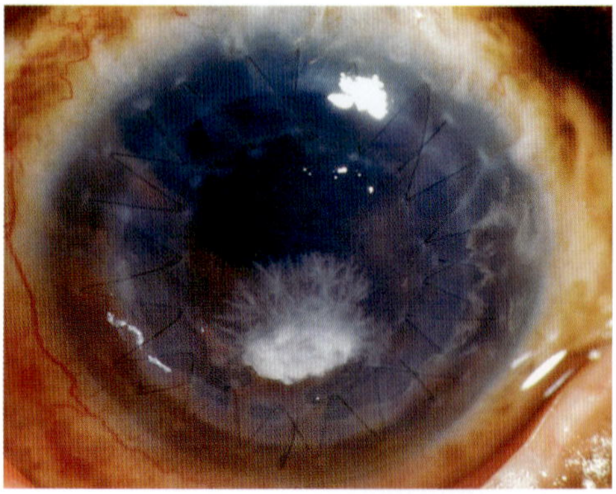

Figure 16-7 Slit-lamp photograph showing infectious crystalline keratopathy after PK. *(Courtesy of Stephen E. Orlin, MD.)*

Microbial keratitis

The following factors predispose the patient to infectious keratitis sometimes caused by unusual organisms:

- long-term use of topical corticosteroids
- loss of corneal sensation after transplantation
- uneven tear film
- suture exposure or erosion
- systemic immunosuppression

Culture of the infiltrate and the exposed suture is recommended, and initiation of broad-spectrum antibiotic therapy can help avoid graft failure. A peculiar form of keratitis, infectious crystalline keratopathy (Fig 16-7; also see Chapter 12), is occasionally observed in grafts and other immunocompromised corneas. Branching colonies of organisms proliferate in the deep corneal stroma, with minimal or no inflammatory response. Many organisms have been implicated, but viridans streptococci are the most frequent causative organism.

Late non–immune-mediated endothelial failure

In the absence of acute inflammation or graft rejection, visually significant corneal edema months to years after the procedure may be due to the normal attrition of endothelial cells, which occurs at a rate 4 times greater than in nontransplanted corneas. In the CDS, median endothelial cell density decreased by 70% over the first 5 years following transplantation; by 10 years, it had decreased by 76%. The CDS showed that the 10-year cumulative probability of non–immune-mediated graft failure was higher in patients treated for pseudophakic or aphakic corneal edema than in patients treated for Fuchs endothelial corneal dystrophy (FECD). The higher failure rate may be related to the placement of a poorly designed anterior chamber lens or improper placement of the lens during previous, complex cataract surgery. Such problems may require an exchange of the IOL at the time of PK. In addition, patients with a prior diagnosis of glaucoma—especially those with a history of glaucoma surgery (particularly tube shunt surgery) and, to a lesser extent, those taking glaucoma medications—face a higher probability of graft failure than do patients who have no history of glaucoma.

Bourne WM. Biology of the corneal endothelium in health and disease. *Eye (Lond).* 2003;17(8):912–918.

Lass JH, Benetz BA, Gal RL, et al; Writing Committee for the Cornea Donor Study Research Group. Donor age and factors related to endothelial cell loss 10 years after penetrating keratoplasty. *Ophthalmology.* 2013;120(12):2428–2435.

Sugar A, Gal RL, Kollman C, et al; Writing Committee for the Cornea Donor Study Research Group. Factors associated with corneal graft survival in the Cornea Donor Study. *JAMA Ophthalmol.* 2015;133(3):246–254.

Graft rejection

Corneal allograft rejection rarely occurs within the first month; however, it may occur many years after PK.

CLINICAL PEARL

Prompt recognition and treatment of rejection is critical as ongoing endothelial rejection causes irretrievable endothelial cell loss.

At each visit, it is important to review with the patient the symptoms of graft rejection, which may include pain, redness, photophobia, and decreased vision. Office staff can be trained in how to respond if a keratoplasty patient calls with these symptoms. Most episodes of graft rejection do not cause irreversible graft failure if recognized early and treated aggressively with corticosteroids.

Corneal transplant rejection after PK occurs in 4 distinct clinical forms, which may occur either singly or in combination (Table 16-7). (See BCSC Section 9, *Uveitis and Ocular Inflammation.*)

Epithelial rejection The immune response may be directed entirely at the donor epithelium (Fig 16-8). Lymphocytes cause an elevated, linear epithelial ridge that advances centripetally. Because host cells replace lost donor epithelium, this form of rejection is problematic only in that in occasional cases it may herald the onset of endothelial rejection. Epithelial rejection occurs in a minority of patients experiencing rejection and is usually seen early in the postoperative period. It may be asymptomatic; however, blurred vision can occur if the epithelial ridge is near the visual axis. The donor epithelium is ultimately replaced by the host epithelium.

Subepithelial rejection Corneal transplant rejection may also present as subepithelial infiltrates (Fig 16-9). These may be asymptomatic or may cause glare or reduced vision. It is not known whether these lymphocytic cells are directed at donor keratocytes or at donor epithelial cells.

Easily missed on cursory examination, subepithelial infiltrates can best be seen with broad, oblique illumination. They resemble the infiltrates associated with adenoviral keratoconjunctivitis but are confined to the donor graft. Subepithelial graft rejection may completely resolve if treated, but not uncommonly it may presage the more severe endothelial graft rejection.

Table 16-7 Corneal Transplant Rejection Types and Treatment

Rejection type	Signs and Symptoms	Treatment	Comments
All types	Possible pain/photophobia Injection Decreased vision	Topical corticosteroids Consider if severe or inadequate response: oral, periocular, or intravenous (IV) corticosteroids; topical tacrolimus	Treat promptly and aggressively to avoid endothelial cell loss Remove loose sutures that can trigger rejection
Epithelial	Epithelial rejection line Epithelial haze, defects Blurred vision or photophobia if approaching visual axis	Corticosteroid eyedrops 4 times daily Adjust per response	Self-limited donor epithelium is usually replaced by the host Typically has a benign course
Subepithelial	Subepithelial infiltrates confined to graft Blurred vision or photophobia if near visual axis	Corticosteroid eyedrops 4–8 times daily Adjust per response	May be a harbinger of stromal or endothelial rejection May require maintenance topical corticosteroid
Stromal	Stromal haze/infiltrates Stromal edema Stromal neovascularization Stromal necrosis Anterior chamber cell and flare Redness and pain	Corticosteroid eyedrops every 1–2 hours Adjust per severity and response Consider oral corticosteroids, topical tacrolimus	May accompany or progress to endothelial rejection Close observation Likely will require maintenance topical corticosteroid
Endothelial	Keratic precipitates confined to graft Anterior chamber cell and flare, typically mild Stromal edema Epithelial edema Blurred vision, redness, and pain	Corticosteroid eyedrops every 1–2 hours Adjust per severity and response Consider oral and/or IV corticosteroids, topical tacrolimus Consider periocular corticosteroid injection, unless patient is a steroid responder or has history of herpes simplex or other recent infection	Irreversible endothelial cell loss increases with rejection severity and chronicity Close observation Likely will require maintenance topical corticosteroids

Stromal rejection Isolated stromal rejection is not common after PK; it is seen more commonly after DALK. It may present as stromal infiltrates, neovascularization, or noninfiltrative keratolysis within the graft–host interface that does not extend into the peripheral recipient stroma. In severe or prolonged episodes of stromal rejection, the cornea can become necrotic. Stromal rejection may be accompanied or followed by endothelial rejection and is treated in a similar fashion.

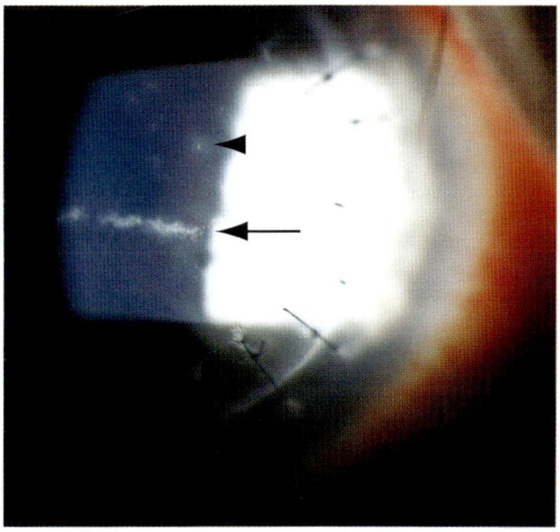

Figure 16-8 Slit-lamp photograph shows an epithelial rejection line *(arrow)* with subepithelial infiltrates *(arrowhead)* after PK. *(Courtesy of Robert W. Weisenthal, MD.)*

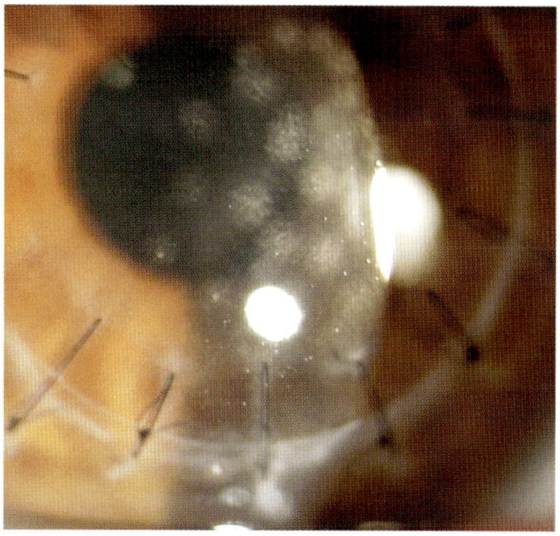

Figure 16-9 Slit-lamp photograph shows corneal graft rejection manifested by subepithelial infiltrates. *(Courtesy of Charles S. Bouchard, MD.)*

Endothelial rejection The most common and serious form of graft rejection is endothelial rejection, because loss of a significant number of endothelial cells leads to graft failure. Inflammatory precipitates are seen on the endothelial surface in fine precipitates, in random clumps, or in linear form underlying or in some cases delineating the area of corneal edema (Khodadoust line; Fig 16-10). Inflammatory cells are usually present in the anterior chamber as well, but anterior uveitis is generally mild. As endothelial function is lost, the corneal stroma thickens with the development of posterior folds, and microcystic or bullous epithelial edema can occur. Patients have symptoms related to inflammation and corneal edema, such as photophobia, redness, irritation, halos around lights, or fogginess of vision.

TREATMENT Frequent administration of corticosteroid eyedrops is the mainstay of therapy for corneal allograft rejection. Prednisolone acetate 1%, dexamethasone 0.1%, or difluprednate ophthalmic emulsion 0.05% eyedrops are used, as often as every hour, depending on the severity of the episode. Close follow-up to monitor for increased IOP is recommended, especially with difluprednate. For steroid responders or recalcitrant rejections, topical tacrolimus ointment 0.03% (Protopic dermatologic) twice per day may be beneficial and is likely more effective than topical cyclosporine drops 4 times per day. For eyes with active herpes simplex epithelial keratitis, oral corticosteroids can be considered, rather than topical corticosteroids; although topical corticosteroid ointment may be used on occasion, the reduced bioavailability of ointment renders it less effective than frequently applied eyedrops.

In cases of endothelial rejection with edema, the use of systemic corticosteroids is recommended either orally (prednisone 60 mg per day, tapered as the graft rejection responds) or intravenously (a 1-time dose of 125–500 mg methylprednisolone), in addition

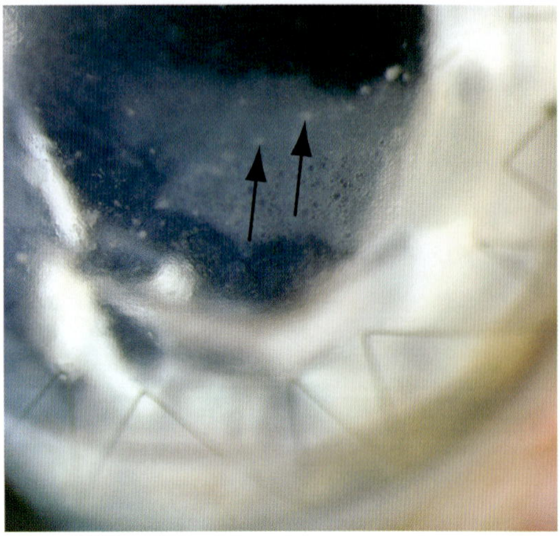

Figure 16-10 Slit-lamp photograph showing corneal endothelial graft rejection with epithelial and stromal edema. Note the Khodadoust line *(arrows)*. *(Courtesy of Robert W. Weisenthal, MD.)*

to topical treatment. Periocular injection of triamcinolone acetonide 0.5 cc of 40 mg/mL or dexamethasone 0.5 cc of 4 mg/mL is recommended for severe rejection episodes or nonadherent patients. Caution is advised in patients who may have steroid-induced elevation of IOP or a history of herpetic keratitis.

Brooks CC, Gupta PK. Diagnosis and management of corneal allograft rejection. In: Mannis MJ, Holland EJ, eds. *Cornea*. Vol 2. 5th ed. Elsevier; 2022:1207–1214.

Hashemian MN, Latifi G, Ghaffari R, et al. Topical tacrolimus as adjuvant therapy to corticosteroids in acute endothelial graft rejection after penetrating keratoplasty: a randomized controlled trial. *Cornea*. 2018;37(3):307–312.

Prevention of graft rejection According to a survey of members of the Cornea Society, prednisolone acetate 1% is the topical corticosteroid of choice for prophylaxis against graft rejection, with dexamethasone as another option. Difluprednate is usually reserved for eyes at high risk of rejection. Loteprednol or fluorometholone may be preferable for steroid responders or phakic eyes. In low-risk cases, the dosage is typically 4 times per day for 3 months; it is then tapered by 1 drop each month until it has been reduced to once per day. If no rejection episodes occur in the first 6 to 12 months, the patient can be switched from prednisolone 1% to fluorometholone 0.1% or loteprednol 0.2%, which reduces the risk of corticosteroid-related complications. The phakic patient may be tapered off corticosteroids or maintained on one of low concentration to minimize the risk of cataract. The pseudophakic or aphakic patient is typically kept on a once-daily steroid regimen. Patients using steroids should continue to be followed for IOP elevation.

In high-risk cases, the use of various immunosuppressive agents, including oral cyclosporine, tacrolimus, and mycophenolate mofetil, has been reported, but these medications require very careful follow-up because of their narrow therapeutic index. Topical tacrolimus has been advocated for use in high-risk patients.

Surgical techniques that avoid proximity to the peripheral cornea and early attention to loosening sutures and infections will minimize the risk of rejection.

Anshu A, Price MO, Price FW Jr. Risk of corneal transplant rejection significantly reduced with Descemet's membrane endothelial keratoplasty. *Ophthalmology*. 2012;119(3):536–540.

Kharod-Dholakia B, Randleman JB, Bromley JG, Stulting RD. Prevention and treatment of corneal graft rejection: current practice patterns of the Cornea Society (2011). *Cornea*. 2015;34(6):609–614.

Magalhaes OA, Marinho DR, Kwitko S. Topical 0.03% tacrolimus preventing rejection in high-risk corneal transplantation: a cohort study. *Br J Ophthalmol*. 2013;97(11):1395–1398.

Ruptured globe

CLINICAL PEARL

Ruptured globe is the most serious postoperative complication of PK, and it remains a lifetime threat in these patients. The scar that forms between graft and host is never as strong as the original corneal tissue. Traumatic wound dehiscence occurs in 5% of eyes following PK, with a visual acuity outcome of 20/200 or worse in the majority of cases.

Patient education includes a discussion of the need for eye protection and lifetime avoidance of activities that present a high risk of ocular trauma.

Elder MJ, Stack RR. Globe rupture following penetrating keratoplasty: How often, why, and what can we do to prevent it? *Cornea*. 2004;23(8):776–780.

Renucci AM, Marangon FB, Culbertson WW. Wound dehiscence after penetrating keratoplasty: clinical characteristics of 51 cases treated at Bascom Palmer Eye Institute. *Cornea*. 2006;25(5):524–529.

Control of Postoperative Corneal Astigmatism and Refractive Error

Keratoplasty success is measured by the achievement of corneal clarity and functional refractive outcome. Severe astigmatism may be associated with decreased visual acuity, anisometropia, aniseikonia, image distortion, and monocular diplopia, rendering an otherwise clear graft poorly functional. In children, visually significant complications or astigmatism may lead to amblyopia.

See the sidebar for methods to reduce corneal astigmatism. Postoperatively, the primary method of reducing astigmatism is to readjust or remove the sutures. However, in addition to suture manipulation, it is essential to optimize the condition of the ocular surface. If a single continuous suture has been placed, the surgeon may redistribute the suture tension at 1 month postoperatively, using corneal topography as a guide. Alternatively, if there is a combination of continuous and interrupted sutures, the interrupted sutures can be removed starting at 1 month (Fig 16-11). If the patient has only interrupted sutures, suture removal should begin at a later stage (eg, ≥3 months) to avoid wound disruption. Clinicians must be cognizant of the slower wound healing in older patients on long-term topical corticosteroid therapy.

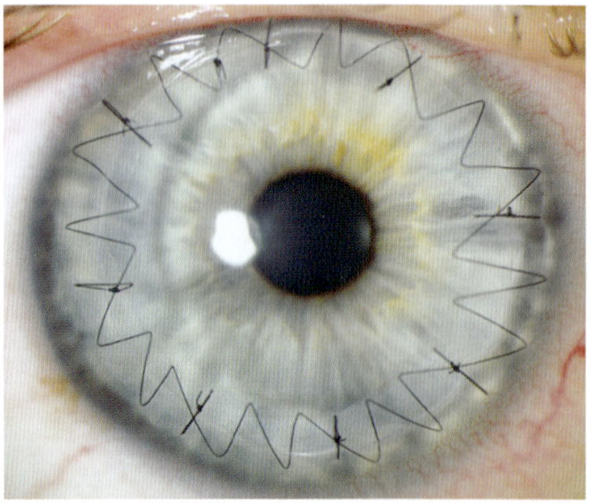

Figure 16-11 Slit-lamp photograph of a full-thickness corneal transplant with interrupted and continuous 10-0 nylon sutures. The interrupted sutures can be removed to control astigmatism. *(Courtesy of Robert W. Weisenthal, MD.)*

SUGGESTED METHODS TO REDUCE CORNEAL ASTIGMATISM

- modification of suturing technique to optimize suture tension
- intraoperative suture adjustments with qualitative keratometry
- improved trephines to better match donor and host
- use of the femtosecond laser (femtosecond laser–assisted keratoplasty [FLAK]) to better match donor and host tissue (long-term clinical studies have not shown that the efficacy of matching the tissue with the femtosecond laser reduces astigmatism)
- postoperative selective suture removal or adjustment of the continuous suture employing corneal topography and tomography
- incisional refractive surgery (can be combined with augmentation sutures in the flat axis)
- ablative surgery with the excimer laser (can be associated with stromal haze)
- wedge resection on one side of the flat axis
- wound revision if significant flattening has occurred in the axis of a wound shift (graft typically shifts anteriorly over the host)
- lens implant surgery after the graft contour has stabilized

Prior to removal of the sutures, the most critical step is to identify the steep axis of astigmatism. Tight sutures while causing focal flattening will induce central steepening in the axis of the suture. The use of corneal topography, tomography, photokeratoscopy, or manual keratometry (see Chapter 2) is essential for evaluating the corneal contour. A power map may show an asymmetric bow tie oriented in the steep axis, while an anterior elevation map will typically show focal depression in the area of a tight suture. In Figure 16-12, the simulated keratometry readings from the power map show a steep axis of 49.93 diopters (D) at 11° and a flat axis of 44.06 D at 101°. The photokeratoscopic image shows clear oval rings, with the horizontal short axis corresponding to the steep axis of corneal astigmatism and the axis of plus cylinder with manifest refraction. Sutures in the steep axis may be selectively removed to improve regular and/or irregular astigmatism, though sometimes with

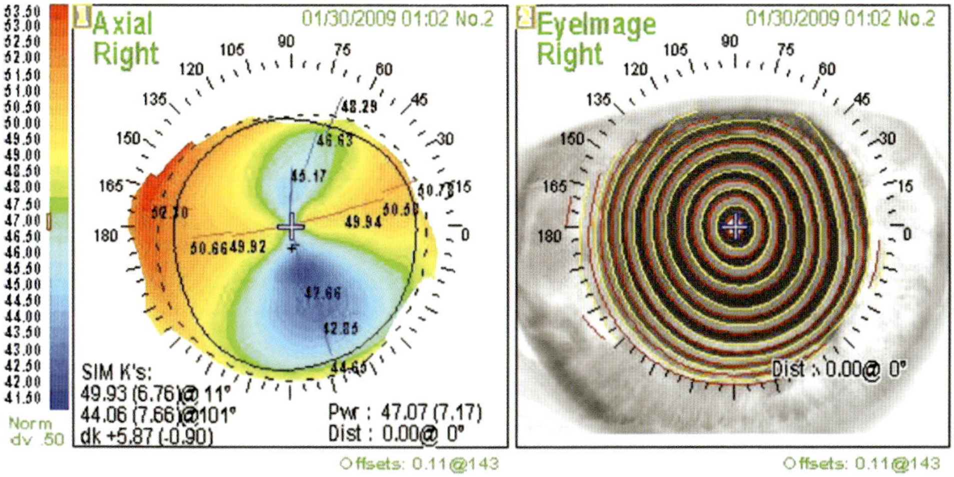

SPH	CYL	AXIS	SimK1	SimK2	dK	e(Q)	SA@4.0	Pupil
-9.00	6.75	4 E	49.93(6.76)@ 11	44.06(7.66)@101	+5.87(-0.90)	-0.58(0.33)	0+0.184 C+0.135	6.33

Figure 16-12 Post-PK corneal topography showing against-the-rule astigmatism in a power map *(left)* and keratoscopic image *(right)*. *(Courtesy of Robert W. Weisenthal, MD.)*

unpredictable results. Rings that appear distorted or indistinct may indicate irregular astigmatism. Surface disruption may distort keratoscopic mires, but a drop of a tear supplement can temporarily make the mires more distinct and assist in the choice of which sutures to remove.

Manifest refraction can aid in confirming the steep axis (plus cylinder). The autorefraction in Figure 16-12 is −9.00 + 6.75 at 4°. The manifest refraction is −7.00 + 5.00 at 4°, achieving 20/25 visual acuity. Removing the interrupted sutures on 1 or both sides of the 4° meridian or adjusting the continuous suture will help reduce the corneal astigmatism. After manipulation or removal of the sutures, a topical antibiotic is recommended for 4 days with a return visit in 1 month for repeat corneal topography and manifest refraction.

The patient can be fitted with a scleral or corneal rigid gas-permeable contact lens to improve symptoms related to anisometropia and high or irregular astigmatism. Corneal neovascularization associated with contact lens wear is less likely to occur or progress once all sutures have been removed. The optimal time for contact lens visual rehabilitation is following suture removal, once topography is stable (usually within several months of final suture removal).

Relaxing keratotomy, performed with a metal or diamond knife or a femtosecond laser, can be effective in reducing astigmatism in patients with poorly tolerated astigmatism, following complete suture removal. The arcuate incisions are placed either in the donor cornea anterior to the graft–host junction or in the graft–host interface at the steep (plus cylinder) meridian. Suture placement at the flat meridian can augment the effect. Laser in situ keratomileusis (LASIK) and photorefractive keratectomy (PRK) have also been used to manage residual anisometropia and astigmatism after transplantation (see BCSC Section 13, *Refractive Surgery*).

If the patient has a visually significant cataract following PK, cataract extraction with appropriate IOL power selection is best performed after all sutures are out and contour has stabilized. If the patient has visually significant regular, stable astigmatism, and a healthy, stable endothelial cell count, a toric IOL is a good option.

Rowsey JJ. Ten caveats in keratorefractive surgery. *Ophthalmology.* 1983;90(2):148–155.

Lamellar Keratoplasty

With advances in surgical instruments and techniques, cornea surgeons are now able to selectively remove the diseased or scarred part of the cornea, preserving the healthy part. The process of removing and replacing select layers of the cornea is called lamellar keratoplasty (LK). The general ophthalmologist should be familiar with the indications, limitations, and common complications associated with various types of lamellar surgery, including ALK, DALK, DSEK, and DMEK (see Table 16-6).

Anterior Lamellar Keratoplasty and Deep Anterior Lamellar Keratoplasty

Anterior lamellar keratoplasty

ALK is the first-line corneal transplant procedure when the pathology does not involve the endothelium. The abnormal stroma is replaced with partial-thickness donor tissue, retaining the healthy host tissue. When the graft involves the central cornea, the best vision outcome is achieved by removing as much stroma as possible. ALK is performed for conditions such as keratoconus, postrefractive corneal ectasia, pellucid marginal degeneration, Terrien marginal degeneration, descemetocele formation (Fig 16-13), superficial corneal tumors, and peripheral ulcerative keratitis with significant keratolysis. See Table 16-6 for additional information.

Deep anterior lamellar keratoplasty

DALK is a version of ALK in which full-depth (or close to full-depth) host stromal replacement is achieved. DALK has become the ALK procedure of choice since the advent of surgical advances such as the "big-bubble" technique, particularly for central or paracentral

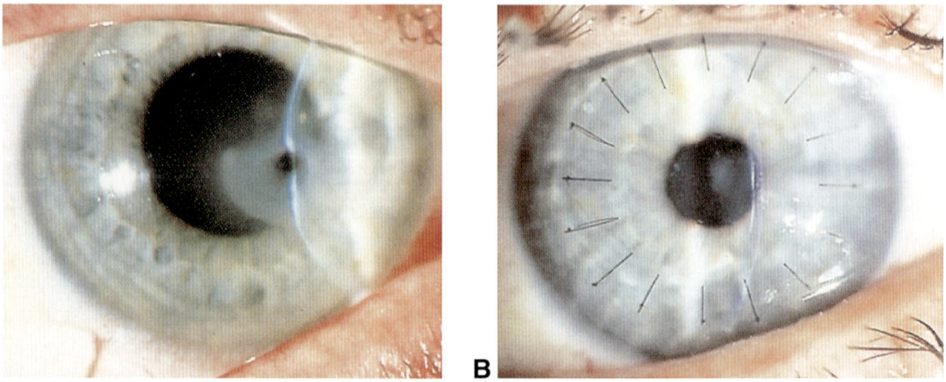
A B

Figure 16-13 Anterior lamellar keratoplasty (ALK) for descemetocele. **A,** Descemetocele. **B,** Postoperative ALK in the same eye. *(Courtesy of Woodford S. Van Meter, MD.)*

pathology. The goal in DALK is to remove at least 85% of the stroma, ideally with complete stromal removal facilitated by creating a cleavage plane at Descemet membrane. In comparison to limited stromal removal, DALK provides a more uniform depth dissection and a smoother lamellar interface, which in turn leads to better postoperative vision.

Full-depth stromal removal is referred to as Descemetic DALK (dDALK). When stromal dissection is deep but not complete, it is called pre-Descemetic DALK (pdDALK). In an OCT study of patients who underwent DALK, 20 μm of residual stromal bed was not visually significant; however, 80 μm of residual tissue was associated with a reduction in vision. There are many techniques for dissecting stromal tissue to expose Descemet membrane, including the Anwar big-bubble technique, the Melles technique, and the use of the femtosecond laser. The reader is encouraged to consult the references at the end of this section and Videos 16-3 through 16-5.

VIDEO 16-3 Deep anterior lamellar keratoplasty (DALK) for keratoconus.
Courtesy of Robert W. Weisenthal, MD.

VIDEO 16-4 DALK.
Courtesy of David D. Verdier, MD. Deep anterior lamellar keratoplasty. In: Copeland RA Jr, Afshari NA, eds. Copeland and Afshari's Principles and Practice of Cornea. *Jaypee Brothers Medical Publishers; 2013.*

VIDEO 16-5 Formation of the big bubble in DALK.
Courtesy of Dasa Gangadhar, MD.

In the big-bubble technique, air is injected into the stroma to create a cavity and separate the stroma from Descemet membrane. Two types of big-bubble formation have been described. The type created depends on the location of Dua layer following air injection. Dua layer is a compact, tough, posterior stromal collagen layer 6 to 15 μm in thickness, just anterior to Descemet membrane, that contains few keratocytes and is relatively impervious to air injection. A type 1 bubble is formed by cleavage between the overlying stroma and Dua layer attached to Descemet membrane. A type 2 bubble occurs when Dua layer is separated from underlying Descemet membrane. Type 2 bubbles are less common than type 1 but are much more delicate and prone to perforation. They are typically recognized by their increased transparency and tendency to extend beyond the central 8 mm of the cornea. Mixed, or hybrid, type 1 and 2 bubbles can also occur; like type 2 bubbles, they require extreme caution to avoid perforation.

Even for experienced surgeons, it may not always be possible to expose Descemet membrane using these techniques. In such cases, manual dissection is generally preferable to PK, but it poses a risk of reduced best-corrected visual acuity due to incomplete removal of the host stromal tissue and secondary interface haze.

Anwar M, Teichmann KD. Big-bubble technique to bare Descemet's membrane in anterior lamellar keratoplasty. *J Cataract Refract Surg.* 2002;28(3):398–403.

Anwar M, Teichmann KD. Deep lamellar keratoplasty: surgical techniques for anterior lamellar keratoplasty with and without baring of Descemet's membrane. *Cornea.* 2002;21(4):374–383.

Ardjomand N, Hau S, McAlister JC, et al. Quality of vision and graft thickness in deep anterior lamellar and penetrating corneal allografts. *Am J Ophthalmol.* 2007;143(2):228–235.e1.

Chen G, Tzekov R, Wensheng L, Jiang F, Mao S, Tong Y. Deep anterior lamellar keratoplasty versus penetrating keratoplasty: a meta-analysis of randomized controlled trials. *Cornea.* 2016;35(2):169–174.

Cohen AW. Deep anterior lamellar keratoplasty (DALK). In: Hausheer JR, ed. *Basic Techniques of Ophthalmic Surgery.* 3rd ed. American Academy of Ophthalmology; 2019:149–152.

Dua HS, Faraj LA, Said DG, Gray T, Lowe J. Human corneal anatomy redefined: a novel pre-Descemet's layer (Dua's layer). *Ophthalmology.* 2013;120(9):1778–1785.

Reinhart WJ, Musch DC, Jacobs DS, Lee WB, Kaufman SC, Shtein RM. Deep anterior lamellar keratoplasty as an alternative to penetrating keratoplasty: a report by the American Academy of Ophthalmology. *Ophthalmology.* 2011;118(1):209–218.

Sarnicola E, Sarnicola C, Sarnicola V. Techniques of anterior lamellar keratoplasty. In: Mannis MJ, Holland EJ, eds. *Cornea.* Vol 2. 5th ed. Elsevier; 2022:1256–1262.

Verdier DD. Deep anterior lamellar keratoplasty. In: Copeland RA Jr, Afshari NA, eds. *Copeland and Afshari's Principles and Practice of Cornea.* Jaypee Brothers Medical Publishers; 2013:1107–1117.

Advantages

ALK has many advantages over PK. It eliminates a full-thickness corneal incision into the anterior chamber, thereby avoiding the risks of glaucoma, cataract, retinal detachment, cystoid macular edema, expulsive hemorrhage, and endophthalmitis. Because the endothelium is not replaced, it also eliminates the risk of endothelial rejection and, consequently, decreases the need for long-term topical corticosteroids. The incidence and severity of a ruptured globe is reduced in ALK. In comparison to PK, DALK offers equivalent or near-equivalent vision. The dramatic loss of endothelial cells over time following PK does not occur with DALK.

Disadvantages

ALK does not replace damaged endothelium. Also, the procedure is more technically demanding and time-consuming than PK. It may be associated with irregular or significant regular astigmatism and with opacification and vascularization of the graft–host interface. Stromal rejection is still possible and may be problematic.

Complications

Allograft rejection Because the corneal endothelium is not replaced, endothelial rejection cannot take place; however, epithelial rejection, subepithelial infiltrates, and stromal rejection can still occur. Fortunately, corticosteroid therapy can be effective in this situation. Stromal rejection, characterized by significant haze and deep vascularization, can lead to corneal opacification and is more common after ALK than PK (Fig 16-14).

Opacification and vascularization of the interface Meticulous dissection of the lamellar plane during ALK is essential for the creation of a smooth, clear interface. Irrigation and cleaning of the lamellar bed at the time of surgery reduce the likelihood of postoperative opacification. Retained interface debris, secondary vascularization, microbial infections, or wrinkling of

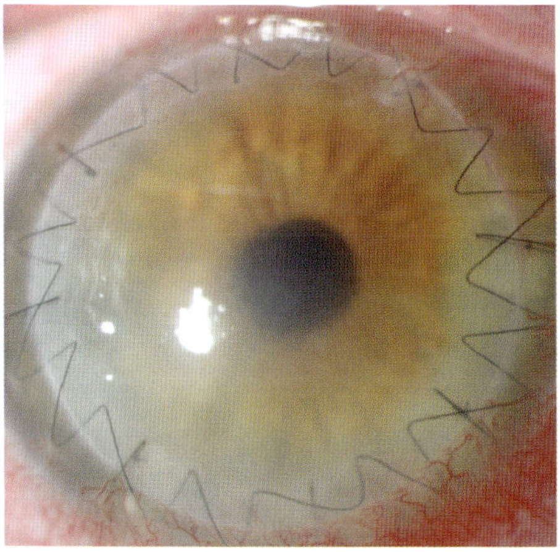

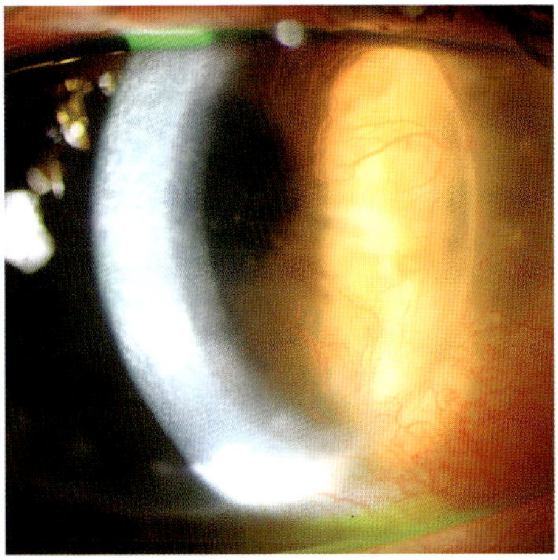

Figure 16-14 Postoperative deep anterior lamellar keratoplasty (DALK). **A,** Diffuse stromal haze worse inferiorly. **B,** Deep stromal vascularization. *(Courtesy of Robert W. Weisenthal, MD.)*

Descemet membrane can reduce vision or prolong vision rehabilitation. Neovascularization can increase the risk of lipid keratopathy, leading to further corneal opacification.

Rupture of Descemet membrane If the rupture is small, the procedure can usually be completed but may result in Descemet detachment. If there is a large perforation, conversion to PK may be necessary.

Double anterior chamber or Descemet detachment Descemet detachment or double (pseudo-) anterior chambers can occur because of fluid in the interface, which results from a host perforation or retained viscoelastic material. Injection of intracameral air can facilitate reattachment.

Additional complications associated with ALK Just as in PK, patients can experience high and/or irregular corneal astigmatism, prolonged healing due to ocular surface disease, suture erosion and abscess, infectious keratitis, neovascularization, graft rejection, and graft failure. In contrast to PK, endophthalmitis and peripheral anterior synechiae formation are rare.

Endothelial Keratoplasty

In 1998, Melles introduced the concept of posterior lamellar surgery for endothelial dysfunction through a procedure called deep lamellar endothelial keratoplasty (DLEK). Melles modified the technique to include stripping of the host Descemet membrane and endothelium (descemetorhexis) and insertion of a hand-dissected posterior lamellar donor button, which was positioned against the host with an air bubble in the anterior chamber; the revised technique is known as Descemet stripping endothelial keratoplasty (DSEK). Gorovoy later automated the lamellar dissection of the donor tissue by using a microkeratome, giving rise to Descemet stripping automated endothelial keratoplasty (DSAEK). Over time, the term DSEK has been adopted for these automated procedures; in this book, the term DSEK is similarly used.

Melles further modified the DSEK procedure by using only donor Descemet membrane and endothelium in a procedure termed Descemet membrane endothelial keratoplasty (DMEK). Further innovations in the technique used to insert and unscroll the tissue, the adoption of an "S" stamp for graft orientation, and the use of sulfur hexafluoride (SF_6) gas to extend the duration of the gas bubble have significantly reduced the incidence of postoperative complications and increased the use and success of DMEK. In addition, the availability of eye bank–prepared, prestamped, and preloaded tissue for DSEK and DMEK has increased the safety and popularity of both procedures.

EK is now the preferred technique for treatment of patients with corneal endothelial dysfunction in the absence of stromal scarring. Due to the success of and rapid rehabilitation observed with EK, the indications for this procedure have expanded to include patients with visually significant cornea guttae in the absence of stromal edema and for endothelial graft failure following PK.

Table 16-8 shows the increased use of DSEK and DMEK in the United States since 2015; EK use surpassed PK use in 2012. DSEK is currently the most performed endothelial keratoplasty procedure, but there has been a steady shift toward DMEK since its introduction. Clinical and patient satisfaction results are similar but not identical for these 2 procedures (Table 16-9). Videos 16-6 through 16-12 show the DSEK and DMEK procedures. Comparisons of PK and endothelial surgery and results are provided in Table 16-10 (also see Table 16-6).

VIDEO 16-6 Descemet stripping endothelial keratoplasty (DSEK).
Courtesy of Robert W. Weisenthal, MD.

VIDEO 16-7 DSEK with alternative lenticule unfolding.
Courtesy of David D. Verdier, MD.

VIDEO 16-8 DSEK combined with phacoemulsification and IOL implantation.
Courtesy of Robert W. Weisenthal, MD.

Table 16-8 Statistics for DSEK and DMEK Procedures Performed in the United States, 2015–2019

	2015	%	2016	%	2017	%	2018	%	2019	%
Total EK procedures	27,208		28,327		28,991		30,336		30,650	
DSEK	22,514	83	21,868	77	21,337	74	19,526	64	17,428	57
DMEK	4694	17	6459	23	7628	26	10,773	36	13,215	43

DMEK = Descemet membrane endothelial keratoplasty; DSEK = Descemet stripping endothelial keratoplasty; EK = endothelial keratoplasty.

Modified with permission from the Eye Bank Association of America (EBAA). *2019 Eye Banking Statistical Report.* EBAA; 2020.

Table 16-9 DSEK Versus DMEK Outcomes

	DSEK Superior	DMEK Superior	DSEK/DMEK Equivalent
Vision outcomes			
BSCVA		+	
Recovery time		+	
Induced refractive error		+	
Graft outcomes			
Primary graft failure			=
Endothelial cell loss			=
Graft success at 5 years			=
Intraoperative complications			
High-risk eyes[a] ease of surgery	+		
Non–high-risk eyes			=
Postoperative complications			
Dislocation/rebubbling rate			=
Rejection		+	
Glaucoma			=

BSCVA = best spectacle-corrected visual acuity; DMEK = Descemet membrane endothelial keratoplasty; DSEK = Descemet stripping endothelial keratoplasty.

[a] Prior vitrectomy, tube shunt, anterior chamber intraocular lens, aphakia, aniridia, poor surgical view through cloudy cornea.

VIDEO 16-9 Descemet membrane endothelial keratoplasty (DMEK).
Courtesy of Robert W. Weisenthal, MD.

VIDEO 16-10 Phakic DMEK.
Courtesy of David D. Verdier, MD.

VIDEO 16-11 DMEK combined with phacoemulsification and IOL implantation.
Courtesy of Robert W. Weisenthal, MD.

VIDEO 16-12 DMEK graft unfolding and positioning tips.
Courtesy of Michael D. Straiko, MD.

American Academy of Ophthalmology Cornea/External Disease Panel. Preferred Practice Pattern Guidelines. *Corneal Edema and Opacification.* American Academy of Ophthalmology; 2018. www.aao.org/ppp

Chen S-Y, Terry MA. Step-by-step Descemet's membrane endothelial keratoplasty surgery. *Taiwan J Ophthalmol.* 2019;9(1):18–26.

Deng SX, Lee WB, Hammersmith KM, et al. Descemet membrane endothelial keratoplasty: safety and outcomes: a report by the American Academy of Ophthalmology. *Ophthalmology.* 2018;125(2):295–310.

Table 16-10 Comparison of Results for Different Surgical Techniques for Corneal Edema (FECD and PBK)

	PK	DSAEK	DMEK
Dislocation rate[a]	0.0%	14.5%–19.0%	5.9%–28.8%
Wound dehiscence	1.3%–5.8%		
Donor failure within 60 days	0.3%	3.4%–5.0%	2.2%–8.0%
Rejection rate at:			
1 year	17.0%	2.0%–9.0%	0.7%–3.0%
2 years	9.7%–13.0%	3.6%–14.0%	
5 years	22.2%	7.9%	2.6%
Graft success rate at 5 years	95% for FECD 73% for PBK	93% 95% for FECD 76% for PBK	93%
BSCVA:			
% 20/40 or better at 1 year	65.0%–84.0% with selective suture removal	38.0%–90.0%	94.0% at 6 months 97.0% 20/30 or better at 1 year
% 20/20 or better		At 5 years: 20.0% 20/20 57.0% 20/25	At 6 months: 17%–67%
Time to BCVA	6–15 months with selective suture removal	Continuing improvement for at least first 5 years	Stable by 6 months
Mean keratometric cylinder			
With sutures in at 1 year	2.50 D		
At 2 years	3.70 ± 3.20 D		
With sutures out	4.40 ± 2.80 D	0.40–0.60 D induced; mean 0.10 D	No significant change
Mean spherical equivalent change	2.80 ± 2.10 D	+1.10 D induced hyperopia	+0.31 D induced hyperopia
Endothelial cell loss at:			
1 year	18%	36%	32%–36%
3 years	39%	38%	40%
5 years	70%	47%	48%
10 years	76%	71%	

BSCVA = best spectacle-corrected visual acuity; BCVA = best-corrected visual acuity; D = diopter; DMEK = Descemet membrane endothelial keratoplasty; DSAEK = Descemet stripping automated endothelial keratoplasty; FECD = Fuchs endothelial corneal dystrophy; PBK = pseudophakic bullous keratopathy; PK = penetrating keratoplasty.

[a]Total and partial detachments, including interface fluid.

Modified from American Academy of Ophthalmology Cornea/External Disease Panel. Preferred Practice Pattern Guidelines. *Corneal Edema and Opacification.* American Academy of Ophthalmology; 2018. www.aao.org/ppp

Endothelial keratoplasty. In: Mannis MJ, Holland EJ, eds. *Cornea.* Vol 2. 5th ed. Elsevier; 2022:1323–1413.

Gorovoy, MS. Descemet-stripping automated endothelial keratoplasty. *Cornea.* 2006;25(8):886–889.

Lee WB, Jacobs DS, Musch DC, Kaufman SC, Reinhart WJ, Shtein RM. Descemet's stripping endothelial keratoplasty: safety and outcomes: a report by the American Academy of Ophthalmology. *Ophthalmology.* 2009;116 (9):1818–1830.

Melles GR. Posterior lamellar keratoplasty: DLEK to DSEK to DMEK. *Cornea.* 2006;25(8):879–881.
Peraza-Nieves J, Baydoun L, Dapena I, et al. Two-year clinical outcome of 500 consecutive cases undergoing Descemet membrane endothelial keratoplasty. *Cornea.* 2017;36(6):655–660.
Price DA, Kelley M, Price FW Jr, Price MO. Five-year graft survival of Descemet membrane endothelial keratoplasty (EK) versus Descemet stripping EK and the effect of donor sex matching. *Ophthalmology.* 2018;125(10):1508–1514.
Stulting RD, Lass JH, Terry MA, et al. Factors associated with graft rejection in the Cornea Preservation Time Study. *Am J Ophthalmol.* 2018;196:197–207.

Advantages

Because the donor tissue is inserted through a small corneal or scleral incision in EK, rather than a large full-thickness incision as in PK, there are many advantages, including

- structural integrity of the eye is preserved, with less risk of ocular injury following trauma to the eye (Fig 16-15)
- reduced incidence of graft rejection because less tissue is transplanted
- reduction in suture-related problems
- preservation of corneal sensation with less ocular surface disruption
- less induced regular and irregular astigmatism
- greater accuracy in IOL power calculations
- more rapid vision rehabilitation

Disadvantages

The main disadvantages of EK include

- increased risk of primary graft failure due to excess intraoperative manipulation or incorrect orientation (eye bank applied "S" stamp has reduced orientation issues)
- risk of pupillary block due to excessive air or gas, or inadequate peripheral iridectomy
- need for surgical interventions postoperatively, such as reinjection of air, known as *rebubbling*
- need for supine positioning postoperatively
- tissue wasted during preparation (minimized with eye bank–prepared tissue)

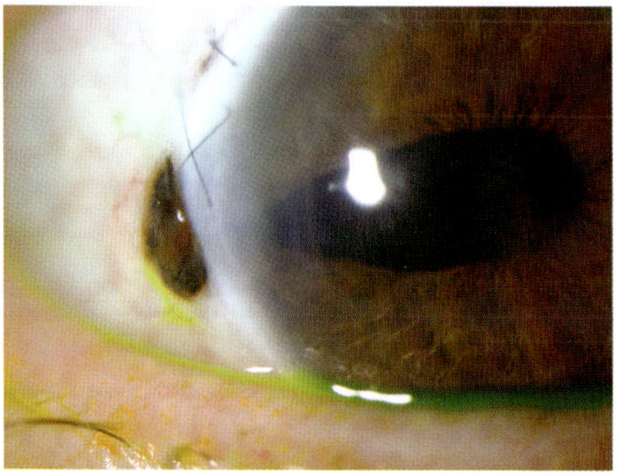

Figure 16-15 Iris prolapse following blunt trauma after Descemet stripping endothelial keratoplasty (DSEK). *(Courtesy of Robert W. Weisenthal, MD.)*

Potential for reduced postoperative visual acuity

Concomitant corneal pathology such as basement membrane changes or subepithelial fibrosis may cause surface irregularity that affects postoperative vision. In some cases, debridement or superficial keratectomy may be beneficial. Preexisting long-standing corneal edema can also cause decreased vision after EK due to light scattering. A prospective evaluation of patients with FECD who underwent DSEK revealed that the corneal light scattering associated with anterior stromal haze progressively improved throughout the 5-year follow-up period, suggesting an ongoing corneal remodeling process. Best spectacle-corrected visual acuity (BSCVA) also continued to improve each year, with 56% of eyes at 20/25 and 20% of eyes at 20/20 5 years postoperatively.

Visual acuity after DMEK reaches its maximum potential by 6 months. On average, patients who have undergone DMEK see 1 Snellen line better than do DSEK patients, with 50% of DMEK eyes at 20/20 after 1 year. The difference in vision outcome between DSEK and DMEK eyes may be related to interface irregularities and alteration of the posterior corneal curvature that occurs with DSEK. In contrast, a nearly normal anatomical restoration of the cornea is achieved with DMEK, which is due to the extremely thin graft tissue used and the exceedingly smooth interface created.

Nevertheless, some surgeons prefer DSEK for routine EK because manipulation and placement of tissue are easier. DSEK is particularly useful in patients with disorganized anterior segments or with anterior chamber IOLs and in patients who have undergone vitrectomy or tube shunt surgery or other glaucoma procedures. Some surgeons advocate using thinner donor grafts (between 50 and 120 μm) to improve the vision outcome after DSEK (a variation called *ultrathin DSEK*). However, a meta-analysis of 23 series found that there may be a weak correlation but, overall, insufficient evidence to conclude that graft thickness is clinically important with respect to BCVA after DSEK. More recently described nanothin (≤50 μm) DSEK grafts have yielded vision and complication rates comparable to those of DMEK.

Dickman MM, Kruit PJ, Remeijer L, et al. A randomized multicenter clinical trial of ultrathin Descemet stripping automated endothelial keratoplasty (DSAEK) versus DSAEK. *Ophthalmology.* 2016;123(11):2276–2284.

Hamzaoglu EC, Straiko MD, Mayko ZM, Sáles CS, Terry MA. The first 100 eyes of standardized Descemet stripping automated endothelial keratoplasty versus standardized Descemet membrane endothelial keratoplasty. *Ophthalmology.* 2015;122(11):2193–2199.

Kurji KH, Cheung AY, Eslani M, et al. Comparison of visual acuity outcomes between nanothin Descemet stripping automated keratoplasty and Descemet membrane endothelial keratoplasty. *Cornea.* 2018;37(10):1226–1231.

Wacker K, Baratz KH, Maguire LJ, McLaren JW, Patel SV. Descemet stripping endothelial keratoplasty for Fuchs' corneal endothelial dystrophy: five-year results of a prospective study. *Ophthalmology.* 2016;123(1):154–160.

Wacker K, Bourne WM, Patel SV. Effect of graft thickness on visual acuity after Descemet stripping endothelial keratoplasty: a systematic review and meta-analysis. *Am J Ophthalmol.* 2016;163:18–28.

Intraoperative Complications

Complications that can occur during DSEK or DMEK include improper orientation during placement of the donor tissue; graft failure due to excessive manipulation of the donor tissue, tearing of the donor tissue, or retention of viscoelastic in the interface; and vitreous or blood in the interface (Fig 16-16). See Table 16-6 for other intraoperative complications associated with EK. Intraoperative anterior segment OCT (AS-OCT), if available, enables the surgeon to check the entire graft for adherence and may reduce the incidence of incomplete attachment intraoperatively (Fig 16-17).

Postoperative Care and Complications

Dislocation or decentration of the donor graft

In DSEK and DMEK, the donor tissue should be well centered over the pupil, without fluid in the interface. To promote tissue adherence over the ensuing days, 40%–60% of the air bubble

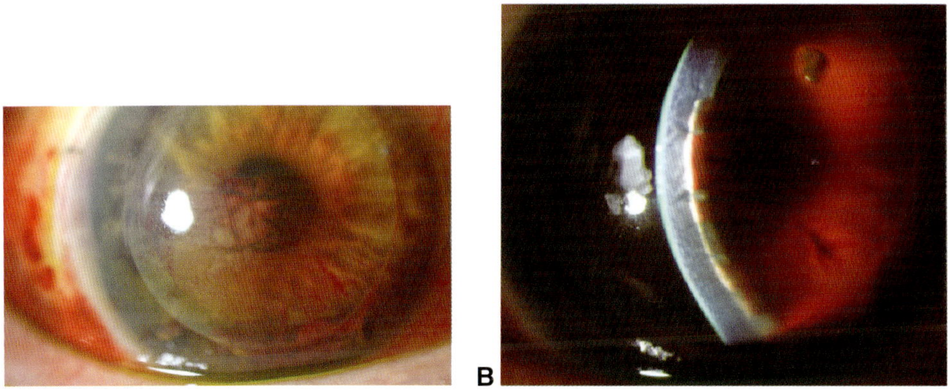

A B

Figure 16-16 DSEK complications. **A,** Hemorrhage in the interface after DSEK. **B,** Slit-lamp photograph showing blood in the interface. *(Courtesy of Robert W. Weisenthal, MD.)*

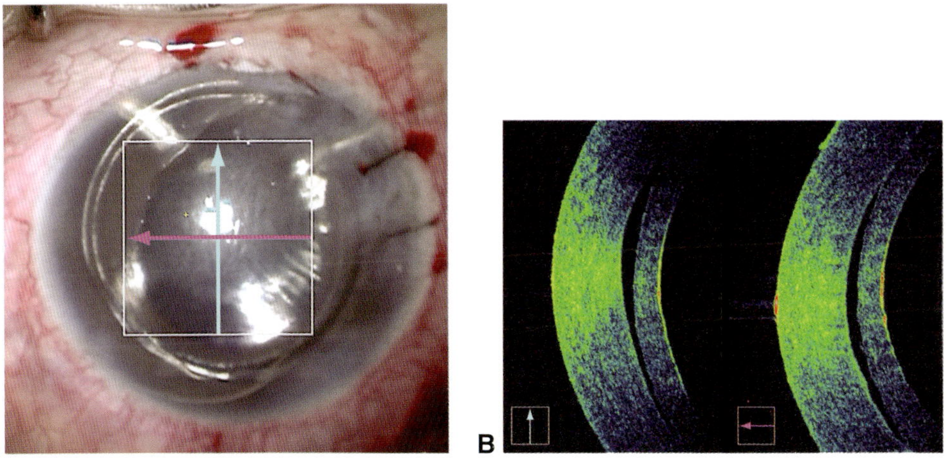

A B

Figure 16-17 Intraoperative anterior segment optical coherence tomography (AS-OCT) of DSEK graft detachment in a patient with 2 tube shunts. **A,** View through the operating microscope. **B**, Intraoperative AS-OCT images of graft detachment noted in both vertical *(blue)* and horizontal *(pink)* meridians. *(Courtesy of Robert S. Feder, MD.)*

injected intraoperatively should remain after DSEK on postoperative day 1 (Fig 16-18), and 80% of the gas (20% SF_6) or air bubble should remain after DMEK on day 1 (Fig 16-19). The air bubble resorbs within 2–4 days, and SF_6 resorbs within 4–7 days. The rate of dislocation of donor tissue decreases for both DSEK and DMEK as surgeon experience increases. See Table 16-10 for dislocation rates for DSAEK and DMEK.

DSEK Dislocation or decentration of the donor graft (Fig 16-20) typically occurs within the first 24 hours after DSEK. A soft eye due to preexisting tube shunt surgery or uncontrolled release of the air increases the likelihood of a decentered or dislocated graft. Retained viscoelastic or the presence of vitreous in the interface may prevent proper adherence of the graft. If the graft remains attached on postoperative day 1, subsequent dislocation is unlikely, although inadvertent trauma or eye rubbing during the first week may displace the donor tissue. Wearing glasses or a shield to protect the eye is recommended, along with exercising caution during instillation of eyedrops.

It is still not clear how long the air bubble should be retained after DSEK; some surgeons remove the air completely on the day of surgery without an increased incidence of tissue dislocation. This raises the possibility that long-term retention of an air bubble is not necessary for graft adherence in DSEK. Also unclear are the role and length of time for

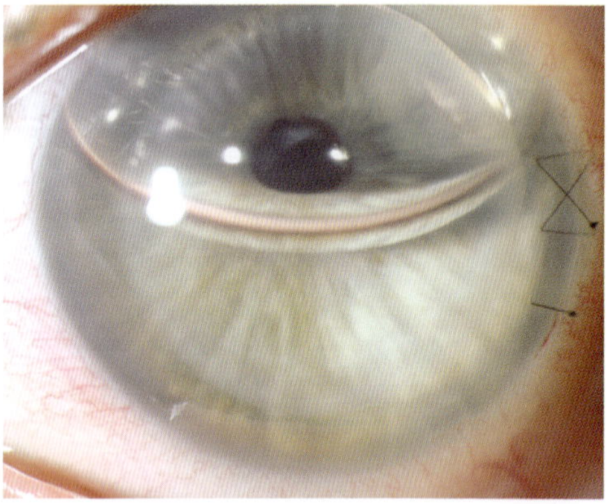

Figure 16-18 Residual air bubble following DSEK (1 day postoperatively). *(Courtesy of Robert W. Weisenthal, MD.)*

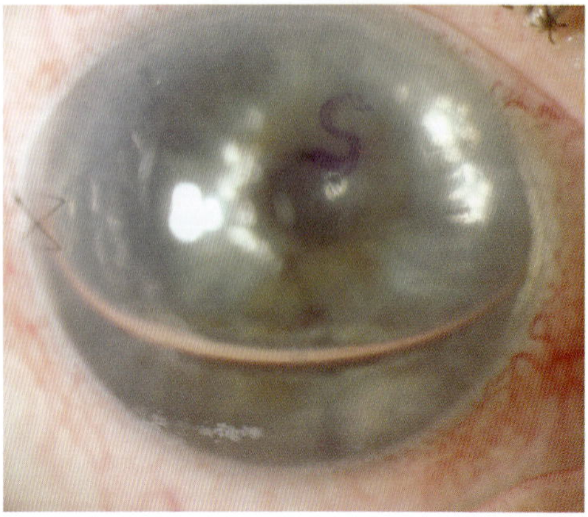

Figure 16-19 Residual air bubble after Descemet membrane endothelial keratoplasty (DMEK) (1 day postoperatively). The "S" stamp indicating proper orientation is seen. *(Courtesy of Robert W. Weisenthal, MD.)*

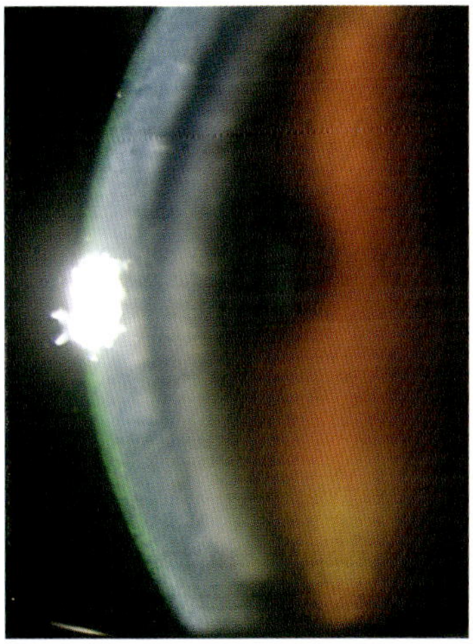

Figure 16-20 Slit-lamp photograph of a detached donor corneal button following DSEK. *(Courtesy of Robert W. Weisenthal, MD.)*

supine positioning following surgery to promote and retain graft adherence. Most surgeons advocate supine positioning for at least 1 hour following surgery; some recommend up to 4 days, at least part-time. Supine positioning may be more important for DMEK than DSEK.

DMEK In DMEK, the donor tissue is more delicate, and as a result, peripheral or central detachments are more common (Fig 16-21). Strategies to reduce DMEK graft detachment include the use of isoexpansile 20% SF_6 gas, which resorbs more slowly than air. The presence of an inferior peripheral iridectomy allows placement of a larger bubble with reduced concern of pupillary block glaucoma. For anticoagulated patients, the surgeon may consider performing a peripheral iridotomy with a YAG laser prior to EK surgery.

In addition to intraoperative AS-OCT (see Fig 16-17), postoperative AS-OCT (Fig 16-22) can be used to identify and follow graft detachment. Small peripheral detachments that do not involve the visual axis can be observed over several weeks to ensure there is no progression. They usually seal without adverse impact.

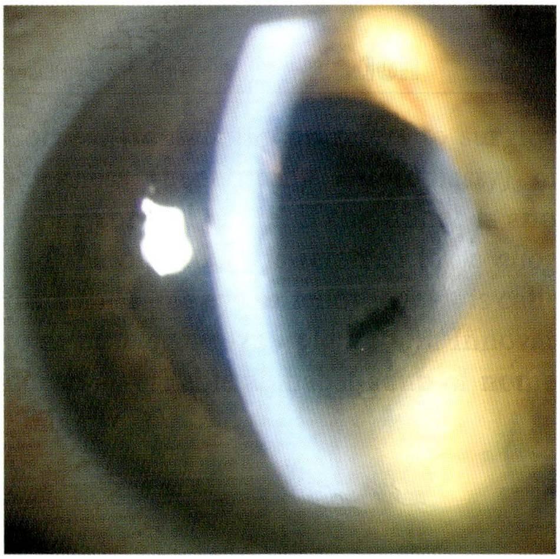

Figure 16-21 Slit-lamp photograph shows corneal edema due to a peripheral detachment of a DMEK graft. *(Courtesy of Robert W. Weisenthal, MD.)*

The surgeon may wish to consider rebubbling if

- graft detachment extends into the visual axis
- greater than one-third of the graft area is involved
- rolled edges are present

Significant reduction in endothelial cell counts were reported at 5-year follow-up in patients with clinically significant graft detachments that were managed without rebubbling; this reduction led to a higher rate of late graft failure. In some cases, permanent stromal haze developed secondary to chronic corneal edema, worsening the vision outcome after repeated DMEK. Thus, early rebubbling seems to be the best course in these cases. If rebubbling is necessary, it can be performed at the slit lamp (Video 16-13).

VIDEO 16-13 Rebubbling a DMEK graft at the slit lamp.
Courtesy of Christopher S. Sáles, MD; Michael D. Straiko, MD; and Mark A. Terry, MD.

If after 2 months the graft is attached but the cornea still has visually significant edema, repeated surgery is indicated prior to the development of chronic corneal edema, which can lead to bullous keratopathy, epithelial breakdown, and scarring or possible secondary infection. Repeated EK, either DMEK or DSEK, before the development of permanent corneal changes has a vision prognosis similar to the original procedure.

Baydoun L, Ham L, Borderie V, et al. Endothelial survival after Descemet membrane endothelial keratoplasty. Effect of surgical indication and graft adherence status. *JAMA Ophthalmol.* 2015;133(11):1277–1285.

Baydoun L, van Dijk K, Dapena I, et al. Repeat Descemet membrane endothelial keratoplasty after complicated primary Descemet membrane endothelial keratoplasty. *Ophthalmology.* 2015;122(1):8–16.

Dirisamer M, van Dijk K, Dapena I, et al. Prevention and management of graft detachment in Descemet membrane endothelial keratoplasty. *Arch Ophthalmol.* 2012;130(3):280–291.

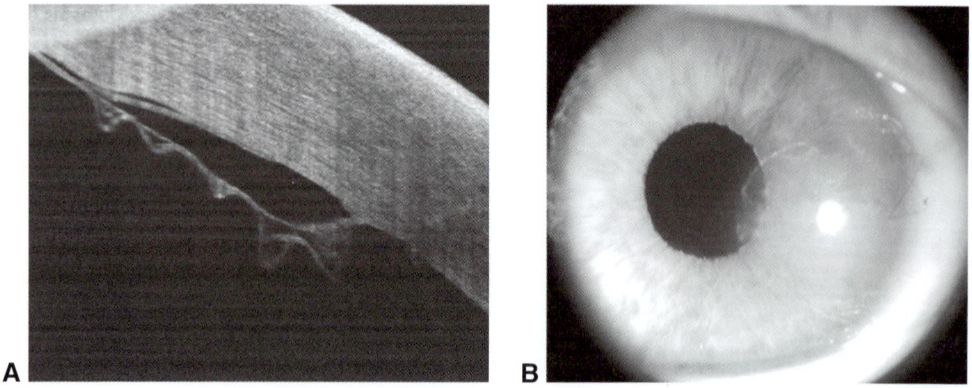

Figure 16-22 Peripheral detachment following DMEK. **A,** Postoperative anterior segment OCT image. **B,** Clinical photograph shows corneal edema in the area of detachment. *(Courtesy of Robert W. Weisenthal, MD.)*

Lehman RE, Copeland LA, Stock EM, Fulcher SF. Graft detachment rate in DSEK/DSAEK after same-day complete air removal. *Cornea.* 2015;34(11):1358–1361.

Price FW Jr, Price MO. To intervene or not to intervene: That is the question. *Ophthalmology.* 2015;122(1):6–7.

Sáles CS, Straiko MD, Terry MA. Novel technique for rebubbling DMEK grafts at the slit lamp using intravenous extension tubing. *Cornea.* 2016;35(4):582–585.

Pupillary block

Anterior pupillary block or iris bombé may occur if the anterior chamber bubble migrates posteriorly, preventing aqueous flow through the pupil. Figures 16-23 and 16-24 show such a block after DSEK and DMEK, respectively. The resultant acute rise in IOP results in pain and can exacerbate preexisting optic nerve damage. Pupillary block may also lead to iridocorneal adhesion, damaging the graft and increasing the risk of rejection. Pupil dilation and supine positioning may relieve the pupil block; if this fails, some air should be

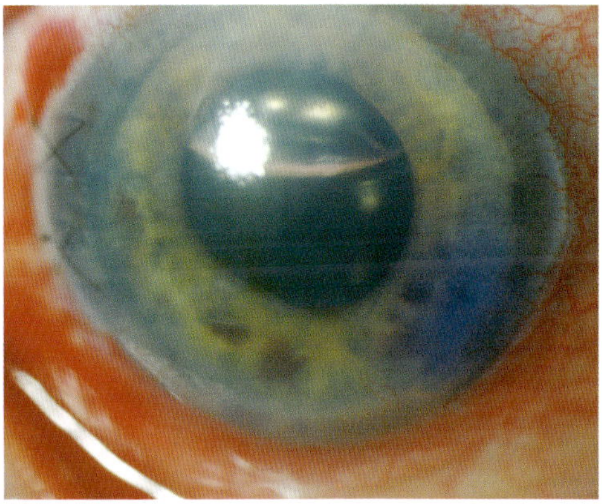

Figure 16-23 Slit-lamp photograph showing pupillary block following DSEK. Air can be seen behind the iris. *(Courtesy of Robert W. Weisenthal, MD.)*

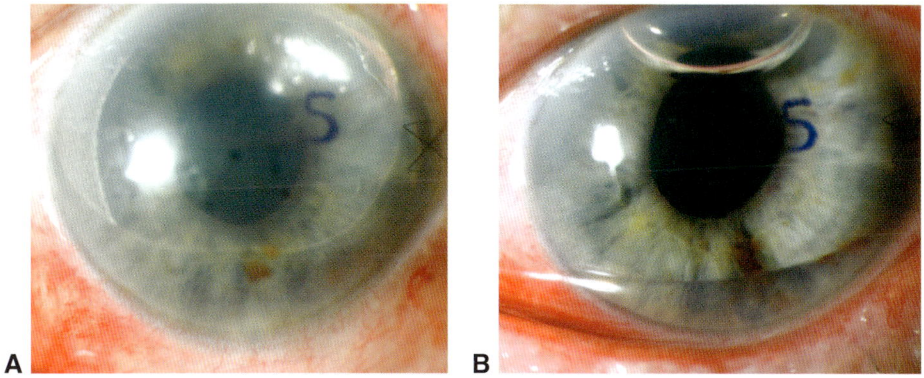

Figure 16-24 Pupillary block following DMEK. **A,** Slit-lamp photograph of pupillary block. **B,** The same patient after the release of air, leading to resolution of the block. *(Courtesy of Robert W. Weisenthal, MD.)*

removed. An inferior iridectomy performed prior to or at the time of the surgery reduces the likelihood of this scenario.

Epithelial ingrowth

Epithelial ingrowth following DSEK is visible as a gray-white deposit within the graft–host interface (Fig 16-25). It typically remains stable and is asymptomatic unless it involves the visual axis. The ingrowth may

- come from either the host or the donor
- be pushed through the wound, side ports, or venting incisions used to drain interface fluid
- enter the eye through a fistulous track
- adhere to the donor corneal button as a result of eccentric trephination beyond the microkeratome incision

In rare cases, epithelial ingrowth leads to graft failure that is missed on clinical examination but recognized on histologic examination of the tissue after removal. In a large series of cases, the majority of patients with epithelial ingrowth were simply observed and continued to see well without further intervention. In the atypical cases that resulted in graft failure, a second DSEK or PK produced a good outcome without recurrent ingrowth. This contrasts with the progressive and devastating course of intraocular epithelial downgrowth associated with intracapsular cataract extraction or full-thickness PK. One case of epithelial ingrowth has recently been reported in DMEK. Fungal or bacterial interface infection can be similar in appearance to epithelial ingrowth.

Dalal RR, Raber I, Dunn SP, et al. Epithelial ingrowth following endothelial keratoplasty. *Cornea.* 2016;35(4):465–470.

Suh LH, Shousha MA, Ventura RU, et al. Epithelial ingrowth after Descemet stripping automated endothelial keratoplasty: description of cases and assessment with anterior segment optical coherence tomography. *Cornea.* 2011;30(5):528–534.

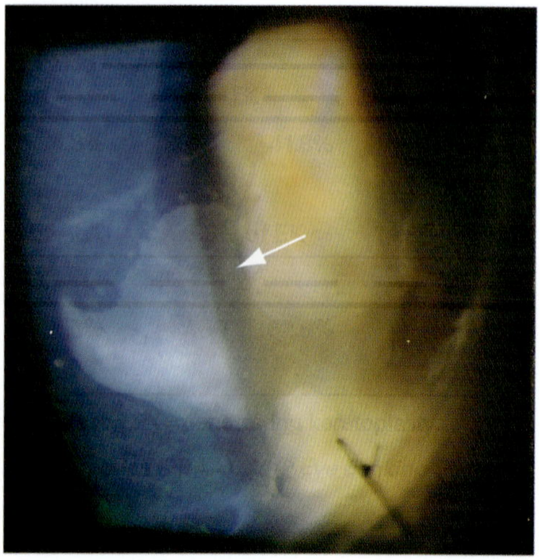

Figure 16-25 Slit-lamp photograph of epithelial ingrowth *(arrow)* in the graft–host interface after DSEK. *(Courtesy of Robert W. Weisenthal, MD.)*

Other interface pathology

Infections can occur in the graft–host interface as a result of pathogens passing through venting incisions, contaminated donor tissue, or bacteria from the ocular surface dragged into the eye during insertion. The incidence of postoperative fungal infections is significantly higher for EK than PK. These infections have occurred primarily in eyes that have undergone DSEK, but there are case reports of infections after DMEK as well. It is possible that these infections are related to the tissue warming that occurs during preparation of donor tissue for EK. Over the past 10 years, the Eye Bank Association of America (EBAA) has reported EK fungal infection rates ranging from 0.011% to 0.052%, peaking in 2013 and decreasing to 0.013% in 2018. Donor rims that are culture positive for fungus have predictive value. In the CPTS, the overall rate of positive donor rim fungal cultures was 1.9%, with postoperative recipient fungal infection occurring in 6.7%, similar to other recent studies. Using a double application of povidone-iodine during tissue procurement, before and after conjunctival peritomy, may help to reduce tissue contamination.

Textural interface opacity (TIO) describes interface irregularity that results from retained viscoelastic or from the shearing of stromal fibrils during an irregular microkeratome donor preparation. The opacity has 2 forms: elongated (a lacy honeycomb pattern of deposits with intervening clear zones) (Fig 16-26) and punctate (small, discrete deposits). Textural interface opacity may be associated with reduced vision, but it typically improves or disappears completely over many months. There have been no reports of textural interface problems after DMEK. Meticulous removal of viscoelastic prior to graft insertion

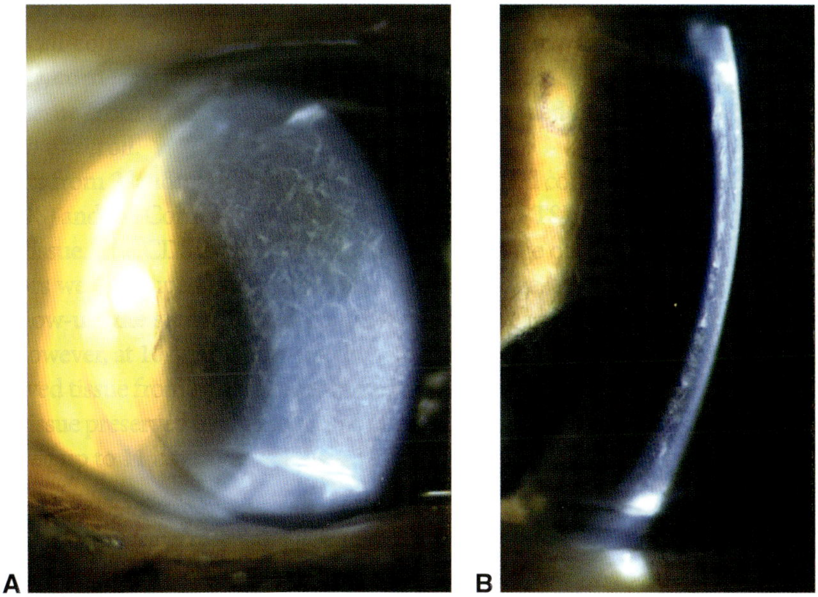

Figure 16-26 Textural interface opacity. **A,** Postoperative DSEK seen in the broad slit-beam view. **B,** Fine slit-beam image. *(Courtesy of David D. Verdier, MD.)*

may reduce the risk of TIO. Interface opacification may also occur because of retention of fibers, incomplete removal of Descemet membrane, and persistence of interface fluid.

Eye Bank Association of America (EBAA). *2018 OARRS Report.* EBAA; 2019.

Mian SI, Aldave AJ, Tu EY, et al. Incidence and outcomes of positive donor rim cultures and infections in the Cornea Preservation Time Study. *Cornea.* 2018;37(9):1102–1109.

Vira S, Shih CY, Ragusa N, et al. Textural interface opacity after Descemet stripping automated endothelial keratoplasty: a report of 30 cases and possible etiology. *Cornea.* 2013;32(5):e54–59.

Wilhelmus KR, Hassan SS. The prognostic role of donor corneoscleral rim cultures in corneal transplantation. *Ophthalmology.* 2007;114(3):440–445.

Progression of cataracts

EK performed in a phakic eye may induce cataract progression, particularly in patients with shallower anterior chambers (<3.0 mm); therefore, EK with lens extraction has been recommended in patients older than 50 years or in the presence of mild to moderate cataract. DSEK or DMEK combined with cataract extraction does not increase the risk of graft dislocation, endothelial cell loss, or other non–cataract-related complications.

Burkhart ZN, Feng MT, Price FW Jr, Price MO. One-year outcomes in eyes remaining phakic after Descemet membrane endothelial keratoplasty. *J Cataract Refract Surg.* 2014;40(3):430–434.

Terry MA, Shamie N, Chen ES, et al. Endothelial keratoplasty for Fuchs' dystrophy with cataract: complications and clinical results with the new triple procedure. *Ophthalmology.* 2009;116(4):631–639.

Tsui JYM, Goins KM, Sutphin JE, Wagoner MD. Phakic Descemet stripping automated endothelial keratoplasty: prevalence and prognostic impact of postoperative cataracts. *Cornea.* 2011;30(3):291–295.

Primary graft failure

In published reports, primary graft failure rates for DSEK and DMEK range from 2.2% to 8.0%; more recent studies of procedures performed by experienced surgeons show rates of 2% or less (see Table 16-10). The lower rates probably reflect better surgical technique, which results in less tissue manipulation and a lower rate of graft dislocations and thus less endothelial trauma.

Graft rejection

The clinical presentation of graft rejection in EK patients differs from that in PK patients. The classic endothelial rejection line of PK is not commonly seen; rather, multiple keratic precipitates scattered across the cornea are typically noted (Fig 16-27).

The incidence of corneal graft rejection following EK is lower than that after PK. When DSEK patients were maintained on topical corticosteroids indefinitely, the rejection rate was 2% after 5 years in 51 eyes. The rate of graft rejection after DMEK is even lower than after DSEK. Prospective studies from the Price group demonstrated a rejection rate of <1% in DMEK eyes followed for 1 year. The dosing recommendations used in these studies, which are followed by many EK surgeons, are described in Table 16-11.

Long-term prophylaxis with a topical corticosteroid once daily, regardless of the strength, is important in reducing the incidence of graft rejection. In a prospective study

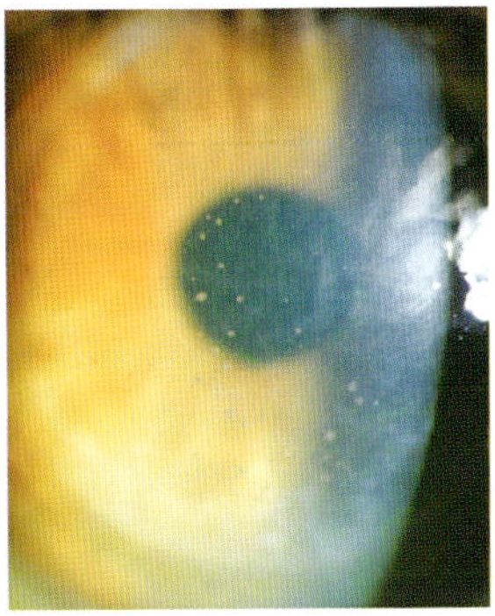

Figure 16-27 Slit-lamp photograph shows endothelial graft rejection after DSEK, characterized by scattered keratic precipitates without an endothelial rejection line. *(Courtesy of Robert W. Weisenthal, MD).*

Table 16-11 Guidelines for Graft Rejection Prophylaxis Following Endothelial Keratoplasty

Postoperative time interval[a]	Medication frequency	Topical medication
Month 1	4 times daily	Prednisolone 1% suspension
Months 2 and 3	4 times daily	Loteprednol 0.5% gel or prednisolone 1% suspension
Month 4	3 times daily	Loteprednol 0.5% gel[b] or prednisolone 1% suspension
Month 5	2 times daily	Loteprednol 0.5% gel[b] or prednisolone 1% suspension
Months 6 through 12	1 time daily	Loteprednol 0.5% gel[b] or prednisolone 1% suspension
After 12 months	1 time daily	Loteprednol 0.5% gel[b]

[a]Periodic intraocular pressure measurement is recommended for all patients on topical corticosteroids.
[b]Acceptable alternatives: fluorometholone 0.1% suspension; loteprednol 0.2% suspension.

of 400 DMEK eyes followed for 24 months, rejection occurred in 6% in eyes after corticosteroids were discontinued at 1 year, versus 0% in eyes continued on a daily corticosteroid eyedrop. It is important to discuss the potential for elevated IOP, infection, and cataract with long-term corticosteroid use with the patient.

Hos D, Matthaei M, Bock F, et al. Immune reactions after modern lamellar (DALK, DSAEK, DMEK) versus conventional penetrating corneal transplantation. *Prog Retin Eye Res.* 2019;73:100768.

Price MO, Feng MT, Scanameo A, Price FW Jr. Loteprednol etabonate 0.5% gel vs. prednisolone acetate 1% solution after Descemet membrane endothelial keratoplasty: prospective randomized trial. *Cornea.* 2015;34(8):853–858.

Price MO, Scanameo A, Feng MT, Price FW Jr. Descemet's membrane endothelial keratoplasty: risk of immunologic rejection episodes after discontinuing topical corticosteroids. *Ophthalmology.* 2016;123(6):1232–1236.

Ratanasit A, Gorovoy MS. Long-term results of Descemet stripping automated endothelial keratoplasty. *Cornea.* 2011;30(12):1414–1418.

Wu EI, Ritterband DC, Yu G, Shields RA, Seedor JA. Graft rejection following Descemet stripping automated endothelial keratoplasty: features, risk factors, and outcomes. *Am J Ophthalmol.* 2012;153(5):949–957.e1.

Endothelial cell loss

Several maneuvers may contribute to early endothelial cell loss in EK patients, including

- manipulation of tissue entailed in the preparation of donor tissue
- placement and orientation of the tissue within the anterior chamber
- primary injection of air to facilitate graft adherence
- rebubbling and tissue manipulation to treat dislocated grafts

At 1 year postoperatively, endothelial cell loss for both DSEK and DMEK is reported to be approximately 35%. In a follow-up study of 95 eyes, the median DSEK endothelial cell loss was 53% at 5 years and 71% at 10 years. These rates compare favorably to results for PK in the CDS, which showed a mean cell loss of 70% at 5 years and 76% at 10 years. Long-term viability of the endothelial cells is influenced by ocular comorbidities such as previous filtering surgery and, in particular, tube shunt surgery. Long-term prospective trials on DMEK and DSEK are necessary to better understand the clinical biology of the corneal endothelium and the impact of endothelial cell loss on graft viability.

Ni N, Sperling BJ, Dai Y, Hannush SB. Outcomes after Descemet stripping automated endothelial keratoplasty in patients with glaucoma drainage devices. *Cornea.* 2015;34(8):870–875.

Price DA, Kelley M, Price FW Jr, Price MO. Five-year graft survival of Descemet membrane endothelial keratoplasty (EK) versus Descemet stripping EK and the effect of donor sex matching. *Ophthalmology*. 2018;125(10):1508–1514.

Price MO, Calhoun P, Kollman C, Price FW Jr, Lass JH. Descemet stripping endothelial keratoplasty: ten-year endothelial cell loss compared with penetrating keratoplasty. *Ophthalmology.* 2016;123(7):1421–1427.

Emerging Methods for Treatment of Endothelial Dysfunction

Descemet stripping only (DSO) is an evolving procedure in which a central descemetorhexis is performed for treatment of FECD and possibly other causes of endothelial cell loss. Removing thickened Descemet membrane and cornea guttae characteristic of FECD may allow peripheral endothelial cells to migrate centrally and restore endothelial function (Fig 16-28, Video 16-14). DSO is unlikely to succeed in FECD eyes with peripheral endothelial cell counts less than 1000 cells/mm^2, or in eyes with other conditions associated with diffuse endothelial cell loss, such as pseudophakic or aphakic corneal edema. In a recent prospective trial, 18 FECD patients were treated with a 4–5-mm descemetorhexis; 8 patients were also given topical ripasudil 0.4% (a Rho kinase inhibitor) 4 times daily for 2 months. At 1-year follow-up, visual acuity was 20/25 or better in 16 patients, 20/30 in 1 patient, and 20/200 in 1 patient who later underwent successful DMEK. The topical ripasudil group had more rapid recovery to 20/40 (4.6 vs 6.5 weeks), higher endothelial cell density at 1 year (1086 vs 736 cells/mm^2), and less loss of peripheral endothelial cells (1142 vs 1233 cells/mm^2). These results, along with results from other studies, suggest that use of ripasudil or other Rho kinase inhibitors might promote corneal endothelial regeneration.

VIDEO 16-14 Descemet stripping only.
Courtesy of David D. Verdier, MD.

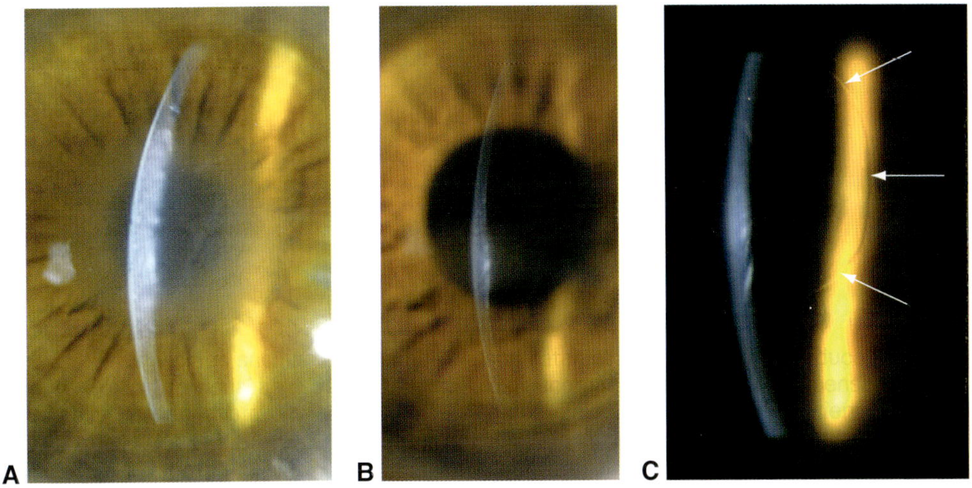

Figure 16-28 Descemet stripping only (DSO). **A,** Slit-lamp photograph of a DSO eye 5 days postoperatively. **B, C,** The same eye 6 weeks postoperatively. The border *(arrows)* of the 4.5 mm descemetorhexis is seen in retroillumination. *(Courtesy of David D. Verdier, MD.)*

Treatment of corneal endothelial disease with cultured human endothelial cells, either by injection or via a cell carrier using techniques similar to DMEK, has with few exceptions been confined to the laboratory. In a study of 11 patients with severe endothelial cell loss, all patients received an injection of cultured human endothelial cells supplemented with a Rho kinase inhibitor into the anterior chamber, then remained prone for 3 hours. At 2-year follow-up, all corneas were clear, with a mean endothelial cell density of 1534 cells/mm^2.

Borkar DS, Veldman P, Colby KA. Treatment of Fuchs endothelial dystrophy by Descemet stripping without endothelial keratoplasty. *Cornea.* 2016;35(10):1267–1273.

Kinoshita S, Koizumi N, Ueno M, et al. Injection of cultured cells with a ROCK inhibitor for bullous keratopathy. *N Engl J Med.* 2018;378:995–1003.

Koenig SB. Planned descemetorhexis without endothelial keratoplasty in eyes with Fuchs corneal endothelial dystrophy. *Cornea.* 2015;34(9):1149–1151.

Macsai MS, Shiloach M. Use of topical Rho kinase inhibitors in the treatment of Fuchs dystrophy after Descemet stripping only. *Cornea.* 2019;38(5):529–534.

Moloney G, Petsoglou C, Ball M, et al. Descemetorhexis without grafting for Fuchs endothelial dystrophy—supplementation with topical ripasudil. *Cornea.* 2017;36(6):642–648.

Pediatric Corneal Transplantation

Better understanding of the special problems associated with pediatric grafts, advances in preoperative diagnostic techniques and in surgical methods, and improved postoperative management have enhanced the vision prognosis for children undergoing corneal transplantation. Furthermore, improvements in pediatric anesthesia and the recognition of the risk of amblyopia have led to earlier surgical intervention. The success rate of pediatric corneal transplantation depends on the extent of coexisting ocular abnormalities.

For example, one of the most common indications for pediatric keratoplasty is Peters anomaly (see Chapter 6). For type 1 disease, characterized by a central corneal opacity with possible iridocorneal adhesions, the survival rate for a clear graft was 83%–90% in one large series (mean follow-up time of 78 months), depending on the age of the patient at the time of surgery. In contrast, in another large series of patients with either type 1 or type 2 Peters anomaly, the outcomes were significantly worse: only 56% of grafts remained clear at 6 months, and 44% at 3 years. This discrepancy was attributed to more severe anterior segment findings, characteristically including adhesions to the cornea by the iris and/or lens; corneal neovascularization; glaucoma; cataract; and corneal staphyloma. With more extensive surgery, the survival rate of the grafts decreased.

Selective lamellar surgery may be very beneficial for pediatric eyes. In a study of 105 unilateral keratoplasty procedures in patients age 16 years and under, graft survival rates at 4-year follow-up ranged from 84% to 90%. For treatment of endothelial disease such as congenital hereditary endothelial dystrophy, EK has been reported to provide good outcomes.

Corneal grafting in children younger than 2 years is associated with rapid neovascularization, especially along the sutures. As the wound heals, erosions may occur along the sutures, leading to eye rubbing, epithelial defects, mucus accumulation, and possible infection. Suture erosion can occur as early as 2 weeks postoperatively in infants and necessitates urgent and frequent examination under anesthesia in the operating room to evaluate the transplant and facilitate suture removal. Removal of any loose or eroded sutures is critical to avoid rejection, which can be sudden and severe, especially in infants and young children. Early fitting with a contact lens (as early as the time of PK) and ocular occlusive therapy may be necessary to stem development of amblyopia in children.

Critical to a successful outcome is the family's (or caregiver's) dedication to following a rigorous postoperative regimen, which includes repeated examinations under anesthesia and adherence to the medication regimen. Rejection, postoperative glaucoma, strabismus, and self-induced trauma are common. As part of obtaining informed consent from the family, the physician must discuss the many difficult issues associated with the surgery, including the

- complicated postoperative course
- guarded long-term vision prognosis
- risk of amblyopia
- anesthesia risk including repeated exams under anesthesia
- extensive ongoing care required for the child
- disruption of home life
- reduced time to devote to other dependents
- loss of time from work (with associated loss of income)

Busin M, Beltz J, Scorcia V. Descemet-stripping automated endothelial keratoplasty for congenital hereditary endothelial dystrophy. *Arch Ophthalmol.* 2011;129(9):1140–1146.

Low JR, Anshu A, Tan ACS, Htoon HM, Tan DTH. The outcomes of primary pediatric keratoplasty in Singapore. *Am J Ophthalmol.* 2014;158(3):496–502.

Nischal KK. Pediatric keratoplasty. In: Mannis MJ, Holland EJ, eds. *Cornea.* Vol 2. 5th ed. Elsevier; 2022:1277–1294.

Rao KV, Fernandes M, Gangopadhyay N, Vemuganti GK, Krishnaiah S, Sangwan VS. Outcome of penetrating keratoplasty for Peters anomaly. *Cornea.* 2008;27(7):749–753.

Yang F, Hong J, Xiao G, et al. Descemet stripping endothelial keratoplasty in pediatric patients with congenital hereditary endothelial dystrophy. *Am J Ophthalmol.* 2020;209:132–140.

Zaidman GW, Flanagan JK, Furey CC. Long-term visual prognosis in children after corneal transplant surgery for Peters anomaly type I. *Am J Ophthalmol.* 2007;144(1):104–108.e1.

Corneal Autograft Procedures

The greatest advantage of a corneal autograft is the elimination of allograft rejection. Clinical circumstances appropriate for autograft are uncommon, but an astute ophthalmologist who recognizes the potential for a successful autograft procedure can spare the patient the risks associated with long-term topical corticosteroid use and the need for lifelong vigilance against rejection.

A *rotational autograft* can be used to reposition a localized corneal scar that involves the pupillary axis. By making an eccentric trephination and rotating the host corneal button before resuturing, the surgeon can place a paracentral zone of clear cornea in the pupillary axis (Fig 16-29). The procedure is particularly useful in children, in whom the prognosis for PK due to rejection is poorer, and in locations where suitable tissue is scarce. It is important that the graft–host junction not be too close to the visual axis, because image distortion and irregular astigmatism could result.

A *contralateral autograft* is reserved for patients who have a corneal opacity in 1 eye with a favorable vision prognosis and a clear cornea in the opposite eye with coexisting severe dysfunction of the afferent system (eg, retinal detachment, severe amblyopia). The clear host cornea button is removed and replaced with an allograft. The clear host button is then transplanted into the fellow eye. If an eye with a clear cornea is to be enucleated or eviscerated, the cornea can be used as a donor for keratoplasty in the fellow eye.

Chan CC, Perez Velasquez MA, Verdier DD. Penetrating keratoplasty: the fundamentals. In: Mannis MJ, Holland EJ, eds. *Cornea.* Vol 2. 5th ed. Elsevier; 2022:1162–1173.

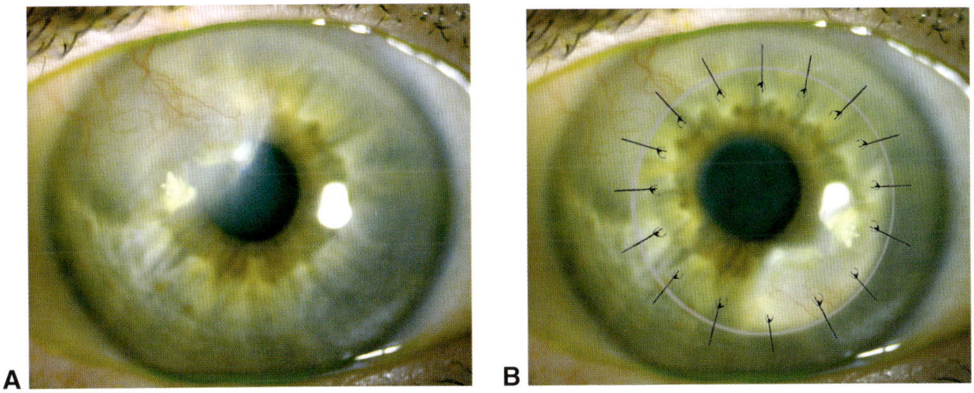

Figure 16-29 Rotational autograft. **A,** Neovascular scar extends into central visual axis. **B,** Eccentric trephination with host button rotated 180° and sutured. *(Courtesy of David D. Verdier, MD.)*

Keratoprosthesis

In some patients, corneal transplantation is associated with an extremely guarded prognosis because of a history of multiple graft failures or associated ocular surface disease, such as chronic bilateral ocular surface disease from Stevens-Johnson syndrome or mucous membrane pemphigoid. These patients may be good candidates for a synthetic keratoprosthesis. High-risk patients can be divided into 2 groups: those with a good blink reflex and adequate tear function and those with significant conjunctival scarring, dry eye, and exposure. In the first group of patients, the type I Boston keratoprosthesis (KPro; Massachusetts Eye and Ear Infirmary) works well (Fig 16-30). For patients with end-stage dry eye disease, the type II Boston keratoprosthesis is an option. Other types of keratoprostheses for these high-risk patients are more popular in Europe and include the TKPro, which uses tibia bone tissue, and the osteo-odonto-keratoprosthesis, which uses dentine and alveolar bone tissue.

Some surgeons have expanded the indications for a keratoprosthesis to include the treatment of ocular trauma, advanced quiescent herpetic disease, aniridia, and congenital corneal opacification.

The vision prognosis for keratoprosthesis implantation has improved because of innovations in the design of keratoprostheses and improvements in postoperative management. The use of a soft contact lens and long-term prophylactic antibiotics has reduced the incidence of infection and necrosis around the keratoprosthesis. A review of the literature on KPro results published by the American Academy of Ophthalmology revealed that a BCSVA of 20/200 or better occurred in 45%–89% of eyes, and a BCSVA of 20/40 or better occurred in 11%–39% of eyes after implantation. In a large, multicenter study of 300 eyes followed for 17.1 ± 14.8 months after implantation of the KPro, there was significant improvement in vision, although only 6% of eyes had visual acuity of 20/60 or better. The retention rate with the KPro ranged from 65% to 100%. Loss of vision resulted from corneal melts due to exposure keratopathy, endophthalmitis, infectious keratitis, or corneal ulceration.

The most common complications following keratoprosthesis implantation (Table 16-12) include

- persistent epithelial defects
- retroprosthetic membrane formation
- stromal necrosis
- elevated IOP, often associated with glaucoma

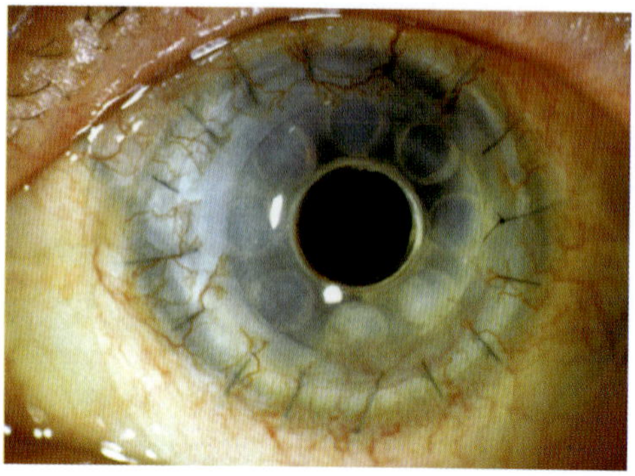

Figure 16-30 Boston keratoprosthesis type I. *(Courtesy of James J. Reidy, MD.)*

Table 16-12 Complications of Keratoprosthesis

Complication	Incidence
Glaucoma	Preexisting in 72.0%–86.0%
Retroprosthetic membrane formation	25.0%–55.0%
Persistent epithelial defects	38.0%
Stromal necrosis	16.0%
Endophthalmitis	12.5%
Cystoid macular edema	8.7%
Infectious keratitis	8.0%
Extrusion of implant	0%–12.5%

Reproduced from American Academy of Ophthalmology Cornea/External Disease Panel. Preferred Practice Pattern Guidelines. *Corneal Edema and Opacification.* American Academy of Ophthalmology; 2018. www.aao.org/ppp

Glaucoma is a major cause of vision loss and can silently and quickly progress in keratoprosthesis eyes. Because of the difficulty of obtaining accurate IOP measurements, optic nerve function should be closely monitored with visual field, OCT nerve fiber layer testing, and direct observation for cupping changes. Prophylactic tube shunt surgery during or prior to keratoprosthesis surgery can be considered in eyes treated or at increased risk for glaucoma.

Aravena C, Yu F, Aldave AJ. Long-term visual outcomes, complications, and retention of the Boston type I keratoprosthesis. *Cornea.* 2018;37(1):3–10.

Chang H-YP, Luo ZK, Chodosh J, Dohlman CH, Colby KA. Primary implantation of type I Boston keratoprosthesis in nonautoimmune corneal disease. *Cornea.* 2015;34(3):264–270.

Charoenrook V, Michael R, de la Paz MF, Temprano J, Barraquer RI. Comparison of long-term results between osteo-odonto-keratoprosthesis and tibial bone keratoprosthesis. *Ocul Surf.* 2018;16(2):259–264.

Fung SSM, Jabbour S, Harissi-Dagher M, et al. Visual outcomes and complications of type I Boston keratoprosthesis in children. A retrospective multicenter study and literature review. *Ophthalmology.* 2018;125(2):153–160.

Lee WB, Shtein RM, Kaufman SC, Deng SX, Rosenblatt MI. Boston keratoprosthesis: outcomes and complications: a report by the American Academy of Ophthalmology. *Ophthalmology.* 2015;122(7):1504–1511.

Part XII, Keratoprosthesis. In: Mannis MJ, Holland EJ, eds. *Cornea.* Vol 2. 5th ed. Elsevier; 2022:1558–1593.

Rudnisky CJ, Belin MW, Guo R, Ciolino JB; Boston Type 1 Keratoprosthesis Study Group. Visual acuity outcomes of the Boston keratoprosthesis type 1: multicenter study results. *Am J Ophthalmol.* 2016;162:89–98.e1.

Sayegh RR, Afshari NA, Chang HP, Lou ZK, Chodosh J. An overview of keratoprosthesis. *Focal Points: Clinical Modules for Ophthalmologists.* American Academy of Ophthalmology; 2014, module 6.

Additional Materials and Resources

Related Academy Materials

The American Academy of Ophthalmology is dedicated to providing a wealth of high-quality clinical education resources for ophthalmologists.

Print Publications and Electronic Products

For a complete listing of Academy clinical education products, visit our online store at https://store.aao.org/clinical-education.html. Or call Customer Service at 866.561.8558 (toll free, US only) or +1 415.561.8540, Monday through Friday, between 8:00 AM and 5:00 PM (PST).

Online Resources

Visit the Ophthalmic News and Education (ONE®) Network at https://www.aao.org/cornea-external-disease to find relevant videos, online courses, journal articles, practice guidelines, self-assessment quizzes, images, and more. The ONE Network is a free Academy-member benefit.

Access free, trusted articles and content with the Academy's collaborative online encyclopedia, EyeWiki, at aao.org/eyewiki.

Get mobile access to the *Wills Eye Manual,* watch the latest 1-minute videos, and set up alerts for clinical updates relevant to you with the AAO Ophthalmic Education App. Download today: Search for "AAO Ophthalmic Education" in the Apple app store or in Google Play.

Basic Texts and Additional Resources

Albert DM, Miller JW, Azar DT, Blodi BA, eds. *Albert & Jakobiec's Principles and Practice of Ophthalmology.* 3rd ed. 4 vols. Saunders; 2008.

Arffa RC, Grayson M, eds. *Grayson's Diseases of the Cornea.* 4th ed. Mosby; 1997.

Brightbill FS, McDonnell PJ, McGhee CN, Farjo AA, Serdarevic O. *Corneal Surgery: Theory, Technique and Tissue.* 4th ed. Mosby; 2009.

Copeland RA Jr, Afshari NA, eds. *Copeland and Afshari's Principles and Practice of Cornea.* Jaypee Brothers; 2013.

Feder RS, ed. *The LASIK Handbook: A Case-based Approach.* 2nd ed. Lippincott Williams & Wilkins; 2013.

Jorgensen JH, Pfaller MA, Carroll KC, Funke G, Landry ML, Richter SS, Warnock DW, eds. *Manual of Clinical Microbiology.* 11th ed. 2 vols. ASM Press; 2015.

Krachmer JH, Palay DA. *Cornea Atlas.* 3rd ed. Elsevier; 2013.

Laver NV, Specht CS, eds. *The Infected Eye: Clinical Practice and Pathological Principles.* Springer International Publishing; 2016.

Levin LA, Nilsson SFE, Ver Hoeve J, Wu SM, Alm A, Kaufman PL, eds. *Adler's Physiology of the Eye.* 11th ed. Saunders; 2011.

Mannis MJ, Holland EJ, eds. *Cornea.* 5th ed. 2 vols. Elsevier; 2021.

Seal DV, Pleyer U. *Ocular Infection: Investigation and Treatment in Practice.* 2nd ed. Informa Healthcare; 2007.

Spalton DJ, Hitchings RA, Hunter P. *Atlas of Clinical Ophthalmology.* 3rd ed. Elsevier/Mosby; 2005.

Requesting Continuing Medical Education Credit

The American Academy of Ophthalmology is accredited by the Accreditation Council for Continuing Medical Education (ACCME) to provide continuing medical education for physicians.

The American Academy of Ophthalmology designates this enduring material for a maximum of 15 *AMA PRA Category 1 Credits*™. Physicians should claim only the credit commensurate with the extent of their participation in the activity.

To claim *AMA PRA Category 1 Credits*™ upon completion of this activity, learners must demonstrate appropriate knowledge and participation in the activity by taking the posttest for Section 8 and achieving a score of 80% or higher.

This activity meets the Self-Assessment CME requirements defined by the American Board of Ophthalmology (ABO). Please be advised that the ABO is not an accrediting body for purposes of any CME program. ABO does not sponsor this or any outside activity, and ABO does not endorse any particular CME activity. Complete information regarding the ABO Self-Assessment CME Maintenance of Certification requirements is available at https://abop.org/maintain-certification/cme-self-assessment/.

To take the posttest and request CME credit online:

1. Go to www.aao.org/cme-central and log in.
2. Click on "Claim CME Credit and View My CME Transcript" and then "Report AAO Credits."
3. Select the appropriate media type and then the Academy activity. You will be directed to the posttest.
4. Once you have passed the test with a score of 80% or higher, you will be directed to your transcript. *If you are not an Academy member, you will be able to print out a certificate of participation once you have passed the test.*

CME expiration date: June 1, 2024. *AMA PRA Category 1 Credits*™ may be claimed only once between June 1, 2021, and the expiration date.

For assistance, contact the Academy's Customer Service department at 866.561.8558 (US only) or + 1 415.561.8540 between 8:00 AM and 5:00 PM (PST), Monday through Friday, or send an e-mail to customer_service@aao.org.

Study Questions

Please note that these questions are not part of your CME reporting process. They are provided here for your own educational use and identification of any professional practice gaps. The required CME posttest is available online (see "Requesting Continuing Medical Education Credit"). Following the questions are answers with discussions. Although a concerted effort has been made to avoid ambiguity and redundancy in these questions, the authors recognize that differences of opinion may occur regarding the "best" answer. The discussions are provided to demonstrate the rationale used to derive the answer. They may also be helpful in confirming that your approach to the problem was correct or, if necessary, in fixing the principle in your memory. The Section 8 faculty thanks the Resident Self-Assessment Committee for drafting these self-assessment questions and the discussions that follow.

1. What is a normal central endothelial cell count?
   a. 250–350 cells/mm^2
   b. 500–1000 cells/mm^2
   c. 2000–3000 cells/mm^2
   d. 5000–6000 cells/mm^2

2. What is the best noninvasive way to visualize the cysts pathognomonic of *Acanthamoeba* keratitis?
   a. anterior segment optical coherence tomography (AS-OCT)
   b. confocal microscopy
   c. sclerotic scatter
   d. specular microscopy

3. Subtle abnormalities in posterior corneal contour are best evaluated by what diagnostic tool?
   a. confocal microscopy
   b. Placido-disk imaging
   c. Scheimpflug tomography
   d. slit-lamp microscope

4. A 70-year-old man presents with chronic unilateral crusting and discharge from the right lateral canthus. Gram stain of the discharge reveals numerous gram-negative cocci in pairs. What pathogen is the most likely cause of the patient's symptoms?
   a. *Chlamydia trachomatis*
   b. *Haemophilus influenzae*
   c. *Moraxella lacunata*
   d. *Pseudomonas aeruginosa*

5. What organism is most commonly associated with phlyctenulosis in low-income countries?
   a. *Candida albicans*
   b. *Chlamydia trachomatis*
   c. *Mycobacterium tuberculosis*
   d. *Staphylococcus aureus*

6. Which type of topical glaucoma medication is most likely to cause aqueous tear deficiency?
   a. α_2-adrenergic agonists
   b. β-blockers
   c. carbonic anhydrase inhibitors
   d. prostaglandin analogues

7. What is the primary cause of exposure keratopathy in patients with Parkinson disease?
   a. cicatricial ectropion
   b. decreased blink frequency
   c. proptosis
   d. upper-eyelid retraction

8. A 58-year-old obese man presents with chronic ocular irritation and inflammation. On examination, the clinician notes significant eyelid laxity; in addition, the upper tarsus everts with minimal upward force. What systemic workup is indicated?
   a. buccal mucosal biopsy
   b. magnetic resonance imaging (MRI) of the brain
   c. sleep study
   d. thyroid function tests

9. After surgical removal of a pterygium, what is the best adjunctive treatment option to minimize the risk of recurrence and avoid any late-term complications?
   a. amniotic membrane transplant
   b. bevacizumab injection
   c. conjunctival autograft
   d. mitomycin-C (MMC) injection

10. What is the most common complication of a conjunctival flap?
    a. epithelial inclusion cysts
    b. flap retraction
    c. hemorrhage beneath the flap
    d. ptosis

11. In addition to antibiotics, what is the most appropriate management for a 3-mm central corneal perforation caused by *Neisseria gonorrhoeae*?
    a. application of cyanoacrylate glue
    b. corneal patch graft
    c. multi-layered amniotic membrane graft
    d. primary closure with 10-0 nylon sutures

12. In cases of untreated congenital syphilis, at what age does the onset of interstitial keratitis typically occur?
    a. 1–3 months
    b. 1–2 years
    c. 6–12 years
    d. 20–40 years

13. How can posterior keratoconus be distinguished from Peters anomaly anatomically?
    a. Descemet membrane is present in posterior keratoconus but absent in Peters anomaly.
    b. Descemet membrane is present in Peters anomaly but absent in posterior keratoconus.
    c. A thin layer of uveal tissue lining the posterior cornea is present in posterior keratoconus but absent in Peters anomaly.
    d. A thin layer of uveal tissue lining the posterior cornea is absent in posterior keratoconus but present in Peters anomaly.

14. What is the treatment for symptomatic conjunctival concretions?
    a. oral azithromycin
    b. removal of lesions with a 25-gauge needle
    c. topical steroids
    d. warm compresses

15. What is the composition of the deposits in spheroidal degeneration?
    a. carbohydrate
    b. glycosaminoglycan
    c. lipid
    d. protein

16. A 73-year-old woman with hyperparathyroidism reports chronic ocular irritation and foreign body sensation. There is a white, horizontal plaque in the interpalpebral zone of the cornea bilaterally. Her corneal condition primarily affects what layer of the cornea?
    a. epithelium
    b. Bowman layer
    c. anterior stroma
    d. deep stroma

17. What is the appropriate surgical therapy for visually significant Salzmann nodular degeneration?
    a. cauterization
    b. cryotherapy
    c. deep anterior lamellar keratoplasty (DALK)
    d. superficial keratectomy

18. A 54-year-old man who has been taking amiodarone for cardiac arrhythmia has developed deposits in a whorl-like pattern in the inferocentral corneal epithelium of both eyes. What is the most appropriate management of the corneal deposits?
    a. discontinuation of the amiodarone
    b. observation
    c. reduction of the dose of amiodarone
    d. superficial keratectomy with excimer laser

19. A 55-year-old woman with a history of multiple episodes of severe eye pain upon awakening reports that both eyes have been affected, although not always simultaneously. What corneal findings are most likely to be present on slit-lamp examination?
    a. basement membrane fingerprint lines
    b. epithelial filaments
    c. punctate epithelial erosions
    d. subepithelial infiltrates

20. What condition is characterized by bilateral dysfunctional corneal endothelial cells that demonstrate epithelial-like behavior?
    a. congenital hereditary endothelial dystrophy
    b. Fuchs endothelial corneal dystrophy (FECD)
    c. iridocorneal endothelial (ICE) syndrome
    d. posterior polymorphous corneal dystrophy

21. A 57-year-old woman has confluent guttae in both eyes. She reports intermittent, transient blurred vision in her left eye on waking. At 8 AM, her best-corrected visual acuity is 20/25 OD and 20/30 OS. What is the appropriate course of management?
    a. bandage soft contact lens
    b. hypertonic sodium chloride ointment in the left eye at night
    c. topical corticosteroids 4 times daily
    d. penetrating keratoplasty (PK)

22. What behavioral modification can lower the risk of keratoconus progression?
    a. avoidance of eye rubbing
    b. increased dietary consumption of omega-3 fatty acids
    c. smoking cessation
    d. reduction of alcohol use

23. Where does corneal thinning usually occur in eyes with pellucid marginal degeneration?
    a. centrally
    b. inferior periphery
    c. nasal and temporal periphery
    d. superior periphery

24. A 42-year-old man is referred for evaluation of red and irritated eyes. Examination reveals severe punctate erosions on the cornea and conjunctiva. A foamy appearing patch is noted on the temporal bulbar conjunctiva of the right eye. Tears bead along the conjunctival surface in small, individual droplets. The patient's medical history is significant for morbid obesity, for which he underwent gastric bypass surgery 6 months prior. Abnormalities in what cell type are responsible for the patient's symptoms and examination findings?
    a. goblet cells
    b. keratocytes
    c. lymphocytes
    d. squamous epithelial cells

25. A young child with cognitive impairment and hyperkeratotic lesions of the palms and soles is treated for recurrent episodes of corneal erosions and pseudodendrites that don't stain well with fluorescein or rose bengal dye. What treatment is indicated?
    a. high-dose oral ascorbic acid
    b. oral and/or topical cysteamine
    c. oral penicillamine
    d. restriction of tyrosine and phenylalanine intake

26. A 32-year-old man visits a clinic for a routine examination. He has a history of thyroid cancer and uncontrolled hypertension. The anterior segment examination reveals enlarged corneal nerves. What additional finding is most likely present in this patient?
    a. angioid streaks
    b. marfanoid body habitus
    c. microspherophakia
    d. preauricular skin tags

27. A 15-year-old adolescent girl with a history of renal transplant reports experiencing a right-sided headache for 2 days. Examination reveals redness of the right forehead, right upper eyelid, and nose, with a few clear vesicles. Slit-lamp examination shows conjunctival hyperemia and superficial punctate keratitis without deeper corneal involvement or iritis. What is the preferred management?
    a. systemic antiviral medications
    b. topical antiviral medications
    c. oral corticosteroids
    d. topical corticosteroids

28. A 34-year-old woman was treated for herpes simplex virus (HSV) epithelial keratitis with topical trifluridine 8 times daily for 2 weeks. She reports that the ocular discomfort improved but that shortly afterward, she developed a new onset of redness, tearing, and discomfort. What is the most likely cause of her newer symptoms?
    a. recurrent HSV keratitis
    b. superimposed bacterial conjunctivitis
    c. toxic epithelial keratopathy
    d. trichiasis

29. Who should receive the recombinant zoster vaccine (Shingrix)?
    a. immunocompetent adults aged 50 years and older
    b. immunocompetent adults aged 65 years and older
    c. immunocompetent adults who have not had chickenpox
    d. immunosuppressed adults aged 18 and older

30. A 7-year-old boy presents with a 2-day history of unilateral purulent conjunctivitis with diffuse subconjunctival hemorrhage. Gram stain shows numerous gram-negative bacilli. What is the most likely causative pathogen?
    a. *Haemophilus influenzae*
    b. *Moraxella catarrhalis*
    c. *Neisseria gonorrhoeae*
    d. *Streptococcus pneumoniae*

31. A 27-year-old patient has 24-hour duration of severe, hyperpurulent conjunctival discharge without a corneal ulcer. Conjunctival Gram stain reveals numerous neutrophils with gram-negative intracellular diplococci (GNID). What is the most appropriate treatment?
    a. intramuscular ceftriaxone
    b. intravenous penicillin G
    c. oral azithromycin
    d. topical gentamicin ointment

32. For acute Stevens-Johnson syndrome (SJS) with a conjunctival defect, what intervention has the greatest long-term benefit?
    a. amniotic membrane transplantation
    b. placement of a symblepharon ring
    c. repeated forniceal debridement with a glass rod
    d. temporary tarsorrhaphy

33. A patient presents with bilateral stromal infiltrates without epithelial ulceration. During the review of systems, the patient reports a recent viral upper respiratory tract infection and difficulty with balance and tinnitus. Rapid plasma reagin (RPR) test and microhemagglutination assay (fluorescent treponemal antibody absorption; FTA-ABS) results are negative. What systemic treatment is indicated as part of the typical therapeutic regimen for this condition?
    a. systemic antibiotic
    b. systemic antiviral medication
    c. systemic corticosteroid
    d. systemic nonsteroidal anti-inflammatory drug

34. What systemic disease is most frequently associated with peripheral ulcerative keratitis?
    a. granulomatosis with polyangiitis (Wegener granulomatosis)
    b. rheumatoid arthritis
    c. systemic lupus erythematosus
    d. ulcerative colitis

35. Conjunctival melanoma in what location is associated with the best long-term prognosis?
    a. bulbar conjunctiva
    b. caruncle
    c. fornix
    d. palpebral conjunctiva

36. A 32-year-old man is diagnosed with ocular surface squamous neoplasia (OSSN). A serologic test should be performed to look for what condition?
    a. herpes simplex virus
    b. HIV
    c. human herpesvirus 8
    d. varicella-zoster virus

37. In a patient with primary acquired melanosis (PAM), what clock-hour extent of conjunctival involvement is an indication to remove the lesion?
    a. more than 1 clock-hour
    b. more than 2 clock-hours
    c. more than 3 clock-hours
    d. more than 6 clock-hours

38. What physical examination finding is the best predictor of late corneal neovascularization in a patient with a chemical injury?
    a. amount of scleral and limbal ischemia
    b. degree of corneal edema
    c. extent of skin and eyelid burns
    d. presence of particulate chemical matter in the fornices

39. Why is tissue from donors younger than 2 years generally not used in corneal transplantation?
    a. The corneal endothelial cells are not sufficiently developed.
    b. The corneal stroma is too thin.
    c. The tissue is steeply curved and flaccid.
    d. There are ethical concerns about using tissue from infants and very young children.

40. In US eye banks, how long can corneal tissue remain viable once preserved in the storage medium?
    a. 24–48 hours
    b. 3–5 days
    c. 11–14 days
    d. 25–35 days

41. What type of rejection is more common in DALK than PK?
    a. endothelial rejection
    b. epithelial rejection
    c. stromal rejection
    d. subepithelial rejection

Answers

1. **c.** Normal central endothelial cell count is between 2000 and 3000 cell/mm^2. Central endothelial cell density decreases with age at an average rate of approximately 0.6% each year, diminishing from approximately 3400 cells/mm^2 at age 15 years to approximately 2300 cells/mm^2 at age 85 years. Eyes with an endothelial cell count below 500 cells/mm^2 may be at risk for developing corneal edema.
2. **b.** Confocal microscopy has demonstrated efficacy in the early diagnosis of patients with *Acanthamoeba* keratitis. It allows rapid identification of *Acanthamoeba* cysts with a relatively high sensitivity and specificity, although it requires a skilled observer to interpret the images. Anterior segment optical coherence tomography (AS-OCT) can provide cross-sectional information about corneal pathology but the resolution of the images obtained with AS-OCT is inadequate for detecting microscopic structures the size of *Acanthamoeba* cysts. Sclerotic scatter is useful for demonstrating subtle anterior corneal pathology such as mild central corneal edema but is not capable of resolving pathology at the microscopic level. Specular microscopy allows imaging of the corneal endothelium but is not considered useful in the diagnosis of *Acanthamoeba* keratitis.
3. **c.** The posterior contour is best evaluated using a Scheimpflug imaging system, a rotating scanning slit-beam device. This technology is particularly useful for evaluating subtle changes in the posterior corneal curvature and elevation that can indicate a higher risk for keratoconus or corneal ectasia in patients undergoing refractive corneal surgery. Although confocal microscopy provides an in vivo highly magnified view of the corneal epithelium, stroma, and endothelium, it does not provide contour information. Placido-disk imaging employed in corneal topography only provides information about the anterior corneal surface. A slit-lamp microscope is not sensitive enough to enable the clinician to identify subtle corneal curvature changes.
4. **c.** The patient's symptoms are consistent with those associated with angular blepharitis, a relatively uncommon entity that may be mistaken for other forms of chronic eyelid margin inflammation. Although *Staphylococcus aureus* and herpes simplex virus are possible etiologies, angular blepharitis is classically caused by *Moraxella lacunata* (which produces the Gram stain result of gram-negative cocci in pairs). *Chlamydia trachomatis* is a potential cause of chronic follicular conjunctivitis, but it is not associated with angular blepharitis. *Pseudomonas aeruginosa* and *Haemophilus influenzae* can cause acute conjunctivitis, but they are not known to cause angular blepharitis and do not demonstrate gram-negative cocci in pairs.
5. **c.** Phlyctenules are hyperemic, focal nodules consisting of chronic inflammatory cells. Phlyctenulosis is believed to represent a T-cell–mediated, or delayed hypersensitivity (type IV) response induced by microbial antigens. Phlyctenulosis is most frequently associated with *Staphlylococcus aureus* in high-income countries and is classically associated with *Mycobacterium tuberculosis* infection affecting malnourished individuals in tuberculosis-endemic areas of the world. Phlyctenulosis is not an ocular manifestation of *Candida albicans* or *Chlamydia trachomatis* infection.
6. **b.** Multiple medications have been associated with aqueous tear deficiency (ATD). Common systemic medications implicated in ATD include diuretics, antihistamines, anticholinergics, and psychotropic drugs. Among topical medications, β-blockers are most

commonly associated with ATD. Although α_2-adrenergic agonists, such as brimonidine, may cause follicular conjunctivitis, they do not cause ATD. Prostaglandin analogues can be associated with intraocular inflammation, and carbonic anhydrase inhibitors may affect endothelial function, but neither causes ATD.

7. **b.** Reduced blink frequency is the major cause of exposure keratopathy in patients with Parkinson disease. Certain medications used in the management of Parkinson disease may also reduce tear production. Although progressive facial paralysis does occur in patients with Parkinson disease, cicatricial ectropion is not the mechanism of exposure. Proptosis and upper-eyelid retraction are associated with thyroid eye disease, not Parkinson disease.
8. **c.** Floppy eyelid syndrome is characterized by chronic ocular irritation, inflammation, and eyelid laxity. Upper eyelid eversion occurs with minimal upward force. It is most frequently seen in obese patients and is associated with obstructive sleep apnea, which can be diagnosed with a sleep study. Floppy eyelid syndrome is not associated with abnormal results from brain imaging, abnormal results from a buccal mucosa biopsy, or abnormalities in thyroid function.
9. **c.** The risk of recurrence after pterygium excision is lower if a conjunctival autograft, rather than an amniotic membrane transplant, is used. If the defect created following dissection of the pterygium is considerably larger than the area that can be covered with an autologous conjunctival graft, an amniotic membrane graft or simple limbal epithelial transplantation (SLET) are viable techniques to cover the entire area of resection. Although there is evidence that mitomycin C (MMC) applied topically in conjunction with conjunctival autografting reduces the pterygium recurrence rate after surgical excision, topical MMC can be toxic and may cause visually significant complications. Bevacizumab has no effect on the recurrence rate after pterygium excision.
10. **b.** Retraction is the most common complication of conjunctival flaps, occurring in approximately 10% of cases. Other, less common complications include hemorrhage beneath the flap and epithelial inclusion cysts. Ptosis, usually due to levator dehiscence in elderly patients, may also occur postoperatively and may or may not be related to the flap itself.
11. **b.** Corneal perforations of 3 mm typically require emergent surgical closure with a corneal patch graft. Primary closure with nylon sutures is generally not feasible, particularly in eyes with acute infectious keratitis in which the surrounding tissue is also likely necrotic. Amniotic membrane grafts and cyanoacrylate glue are best suited for impending perforations or small perforations ($\leq$1 mm). They are unlikely to provide watertight closure of a large perforation.
12. **c.** Congenital syphilis is acquired in utero and caused by infection with the spirochete *Treponema pallidum*. In children with untreated congenital syphilis, onset of interstitial keratitis is typically between 6 and 12 years of age and is not present at birth.
13. **a.** Posterior keratoconus may be a variant of Peters anomaly, but these conditions can be differentiated by the presence of Descemet membrane, which is absent in Peters anomaly. Peters anomaly is characterized by the presence, at birth, of a central or paracentral corneal opacity (leukoma), which is due to the localized absence of the corneal endothelium and Descemet membrane beneath the area of opacity. Posterior keratoconus is characterized by a typically localized central or paracentral indentation of the posterior cornea without protrusion of the anterior corneal surface. Keratectasia differs from congenital anterior staphyloma histologically by the absence of a thin layer of uveal tissue lining the posterior cornea, which is present in congenital anterior staphyloma.

14. **b.** Conjunctival concretions are epithelial inclusion cysts filled with epithelial and keratin debris, as well as mucopolysaccharide and mucin. The majority of conjunctival concretions are asymptomatic. If they erode the conjunctival epithelium and cause symptoms of persistent foreign body irritation, they can be removed with a fine-gauge needle. Oral azithromycin, warm compresses, and topical steroids are not effective treatments for conjunctival concretions.
15. **d.** Spheroidal degeneration is characterized by the appearance of translucent, golden-brown, spheroidal deposits in the superficial stroma and Bowman layer. Despite its appearance, the brown deposit is proteinaceous in nature, rather than lipid. In contrast to spheroidal degeneration, lipid keratopathy most often occurs in association with stromal neovascularization. It can occur in the mid and deep stroma and is creamy white in color. Glycosaminoglycan deposition is found in multiple lysosomal storage diseases. Carbohydrate deposits are not associated with this corneal opacification.
16. **b.** Calcific band keratopathy is a degeneration of the superficial cornea that involves mainly Bowman layer. The degeneration begins as fine, dustlike, basophilic deposits in at the level of Bowman layer, usually first seen peripherally in the 3- and 9-o'clock positions. Eventually, the deposits may coalesce to form a dense horizontal band of calcific plaques across the interpalpebral zone of the cornea. Numerous systemic diseases, including hyperparathyroidism, chronic renal failure, sarcoidosis, and gout are risk factors for band keratopathy.
17. **d.** Salzmann nodular degeneration refers to grayish subepithelial nodules that occur primarily or secondary to previous inflammatory or mechanical insult to the cornea. These changes are typically confined to the very superficial anterior stroma and are amenable to debridement with superficial keratectomy. Deep anterior lamellar keratoplasty (DALK) is unnecessarily invasive for this superficial condition. Cauterization and cryotherapy are not effective treatments for Salzmann nodular degeneration.
18. **b.** Cornea verticillata, or vortex keratopathy, manifests as a whorl-like pattern of golden-brown or gray deposits in the inferior interpalpebral aspect of the cornea. The antiarrhythmic medication amiodarone is the most common cause of corneal verticillata. Because it is unusual for these deposits to result in reduction of vision or ocular symptoms, treatments such as superficial keratectomy with excimer laser are not necessary. It is acceptable for the patient to continue taking the recommended dose of systemic medication. The patient should be monitored by the ophthalmologist.
19. **a.** Recurrent corneal erosions typically occur in eyes that have suffered prior ocular surface trauma, usually an abrading injury with shearing force, such as a fingernail injury. Approximately 50% of patients with recurrent corneal erosions are believed to have underlying epithelial basement membrane dystrophy (EBMD), although only 10% of patients with EBMD will develop recurrent corneal erosions. Patterns of corneal epithelial findings evident on slit-lamp examination in eyes with EBMD include fingerprint lines, maps, dots, and a bleb pattern. Filamentary keratitis is more characteristically associated with dry eye disease and superior limbic keratoconjunctivitis than with recurrent corneal erosions. Punctate epithelial erosions are associated with corneal surface dryness from dry eye disease, but they are not a hallmark of recurrent corneal erosions. Subepithelial infiltrates are most typically seen in epidemic keratoconjunctivitis.
20. **d.** Posterior polymorphous corneal dystrophy (PPCD) is characterized by bilateral (can be asymmetric) vesicular or scalloped areas of abnormal endothelium that demonstrates

epithelial characteristics. The abnormal epithelium typically produces progressive or episodic corneal edema and may produce peripheral anterior synechiae or iridocorneal adhesions that cause corectopia. Although iridocorneal endothelial (ICE) syndrome can mimic all of these features, it is characteristically a unilateral condition. Fuchs endothelial corneal dystrophy (FECD) and congenital hereditary endothelial dystrophy (CHED) both cause bilateral endothelial dysfunction, but the endothelium in eyes with these dystrophies does not have the epithelial properties seen in eyes with PPCD.

21. **b.** The signs and symptoms are typical of the early stages of FECD. The most commonly used treatments for early FECD are hyperosmotic agents (5% sodium chloride); eyedrops used during the day and ointment applied at night may reduce edema upon awakening. Another option is a hair dryer used on the cool setting. Bandage soft contact lenses may be used to treat painful erosions and ruptured bullae but are not routinely used to treat early morning edema. In cases of more advanced disease, surgical options can be considered; the first-line therapy is endothelial keratoplasty in patients without significant stromal scarring. Penetrating keratoplasty (PK) is reserved for patients with endothelial failure and significant corneal scarring.

22. **a.** Patients with keratoconus should be cautioned against eye rubbing because it can contribute to the progression of keratoconus and increases the risk of hydrops in advanced cases. Smoking, alcohol use, and reduced omega-3 fatty acid intake do not increase the risk of keratoconus progression.

23. **b.** Pellucid marginal degeneration is characterized by protrusion above a band of inferior peripheral thinning in the absence of inflammation. In contrast, in eyes with keratoconus, typically there is inferior paracentral thinning at the apex of the cone. Mooren ulcer is an inflammatory condition with associated stromal thinning that starts in the nasal or temporal periphery. Terrien degeneration typically begins with superior peripheral thinning associated with corneal neovascularization that crosses the thinned area and lipid deposition at the central edge.

24. **a.** Vitamin A deficiency is associated with the loss of mucus production by goblet cells. This results in xerosis, abnormal dryness of the conjunctival surface. In impoverished regions of the world, vitamin A deficiency results from low dietary intake. Gastric bypass surgery can also result in vitamin A deficiency due to malabsorption. Vitamin A deficiency can also result in reduced night vision. Abnormalities in keratocytes, lymphocytes, and squamous cells are not associated with the conjunctival lesion or tear findings.

25. **d.** Tyrosinemia type II (Richner-Hanhart syndrome) is an autosomal recessive disorder resulting from defective tyrosine aminotransferase, which leads to excess tyrosine in the blood and urine. Signs and symptoms include marked photophobia, tearing, conjunctival injection, and tarsal papillary hypertrophy. Affected patients experience recurrent episodes of corneal erosions and pseudodendrites. Patients with tyrosinemia type II may show hyperkeratotic lesions of the palms, soles, and elbows, as well as cognitive impairment. Restriction of dietary intake of tyrosine and phenylalanine can reduce the severity of both the corneal and systemic changes. High-dose ascorbic acid may reduce arthropathy in patients with alkaptonuria, not tyrosinemia. Oral and/or topical cysteamine is the treatment for cystinosis, and oral penicillamine is used to treat Wilson disease.

26. **b.** Enlarged corneal nerves are associated with multiple endocrine neoplasia type 2B (MEN 2B), a condition that is also characterized by pheochromocytoma, medullary carcinoma of the thyroid, mucosal neuromas, and a marfanoid body habitus. Angioid streaks may

be seen in a number of conditions, including pseudoxanthoma elasticum, Ehlers-Danlos syndrome, Paget disease of bone, and sickle cell disease. Microspherophakia is seen in Weill-Marchesani syndrome, a condition also associated with short stature, ectopia lentis, and brachydactyly. Preauricular skin tags may be seen in individuals with Goldenhar-Gorlin syndrome, also known as oculoauriculovertebral syndrome.

27. **a.** Herpes zoster virus infection occurs when dormant varicella-zoster virus in the dorsal root and cranial nerve (CN) ganglia reactivates. Pain in a sensory nerve distribution may be the first sign of reactivation. A unilateral vesicular rash that follows a dermatomal distribution is characteristic. Postherpetic neuralgia may follow resolution. When CN V_1 is involved, the condition is called herpes zoster ophthalmicus (HZO). The current treatment recommendation for all patients with HZO is systemic antiviral therapy. Topical antiviral medications are effective only in the treatment of epithelial mucoid plaques or more chronic epithelial disease. Topical corticosteroids are indicated for treatment of keratouveitis. Oral corticosteroids, a controversial treatment aimed at reducing postherpetic neuralgia, are contraindicated in immunocompromised patients.

28. **c.** Although trifluridine is effective in treating herpes simplex virus (HSV) epithelial keratitis, continued use of trifluridine may lead to toxicity of the ocular surface, which can manifest with symptoms similar to those of the original HSV episode. The most common corneal finding associated with toxicity is diffuse punctate epithelial erosions. Oral acyclovir has been reported to be as effective as topical antiviral medications for the treatment of epithelial keratitis and does not cause ocular toxicity. For this reason, oral therapy is preferred by an increasing number of ophthalmologists. Recurrent HSV keratitis would be unlikely, given that the patient was still on topical antiviral treatment. Superimposed bacterial conjunctivitis is quite unlikely, particularly in the absence of purulent discharge. Trichiasis, while possible, is far less likely than toxic keratopathy.

29. **a.** Although there are 2 vaccines for prevention of shingles, Zostavax and Shingrix, Zostavax is no longer available in the United States. The recombinant zoster vaccine Shingrix, which has been available since 2017, is recommended by the CDC as the preferred shingles vaccine, with 2 doses separated by 2 to 6 months for immunocompetent adults aged 50 year and older.

30. **a.** Acute purulent conjunctivitis in a child can be caused by a number of pathogens. In this case, the associated subconjunctival hemorrhage and the result of the Gram stain make *Haemophilus influenzae* the most likely etiology. *Streptococcus pneumoniae* can produce a purulent conjunctivitis, but the Gram stain would demonstrate gram-positive cocci. *Moraxella catarrhalis* generally causes a chronic, low-grade conjunctivitis, which may have associated angular blepharitis. Subconjunctival hemorrhages are not typically present, and the Gram stain would reveal gram-negative diplococci. *Neisseria gonorrhoeae* typically presents as a hyperacute purulent conjunctivitis in sexually active adults. The Gram stain would reveal gram-negative intracellular diplococci (GNID).

31. **a.** Hyperacute conjunctivitis with GNID is diagnostic of gonococcal conjunctivitis caused by *Neisseria gonorrhoeae*. If corneal ulceration is present, the patient should be admitted to the hospital to receive intravenous ceftriaxone. In the absence of corneal involvement, outpatient therapy with intramuscular ceftriaxone 1 g and close observation is appropriate. Intravenous penicillin G is indicated for treatment of neurosyphilis. Oral azithromycin is indicated for the treatment of chlamydial conjunctivitis. Although topical gentamicin ointment can be used as an adjunctive treatment for gonococcal conjunctivitis, the mainstay of treatment is systemic ceftriaxone.

32. **a.** Early amniotic membrane transplantation (within the first 3–7 days) has been shown to reduce the formation of symblepharon and minimize long-term ocular surface complications for patients with conjunctival inflammation from Stevens-Johnson syndrome (SJS). Symblepharon rings and forniceal debridement have been largely supplanted by amniotic membrane grafting. Repeated forniceal debridement may even worsen conjunctival scarring due to mechanical trauma. Temporary tarsorrhaphy may be indicated for nonhealing epithelial defects, but it is not directly beneficial to preventing symblepharon formation.

33. **c.** Bilateral nonulcerative stromal inflammation is suggestive of interstitial keratitis, an inflammatory, nonulcerative condition that primarily involves the corneal stroma. Herpes simplex and syphilis are the most common etiologies of interstitial keratitis in the United States. In this case, the negative rapid plasma reagin (RPR) and fluorescent treponemal antibody absorption (FTA-ABS) test results and the vestibuloauditory pathology suggested by the review of systems are consistent with Cogan syndrome, a rare autoimmune disease often precipitated by a viral illness, with features that overlap with polyarteritis nodosa. Cogan syndrome can be associated with vertigo and can lead to permanent deafness if not treated promptly with systemic corticosteroids. A systemic antibiotic would not be appropriate with a negative syphilis serology. A systemic antiviral medication could be considered if herpes simplex was being considered. A systemic nonsteroidal anti-inflammatory drug would not be the best choice for a patient with Cogan syndrome.

34. **b.** Rheumatoid arthritis is the condition most frequently associated with peripheral ulcerative keratitis. Testing for rheumatoid factor (RF) is warranted as part of the systemic evaluation. Systemic lupus erythematosus, granulomatosis with polyangiitis (Wegener granulomatosis), and ulcerative colitis are also associated with peripheral ulcerative keratitis but are less commonly present.

35. **a.** Conjunctival melanoma–related mortality at 10 years ranges from 13% to 38%. Involvement of the caruncle, palpebral conjunctiva, or conjunctival fornix are all associated with a twofold or greater risk for mortality than is bulbar conjunctival involvement alone.

36. **b.** Risk factors associated with ocular surface squamous neoplasia (OSSN) include older age, ultraviolet light exposure, prior skin cancer, male sex, smoking, fair complexion, human papillomavirus (HPV) infection, HIV infection, and systemic immunosuppression. In a young adult, OSSN should prompt consideration of a serologic test for HIV. Rapid growth of lesions may occur in a person with AIDS. Neither herpes simplex virus nor varicella-zoster virus is considered a risk factor for OSSN. Human herpesvirus 8 is the etiology of Kaposi sarcoma.

37. **b.** Primary acquired melanosis (PAM) is an acquired, noncystic, flat, patchy or diffuse, tan to brown pigmentation of the conjunctival epithelium. PAM is usually unilateral or asymmetric if bilateral and is most often seen in individuals with fair skin. Two clock-hours or less of conjunctival involvement is associated with a lower risk of malignant transformation; involvement of more than 2 clock-hours is an indication to remove the lesion for histologic diagnosis.

38. **a.** Although all these clinical features are pertinent when documenting the extent of ocular surface injury resulting from chemical trauma, the degree of limbal ischemia is the most important predictor of progression to limbal stem cell deficiency (which results in corneal neovascularization). Treatments to improve prognosis include those intended to minimize ongoing exposure to the agent (eg, immediate irrigation with water or saline,

removal of any particulate matter), decrease inflammation (topical corticosteroids, oral tetracyclines), and promote healing (oral vitamin C, amniotic membrane transplantation).

39. **c.** Most eye banks accept corneal tissue from donors 2 to 75 years of age. Tissue from donors younger than 2 years is typically not used because of the extremely steep curvature and flaccid nature of the tissue, which makes the tissue difficult to handle. This poses challenges for the surgeon in creating a watertight closure and achieving a predictable outcome.

40. **c.** In the United States, the most commonly used storage media used for corneal tissue are Optisol GS (Bausch + Lomb) and Life4°C (Numedis). Both contain chondroitin sulfate, dextran, gentamycin, and streptomycin; Life4°C also contains insulin. Tissue is stored at 2° to 8°C and can remain viable for up to 14 days. In Europe, donor corneal tissue is incubated in organ culture storage that allows tissue to be stored for up to 35 days, but this requires a culture at the end of storage to confirm sterility, which can be complex, expensive, and labor intensive.

41. **c.** Stromal rejection, characterized by significant haze and deep vascularization, can lead to corneal opacification and is more common after DALK than PK. In DALK, the corneal endothelium is not transplanted; therefore, endothelial rejection cannot take place. Epithelial rejection and subepithelial infiltrates tend to be less visually significant and are possible in both DALK and PK.

Index

(*f* = figure; *t* = table)

Ablation. *See* Excimer laser ablation
Abrasions
  blunt trauma sign, 437, 438
  differential diagnosis, 438
  foreign bodies and, 447, 448*f*
  mucous membrane pemphigoid sign, 370
  recurrent erosion syndrome association, 97, 97*f*
  treatment, 438, 451
Abscesses
  chalazia association, 84
  hordeola association, 84
  postoperative complication, 479, 479*f*
  transplant complication, 491
Acanthamoeba keratitis
  about, 344
  corticosteroid precaution, 340
  differential diagnosis, 53*t*, 290*t*, 292*t*, 293, 319*t*, 337, 350, 382
  laboratory evaluation, 320–321*t*, 321, 345–346, 345*f*
  neurotrophic keratopathy cause, 95*t*
  pathogenesis, 320, 345
  postoperative transplant complication, 478
  prominent corneal nerves association, 276*t*
  signs and symptoms, 53*t*, 344–345, 344*f*
  treatment, 346
Acanthamoeba scleritis, 350
Accelerated corneal crosslinking, 245
Acetic acid, 424*t*
Acetylcysteine, 69, 374, 384, 386
Achondroplasia, 138*t*, 141
Acid burns, 424–427*t*, 425, 429–431*f*, 429–432
ACL (acromegaly, cutis verticis gyrata, corneal leukoma) syndrome, 152
Acne rosacea. *See* Rosacea
Acrocephalopolysyndactyly type II (Carpenter syndrome), 267*t*
Acromegaly, cutis verticis gyrata, corneal leukoma (ACL) syndrome, 152
Actinic keratopathy (spheroidal degeneration), 163–165, 164*f*, 169, 260
Actinomyces spp, 319*t*, 337*t*
Acute hemorrhagic conjunctivitis (AHC), 315
Acute retinal necrosis (ARN), 301
Acyclovir (intravenous therapy), 302
Acyclovir (oral), 287*t*, 291, 294–295*t*, 294–296, 299, 302
Acyclovir (topical), 287*t*, 291
Adaptive immunity classification, 354
Adenovirus infections
  about, 282, 306
  conjunctivitis, 50*t*, 53*t*, 307, 315, 332
  diagnosis, 283*t*, 309
  differential diagnosis, 284–285, 290*t*, 303
  disinfection, 308
  epidemic keratoconjunctivitis, 53*t*, 307–308, 307–309*f*
  keratitis, 53*t*, 308–309, 309*f*, 332
  pathogenesis, 308–309
  Stevens-Johnson syndrome and, 367
  transmission, 308, 310
  treatment, 309–310
Adolescents
  benign lymphoid folliculosis in, 49, 51*f*
  chlamydial infections and, 332
  cystinosis in, 258
  Fuchs superficial marginal keratitis and, 173
  herpes simplex virus and, 285
  keratoconjunctivitis in, 358–359, 362*t*
  keratoconus treatment for, 228
  lice infestations and, 323
  osteogenesis imperfecta in, 270
  rosacea in, 76
Adrenochrome deposition, 166*t*
Adult cystinosis (nonnephropathic cystinosis), 258
Advancement flap, 116, 117*f*
Afferent pupillary defect, 451
Afipia felis, 333
Aging
  conjunctival signs of, 157, 158, 160
  corneal signs of, 162, 171, 177–178
  donor-cornea selection and, 467
  dry eye risk factor, 56*t*
  endothelial cell density and, 40–41
  lymphoid malignancy risk factor, 63
  scleral signs of, 178–179
AHC. *See* Acute hemorrhagic conjunctivitis
AIDS. *See* HIV and AIDS-related ocular disorders
Air bubble retention, 497–499, 498*f*
AKC. *See* Atopic keratoconjunctivitis
Alagille syndrome (arteriohepatic dysplasia), 139*t*, 146
Albendazole (oral), 349
Albright hereditary osteodystrophy, 267*t*
ALK. *See* Anterior lamellar keratoplasty
Alkali burns, 104, 123*f*, 423–425, 424–427*t*, 428*f*, 431
Alkaptonuria, 166*t*, 257*t*, 260–261, 271*t*
Allergic conjunctivitis. *See* Conjunctivitis (immune-related)
Allografts
  defined, 463
  indications, 108*t*
  limbal stem cell deficiency treatment, 101–102
  limbal transplantation, 108*t*, 120*t*, 121, 122–124
  rejections, 481–485, 482*t*, 483–484*f*, 490, 491*f*
Allopurinol, 264, 367
α-adrenergic agents, 354
α-galactosidase A deficiency, 252*t*, 253–254
α-hemolytic *Streptococcus* spp, 335, 336*f*
Alport syndrome, 138*t*, 142
Amblyopia, 444, 461, 470, 485, 508
Amebic keratitis. *See Acanthamoeba* keratitis
Amino acid metabolism disorders, 257–260, 257*t*

Aminocaproic acid, 445
Aminoglycosides (intravenous), 458
Aminoglycosides (topical), 103*t*, 104, 326, 346, 354
Amiodarone, 66*t*, 179, 180, 253, 271*t*
Ammonia, 424*t*
Amniotic membrane grafts
about, 119–120, 130
for bare sclera coverage, 110, 112
chemical injury treatment, 428*f*, 431–432
congenital corneal anesthesia treatment, 153
conjunctivitis treatment, 364
conjunctivochalasis treatment, 92
epithelial defect treatment, 96, 477
herpetic eye disease treatment, 298
indications overview, 108*t*
keratoconjunctivitis treatment, 91*t*
for limbic stem cell transplantation, 120*t*, 121
melt treatment, 130
for mucous membrane grafting, 124
pterygium treatment, 109*t*
radiation injury treatment, 434
for scleral reinforcement, 394
SJS/TEN treatment, 367
thermal burn treatment, 433
ulcer treatment, 297, 361
Amphotericin B (injectable), 343
Amphotericin B (topical), 343
Amyloid depositions
amyloidosis and, 261–264, 262*t*, 263*f*, 419, 437
corneal dystrophies and, 196–197, 198*f*, 199*t*, 201
gelatinous droplike corneal dystrophy sign, 191
polymorphic amyloid degeneration, 172, 172*f*
Androgen, 15–16*f*
Androgen deficiency, 56*t*, 64*t*
Anesthetics (topical)
abuse of, 53*t*, 105–106, 106*f*, 293
dry eye cause, 59
toxic reactions to, 95*t*, 103
Aneurysms (conjunctiva), 253
Angiokeratoma corporis diffusum (Fabry disease), 180, 251, 252*t*, 253–254, 290
Angle anomalies, 45, 139*t*
Angle-closure glaucoma, 141, 143, 177*t*, 213, 342
Angle kappa, 34
Aniridia, 100, 102*t*, 108*t*, 146, 147, 219*t*
Ankyloblepharon, 278, 369, 370*f*
Ankylosing spondylitis, 389
Annular keratopathy, 437
Anterior basement membrane dystrophy. *See* Epithelial basement membrane dystrophy
Anterior ciliary arteries, 8
Anterior lamellar keratoplasty (ALK)
about, 464, 465, 488, 488*f*
comparisons, 465, 473–475*t*
indications, 466*t*, 469*t*, 473*t*, 475*t*, 490–491
intraoperative complications, 473*t*
Mooren ulcer treatment, 386, 386*f*
postoperative complications, 474*t*
tattooing with, 134*f*, 135
Anterior lens capsule, 45, 181, 273
Anterior megalocornea, 233*t*
Anterior scleritis, 389–390, 389–390*f*, 389*t*, 391, 391*f*, 392
Anterior segment dysgenesis, 141, 145–151, 146–148*f*, 150–151*f*
Anterior segment examination, 21–26, 39, 44–45
Anterior segment optical coherence tomography (AS-OCT)
about, 37, 44, 44*f*
for conjunctival degeneration evaluation, 159, 159*f*
for corneal dystrophy evaluation, 194, 195*f*, 196*t*
for keratoconus evaluation, 224–225
for ocular surface squamous neoplasia evaluation, 159, 405, 405*f*
for transplantation imaging, 497, 497*f*, 499, 500*f*
Anterior stromal puncture (ASP)
corneal dystrophy treatment, 190, 211, 214
recurrent corneal erosions treatment, 99, 126–127, 127*f*
Anterior uveitis
about, 439
etiology, 305, 314, 432, 435, 439
prophylaxis, 303
reactive arthritis association, 376
treatment, 294–295*t*, 439
Antibiotics (fortified), 339
Antibiotics (intravenous), 458
Antibiotics (oral)
burn treatment, 433
cellulitis treatment, 85
conjunctivitis treatment, 326, 327, 328
corneal perforation treatment, 130
keratitis treatment, 339
perforating injury treatment, 451
Antibiotics (topical)
adenovirus infection treatment, 309–310
band keratopathy treatment, 168
blepharitis treatment, 81
burn treatment, 433
conjunctivitis treatment, 326, 327
corneal abrasion treatment, 438
corneal perforation treatment, 130
descemetocele treatment, 130
dry eye treatment, 74
foreign bodies treatment, 449
keratitis treatment, 337
perforating injury treatment, 451
phlyctenulosis treatment, 84
postoperative use, 113, 458–459, 476
post-trauma use, 435, 436
precautions, 74
RES treatment, 99
SJS/TEN treatment, 367
Antibody-mediated cytotoxic (type II) reactions, 353
Anticholinergic drugs, 56*t*, 66
Anticoagulant drugs, 75, 163*t*, 437, 499
Anticonvulsant drugs, 366
Antidepressant drugs, 56*t*, 66*t*
Antifibrinolytic drugs, 445

Antigen-presenting cells (APCs), 16, 16*f*, 17, 380
Antihistamines
atopic dermatitis treatment, 356
conjunctivochalasis treatment, 92
contact dermatoblepharitis treatment, 355
dry eye risk factor, 56*t*
keratoconjunctivitis treatment, 360
loiasis treatment, 349
Antihypertensive drugs, 56*t*, 66*t*, 354, 445
Antiplatelet drugs, 437
Anti–TNF-α drugs, 373, 373*t*, 393
Antiviral drugs
adverse effects, 104, 354
for herpes simplex virus infections, 286, 287, 287*t*, 288, 290–291, 294–295*t*, 294–298
mechanism of action, 282
postoperative use of, 297–298
for varicella-zoster virus infections, 302–304
Anxiolytics, 56*t*
APCs. *See* Antigen-presenting cells
Apert syndrome, 267*t*
Aphakic corneal edema, 480, 484
Apical scarring, 220, 222*f*, 226, 228
Apocrine sweat glands, 4
Apoptosis (programmed cell death), 57, 63
Aqueous tear deficiency (ATD)
chlamydia association, 329
differential diagnosis, 30, 67
dry eye and, 67
pathogenesis, 57–58, 62–63
signs and symptoms, 30, 59–63, 61–62*t*, 67, 67*f*
Sjögren syndrome association, 62–63, 62*t*, 367–368
SLK-association, 90
treatment, 67–71, 67*f*, 68*t*, 71*f*
Arachnid injuries, 435, 435*f*
Arcus juvenilis, 138*t*, 142, 171
Arc welding, 433
Argyriasis, 166*t*
Arlt line, 329, 330*f*
ARN (acute retinal necrosis), 301
Arteriohepatic dysplasia (Alagille syndrome), 139*t*, 146
Artificial tears
ATD treatment, 68
conjunctivitis (allergic) treatment, 357
dellen treatment, 100
exposure keratopathy treatment, 94
keratitis treatment, 377
keratoconjunctivitis treatment, 91*t*
postherpetic neuralgia treatment, 303
pterygium treatment, 159
for radiation injuries, 434
SJS/TEN treatment, 367
Ascorbic acid, 260, 431
AS-OCT. *See* Anterior segment optical coherence tomography
ASP. *See* Anterior stromal puncture
Aspergillus spp, 319*t*, 343
Aspirin, 437
Astigmatism
birth trauma association, 154
contact lenses for, 470
corneal degeneration sign, 231*t*
corneal dystrophy sign, 184, 188
etiology, 152
Goldenhar-Gorlin syndrome sign, 271
herpetic eye disease complication, 297
keratoconus association, 149, 220, 222–223, 225*f*, 227
megalocornea association, 143
pellucid marginal degeneration sign, 229, 231*t*
postoperative complication, 455
postoperative control of, 485–488, 486–487*f*
post-transplant complication, 475*t*, 479, 490, 491, 509
post-transplant management, 485–488, 486–487*f*
signs and symptoms, 33, 35
surgical management, 107, 108*f*, 161*f*, 173, 461
with-the-rule astigmatism, 35*f*, 108*f*, 143
Ataxia-telangiectasia (Louis-Bar syndrome), 417
ATD. *See* Aqueous tear deficiency
Atopic dermatitis, 355–356, 356*f*, 362
Atopic keratitis, 292*t*
Atopic keratoconjunctivitis (AKC)
differential diagnosis, 53*t*, 88, 362*t*
pathogenesis, 362
signs and symptoms, 53*t*, 361–362, 362*t*, 363*f*
treatment, 362–363
ATP7B gene, 265
Atropine (topical), 103, 354
Atypical granular corneal dystrophy (Reis-Bücklers corneal dystrophy), 186*t*, 192–194, 193*f*, 195, 196*t*
Atypical mycobacteria. *See Mycobacterium* spp
Autografts
complications, 113–114, 113*f*
conjunctiva, 108*t*, 109*t*, 110, 110–111*f*, 112
conjunctival-limbal, 109*t*, 112
defined, 463
of limbal stem cells, 101, 121, 122–123*f*
postoperative care, 113
technique, 110, 110*f*
types of, 509, 509*f*
Autoimmune-related keratitis, 375, 376
Autologous serum solutions, 69, 91*t*, 96, 297, 375
Autologous transplantation
for bare sclera coverage, 108, 112
chemical injury treatment, 432
conjunctival, 108, 112, 114, 432
defined, 463
of limbal stem cells, 101, 120*t*, 432
radiation injury treatment, 434
Avellino corneal dystrophy (granular corneal dystrophy type 2), 199*t*, 201, 201*f*
Axenfeld-Rieger syndrome (Axenfeld anomaly [syndrome] or Rieger anomaly [syndrome]), 139*t*, 146, 147*f*, 215*t*
Axial curvature power map, 34, 35–36*f*
Azelaic aid, 78

Azithromycin (oral)
conjunctivitis treatment, 331, 332, 333
dry eye treatment, 75, 78
rosacea treatment, 78
Azithromycin (topical), 74, 81

Bacillus spp, 318*t*, 453
Bacitracin, 81, 326, 327
Bacterial infections
conjunctivitis, 323–333, 324*t*. *See also under* Conjunctivitis
differential diagnosis, 436
keratitis, 334–341, 335–336*f*, 337–338*t*. *See also* Bacterial keratitis
pathogenesis, 318–322, 319*t*
specimen collection and evaluation, 320–321*t*, 322*f*
Bacterial keratitis
about, 334
atypical mycobacteria etiology, 341, 341*f*
differential diagnosis, 53*t*, 293
etiology, 337*t*
intrauterine keratitis, 151–152
laboratory evaluation, 336–337
pathogenesis, 335–336
postoperative complication, 480
postoperative transplant complication, 478
risk factors, 334
signs and symptoms, 53*t*, 334–335, 335–336*f*
transplant complication, 491
treatment, 337–341, 338*t*
BAK. *See* Benzalkonium chloride
Baltimore virus classification, 282, 283*f*
Bandage soft contact lenses (BSCLs)
band keratopathy treatment, 167–168
for bare sclera coverage treatments, 110*f*, 113–114
chemical injury treatment, 431–432
corneal abrasion treatment, 438, 451
dellen treatment, 100
descemetocele treatment, 130
epithelial defect treatment, 128–129, 477
foreign bodies treatment, 449
graft-vs-host disease treatment, 374
keratitis treatment, 377, 384
melting treatment, 384
perforating injury treatment, 451
precautions, 94
radiation injury treatment, 434
RES treatment, 99
shield ulcer treatment, 361
SLK treatment, 91*t*
Band keratopathy
ATD sign, 60
Cockayne syndrome sign, 267*t*
differential diagnosis, 191, 192*f*
etiology, 167, 168*t*, 264
hypophosphatasia sign, 268*t*
ichthyosis sign, 278
parathyroid disease and, 277
signs and symptoms, 165–167, 167*f*
treatment, 167–168
Bark, 448
Bartonella species, 333
Basic secretion test, 30
Bassen-Kornzweig syndrome, 256
B-cell non-Hodgkin lymphoma, 420
BCVA. *See* Best-corrected visual acuity
Bee stings, 435
Bence Jones proteins, 275
Benign monoclonal gammopathy, 259*t*, 273, 274
Benzalkonium chloride (BAK), 103
Best-corrected visual acuity (BCVA; corrected distance visual acuity), 237–238
β-blockers, 56*t*, 68, 354
β-galactosidases deficiency, 250*t*, 253
Bevacizumab, 113
Biber-Haab-Dimmer (lattice corneal dystrophy type 1) and variants, 186*t*, 196–199, 187–199*f*, 199*t*, 201, 261, 478
Bietti nodular dystrophy (spheroidal degeneration), 163–165, 164*f*, 169, 260
"Big bubble" technique, 488–489
Biguanides, 346
Biliary cirrhosis, 166*t*, 265
Biopsy
conjunctiva
about, 118
conjunctival papilloma treatment, 401
cystinosis evaluation, 258
Fabry disease evaluation, 253
lymphoid hyperplasia evaluation, 419
map biopsies, 407, 413
MPM evaluation, 371–372, 372*f*
of nevus, 412
primary acquired melanosis evaluation, 413
sebaceous carcinoma evaluation, 407
tyrosinemia evaluation, 260
cornea, 125, 315, 321
sclera, 350
Bipedicle flap, 116, 117*f*
Birth trauma, 154–155, 155*f*, 177*t*
Bitôt spot, 272, 272*f*
Blast injuries, 448
Bleb pattern, 188, 190, 190*f*
Blepharitis
bacterial, 81, 321
differential diagnosis, 53*t*, 85
ectodermal dysplasia association, 278
etiology, 319*t*
meibomian gland disease association, 73*t*, 80*t*
parasitic, 73*t*, 79, 322–323, 323*f*
rosacea association, 76
signs and symptoms, 53*t*, 79, 79–80*f*, 80*t*, 81–82, 84*f*, 354, 355*f*
treatment, 81, 354–355, 373
types of, 78–82, 80*t*. *See also specific disorders*
Blepharoconjunctivitis
bacterial, 81–82, 83*f*, 325
differential diagnosis, 407
marginal keratitis risk factor, 381
viral, 284, 284–285*f*, 287

Blepharoplasty, 91, 94
Blepharospasm, 90, 154
Blindness
  about, 272
  bacterial etiology, 329
  immune-related etiology, 379
  snow blindness, 433
  surgical treatment, 374
  viral etiology, 286, 314
  vitamin A deficiency and, 272
Blinking (reflex), 3, 6, 20, 32
Blink rate, 32, 58*f*, 477
Blue sclera
  differential diagnosis, 267–268*t*, 271*t*
  Ehlers-Danlos syndrome association, 266, 269
  keratoglobus association, 140*t*, 232
  Marfan syndrome association, 269
  osteogenesis imperfecta association, 270, 270*f*
Blunt trauma
  anterior uveitis cause, 439
  conjunctival involvement, 436–437, 437*f*
  corneal involvement, 154–155, 155*f*, 177*t*, 437–438, 437*f*
  cyclodialysis cause, 440, 442*f*
  hyphema cause, 439, 440–446, 442–444*f*
  iridodialysis cause, 439, 442–444*f*
  miosis cause, 439
  mydriasis cause, 439, 439*f*
  subconjunctival hemorrhage, 436–437, 436*f*
B lymphocytes (plasma cells), 274–275
Borrelia burgdorferi, 378
Boston keratoprosthesis, 464, 510, 510*f*
Botulinum toxin A, 133
Bowman layer
  dystrophies of, 186*t*, 192–194, 193*f*, 195*f*, 196*t*
  structure and function, 9*f*, 10–11
Bow-tie pattern, 223, 223–224*f*
Breast cancer, 75
Breastfeeding, 75
Brittle cornea, 266, 267*t*, 269, 270
BSCLs. *See* Bandage soft contact lenses
Buffer solutions, 429
Bulbar conjunctiva
  Bitôt spot, 272, 272*f*
  cysts of, 160
  donor site, 110–112, 111*f*, 122*f*
  keratoconjunctivitis, 90–91, 91*t*
  neoplastic disorders of, 403, 410, 413*f*, 414, 415*f*, 417
  pinguecula, 158
  structure and function, 7–8
Bulbar follicles, 104, 104*f*
Bulla, 48*t*, 49*t*
Bullous keratopathy, 99, 114, 210, 297, 500
Bullous pemphigoid, 265
Buphthalmos, 142, 143, 154
Burns
  chemical, 423–432, 424–427*t*
  limbal stem cell deficiency cause, 100, 101*f*
  thermal, 432–433, 433*f*
Cactus spines, 436, 447
Calcific band keratopathy, 165–168, 166*t*, 167*f*, 168*t*
Calcitonin, 276–277
Calcium deposition
  ATD sign, 60
  corneal, 165–168, 167*f*, 168*t*, 172
  hypophosphatasia sign, 268*t*
  parathyroid disease and, 277
  scleral, 178–179
Calcium hydroxide lime, 424*t*
Calcium oxalate crystals, 436
CALT. *See* Conjunctiva-associated lymphoid tissue
CAM. *See* Complexion-associated melanosis
Canaliculitis, 71, 82, 319*t*
Candida spp, 319*t*, 342–343
Capillary hemangioma, 416
Carbon deposition, 166*t*
Carbon fragments, 447–448
Carbonic anhydrase inhibitors, 95*t*, 211, 430, 445
Cardiac arrhythmia, 75
Carotid artery disease, 171
Carpenter syndrome (acrocephalopolysyndactyly type II), 267*t*
Caruncle, 7–8, 407, 410
Cataracts
  chemical injuries and, 425
  congenital, 138*t*, 139*t*, 141, 142
  graft-vs-host disease association, 375
  post-transplant, 487–488, 504
  scleritis complication, 391
  spokelike, 253
  sunflower cataract, 265, 273
  surgical management, 143, 160, 212, 432–433
  systemic disorders associated with, 265, 269, 278
  viral etiology, 314
Caterpillar hairs, 435
"Cat-scratch" disease, 333, 388
Caustic soda, 424*t*
Cauterization
  about, 119
  conjunctival papilloma treatment, 401
  conjunctivochalasis treatment, 92, 119
  keratoconjunctivitis treatment, 91*t*
  postoperative epithelial defect treatment, 477
Cavernous hemangiomas, 417
CDS. *See* Cornea Donor Study
CDVA. *See* Corrected distance visual acuity
Ceftriaxone (injectable), 327, 328, 338*t*
Cell-mediated (delayed hypersensitivity) (type IV) reactions, 353, 354–355, 356, 360, 362, 367
Cenegermin, 96, 297, 303
Central cloudy dystrophy, 138*t*, 207
Cephalosporins, 327, 458
Ceruloplasmin, 265
Cevimeline hydrochloride, 70
Chalasis, 48*t*
Chalazia, 76, 84–85, 407, 408*f*
Chalcosis, 166*t*, 265
Chandler syndrome, 175, 177*t*

CHED. *See* Congenital hereditary endothelial dystrophy
Chemical injuries
  about, 423, 424–427*t*
  acid burns, 424–427*t*, 425, 429–431*f*, 429–432
  alkali burns, 104, 123*f*, 423–425, 424–427*t*, 428*f*, 431
  classification and grading schemes, 425–427*t*
  limbal stem cell deficiency cause, 100, 101*f*
  treatment, 429–432, 431*f*
Chemosis, 8, 48*t*, 354, 355*f*
Chemotherapy (systemic), 419, 421
Chemotherapy (topical)
  about, 398–399, 399–400*f*
  Kaposi sarcoma treatment, 419
  lymphoma treatment, 421
  melanoma treatment, 415
  ocular surface neoplasia treatment, 406–407
  primary acquired melanosis treatment, 414
Cherry-red spot, 253, 254
Chicken pox, 298–299
Children
  amblyopia risk factors in, 485
  atopic dermatitis in, 355, 356*f*
  benign lymphoid folliculosis in, 49, 51*f*
  conjunctivitis in, 323–333
  corneal blood staining and, 444
  corneal transplantation for, 507–509
  cytomegalovirus and, 305
  dry eye treatment, 75
  endothelial cell density in, 40
  human papillomaviruses and, 401
  keratitis and, 152, 173, 376
  keratoconjunctivitis in, 358–359, 362*t*
  myopia treatment for, 234
  nevi and, 411
  osteogenesis imperfecta and, 270
  rosacea in, 76
  sphingolipidoses and, 253
  systemic mucopolysaccharidoses and, 248
  tetracycline contraindication, 75
  tyrosinemia and, 259
  viral infections, 298, 299, 314, 378
  vitamin A deficiency and, 272, 314
Chlamydial infections
  conjunctivitis and, 81, 328–333, 328*t*
  neonatal conjunctivitis, 332–333
  pathogenesis, 320
  specimen collection and evaluation, 320*t*, 322*f*
  trachoma, 329–331, 330*f*
Chlamydia trachomatis, 376, 378
Chlorhexidine, 346
Chloroquine, 179, 253
Chlorpromazine, 181
Chocolate cyst, 417
Cholesterol depositions, 199*t*, 204, 256
Cholinergic agonists, 70
Choristomas, 270–271
Choroiditis, 301
Chronic conjunctivitis, 118
Chronic follicular conjunctivitis, 420, 420*f*
Chrysiasis, 166*t*
Cicatricial disorders
  conjunctivitis, 118, 368, 370, 371*t*
  differential diagnosis, 50*t*
  ectropion, 278
  entropion, 89
  treatment, 124
Cigarettes and smoking
  dry eye risk factor, 58, 68
  thermal burns and, 432, 433*f*
Ciliary body, 45, 440, 442*f*
Ciliary spasm, 438
Cimetidine, 313, 401
CIN (conjunctival intraepithelial neoplasia). *See* Ocular surface squamous neoplasia
CIPA. *See* Congenital insensitivity to pain with anhidrosis
Ciprofloxacin (oral), 327
Ciprofloxacin (topical), 181, 181*f*, 327
Classic granular dystrophy (granular corneal dystrophy type 1), 199–200, 199*t*, 200*f*
CLET. *See* Cultivated limbal epithelial transplantation
Climatic droplet keratopathy (spheroidal degeneration), 163–165, 164*f*, 169, 260
Clindamycin, 453
CLK. *See* Contact lens–induced keratoconjunctivitis
Clofazimine, 181
Clopidogrel, 437
Clotrimazole, 346
Clotting disorders, 443
Coats white ring, 162–163, 164*f*
Coccidioidomycosis, 333
Cochet-Bonnet esthesiometer, 20–21
Cockayne syndrome, 267*t*
Coconut shell, 436
Cogan microcystic epithelial dystrophy. *See* Epithelial basement membrane dystrophy
Cogan plaque (senile plaque), 179, 179*f*
Cogan-Reese (iris nevus) syndrome, 175, 176*f*
Cogan syndrome, 53*t*, 292*t*, 379–380
COL1A1 and *COL1A2* genes, 270
Cold injuries, 433
Collagen, 11, 270
Collagenase inhibitors, 384
Collagenolysis, 92, 431
Collagen punctal plug, 70
Collagen vascular diseases, 53*t*
Colobomas, 134, 135*f*, 138*t*, 143, 267–268*t*, 270
Complete Moisture Plus multipurpose solution, 344
Complexion-associated melanosis (CAM; racial melanosis), 411*t*, 412, 412*f*
Compound nevi, 410–411
Computer use, 56*t*, 58
Confocal microscopy, 40, 42–43, 43*f*
Congenital anomalies. *See also specific anomalies*
  about, 137, 138–140*t*
  anterior segment dysgenesis, 141, 145–151, 146–148*f*, 150–151*t*

corneal edema differential diagnosis, 177*t*
cornea size and shape anomalies, 137, 141–142*f*, 141–145, 144*f*
secondary corneal abnormalities, 151–155, 153–155*f*
Congenital anterior staphyloma, 140*t*, 150–151, 151*f*
Congenital cataracts, 138*t*, 139*t*, 141, 142
Congenital corneal anesthesia, 153
Congenital corneal keloid, 152
Congenital glaucoma, 139*t*, 142, 147, 154, 155*f*, 233*t*
Congenital hereditary endothelial dystrophy (CHED), 177*t*, 214–216, 215*f*
Congenital insensitivity to pain with anhidrosis (CIPA), 153
Congenital iris colobomas, 134, 135*f*
Congenital melanosis, 409, 409*f*
Congenital stromal corneal dystrophy (CSCD), 206, 206*f*
Congenital syphilis, 151–152, 378
Conjunctiva. *See also specific disorders*
biopsy evaluation, 118. *See also under* Biopsy
chemical injuries, 424–425, 425*t*, 428*f*, 429–432
cysts of, 160–162, 161–162*f*
defense mechanisms, 8, 16–17
degenerations and depositions, 157–162, 158–162*f*, 164*f*
epithelium, 8, 16, 16*f*
examination, 26, 60
immune-related disorders of, 356–376. *See also under* Conjunctivitis
keratinization of, 370, 370*f*
normal flora of, 317–318, 317*t*
OSD sign, 48*t*, 60, 60*f*
radiation injuries, 434–435
reconstruction techniques, 107–124. *See also specific interventions*
structure and function, 7–8, 16
surface disorders of, 90–92
traumatic injuries, 436–437, 439, 446–448. *See also* Traumatic injuries
tumors of. *See* Neoplastic disorders
vascular conditions of, 162, 163*t*
Conjunctiva-associated lymphoid tissue (CALT), 8
Conjunctival concentrations, 160, 161*f*
Conjunctival fixation (plication), 91*t*, 119
Conjunctival flaps, 114–118, 115–117*f*, 153, 384–385, 434
Conjunctival injection, 49, 63, 90, 288, 334
Conjunctival intraepithelial neoplasia (CIN). *See* Ocular surface squamous neoplasia
Conjunctival papilloma, 400–402, 401*f*
Conjunctivitis
bacterial
acute purulent conjunctivitis, 324–326, 325*f*
chlamydial, 329–333, 330*f*
classification, 324*t*
differential diagnosis, 88
gonococcal conjunctivitis, 324*t*, 326–327*f*, 326–328, 328*t*
neonatal, 324*t*, 328–329, 332–333
pathogenesis, 323–324
signs and symptoms, 323, 324*t*
chronic, 118, 420, 420*f*
differential diagnosis, 50*t*, 81
eyelid conditions associated with, 76, 79
follicular
acute hemorrhagic conjunctivitis association, 315
differential diagnosis, 50*t*, 420, 420*f*
etiology, 103*t*, 104, 303, 307, 313*t*, 314
molluscum contagiosum and, 311*f*
OSD and, 49–52, 51–52*f*
pathogenesis, 104
immune-related
atopic keratoconjunctivitis, 361–364, 362*t*, 363*f*
autoimmune, 374, 375
diagnosis, 30
dry eye and, 56*t*, 58
graft-vs-host disease, 374–375, 375*f*
ligneous conjunctivitis, 364–365, 364*f*
misdiagnosis, 59
mucous membrane pemphigoid, 368–374, 369–372*f*, 371*t*, 373*t*
reactive arthritis association, 375–376
seasonal allergic conjunctivitis, 356–358, 358*t*
Stevens-Johnson syndrome, 365–368, 366*f*
toxic epidermal necrolysis, 365–368
treatment, 358*t*
vernal keratoconjunctivitis, 358–361, 359–360*f*
inflammation signs, 47–51, 50–52*f*, 50*t*
papillary, 47, 48*t*, 49, 50–51*f*, 50*t*, 375–376
viral
adenovirus, 50*t*, 53*t*, 307, 315, 332
Epstein-Barr virus, 303
HIV, 315
RNA viruses, 313
sexually transmitted, 328
signs and symptoms, 323
Conjunctivochalasis (lax conjunctiva), 67, 91, 92, 93*f*, 119–120
Connective tissue and skeletal disorder manifestations, 266–271, 267–268*t*
Contact dermatoblepharitis, 354–355, 354*f*
Contact lens fitting, 33
Contact lens–induced keratoconjunctivitis (CLK), 91
Contact lens wear
dry eye and, 56*t*, 59
epithelial defects and, 438
keratitis and, 334, 342, 381
keratopathy risk factor, 336
limbal stem cell deficiency cause, 100, 101*f*
procedures for increasing tolerance of, 237
tear film instability and, 58
toxic reactions to, 104
Contralateral autograft, 509
Copper deposition, 264–265, 265*f*, 273
Corectopia, 146, 176
Cornea
abrasions, 438. *See also* Abrasions
animal injuries of, 435, 435*f*
biomechanics of, 40
biopsy evaluation, 125, 315, 321

chemical injuries of, 423–432, 424*t*. *See also* Chemical injuries
congenital anomalies, 137, 138–141*t*, 141–155. *See also* Congenital anomalies
defense mechanisms, 14–17, 15–16*f*
degenerations and depositions, 35, 162–178, 163*t*, 166*t*. *See also specific degenerations and depositions*
dimensions, 141*t*
dystrophies, 163*t*, 183–216. *See also* Dystrophies
ecstatic diseases of, 217–246. *See also* Ectasias
examination of, 19–45. *See also* Examination approaches
foreign bodies and, 448–450, 449–450*f*
immune-related disorders of, 376–386. *See also specific diseases*
plant injuries, 436, 447, 448
radiation injuries of, 433–435
reconstruction techniques, 125–135. *See also specific interventions*
structure and function, 8–13, 9–12*f*
surface disorders of, 93–106. *See also* Ocular surface disease
thermal injuries, 432–433, 433*f*
traumatic injuries of, 437–438, 437*f*, 446–461. *See also* Penetrating and perforating trauma
tumors of. *See* Neoplastic disorders
Cornea Donor Study (CDS), 467, 480
Cornea farinata, 178, 178*f*
Corneal anesthesia, 153, 301
Corneal apex, 10, 11*f*
Corneal arcus
complexion-associated melanosis association, 412*f*
description, 170–171, 171*f*, 205*f*
as developmental anomaly, 138*t*, 142, 171
furrow degeneration association, 172
lysosomal storage diseases as cause of, 256
ocular associations, 231*t*
Schnyder corneal dystrophy association, 204, 205*f*
Corneal blood staining, 443–444, 444*f*, 445, 446*t*
Corneal clarity (transparency), 10, 11, 13, 247
Corneal clouding
corneal dystrophies and, 206, 206*f*, 214–215
lysosomal storage diseases and, 248, 249–250*t*, 251*f*, 254–256
Corneal conjunctivalization, 120–123, 120*t*, 122–123*f*
Corneal contour evaluation
corneal tomography, 36–39, 38–39*f*, 38*t*
corneal topography, 33–35, 35–37*f*
keratometry, 32–33, 33*f*
keratoscopy, 33, 34*f*
Corneal crosslinking (CXL), 36, 228, 241–246
Corneal dermoids, 125, 270–271
Corneal dystrophy of Bowman layer type 1 (Reis-Bücklers corneal dystrophy), 186*t*, 192–194, 193*f*, 195, 196*t*
Corneal endothelium
birth trauma and, 154
cell density, 40–41, 162
coefficient of variation (CV), 41
depositions and degenerations, 166*t*, 175–177
dystrophies of, 185–186*t*, 210–216
examination, 23–24, 24–25*f*, 40–42, 41*f*
hexagonal cell percentage, 41
OSD sign, 53–54
structure and function, 9*f*, 13, 40–41, 42
thickness assessment, 42, 44, 210–211, 215, 215*f*
Corneal epithelium
dystrophies of, 185*t*, 187–202
iron depositions, 159, 160*f*, 165, 165*f*, 166*t*
OSD sign, 52, 54*f*
structure and function, 9*f*, 10, 24*f*
TGFBI dystrophies, 185–186*t*, 192–202
viral infection of, 287*t*, 288–290*f*, 288–291, 290*t*
Corneal facets, 163
Corneal haze, 314
Corneal hysteresis, 40
Corneal inflammation, 52–54, 53*t*, 54–55*f*
Corneal intraepithelial neoplasia (CIN). *See* Ocular surface squamous neoplasia
Corneal keloids, 152, 174
Corneal leukoma, 267*t*
Corneal melting, 383, 384, 425
Corneal nerves
evaluation, 43, 43*f*
prominent, 276, 276*t*, 277*f*
Corneal perforation
ATD sign, 60
evaluation, 28–29, 29*f*
exposure keratopathy and, 93
traumatic, 448–450, 449–450*f*
treatment, 130–132, 131*f*
Corneal resistance factor (CRF), 40
Corneal sensation
evaluation, 20–21, 471
postoperative complication risk factor, 477
Corneal stem cell deficiency, 120–123, 120*t*, 122–123*f*
Corneal tattooing, 134–135, 134–135*f*, 166*t*
Corneal thinning
ATD sign, 60
corneal dystrophies and, 202*f*, 203
differential diagnosis, 231*t*
evaluation, 23
furrow degeneration association, 231*t*
keratoconus sign, 217, 218*f*, 223–224, 223*f*, 225*f*
keratoglobus sign, 218*f*, 232, 233*f*
mooren ulcer sign, 231*t*
pellucid marginal degeneration sign, 218*f*, 229, 230*f*
Terrien marginal degeneration sign, 231*t*
treatment, 129–130, 129–130*f*
Corneal transplantation
about, 463–465, 463*t*, 466*t*
autograft procedures, 509, 509*f*
disease transmission from, 469*t*
donor-cornea selection, 467, 468*t*
emerging treatment alternatives, 506–507, 507*f*
endothelial keratoplasty, 491–507, 492–494*t*. *See also* Endothelial keratoplasty
graft failure sign, 177*t*
indications, 465, 466*t*

keratoprosthesis, 510–511, 510*f*, 511*t*
lamellar keratoplasty, 473–475*t*, 488–491. *See also* Lamellar keratoplasty
milestones, 464
patient history considerations, 470
pediatric transplantation, 507–509
penetrating keratoplasty, 473–475*t*, 476–488. *See also* Penetrating keratoplasty
Peters anomaly treatment, 148
preoperative evaluation and preparation of patient, 470–472, 471*f*
procedure of choice, 469–470, 469*t*
rejection sign, 177*t*
tissue processing and preservation, 465–467
trends, 464–465, 464*t*, 466*t*
Corneal vertex, 10, 11*f*
Corneal xerosis, 272
Cornea plana, 138–139*t*, 141*t*, 143–144, 208
Cornea Preservation Time Study (CPTS), 467
Cornea stroma. *See* Stroma (corneal)
Cornea verticillata
differential diagnosis, 180
etiology, 179–180, 180*t*, 251, 253*f*
evaluation, 25
signs and symptoms, 179, 180, 180*f*
Coronavirus disease 2019 (COVID-19), 313–314
Coronaviruses, 313–314
Corrected distance visual acuity (CDVA; best-corrected visual acuity), 237–238
Corticosteroids (injectable), 85, 361, 416, 418
Corticosteroids (oral)
animal injury treatment, 435
dry eye treatment, 368
graft rejection treatment, 483–484
herpes zoster ophthalmic treatment, 302–303
hyphema treatment, 444
loiasis treatment, 349
melting treatment, 384
MPM treatment, 372–373
scleritis treatment, 393
viral infections and use of, 291, 294*t*
Corticosteroids (topical)
adenovirus infection treatment, 309–310
animal injury treatment, 435
anterior uveitis treatment, 439
atopic dermatitis treatment, 356
atopic keratoconjunctivitis treatment, 363
bacterial conjunctivitis treatment, 326
band keratopathy treatment, 168
chemical injury treatment, 430–431
Cogan syndrome treatment, 380
complications, 326
conjunctivochalasis treatment, 92
contact dermatoblepharitis treatment, 355
contraindications, 291, 448
descemetocele treatment, 130
dry eye treatment, 74, 368
graft rejection prophylaxis, 484, 504–505, 505*f*
graft rejection treatment, 483–484
hemangioma treatment, 416
herpes zoster ophthalmic treatment, 302
herpetic keratitis treatment, 295, 296
hyphema treatment, 444
infectious crystalline keratopathy risk factor, 336
keratitis precautions, 339–340, 342, 346, 377, 478
ligneous conjunctivitis treatment, 364
limbal stem cell deficiency treatment, 101
lymphoid hyperplasia treatment, 419
marginal keratitis treatment, 381–382
miosis treatment, 439
penetrating keratoplasty postoperative care, 476
phlyctenulosis treatment, 84
pingueculitis treatment, 158
plant injury contraindications, 436
postoperative, 113, 459
precautions, 74, 81, 306
pyogenic granuloma treatment, 418
RES treatment, 99
SJS/TEN treatment, 367
staphylococcal blepharitis treatment, 81
syphilitic keratitis treatment, 379
thermal burn treatment precautions, 433
Thygeson superficial punctate keratitis treatment, 377
toxic reactions to, 103
ulcerative keratitis treatment, 78
vernal keratoconjunctivitis treatment, 360
Corynebacterium spp, 337*t*
Corynebacterium xerosis, 272
COVID-19 (coronavirus disease 2019), 313–314
Coxsackievirus, 315
CPTS. *See* Cornea Preservation Time Study
"Crab claw" pattern, 229, 232*f*
Cranial nerve III (oculomotor nerve), 301
Cranial nerve V (trigeminal nerve), 6*f*, 70, 95, 286, 300, 409, 433
Craniosynostosis, 138*t*, 142
CRF. *See* Corneal resistance factor
Crocodile shagreen (mosaic degeneration), 171–172
Crouzon syndrome, 267*t*
Cryoglobulinemia, 259*t*
Cryoglobulins, 274
Cryotherapy, 89, 401, 406, 414–415, 419
Cryptococcal optic neuritis, 315
Crystalline deposition, 25, 258, 259*t*, 273–275, 274*f*
CSCD. *See* Congenital stromal corneal dystrophy
Cultivated limbal epithelial transplantation (CLET), 121
Cutaneous keloids, 152
CXL. *See* Corneal crosslinking
Cyanoacrylate glue, 130–132, 133, 384
Cyclodialysis, 440, 442*f*
Cyclophosphamide, 371*f*, 373, 384
Cycloplegic agents (topical)
adverse effects, 354
animal injury treatment, 435
anterior uveitis treatment, 439
band keratopathy treatment, 168
chemical injury treatment, 430
corneal abrasion treatment, 438
gonococcal conjunctivitis treatment, 329
herpes zoster ophthalmic treatment, 302

hyphema treatment, 444
keratitis treatment, 379
miosis treatment, 439
plant injury treatment, 436
thermal burn treatment, 433
Cyclosporine (oral), 384
Cyclosporine (topical)
adenovirus infection treatment, 310
aqueous tear deficiency treatment, 69
atopic keratoconjunctivitis treatment, 363
graft-vs-host disease treatment, 374–375
keratitis treatment, 377
ligneous conjunctivitis treatment, 364
limbal stem cell deficiency treatment, 101
melting treatment, 384
SLK treatment, 91*t*
vernal keratoconjunctivitis treatment, 361
Cylindrical dandruff (eyelash sleeves), 79, 79–80*f*
Cysteamine (oral), 258–259
Cysteamine (topical), 258
Cysteine, 257–258
Cystinosis, 257–259, 257*t*, 258*f*, 259*t*
Cysts
of bulbar conjunctiva, 160
of ciliary body, 45
of conjunctiva, 160–162, 161–162*f*
epithelial inclusion cysts, 116, 160–162, 162*f*, 411
pars plana proteinaceous cysts, 273
Cytarabine, 104
Cytokines, 16
Cytomegalovirus, 304–306, 305*f*

Dacryoadenitis, 303, 314
DALK. *See* Deep anterior lamellar keratoplasty
Dander, 357
dDALK. *See* Descemetic DALK
Deep anterior lamellar keratoplasty (DALK)
about, 464, 465, 488–490
anatomical landmarks, 12
comparisons, 465, 473–475*t*
cornea plana treatment, 144
herpetic eye disease treatment, 297–298
indications, 466*t*, 469*t*, 473*t*, 475*t*, 490–491
intraoperative complications, 473*t*
keratoconus treatment, 228
modifications of, 489
mucopolysaccharidoses treatment, 251
pellucid marginal degeneration treatment, 230
postoperative complications, 474*t*, 491*f*
stromal dystrophy treatment, 194
Deep lamellar endothelial keratoplasty (DLEK), 491
Defense mechanisms, 14–17, 15–16*f*
Degenerations and depositions
calcium
ATD sign, 60
corneal, 165–168, 167*f*, 168*t*, 172
hypophosphatasia sign, 268*t*
parathyroid disease and, 277
scleral, 178–179
treatment, 125
conjunctival, 157–162, 158–162*f*, 164*f*
copper, 264–265, 265*f*, 273
corneal, 35, 162–178, 163*t*, 166*t*
drug-induced, 179–181, 180*t*
hyaline, 199*t*, 200, 200*f*, 201
iron, 159, 160*f*, 165, 165*f*, 166*t*, 226
scleral, 178–179
Delayed hypersensitivity (type IV, T cell-mediated), 84
Dellen, 100, 129, 129*f*, 437
Demodex brevis, 318
Demodex folliculorum, 318
Demodicosis, 73*t*, 79, 80*f*, 318, 322–323, 323*f*
Demulcent solutions, 68
Dendritic antigen-presenting cells (APCs), 16, 16*f*, 17
Dendritic keratitis. *See* Epithelial (dendritic) keratitis
Dental setting, 448
Depositions. *See* Degenerations and depositions
Dermatoblepharitis, 319*t*, 354–355, 354*f*
Dermoids
corneal, 125, 270–271
limbal, 152, 153*f*, 267*t*, 270, 271, 271*f*
Descemet dystrophy, 278
Descemetic DALK (dDALK), 464*t*, 489
Descemet membrane
birth trauma rupture of, 154
blunt trauma to, 437, 437*f*
congenital absence of, 146, 150
congenital anomalies of, 149
depositions, 166*t*
structure and function, 9*f*, 12, 24*f*
transplant complications of, 491
Descemetocele, 129–130, 129–130*f*, 488, 488*f*
Descemet stripping automated endothelial keratoplasty (DSAEK), 491
Descemet stripping/membrane endothelial keratoplasty (DSEK/DMEK)
about, 491–492, 492*t*
indications, 473*t*
intraoperative complications, 473*t*, 496–497, 497*f*
lamellar keratoplasty comparison, 474–475*t*
outcomes, 493–494*t*
penetrating keratoplasty comparison, 474–475*t*
postoperative complications, 474*t*, 494*t*, 495–496, 497–506, 498–504*f*
trends, 465, 467
ultrathin, 496
visual acuity and, 496
Descemet stripping only (DSO), 506, 507*f*
Dexamethasone (intravenous), 484
Dexamethasone (topical), 310, 483, 484
Diabetes
dry eye probable risk factor, 56*t*
neurotrophic keratopathy treatment recommendations, 96
ocular manifestations of, 275–276
subconjunctival hemorrhage association, 437
tear film instability and, 58
Diabetic keratopathy, 275
Diabetic neuropathy, 95

Diabetic neurotrophic keratitis, 43
Diamidines (topical), 346
Diamond burr superficial keratectomy, 99
Diathesis, 437
Dieffenbachia spp, 436
Dietary supplements, 70, 74
Diethylcarbamazine, 349
Diffuse anterior scleritis, 388*f*, 389
Diffuse scleritis, 388, 388*f*
Diffuse vascular tortuosity, 163*t*
Difluprednate (topical), 476, 483, 484
Diphtheroids, 317
Diplopia, 114
Dirt, 448
Disciform keratitis, 54, 292, 293*f*
Disodium EDTA, 167, 168
Distichiasis, 89, 89*f*
Diuretics, 56*t*
DLEK. *See* Deep lamellar endothelial keratoplasty
DNA viruses, 284–313. *See also* Adenovirus infections; Cytomegalovirus; Epstein-Barr virus; Herpesviruses; Papillomaviruses; Poxviruses; Varicella-zoster virus
Donor-cornea selection, 467, 468–469*t*
Dots, 187–188, 188*f*, 190
Double (pseudo-) anterior chambers, 491
Down syndrome, 138*t*, 142, 219*t*, 221
Doxycycline (oral)
  adverse effects, 75
  chalazia treatment, 85
  chlamydial conjunctivitis treatment, 332
  contraindications, 75
  descemetocele treatment, 130
  dry eye treatment, 74–75, 78
  granular conjunctivitis treatment, 333
  hordeola treatment, 85
  limbal stem cell deficiency treatment, 101
  melting treatment, 384
  precautions, 75
  RES treatment, 99
  rosacea treatment, 78
Dresden protocol. *See* Corneal crosslinking
Drug-induced degenerations and depositions, 179–181, 180*t*
Dry eye
  about, 54–57
  classifications, 59–66, 61*t*. *See also* Aqueous tear deficiency; Evaporative dry eye
  contact lens options, 69
  differential diagnosis, 53*t*, 67, 92, 153
  diseases and conditions associated with, 64*t*, 67
  etiology, 54, 66*t*
  pathogenesis, 57–59, 57*f*
  radiation injuries and, 434
  risk factors, 56*t*
  signs and symptoms, 30–32, 33, 53*t*, 59, 67, 67*f*
  SJS/TEN association, 367–368
  staphylococcal blepharitis as cause of, 321
  treatment, 66–76, 67*f*, 368, 373
  viral etiology, 300
DSAEK. *See* Descemet stripping automated endothelial keratoplasty
DSEK/DMEK. *See* Descemet stripping/membrane endothelial keratoplasty
DSO. *See* Descemet stripping only
Dua (pre-Descemet) layer, 12
Dupilumab (injectable), 356
Dust, 357
Dwarfism, 138*t*, 142, 258
Dye disappearance test, 28
Dysentery, 376
Dysmorphic sialidosis (ML I), 254, 254*t*
Dystrophies
  about, 183–185
  classification, 185*t*
  degeneration comparison, 163*t*
  endothelial, 185–186*t*, 210–216
  epithelial and subepithelial, 185–186*t*, 187–191
  epithelial-stromal *TGFBI*, 185–186*t*, 192–202
  evaluation, 43
  genetics of, 186*t*
  stromal, 185–186*t*, 202–209

EBMD. *See* Epithelial basement membrane dystrophy
Eccrine sweat glands, 4
Ectasias
  atopic keratoconjunctivitis sign, 362
  congenital, 144–145, 149
  evaluation, 22*f*, 35, 36, 38, 38*f*, 40
  keratoconus, 217–229. *See also* Keratoconus
  keratoglobus, 232–234. *See also* Keratoglobus
  pellucid marginal degeneration, 229–232. *See also* Pellucid marginal degeneration
  risk factors, 40, 226
  as surgical complication, 226, 238, 243
  surgical management
    anterior lamellar keratoplasty, 488
    corneal crosslinking, 36, 228, 241–246
    intrastromal corneal ring segments, 235–241
Ectodermal dysplasia, 278
Ectopia lentis, 138*t*, 142, 269, 269*f*
Eczema, 48*t*
Edema
  conjunctival, 48*t*, 113, 434
  corneal
    biomechanics of, 40
    birth trauma and, 154–155, 155*f*
    blunt trauma and, 437–438
    congenital glaucoma sign, 154, 155
    differential diagnosis, 154–155, 175, 177*t*
    dystrophies and, 210–211, 213, 214–215, 215*t*
    evaluation, 23, 26, 40, 42, 49*t*, 53–54
    graft detachment and, 499–500, 499–500*f*
    graft rejection and, 483–484
    iridocorneal endothelial (ICE) syndrome sign, 175, 176*f*
    keratoconus and, 221, 222*f*
    peripheral cornea guttae sign, 178
    postoperative complication, 244, 480, 484, 494*t*
    preoperative evaluation of, 471

recurrent erosion syndrome cause, 99, 128
risk factors, 41
stromal keratitis sign, 292
surgical management of, 212, 214, 216, 469*t*, 494*t*
systemic disorders associated with, 268*t*, 275
traumatic etiology, 175, 435, 437
epithelial, 49*t*, 53
evaluation, 40, 42
of eyelid, 434
macular, 471–472
preoperative evaluation of, 471–472
scleral, 387, 388, 388*f*, 389, 389*f*, 433
EDS. *See* Ehlers-Danlos syndrome
EDTA (ethylenediaminetetraacetic acid), 167, 168, 277
Effector T cells (Teff cells), 15–16*f*
Effusion, choroidal, 461
Ehlers-Danlos syndrome (EDS)
about, 266, 267*t*, 269
cornea plana association, 143
keratoconus association, 219*t*
keratoglobus association, 144–145
microcornea association, 141
EK. *See* Endothelial keratoplasty
EKC. *See* Epidemic keratoconjunctivitis
Electrolysis, 89
Elschnig pearl, 26*f*
Endophthalmitis, 477
Endothelial corneal dystrophy (Fuchs endothelial corneal dystrophy), 41, 44, 210–212, 211*f*, 480, 506, 507*f*
Endothelial keratoplasty (EK)
about, 491–495, 492*t*
comparisons, 473–475*t*, 494*t*, 495
emerging treatment alternatives, 506–507, 507*f*
fungal keratitis risk factor, 342
indications, 466*t*, 469*t*, 473*t*, 475*t*
intraoperative complications, 473*t*, 496–497, 497*f*
outcomes, 493*t*
postoperative complications, 474*t*, 494*t*, 496, 497–506, 498–504*f*
postoperative evaluation, 44
trends, 465, 492
types of. *See* Descemet stripping/membrane endothelial keratoplasty
Endotheliitis (trabeculitis), 177*t*, 292, 305, 305*f*
Enterobacter spp, 337*t*
Enterovirus, 315
Entropion (inturned eyelid), 89, 368, 370
Enucleation, 453–454
Enveloped viruses, 281–282, 282*f*
Environmental issues, 56*t*, 68, 159
Enzyme replacement therapy, 254
Epibulbar dermoids (limbal dermoids), 152, 153*f*, 267*t*, 270, 271, 271*f*
Epidemic keratoconjunctivitis (EKC), 307–308, 307–309*f*
Epinephrine (topical), 166*t*, 370, 408
Epiphora, 48*t*, 154
Episclera, 8
Episcleritis
classification, 387
description, 48*t*
differential diagnosis, 387
herpes zoster ophthalmicus sign, 300
immune-related diseases of, 387–388, 387*f*
OSD sign, 48*t*
reactive arthritis association, 375, 376
rosacea-associated, 77*f*, 78
Stevens-Johnson syndrome sign, 365–366
Epithelial (dendritic) keratitis
adenovirus, 308–309, 309*f*
chlamydia association, 329
cytomegalovirus, 305
differential diagnosis, 290, 290*t*
herpes simplex virus, 284, 285*f*, 287*t*, 288–290*f*, 288–291, 290*t*, 295*t*
herpes zoster, 52, 53*t*, 54*f*, 300–301, 301*f*
measles, 314
treatment, 295*t*
Epithelial basement membrane dystrophy (EBMD; map-dot-fingerprint dystrophy, anterior basement membrane dystrophy, Cogan microcystic epithelial dystrophy)
about, 187
differential diagnosis, 189
genetics, 186*t*, 187
pathogenesis, 190
recurrent corneal erosions association, 98, 98*f*, 189
scarring and, 125
signs and symptoms, 187–189*f*, 187–190
treatment, 125, 190
Epithelial debridement, 99, 101, 291
Epithelial defects
of conjunctiva, 48*t*, 390, 390*f*
of cornea
atopic keratoconjunctivitis sign, 362
chemical injuries, 425, 429*f*
contact lens wear and, 438
gonococcal conjunctivitis association, 327
neurotrophic keratopathy sign, 94–95, 95*f*, 96
plant injury sign, 436
RES sign, 97–98
signs, 27, 49*t*
treatment, 114, 120–123, 128–132, 438, 477
Epithelial inclusion cysts, 160–162, 162*f*, 411
Epithelial keratopathy, 60, 60*f*
Epitheliectomy, 406
Epitheliopathy, 296
Epstein-Barr virus (infectious mononucleosis), 292*t*, 303–304, 304*f*, 378
Erosions, 48*t*, 49*t*, 50*t*. *See also* Punctate epithelial erosions; Recurrent erosion syndrome
Erythromycin (oral), 75, 78, 332, 333
Erythromycin (topical), 81, 327, 329
Escherichia coli, 317
Essential (progressive) iris atrophy, 175, 176*f*
Esthesiometer, 20–21
Ethylenediaminetetraacetic acid (EDTA), 167, 168, 277

Evaporative dry eye
- differential diagnosis, 93
- diseases and conditions associated with, 63, 64*t*, 65, 67, 76–78, 77*f*, 79
- etiology, 31
- examination, 30, 31–32
- pathogenesis, 58
- signs and symptoms, 63–65, 65*f*, 67, 67*f*
- treatment, 67, 67*f*, 72–73*t*, 72–76

Examination approaches
- anterior segment
  - anterior segment optical coherence tomography, 44, 44*f*
  - Scheimpflug-based corneal tomography, 39, 39*f*
  - slit-lamp biomicroscopy, 21–26, 21–26*f*
  - ultrasound biomicroscopy, 45, 45*f*
- cornea
  - anterior segment optical coherence tomography, 44, 44*f*
  - biomechanics, 40
  - confocal microscopy, 42–43, 43*f*
  - contour, 32–39, 33–37*f*, 38*t*, 39*f*
  - endothelial appearance and function, 40–42, 41*f*
  - ocular surface staining, 27–29, 27*t*, 28–29*f*
  - pachymetry, 41–42
  - sensation, 20–21, 471
  - slit-lamp biomicroscopy, 21–26, 22–26*f*
  - specular microscopy, 40–41, 41*f*
  - ultrasound biomicroscopy, 45, 45*f*
- external eye
  - blink response, 20–21
  - eyelids, 20
  - general appearance, 19–20
  - ocular surface staining, 27–29, 27*t*, 28–29*f*
  - slit-lamp biomicroscopy, 21–26, 22–26*f*
  - tear production, 30–32, 31*f*
- ocular surface, 27–29, 27*t*

Excimer laser ablation
- complications following, 183, 226
- corneal astigmatism treatment, 486
- of eyelashes, 89
- for ocular surface disorders, 99, 125–126, 128

Exposure keratopathy, 93–94, 267*t*, 314

External eye
- defense mechanisms of, 14–17, 15–16*f*
- examination of, 19–32. *See also under* Examination approaches
- structures and functions, 3–8, 4–7*f*

External hordeola (styes), 84

Eye banking, 465–467, 466*t*, 468–469*t*, 492

Eyebrows, sparse, 278

Eyelashes
- aberrant, 89, 331
- function of, 3
- loss of, 81, 85
- surface disorders and, 89–90, 89*f*, 278

Eyelash sleeves (cylindrical dandruff), 79, 79–80*f*

Eyelid
- blood supply, 8
- evaluation, 23
- evaporative dry eye signs, 63–64
- examination, 20, 26
- foreign bodies of, 447, 447*f*
- hygiene recommendations, 72, 74
- immune-related disorders of, 354–356. *See also specific disorders*
- infections of, 310, 311*f*, 322–323, 323*f*
- malposition treatments, 71
- neoplastic disorders of, 418
- normal flora of, 317–318, 317*t*
- ocular surface disease conditions, 76–85, 77*f*, 79–80*f*, 80*t*, 83–85*f*
- seborrheic changes, 64
- structure and function, 3–4, 4–5*f*
- surface disorders and, 88–90
- telangiectatic blood vessels, 64
- tumors of, 407, 416

Eyelid taping, 96, 153

Fabry disease (angiokeratoma corporis diffusum), 180, 251, 252*t*, 253–254, 290

Facial anomalies, 138*t*, 142

Facial hemiatrophy, 138*t*, 142

Factitious illness, 82

Famciclovir, 287*t*, 302

Familial amyloidosis (Meretoja syndrome), 196, 262*t*, 263

Familial aniridia, 139*t*, 146

Familial dysautonomia (FD; Riley-Day syndrome), 153

Familial hypobetalipoproteinemia, 256

Familial lecithin-cholesterol acyltransferase (LCAT) deficiency, 256, 256*f*, 259*t*

Fatty acid intake, 56*t*, 58

FBN1 gene, 269

FBS. *See* Foreign-body sensation

FCD. *See* Fleck corneal dystrophy

FD. *See* Familial dysautonomia

FECD. *See* Fuchs endothelial corneal dystrophy

Femtosecond laser, 489

Ferrara rings, 235

Ferry line, 166*t*

FES. *See* Floppy eyelid syndrome

Fetal alcohol syndrome, 138*t*, 141

Fiberglass, 449*f*

Fibrillin synthesis, 269

Fibrin glue, 110, 111*f*, 112

Fibrous histiocytoma, 418

Filamentary keratitis, 59, 60, 60*f*, 69, 90, 343

Filaments, 49*t*, 60, 60*f*

Fingerprint lines (horse's tail), 25, 97, 98*f*, 187, 187*f*, 190

Fish eye disease, 255–256

5-fluorouracil (5-FU), 398, 406–407

Flaps
- complications, 116–117
- Gundersen conjunctival flap surgery, 114–118, 115–117*f*
- removal of, 117–118
- smaller conjunctival flaps, 116, 117*f*

Fleck corneal dystrophy (FCD; François-Neetens speckled corneal dystrophy), 207, 207*f*
Fleischer ring, 165, 166*t*, 220, 221*f*
Floppy eyelid syndrome (FES), 88–89, 88*f*, 219*t*
Fluconazole (oral), 343
Fluorescein stain, 27–29, 27*t*, 28–29*f*, 60, 83
Fluorometholone (topical), 360, 377, 476, 484
Fluoroquinolone (oral), 327, 339
Fluoroquinolone (topical), 326, 329, 337, 348, 453
Follicles, 48*t*, 332
Footprint (ghost opacity), 288, 290*f*
Foreign bodies
  from animals, 435, 435*f*
  complications, 453
  of conjunctiva, 447–448, 447–448*f*
  copper, 166*t*
  of cornea, 125, 448–450, 449–450*f*
  differential diagnosis, 293, 438
  evaluation, 45
  iron as, 166*t*
  penetrating and perforating trauma, 446–461. *See also* Penetrating and perforating trauma
  from plants, 436
  removal of, 457, 458–459*f*
  rust as, 447*f*, 448–449, 449*f*
  treatment overview, 125, 452
Foreign-body sensation (FBS), 63, 88, 90, 93, 97, 160
Forniceal conjunctiva, 7
Fornix shortening, 114, 366, 366*f*, 369, 369*f*
Fortified antibiotics, 339
François-Neetens speckled corneal dystrophy (Fleck corneal dystrophy), 207, 207*f*
Fresh frozen plasma (intravenous), 365
Fresh frozen plasma (topical), 364
Frontal bossing, 138*t*, 142
Frost suture, 132
Frozen globe, 369
Fuchs endothelial corneal dystrophy (FECD; endothelial corneal dystrophy), 41, 44, 210–212, 211*f*, 480, 506, 507*f*
Fuchs superficial marginal keratitis, 173
Fucosidosis, 255
Full-thickness corneal transplantation. *See* Penetrating keratoplasty
Fumagillin (topical), 348, 349
Fungal hyphae, 198
Fungal infections
  corneal abrasion association, 438
  corticosteroid precaution, 340
  differential diagnosis, 436
  of eyelid, 322–323
  granuloma cause, 418
  keratitis, 341–344. *See also* Fungal keratitis
  pathogenesis, 318–322, 319*t*
  postoperative complication, 503
  specimen collection and evaluation, 320–321*t*, 322*f*
Fungal keratitis
  about, 341
  differential diagnosis, 53*t*, 293
  laboratory evaluation, 343
  postoperative complication, 480
  postoperative transplant complication, 478
  risk factors, 342
  signs and symptoms, 53*t*, 54, 342–343, 342*f*
  transplant complication, 491
  treatment, 343–344
Furrow degeneration, 172, 231*t*
Fusarium solani, 343
Fusarium spp, 343

GAGs. *See* Glycosaminoglycans
Galactosialidosis (Goldberg syndrome), 255
Ganciclovir (implants), 306
Ganciclovir (topical), 287*t*, 291, 306
Gangliosides, 251, 252*t*
Gatifloxacin, 453
GCD1. *See* Granular corneal dystrophy type 1
GCD2. *See* Granular corneal dystrophy type 2
GDLD. *See* Gelatinous droplike corneal dystrophy
Gelatinous droplike corneal dystrophy (GDLD; subepithelial amyloidosis, primary familial amyloidosis), 191, 192*f*, 261
Gell and Coombs hypersensitivity reaction classification, 353–354
Gelsolin, 263
Generalized gangliosidosis (GM_1 gangliosidosis type I), 251, 252*t*
Gentamicin (topical), 103*t*, 327, 329, 354
Geographic epithelial keratitis, 288, 289*f*
Ghost opacity (footprint), 288, 290*f*
Ghost vessels, 153, 203, 379
Giant cell arteritis, 389
Giant fornix syndrome, 81
Giant papillary conjunctivitis, 88, 479
Glands of Moll, 4, 4–5*f*
Glands of Zeis, 4, 4–5*f*, 84
Glandular tumors, 407
Glass particles, 438, 447, 448, 449*f*
Glaucoma
  animal injury sign, 435
  Axenfeld-Rieger syndrome association, 146
  chemical injuries as cause of, 425
  congenital, 139*t*, 142, 147, 154, 155*f*, 233*t*
  ectodermal dysplasia sign, 278
  Ehlers-Danlos syndrome sign, 266
  etiology, 175
  graft failure and, 480
  graft failure risk factor, 471
  keratoprosthesis complication, 510–511
  malignant, 45
  megalocornea association, 142
  rebleeding as cause of, 443
  risk factors, 141
  rubella as cause of, 314
  scleritis complication, 391
  secondary, 410, 425, 435
  signs and symptoms, 177*t*, 178
  treatment, 176
Glaucoma medications, 60, 103
Globe rupture, 485, 490

Glycosaminoglycan depositions, 199*t*, 203, 203*f*, 207
Glycosaminoglycans (GAGs; mucopolysaccharides), 248
GM_1 gangliosidosis type I (generalized gangliosidosis), 251, 252*t*
GM_2 gangliosidosis type I (Tay-Sachs disease), 251, 252*t*, 253–254
Goblet cells, 6, 8
Goldberg syndrome (galactosialidosis), 255
Gold depositions, 166*t*
Goldenhar-Gorlin syndrome (oculoauriculovertebral syndrome), 152, 267*t*, 268*t*, 270–271, 271*f*
Goldenhar syndrome, 153
Gold salts, 181
Gold weight implants, 94
Goniodysgenesis, 138*t*, 142
Gout, 168*t*, 259*t*, 264, 389
GPA. *See* Granulomatosis with polyangiitis
Grafts
  allografts. *See* Allografts
  amniotic membrane grafts, 108–109*t*, 110, 112, 119–120, 124, 130
  autografts. *See* Autografts; Autologous transplantation
  bare sclera coverage technique, 110, 110–111*f*, 112
  detachment, 499–500, 499–500*f*
  failure
    ALK complication, 491
    endothelial failure, 476, 476*f*, 480–481
    endothelial keratoplasty complication, 494*t*, 495, 504
    graft rejection and, 481
    risk factors, 470
    transplant indication, 472
  indications, 108*t*
  limbal stem cell transplantation, 120–123, 120*t*, 122–123*f*, 124
  mucous membrane grafts, 108*t*, 123–124
  rejection
    ALK complication, 491
    endothelial keratoplasty complication, 504–505, 505*f*, 505*t*
    endothelial rejection, 54, 305, 482*t*, 483, 484*f*
    epithelial rejection, 481, 482*t*, 483*f*
    penetrating keratoplasty complication, 504
    prevention, 484–485
    signs and symptoms, 54
    stromal rejection, 482, 482*t*
    subepithelial rejection, 481, 482*t*, 483*f*
    transplantation procedures choice and, 474*t*, 481
    treatment, 483–484, 504–505
Graft-vs-host disease (GVHD)
  biopsy evaluation, 118
  chronic, 89
  limbal stem cell deficiency cause, 101
  pathogenesis, 374
  signs and symptoms, 374, 375*f*
  SLK cause, 91
  treatment, 374–375
Granular corneal dystrophy, 478, 478*f*
Granular corneal dystrophy type 1 (GCD1; Groenouw corneal dystrophy type I, classic granular dystrophy), 199–200, 199*t*, 200*f*
Granular corneal dystrophy type 2 (GCD2; Avellino corneal dystrophy), 199*t*, 201, 201*f*
Granulomas, 50*t*, 113, 417–418, 418*f*, 443
Granulomatosis with polyangiitis (GPA, Wegener granulomatosis), 389
Granulomatous conjunctivitis (Parinaud oculoglandular syndrome), 303, 333
Granulomatous iridocyclitis, 296
Groenouw corneal dystrophy type I (granular corneal dystrophy type 1), 199–200, 199*t*, 200*f*
Groenouw corneal dystrophy type II (macular corneal dystrophy), 199*t*, 202–203*f*, 202–204
Gundersen conjunctival flap surgery, 96, 114–118, 115–117*f*
Gunpowder, 447–448
Guttae, 162, 177–178, 202, 210, 211
GVHD. *See* Graft-vs-host disease

Haab striae, 143, 154
HAART (highly active antiretroviral therapy), 419
Haemophilus influenzae, 325, 326
Hallermann-Streiff-François syndrome (oculomandibulodyscephaly), 267*t*
Hamartomas, 443
Handheld (Cochet-Bonnet) esthesiometer, 20–21
Hansen disease (leprosy), 53*t*, 350, 388
Hassall-Henle bodies (peripheral corneal guttae), 162, 177–178
Heat injuries, 432–433, 433*f*
Heavy-chain disease, 275
HEDS. *See* Herpetic Eye Disease Study
Helmholtz keratometer, 32, 33*f*
Hemangiomas, 416–417
Hematologic disorders, 259*t*, 273–275, 273*f*
Heme synthesis, 265–266
Hemifacial microsomia, 267*t*
Hemorrhages
  conjunctival, 163*t*, 315, 436–437, 436*f*
  flap surgery complication, 116
  subconjunctival, 92
HEP. *See* Hepatoerythropoietic porphyria
Heparin (topical), 364, 437
Hepatitis, 166*t*, 265, 386
Hepatoerythropoietic porphyria (HEP), 266
Herbert pits, 329, 330*f*
Herpes simplex virus (HSV)
  background, 284
  blepharoconjunctivitis, 284, 284–285*f*, 287
  characteristics of, 282
  complications of, 296–297
  corneal scarring, 297
  diagnostic techniques, 283*t*, 286
  differential diagnosis, 284–285
  differentiating features, 298*t*
  epitheliopathy, 296
  Herpetic Eye Disease Study (HEDS), 294–295, 294–295*t*

keratitis, 288–296. *See also* Herpetic keratitis
keratoplasty complications and, 470
metaherpetic ulcers, 297
neurotrophic keratopathy, 95, 297
pathogenesis, 285–287
persistent bullous keratopathy, 297
primary infection, 284–285*f*, 284–286
recurrent infections, 286–296
sexually transmitted conjunctivitis, 328, 328*t*
Stevens-Johnson syndrome cause, 367
stromal keratitis, 291–296, 292–293*f*, 292*t*, 294–295*t*
surgical management, 297–298
trabeculitis (endotheliitis), 177*t*
treatment, 287*t*
Herpesviruses, 175, 284–303, 312. *See also* Cytomegalovirus; Epstein-Barr virus; Herpes simplex virus; Varicella-zoster virus
Herpes zoster. *See* Varicella-zoster virus
Herpes zoster ophthalmicus (HZO), 300, 300*f*, 315
Herpetic Eye Disease Study (HEDS), 294–295, 294–295*t*
Herpetic keratitis
differential diagnosis, 153, 290*t*, 345, 438
disciform, 54, 293*f*
endothelial, 53*t*
epithelial, 53*t*, 54*f*, 284, 285*f*, 288–290*f*, 288–291
graft rejection precautions, 483, 484
HIV association, 286
neurotrophic keratopathy association, 95
postoperative complication, 478, 478*f*
stromal, 53*t*, 284, 286, 291–296, 292–293*f*, 292*t*, 294–295*t*, 438
treatment, 290–291
varicella-zoster virus and, 52, 53*t*, 54*f*, 300–301
Heterochromia, 435
Hexamidine (topical), 346
HGD gene, 260
High-frequency ultrasound, 145
Highly active antiretroviral therapy (HAART), 419
HIV and AIDS-related ocular disorders
about, 315
characteristics of, 282
Epstein-Barr viral infections and, 305
keratitis (microsporidial) association, 347
molluscum contagiosum infection in, 310, 311*f*
OSSN risk factor, 402
sexually transmitted conjunctivitis, 328, 328*t*
varicella-zoster viral infections, 300
HLA-B27–related diseases, 376
Hodgkin lymphoma, 420
Holocrine sebaceous glands, 4
Homatropine (topical), 354
Homogentisic acid oxidase (homogentisate 1,2-dioxygenase), 260
Hordeola, 84–85, 85*f*
Hormone therapies, 56*t*, 69
Horner-Trantas dots, 359, 359*f*
Horse's tail (fingerprint lines), 25, 97, 98*f*, 187, 187*f*, 190
HPVs. *See* Human papillomaviruses
HSV. *See* Herpes simplex virus
Hudson-Stähli line, 165, 166*t*
Hughes classification scheme, 425–427*t*
Human papillomaviruses (HPVs), 312–313, 312*f*, 401, 402
Hunter syndrome (MPS II), 248, 249*t*
Hurler-Scheie syndrome (MPS IH/S), 248, 249*t*, 251
Hurler syndrome (MPS IH), 248, 249*t*, 251, 251*f*
Hyaline depositions, 199*t*, 200, 200*f*, 201
Hyaluronic acid solutions, 69
Hydration, 11–12, 13
Hydrochloric acid, 424*t*
Hydrofluoric acid, 424*t*, 425
Hydrops, 173, 177*t*, 221, 222*f*, 228
Hydroxychloroquine, 179
Hydroxypropyl cellulose inserts, 68
Hyfrecation (electrolysis with radiofrequency probe), 89
Hyperacute gonococcal conjunctivitis, 324*t*, 326–327*f*, 326–328, 328*t*
Hypercholesterolemia, 204
Hyperlipidemia, 205
Hyperlipoproteinemia, 205
Hyperopic photorefractive kerectomy, 126, 128
Hyperparathyroidism, 168*t*, 277
Hypertelorism, 138*t*, 142
Hypertension, 437
Hypertonic saline solution, 99
Hyperuricemia, 259*t*, 264
Hyphema, 435, 439, 440–446, 442–444*f*
Hypochlorous acid, 79, 81
Hypocholesterolemia, 256
Hypolipoproteinemias, 255–256, 256*f*, 259*t*
Hypophosphatasia, 268*t*
Hypoplasminogenemia, 364
Hypopyon, 335, 335*f*, 342
Hypotony, postoperative, 460
HZO. *See* Herpes zoster ophthalmicus

Ibuprofen, 393
ICE. *See* Iridocorneal endothelial (ICE) syndrome
Ichthyosis, 277–278
Ichthyosis vulgaris, 278
ICRS. *See* Intrastromal corneal ring segments
Idoxuridine, 354, 370
IgE (immunoglobulin E) microassay, 30
IgG (immunoglobulin G), 273, 304
IgM (immunoglobulin M), 274
IK. *See* Interstitial keratitis
IL-1RA (interleukin 1 receptor antagonist), 7*f*, 15–16*f*
Imidazoles, 346
Immediate hypersensitivity (anaphylaxis) (type I) reactions, 353, 354–355, 355*f*, 357, 362
Immune complex–mediated (type III) reactions, 353
Immune-related disorders. *See also specific disorders*
of conjunctiva, 356–376
of cornea, 376–386
of episcleritis, 387–388
of eyelid, 354–356

hypersensitivity reaction classification, 353–354
pathogenesis, 16
of sclera, 388–394, 389*t*
Immunoglobulin disorders, 259*t*, 273–275
Immunoglobulin E (IgE) microassay, 30
Immunoglobulin G (IgG), 273, 304
Immunoglobulin M (IgM), 274
Immunohistochemical staining, 371–372, 372*f*
Immunosuppression therapy, 102, 373, 373*t*, 393
Inclusion cell disease (ML II), 254, 254*t*
Inclusion cysts, 116, 160–162, 162*f*, 411
Indomethacin, 179, 393
INF-α_{2a} (interferon-α_{2a}), 419
INF-α_{2b} (interferon-α_{2b}), 313, 398, 401, 406, 421
Infants. *See also* Congenital anomalies; *specific congenital disorders*
birth trauma, 154–155, 155*f*, 177*t*
cystinosis and, 257–259
neonatal conjunctivitis, 328–329, 332–333
neonatal gonococcal conjunctivitis, 328–329
normal flora of, 317
osteogenesis imperfecta and, 270
pediatric transplantation, 507–509
vitamin A deficiency and, 272
Infections. *See also* Bacterial infections; Fungal infections; Parasitic infections; Viral infections
defense mechanisms, 14–17, 15–16*f*
evaluation, 30
granuloma cause, 418
pathogenesis, 318–322, 319*t*
specimen collection and evaluation, 320–321*t*, 321–322, 322*f*
Infectious crystalline keratopathy, 335, 336*f*, 480*f*
Infectious mononucleosis (Epstein-Barr virus), 292*t*, 303–304, 304*f*, 378
Inferior tarsal muscle, 3, 5*f*
Inferonasal bulbar conjunctiva, 8
Inflammatory pseudoguttae, 53
Infliximab, 384
Injuries. *See* Burns; Chemical injuries; Radiation; Traumatic injuries
Insect hairs, 435, 435*f*, 447
Instrument cleaning, 308
Intacs, 235, 238
Intellectual disability, 138*t*, 142
Intense Pulsed Light (IPL) therapy, 76
Interferometry, 31, 31*f*
Interferon-α_{2a} (INF-α_{2a}), 419
Interferon-α_{2b} (INF-α_{2b}), 313, 398, 401, 406, 421
Interior tear meniscus, 6
Interleukin 1, 16, 57
Interleukin 1 receptor antagonist (IL-1RA), 7*f*, 15–16*f*
Internal hordeola, 84, 85
International Trachoma Initiative, 331
Interstitial keratitis (IK)
band keratopathy cause, 168*t*
differential diagnosis, 203, 292*t*
herpetic, 292, 292*f*, 295
syphilitic, 151–152, 377–379, 379*f*
Intracanalicular plugs, 70–71
Intraepithelial dysplasia, 190
Intraepithelial nevi, 411
Intraocular lens (IOL) implant, 33, 443
Intraocular pressure (IOP)
about, 40
chemical injuries and, 430
corneal hydration and, 12
hyphemas and, 444–446, 446*t*
keratoprosthesis complication, 510–511
postoperative complication, 477, 478
postoperative monitoring, 460
preoperative transplant evaluation of, 471
rebleeding and, 443–444
RNA viral infection and, 314
Intrastromal corneal ring segments (ICRSs)
background, 235, 235*f*
combined techniques, 245–246
complications, 235, 238–240, 239–240*f*
contraindications, 236
indications, 228, 235–236
instrumentation, 236
keratoconus treatment, 228
outcomes, 237–238
technique, 236–237, 237*f*
Intrauterine keratitis, 151–152
Inturned eyelid (entropion), 89, 368, 370
Inverted conjunctival papilloma, 401
IOL (intraocular lens) implant, 33, 443
Ionizing radiation injuries, 434–435
IOP. *See* Intraocular pressure
IPL (Intense Pulsed Light) therapy, 76
Iridectomy, 340
Iridocorneal endothelial (ICE) syndrome
classification, 175, 175*t*
differential diagnosis, 146, 175, 214, 215*t*
etiology, 175
signs and symptoms, 175, 175*t*, 176–177*f*, 177*t*, 215*t*
treatment, 177–178
Iridocyclitis, 78, 375
Iridodialysis, 440, 440–442*f*, 458
Iridodonesis, 138*t*, 142, 143
Iris
blunt trauma, 439–444*f*, 439–446
defects, 25, 134, 135*f*
evaluation, 23, 25, 45, 45*f*
foreign body trauma, 448
hamartomas, 443
hypoplasia, 138*t*, 142, 146, 314
incarceration postoperatively, 477
prolapse of, 455*f*
prosthesis, 439
retroillumination of, 25
sphincter tears, 439, 439*f*, 440
trauma treatment, 441–442*f*, 451, 451*t*, 454, 455*f*, 458, 459–460*f*
Iris diaphragm contact lenses, 439
Iris nevus (Cogan-Reese) syndrome, 175, 176*f*
Iris strands, 146
Iron depositions, 159, 160*f*, 165, 165*f*, 166*t*, 226
Iron foreign bodies, 447*f*, 448–449, 449*f*

Iron line (Stocker line), 159, 160*f*, 165, 165*f*, 166*t*
Irrigation, 429, 447–448
Ischemic optic neuropathy, 314
Isotretinoin, 56*t*
Itraconazole (oral), 343, 348
Itraconazole (topical), 346
Ivermectin (oral), 79, 349

Javal-Schiøtz keratometer, 32
Junctional nevi, 410–411
Juvenile idiopathic arthritis, 168*t*
Juvenile xanthogranuloma, 418, 443

Kaposi sarcoma, 312, 418–419, 419*f*
Kayser-Fleischer ring, 166*t*, 264–265, 265*f*, 273
KC. *See* Keratoconus
KCS. *See* Keratoconjunctivitis sicca
Keloids, 152, 174
KERA gene, 143, 208
Kerarings, 235
Keratan sulfate proteoglycans, 143
Keratectasia, 140*t*, 150–151, 151*f*, 166*t*
Keratectomy
  ocular surface disease reconstruction technique, 125–126
  photorefractive keratectomy, 44, 59, 99, 226, 245–246
  phototherapeutic keratectomy, 99, 125–126
  Salzmann nodular degeneration treatment, 169–170
Keratic precipitates (KPs), 23, 53–54
Keratinization, 429*f*
Keratitis. *See also specific types of keratitis*
  acanthamoeba, 344–347. *See also Acanthamoeba* keratitis
  adenovirus, 53*t*, 308–309, 309*f*, 332
  animal injury sign, 435*f*
  atopic, 292*t*
  autoimmune-related, 375, 376
  bacterial, 334–341. *See also* Bacterial keratitis
  differential diagnosis, 105–106, 438
  Epstein-Barr virus, 303
  evaluation, 43, 43*f*
  fungal, 341–344. *See also* Fungal keratitis
  gonococcal conjunctivitis association, 326–327
  herpetic, 288–296. *See also* Herpetic keratitis
  infectious crystalline keratopathy, 335, 336*f*, 480*f*
  measles as cause of, 314
  plant injury sign, 436
  postoperative complications, 478, 478*f*, 480, 480*f*
  preoperative transplant evaluation of, 471
  risk factors, 69
  seborrheic blepharitis sign, 79
  systemic infections associated with, 347–349, 347–349*f*
  treatment, 337, 339, 374, 377, 384
Keratoacanthoma, 310
Keratoconjunctivitis, 103*t*, 436
Keratoconjunctivitis sicca (KCS), 71, 105, 315, 374, 384
Keratoconus (KC)
  about, 140*t*, 217–218, 218*f*
  contact lens options, 227–228, 227*f*
  differential diagnosis, 218*f*
  evaluation, 33, 35, 36, 40
  immune disorder associations, 360
  ocular disorder associations, 88, 149, 362
  pathogenesis, 226
  signs and symptoms, 149, 150*f*, 218*f*, 220–225*f*, 220–226
  staging, 226
  systemic associations, 219*t*, 266, 267–268*t*, 270
  treatment, 226–229, 227*f*, 235, 243, 472, 488
Keratocytes, 11, 12*f*
Keratoepithelin-associated (*TGFBI* epithelial-stromal) dystrophies, 185–186*t*, 192–202
Keratoglobus
  about, 140*t*, 144–145
  contact lens options, 233
  differential diagnosis, 218*f*, 233*t*
  pathogenesis, 233
  signs and symptoms, 218*f*, 232, 233–234*f*
  systemic disorder associations, 266, 267*t*
  treatment, 233–234
Keratolimbal allograft, 122
Keratolysis, 382
Keratometry, 32–33, 33*f*
Keratopathy. *See* Keratitis
Keratoplasty
  chemical injury treatment, 425
  cytomegalovirus recurrence and, 306
  indications, 148, 228
  keratitis treatment, 346, 384
  neurotrophic keratopathy cause, 95
  rejection, 53*t*
  trends, 465
  types of, 464*t*. *See also* Endothelial keratoplasty; Lamellar keratoplasty; Penetrating keratoplasty
Keratoprosthesis
  about, 510–511, 510*f*, 511*t*
  chemical injury treatment, 425
  dry eye treatment, 368
  for herpetic eye disease, 298
  limbal stem cell deficiency treatment, 102
  MPM treatment, 374
  SJS treatment, 368
Keratoscopy, 33, 34*f*
Keratosis, 48*t*, 448
Ketoconazole, 343, 346
KPs. *See* Keratic precipitates
Krukenberg spindle, 142–143, 166*t*
Kumquat-like lesions, 191, 192*f*

Labrador keratopathy (spheroidal degeneration), 163–165, 164*f*, 169, 260
Lacerations
  blunt trauma and, 437
  conjunctiva, 446–447
  cornea
    postoperative management, 458–461
    treatment, 453, 454–458, 455–460*f*
  iris, 458, 460*f*
  sclera, 453, 453*f*, 454–458, 455–460*f*

Lacrimal functional unit (LFU), 5–6, 6*f*, 54, 62–63
Lacrimal glands
  dry eye and, 59
  examination, 30
  infiltration, graft-vs-host disease association, 374
  innervation of, 6
  radiation injuries of, 434–435
  tumors of, 407
Lacrimal pump, 3
Lacrimal puncta, 6, 300
Lactoferrin levels, 30
Lacus lacrimalis (lacrimal lake), 8
Lagophthalmos, 93–94
Lamellar keratoplasty (LK)
  about, 488–490, 488*f*
  bacterial keratitis treatment, 340
  comparisons, 474–475*t*, 490, 493*t*
  fungal keratitis treatment, 343
  indications, 473*t*
  intraoperative complications, 473*t*
  keratitis (amebic) treatment, 346
  penetrating keratoplasty comparison, 474–475*t*, 490
  peripheral ulcerative keratitis treatment, 384
  postoperative complications, 474*t*, 490–491, 491*f*
  trends, 464–465
  types of. *See* Anterior lamellar keratoplasty; Deep anterior lamellar keratoplasty
Lamina fusca, 8
Langerhans cells, 16, 16*f*, 17
Laser in situ keratomileusis (LASIK)
  complications, 224*f*, 226, 238, 243
  contraindications, 275–276
  corneal biomechanics following, 40
  dry eye etiology, 59
  neurotrophic keratopathy cause, 95
  postoperative evaluation, 44
  postsurgical infections, 341, 341*f*
  preoperative evaluation, 44
Lash loss (madarosis), 81, 85
LASIK. *See* Laser in situ keratomileusis
Latex (milky sap), 436
Lattice corneal dystrophy type 1 (LCD1; Biber-Haab-Dimmer) and variants, 186*t*, 196–199, 197–199*f*, 199*t*, 201, 261, 478. *See also specific interventions*
Lattice lines, 262, 263, 263*f*
Lax conjunctiva (conjunctivochalasis), 67, 91, 92, 93*f*, 119–120
Layered hyphema, 440, 443*f*
LCAT deficiency. *See* Lecithin-cholesterol acyltransferase (LCAT) deficiency
LCD1. *See* Lattice corneal dystrophy type 1
Leaves, 448
Leber tapetoretinal degeneration, 219*t*
Lecithin-cholesterol acyltransferase (LCAT) deficiency, 255–256, 256*f*, 259*t*
Leiomyosarcoma, 416, 419
Leishmania spp, 378
Lens
  instability, 143
  opacities, 362
  trauma to, 440–446, 442–444*f*
Lenticular opacity, 435
Leprosy (Hansen disease), 53*t*, 350, 388
Leukemia, 443
Leukoma, 134, 134*f*, 146
Levator palpebrae muscle, 3, 4*f*
Levofloxacin, 453
LFU. *See* Lacrimal functional unit
Lice infestations, 323
Lifitegrast (topical), 69
Ligneous conjunctivitis, 364–365, 364*f*
Limbal dermoids (epibulbar dermoids), 152, 153*f*, 267*t*, 270, 271, 271*f*
Limbal paracentesis, 445–446
Limbal stem cell deficiency (LSCD)
  about, 100
  classification, 102*t*
  pathogenesis, 100–101, 101*f*, 296
  signs and symptoms, 100, 101*f*
  treatment, 120–123
Limbal stem cell transplantation
  about, 120
  chemical injury treatment, 425, 432
  dry eye treatment, 368
  indications, 101, 108*t*
  radiation injury treatment, 434–435
  SJS treatment, 368
  types of, 120*t*, 121–123, 122–123*f*
Limbal vernal keratoconjunctivitis, 359, 359*f*
Limbus
  defense mechanisms of, 16*f*, 17
  dendritic cells of, 17
  reconstruction techniques, 109*t*, 112
  scarring, 83
  structure and function, 9, 9–10*f*, 14, 14*f*
  as surgical landmark, 454, 455*f*
Linear IgA dermatosis, 370
Linear nevus sebaceous syndrome, 152
Lipid depositions
  corneal dystrophies and, 199*t*, 204–205, 207
  lipid keratopathy, 174, 174*f*
  sphingolipidoses and, 251–254, 252*t*, 253*f*
  Terrien marginal degeneration sign, 173
Lipid keratopathy, 259*t*, 301, 301*f*
Lipid metabolism disorders, 204, 205, 254–255, 254*t*
LipiFlow Thermal Pulsation System, 75
Lipofuscin, 178
Liposarcoma, 419
Liposomal sprays, 68
Lissamine green stain, 29, 29*f*, 60, 60*f*
Liver disease, 75
LK. *See* Lamellar keratoplasty
Loa loa, 349, 350*f*
Loiasis, 349, 350*f*
Loteprednol, 484
Louis-Bar syndrome (ataxia-telangiectasia), 417
Lowe (oculocerebrorenal) syndrome, 152

Low-water-content bandage contact lenses, 96
LSCD. *See* Limbal stem cell deficiency
Lubricants (topical)
chemical injury treatment, 431
congenital corneal anesthesia treatment, 153
conjunctivochalasis treatment, 92
dellen treatment, 100
limbal stem cell deficiency treatment, 101
pingueculitis treatment, 158
postoperative epithelial defect treatment, 477
Lye, 424*t*
Lyme disease, 53*t*, 292*t*, 347, 378, 388
Lymphangiectasia, 417
Lymphangioma, 437
Lymphangioma (lymphatic malformation), 417
Lymphatic malformation (lymphangioma), 417
Lymphoid hyperplasia (reactive lymphoid hyperplasia), 419–420, 420*f*
Lymphoid tumors, 419–421
Lymphoma, 395, 419, 420, 421*f*
Lysosomal storage diseases, 248, 249–250*t*, 251–256. *See also specific lysosomal storage diseases*
Lys-plasminogen, 365

Macular corneal dystrophy (MCD; Groenouw corneal dystrophy type II), 199*t*, 202–203*f*, 202–204
Macule, 48*t*
Magnesium hydroxide, 424*t*
Malassezia furfur, 323
Malignancies
differential diagnosis, 82, 85
glaucoma, 45
lesions, 395, 411*t*, 414–416
tumors, 395, 410, 418–420
Malignant fibrous histiocytoma, 419
Malignant glaucoma, 45
Malignant melanoma, 395, 411*t*
Manchineel tree, 436
Mandibulofacial dysostosis (Treacher Collins syndrome), 268*t*
Manifest refraction, 487
Mannosidosis, 255
Manual keratometer, 32, 33*f*
Map biopsies, 407, 413
Map-dot-fingerprint dystrophy. *See* Epithelial basement membrane dystrophy
Maps, 33–35, 35–37*f*, 187, 188–189*f*, 190
Marfan syndrome, 138*t*, 142, 268*t*, 269, 269*f*
Marginal keratitis
about, 380–381
rosacea-associated, 76, 77*f*
signs and symptoms, 82–83, 83*f*, 381–382, 381*f*
staphylococcal blepharoconjunctivitis sign, 82
treatment, 83, 381–382
Maroteaux-Lamy syndrome (MPS VI), 248, 250*t*
Mascara, 408
Maskin Meibomian Gland Intraductal Probe, 75
Mast-cell stabilizers, 355, 357, 358*t*, 360
Matrix metalloproteinase 9 (MMP-9), 30
Mature dendritic cell (mDC), 15–16*f*
McCannel technique, 458, 460*f*
MCD. *See* Macular corneal dystrophy
mDC. *See* Mature dendritic cell
Mean curvature power map, 34, 37*f*
Measles (rubeola), 314, 378
MECD. *See* Meesmann epithelial corneal dystrophy
Mechanical epilation, 89
Mechanical keratectomy, 125
Medroxyprogesterone, 384, 431
Meesmann epithelial corneal dystrophy (MECD), 186*t*, 190–191, 190*f*
Megalocornea, 138*t*, 141*t*, 142–143, 142*f*, 233*t*, 270
Meibography (infrared), 31, 31*f*, 64
Meibomian gland carcinoma, 85
Meibomian gland dropout, 31, 31*f*
Meibomian gland dysfunction (MGD)
differential diagnosis, 65
dry eye and, 58
dry eye association, 56*t*, 63, 64, 65*f*
pathogenesis, 63
rosacea-associated, 76
signs and symptoms, 31–32, 31*f*, 64–65, 65*f*
systemic diseases and conditions associated with, 78
treatment, 72, 72–73*t*, 74–76
Meibomian glands
diagnosis and classifications, 72–73*t*
dysfunction. *See* Meibomian gland dysfunction
ectodermal dysplasia and, 278
evaluation, 33
evaporative dry eye signs, 64, 65*f*
examination, 26, 31, 31*f*, 64
expression of, 64, 65*f*
eyelashes emerging form (distichiasis), 89, 89*f*
hordeola of, 84
innervation of, 6
secretions of, 64, 65*f*, 79
structure and function, 4, 4–5*f*, 6
Melanin depositions, 166*t*, 178
Melanin-like pigment depositions, 166*t*
Melanocytic tumors, 399
Melanomas
about, 414
differential diagnosis, 411
ocular melanocytosis as risk factor, 410
risk factors, 413
signs and symptoms, 414, 415*f*
treatment overview, 414–416
Melanosis, 408, 409, 409*f*, 411*t*, 412–413*f*, 412–414
Melles technique, 489, 491–492
Melting
corneal, 383, 384, 425
stromal, 93, 96, 425
MEN. *See* Multiple endocrine neoplasia
Meretoja syndrome (familial amyloidosis), 196, 262*t*, 263
Metals
as foreign bodies, 438, 448
thermal burns and, 432
Metastatic tumors, 421

Methotrexate, 373, 384
Metronidazole, 78
MGD. *See* Meibomian gland dysfunction
Miconazole, 346
Microcornea
  about, 138*t*
  congenital anomaly associations, 141, 147
  cornea plana association, 143
  prognosis, 142
  signs and symptoms, 141*f*, 141*t*
  systemic disorder associations, 267–268*t*
Micropannus, 329, 330*f*, 332
Microphthalmos, 141, 314
Microscopic hyphema, 440, 443*f*
Microsporidial keratoconjunctivitis, 315
Microsporidiosis, 347–349, 347–349*f*
Milk-alkali syndrome, 168*t*, 277
Milky sap (latex), 436
Mineral metabolism disorders, 264–265
Mini scleral design (MSD) lens, 227, 271
Minocycline, 74–75, 78, 166*t*, 384, 408
Miosis, 138*t*, 142, 439
Mites, 357
Mitomycin C (MMC)
  adverse effects, 399
  intraoperative application, 112
  melanoma treatment, 415
  OSSN treatment, 399*f*, 407
  primary acquired melanosis treatment, 414
  toxic reactions to, 103–104
MLs. *See* Mucolipidoses
MMC. *See* Mitomycin C
MMP. *See* Mucous membrane pemphigoid
MMP-9 (matrix metalloproteinase 9), 30
Möbius syndrome, 153
Moisture chamber glasses, 69, 133
Molds, 357
Molecular diagnostics, 321
Moll, glands of, 4, 4–5*f*
Molluscum contagiosum, 81, 310–312, 311*f*, 315
Monoclonal gammopathy, 196, 259*t*, 273, 274
Monocular diplopia, 134, 135*f*
Mononucleosis. *See* Epstein-Barr virus
Mooren ulcer, 53*t*, 231*t*, 373*t*, 385–386
Moraxella lacunata, 82, 324*t*
Moraxella spp, 318*t*, 319*t*, 337*t*
Morquio syndrome (MPS IV), 248, 250*t*
Mosaic degeneration (crocodile shagreen), 171–172
Moxifloxacin, 453, 458
M proteins, 275
MPSs. *See* Mucopolysaccharidoses
MSD (mini scleral design) lens, 227, 271
Mucoepidermoid carcinoma, 404
Mucolipidoses (MLs), 138*t*, 142, 155, 254–255, 254*t*
Mucolytic agent, 91*t*
Mucopolysaccharides (glycosaminoglycans), 248
Mucopolysaccharidoses (MPSs), 155, 203, 248, 249–250*t*, 251, 251*f*
Mucous membrane conjunctivitis, 101
Mucous membrane grafts
  about, 123–124
  indications, 108*t*, 368, 373, 434
Mucous membrane pemphigoid (MMP; ocular cicatricial pemphigoid)
  biopsy evaluation, 118
  differential diagnosis, 105, 370, 371*t*
  keratoprosthesis for, 510
  laboratory evaluation, 371–372, 372*f*
  limbal stem cell deficiency cause, 101
  ocular surface disease treatment, 124
  pathogenesis, 371
  signs and symptoms, 368–371, 369–371*f*
  treatment, 371*f*, 372–374, 373*t*
  trichiasis cause, 89, 90
Mucous plaques, 60
Mucus-fishing syndrome, 81, 105
Mulberry configuration, 191, 192*f*
Müller muscle, 3, 4*f*
Multiple endocrine neoplasia (MEN), 276, 276*t*, 277*f*, 416
Multiple myeloma, 166*t*, 259*t*, 265, 273, 274*f*
Multiple sulfatase deficiency, 251, 252*t*
Mumps, 292*t*, 314
Munson sign, 220, 220*f*
Mycobacterium chelonae, 341
Mycobacterium fortuitum, 341
Mycobacterium leprae, 378
Mycobacterium spp
  keratitis cause, 337*t*, 341, 341*f*, 378
  keratoconjunctivitis cause, 84
  scleritis cause, 350
  specimen collection and evaluation, 321*t*, 322*f*
Mycobacterium tuberculosis, 84, 378
Mycophenolate mofetil, 373
Mycoplasma pneumoniae, 367
Mydriasis, 439, 439*f*
Myopia, 143
Myopic photorefractive keratectomy, 128
Myotonic dystrophy, 138*t*, 141

Nail–patella syndrome (onycho-osteodysplasia), 268*t*
Nanophthalmos, 141
Narrow angles, 45
Nasolacrimal nerve, 70
Nasolacrimal system, 81
Natamycin, 343
Natowicz syndrome (MPS IX), 248, 250*t*
Natural regulatory T cells (nTreg cells), 15–16*f*
Nebulae, 25
Necrosis
  of conjunctiva, 434
  of sclera, 434
  of stroma, 510
Necrotizing keratitis, 292–293, 293*f*, 296
Necrotizing retinitis, 305
Necrotizing scleritis, 48*t*, 265, 390, 390*f*, 391*f*
Neisseria gonorrhoeae, 323, 327, 328*t*
Neisseria meningitidis, 323

Neisseria spp, 337*t*
Neomycin, 346, 354
Neonatal conjunctivitis, 324*t*, 328–329, 332–333
Neonatal gonococcal conjunctivitis, 328–329
Neoplastic disorders
  about, 395–396
  biopsy for, 397
  epithelial tumors, 400–407, 401*t*
  evaluation, 45, 81
  glandular tumors, 407
  lymphoid tumors, 419–421
  malignant lesions, 395, 411*t*, 414–416
  malignant tumors, 395, 410, 418–420
  metastatic tumors, 405, 415, 421
  neuroectodermal tumors, 408–416, 409*t*
  observation period, 397
  signs and symptoms overview, 396
  treatment follow-up, 400
  treatment overview, 397–400, 399–400*f*
  vascular benign lesions, 416–418
Neovascularization and vascularization
  of conjunctiva, 414
  of cornea
    atopic keratoconjunctivitis sign, 362
    etiology, 53, 55*f*
    of herpes zoster ophthalmicus, 301
    ichthyosis sign, 278
    limbal stem cell deficiency sign, 100, 101*f*
    MPM sign, 370, 371*f*
    postoperative complication, 479
    reactive arthritis association, 376
    rosacea association, 77*f*, 78
    tyrosinemia sign, 259
    vernal keratoconjunctivitis sign, 360
  of iris, 25
  of stroma, 105–106, 174, 174*f*, 191
  transplant complication, 491
Nephropathic cystinosis, 258
Neurilemoma, 416
Neuroectodermal tumors, 408–416, 409*t*
Neurofibromas, 416
Neurofibromatosis, 416
Neurogenic tumors, 416
Neuromas, 416
Neurotization, 96
Neurotrophic keratitis
  antiviral drug complication, 297
  causes, 95*t*
  differential diagnosis, 105
  of herpes zoster ophthalmicus, 301
  herpetic eye disease complication, 297, 300
  pathogenesis, 95, 95*t*
  signs and symptoms, 94–95, 95*f*
  treatment, 96, 297
  viral infection sign, 290
Nevi
  of conjunctiva, 409–411*f*, 409–412, 411*t*
  excision complications, 114
  of iris, 175, 175*t*
Nevus flammeus, 417
Nevus of Ota, 409, 410*f*
Night blindness (nyctalopia), 272
Nighttime lagophthalmos, 189–190
Nocardia spp, 337*t*, 350
Nodular anterior scleritis, 389, 389*f*
Nodular episcleritis, 387, 387*f*
Nodular fasciitis, 418
Nodular scleritis, 388, 389, 389*f*
NOMGD. *See* Nonobvious meibomian gland dysfunction
Nonenveloped viruses, 282
Nongonococcal urethritis, 376
Nongranulomatous iridocyclitis, 296
Non-Hodgkin lymphoma, 420
Nonnephropathic cystinosis (adult cystinosis), 258
Nonobvious meibomian gland dysfunction (NOMGD), 64
Nonsteroidal anti-inflammatory drugs (NSAIDs), 103, 367, 388, 393, 437, 438
Nonsuppurative stromal keratitis, 49*t*, 347–349, 347–349*f*
NSAIDs. *See* Nonsteroidal anti-inflammatory drugs
nTreg cells (natural regulatory T cells), 15–16*f*
NTRK1 gene, 153
Nummular keratitis, 301, 301*f*
Nutritional disorder manifestations, 272–273
Nyctalopia (night blindness), 272

OAV. *See* Oculoauriculovertebral (OAV) syndrome
Obstructive meibomian gland dysfunction, 63
Obstructive sleep apnea, 88
Occlusive retinal vasculitis, 301
Ochronosis, 166*t*, 260
OCP. *See* Ocular cicatricial pemphigoid
OCT. *See* Optical coherence tomography
Ocular cicatricial pemphigoid (OCP). *See* Mucous membrane pemphigoid
Ocular immune response, 15–16*f*, 15–17
Ocular melanocytosis, 409–410, 409–410*f*, 411*t*
Ocular surface disease (OSD)
  conjunctival signs, 47–51, 50–52*f*, 50*t*
  corneal signs, 52–54, 53*t*, 54–55*f*
  differential diagnosis, 50*t*
  dry eye, 54–76. *See also* Dry eye
  ectodermal dysplasia and, 278
  evaluation, 43
  eyelid conditions associated with, 76–85, 77*f*. *See also specific conditions*
  signs and symptoms, 47–54, 48–50*t*, 53*t*
  therapeutic interventions, 107–135, 108*t*. *See also* Reconstruction of ocular surface; *specific interventions*
Ocular surface disorders, self-induced, 95*f*, 105–106, 106*f*
Ocular surface squamous neoplasia (OSSN)
  about, 402
  biopsy evaluation, 118
  differential diagnosis, 159, 159*f*, 404
  evaluation, 29, 29*f*

invasive OSSN, 395, 403–404, 404*f*
invasive variants, 404
noninvasive OSSN, 402–403, 403–404*f*
risk factors, 402
treatment, 399, 399–400*f*, 405–406*f*, 405–407
Ocular surface tumors. *See* Neoplastic disorders
Oculoauriculovertebral (OAV) syndrome, 152, 267*t*, 268*t*, 270–271, 271*f*
Oculocerebrorenal (Lowe) syndrome, 152
Oculodento-osseous dysplasia, 268*t*
Oculodermal melanocytosis, 409, 410*f*, 411*t*
Oculomandibulodyscephaly (Hallermann-Streiff-François syndrome), 267*t*
Oculomotor nerve (cranial nerve III), 301
Ofloxacin, 327
OI. *See* Osteogenesis imperfecta
Omega-3 fatty acid supplementation, 70, 74
Omega-6 to omega-3 fatty acid ratio, 56*t*, 58, 70, 74
Onchocerca volvulus (onchocerciasis), 53*t*, 378
Oncocytoma, 407
Onycho-osteodysplasia (nail–patella syndrome), 268*t*
Opacification
atopic keratoconjunctivitis sign, 362
chemical injury sign, 429*f*
corneal transplantation complication, 490–491, 491*f*
diagnostic algorithm, 22*f*
etiology, 52–53
footprint, 288, 290*f*
of herpes zoster ophthalmicus, 301
ichthyosis sign, 278
penetrating keratoplasty indication, 472
syphilitic interstitial keratitis sign, 379
viral infection sign, 288
Open-angle glaucoma, 141, 143, 213, 269
Ophthalmia nodosum, 435, 435*f*
Optical coherence tomography (OCT), 40, 471, 472. *See also* Anterior segment optical coherence tomography
Optical zone, 10
Optic atrophy, 248, 443, 445, 446*t*
Optic nerve hypoplasia, 138*t*, 141
Optic neuritis, 314
Orbicularis oculi muscle, 3, 4–5*f*, 6
Orthokeratology, 334
OSD. *See* Ocular surface disease
OSSN. *See* Ocular surface squamous neoplasia
Osteogenesis imperfecta (OI), 138*t*, 142, 219*t*, 268*t*, 270, 270*f*, 271*t*
Osteo-odonto-keratoprosthesis, 510
Oxalosis, 259*t*

PACD. *See* Posterior amorphous corneal dystrophy
Pachymetry, 41–42
PAD. *See* Polymorphic amyloid degeneration
Palisades of Vogt, 14, 14*f*, 100
Palpebral (tarsal) conjunctiva, 7, 8
Palpebral vernal keratoconjunctivitis, 51*f*, 359, 359*f*
PAM. *See* Primary acquired melanosis
Pannus (vascularized), 53, 55*f*, 65, 121, 122*f*, 173, 329, 330*f*
Papillae, 47, 48*t*, 49, 50–51, 88
Papilledema, 253
Papillitis, 301
Papilloma, 312, 313*f*
Papillomaviruses, 312–313, 312*f*
Papule, 48*t*
Paramyxoviruses, 314
Paraproteins, 275
Parasitic infections
demodicosis, 73*t*, 79, 80*f*, 322–323, 323*f*
of eyelid, 322–323, 323*f*
granuloma cause, 418
Mooren ulcer cause, 386
pathogenesis, 318–322, 319*t*
Parathyroid disease, 276–277
Parinaud oculoglandular syndrome (granulomatous conjunctivitis), 303, 333
Paromomycin, 346
Parry-Romberg syndrome (progressive facial hemiatrophy), 268*t*
Partial-thickness corneal transplantation. *See* Lamellar keratoplasty
Patching (graft), 128, 131*f*, 384
Patching (therapeutic)
conjunctivochalasis treatment, 92
corneal abrasion treatment, 438, 451
dellen treatment, 100
foreign bodies treatment, 449
neurotrophic keratopathy treatment, 96
perforating injury treatment, 451
postoperative epithelial defect treatment, 477
RES treatment, 99
PCG. *See* Primary congenital glaucoma
PCR. *See* Polymerase chain reaction, 321
PDCD. *See* Pre-Descemet corneal dystrophy
pdDALK. *See* Pre-Descemetic DALK
Pediatric multisystem inflammatory syndrome, 314
Pediculus humanus capitis, 323
Pediculus humanus corporis, 323
Pedunculated conjunctival papilloma, 400, 401, 401*f*
PEK. *See* Punctate epithelial keratitis
Pellucid marginal degeneration (PMD)
about, 229
anterior lamellar keratoplasty indication, 488
atopic keratoconjunctivitis sign, 362
contact lens options, 230
differential diagnosis, 218*f*, 231*t*
evaluation, 33
pathogenesis, 229
signs and symptoms, 218*f*, 229, 230*f*, 231*t*, 232*f*
treatment, 230, 235
Pemphigus vulgaris, 118
Penciclovir, 287*t*
Pencil tree, 436
Penetrating and perforating trauma
anesthesia, 453
of conjunctiva, 446–447
of cornea, 448–450, 449–450*f*
corneoscleral laceration repair, 454–458, 455–456*f*
defined, 446

evaluation of, 450–451, 451–452*t*
nonsurgical treatment, 451–452
preoperative management, 452–453
signs and symptoms, 450–451, 451*t*
surgical considerations, 454–455, 454*f*
surgical treatment, 452–461
Penetrating keratoplasty (PK)
bacterial keratitis treatment, 340
comparisons, 465, 473–475*t*, 490, 494*t*, 495
congenital anterior staphyloma and keratectasia treatment, 151
cornea plana treatment, 144
dry eye treatment, 368
for herpetic eye disease, 297–298
indications, 228, 466*t*, 469*t*, 472, 473*t*, 475*t*, 476–488
intraoperative complications, 473*t*
keratitis risk factor, 342
keratitis treatment, 343, 346, 348, 384
MPM treatment, 373–374
mucopolysaccharidoses treatment, 251
outcomes, 494*t*
pellucid marginal degeneration treatment, 230
postoperative astigmatism and refractive error, 485–488, 486–487*f*
postoperative complications, 474*t*, 476–485, 476*f*, 478–480*f*, 482*t*, 483*f*
radiation injury treatment, 435
rosacea precautions, 78
SJS treatment, 368
trends, 464–465
Penicillamine, 265
Penicillin, 379
Penicillin-resistant *Neisseria gonorrhoeae* (PRNG), 327
Perennial allergic conjunctivitis, 356–358, 358*t*
Perforating trauma. *See* Penetrating and perforating trauma
Peripheral corneal guttae (Hassall-Henle bodies), 162, 177–178
Peripheral hypertrophic subepithelial corneal degeneration, 170, 171*f*
Peripheral iridectomy, 340
Peripheral ulcerative keratitis (PUK)
about, 382
anterior lamellar keratoplasty indication, 488
differential diagnosis, 53*t*, 173, 382*t*, 385
evaluation, 30
signs and symptoms, 53*t*, 382–383, 383*f*
systemic immune-mediated diseases associated with, 382–385, 382*t*, 383*f*
Persistent bullous keratopathy, 297
Persistent fetal vasculature (PFV), 138*t*, 139*t*, 141, 142, 147
Peters anomaly (kerato-irido-lenticular dysgenesis), 45, 139*t*, 146–149, 148*f*
Peters-plus syndrome, 149
PFV. *See* Persistent fetal vasculature
Pharyngoconjunctival fever, 307
Phenothiazines, 179
Phenylalanine, 259–260
Phenylephrine, 387
Phlyctenular keratoconjunctivitis (phlyctenulosis), 83–84, 84*f*
Phlyctenule, 48*t*, 82
Phospholipid depositions, 199*t*, 204
Photophobia
anterior uveitis sign, 439
ATD symptom, 59
bacterial keratitis sign, 334
exposure keratopathy symptom, 93
primary congenital glaucoma sign, 154
RES symptom, 97
traumatic injury as cause of, 438
tyrosinemia sign, 259
Photorefractive keratectomy (PRK), 44, 59, 99, 126, 128, 226, 245–246
Photosensitivity, 278
Phototherapeutic keratectomy (PTK), 99, 125–126
Phthiriasis palpebrum, 323
Phthisical eye, 114
Phthisis, 425
Phthisis bulbi, 168*t*
Picornaviruses, 315
Pierre Robin malformation, 268*t*
Pigmentary retinopathy, 314
Pigmentation
about, 408, 409*t*
benign lesions, 409–412
deposition, 260, 261*f*, 265–266
differential diagnosis, 408, 411*t*
dispersion, 45, 138*t*, 142–143
malignant lesions, 414–416
preinvasive lesions, 412–414
Pigment spot of the sclera, 408
Pilocarpine, 70, 370
Pimecrolimus cream, 355, 356
Pinguecula, 114, 158, 158*f*
Pingueculitis, 158
PK. *See* Penetrating keratoplasty
Placido disk–based corneal topography, 33–35, 35–37*f*, 38, 40
Plant injuries, 436, 447, 448
Plasma cells (B lymphocytes), 274–275
Plasminogen, 364
Plasminogen deficiency, 364
Plasminogen gene *(PLG)*, 364
Platinum weight implants, 94
Pleomorphism, 41
Plica semilunaris, 7, 8
Plication (conjunctival fixation), 91*t*, 119
PMD. *See* Pellucid marginal degeneration
PMMA. *See* Polymethyl methacrylate
PMNs. *See* Polymorphonucleocytes
Pneumococci, 317
Poliosis (white lashes), 81
Pollen, 356–357
Polyarteritis nodosa, 389
Polyhexamethylene biguanide (polyhexanide), 346

Polymegethism, 41
Polymerase chain reaction (PCR), 321
Polymethyl methacrylate (PMMA), 235
Polymorphic amyloid degeneration (PAD), 172, 172*f*, 196, 261
Polymorphonucleocytes (PMNs), 430–431
Polymyxin B-trimethoprim, 326
Porphyria, 259*t*, 265–266
Porphyria cutanea tarda, 265
Porphyrins, 265–266
Port-wine birthmark, 417
Posaconazole, 343
Posner-Schlossman syndrome, 177*t*, 305
Posterior amorphous corneal dystrophy (PACD), 208–209, 208*f*
Posterior annular keratopathy, 437
Posterior embryotoxon, 139*t*, 145–146, 146*f*, 268*t*
Posterior keratoconus, 140*t*, 149, 150*f*
Posterior polymorphous corneal dystrophy (PPCD; posterior polymorphous dystrophy, Schlichting dystrophy), 177*t*, 213–214, 213–214*f*, 215*t*
Posterior scleritis, 389*t*, 391, 392, 392*f*
Posterior synechiae, 439
Postherpetic neuralgia, 303
Potassium hydroxide, 424*t*
Povidone-iodine, 310
Power maps, 34–35, 35–37*f*
Poxviruses, 310–312
PPCD. *See* Posterior polymorphous corneal dystrophy
Preauricular appendages, 270, 271*f*
Pre-Descemet (Dua) layer, 12
Pre-Descemet corneal dystrophy (PDCD), 185*t*, 209, 209*f*
Pre-Descemetic DALK (pdDALK), 464*t*, 489
Prednisolone (topical), 295, 476, 483, 484
Prednisone (oral), 361, 384, 393
Pregnancy, 75
Preservatives, in topical preparations, 58, 69, 168*t*, 354
Primary acquired melanosis (PAM), 118, 411*t*, 412–414, 413*f*
Primary congenital glaucoma (PCG), 154, 154*f*, 155
Primary familial amyloidosis (gelatinous droplike corneal dystrophy), 191, 192*f*, 261
Primary hyperparathyroidism, 277
Primary liquid keratopathy, 174
Primary localized amyloidosis, 261, 262*t*, 419
Primary Sjögren syndrome, 63, 64*t*
Primary spheroidal degeneration, 164
Primary systemic amyloidosis, 261–263, 262*t*
PRK. *See* Photorefractive keratectomy
PRNG. *See* Penicillin-resistant *Neisseria gonorrhoeae*
Progesterone cream (topical), 69
Programmed cell death (apoptosis), 57, 63
Progressive (essential) iris atrophy, 175, 176*f*
Progressive facial hemiatrophy (Parry-Romberg syndrome), 268*t*
Prolapse, of iris, 495*f*
Prominent corneal nerves, 276, 276*t*, 277*f*
Propamidine, 346
Propionibacteria spp, 337*t*
Propranolol, 416
Proptosis, 93–94
Protein metabolism disorders, 259*t*, 261–265
Proteoglycans, 11
Proteus spp, 337*t*
Pseudo–anterior chambers, 491
Pseudodendrites, 259, 259*f*
Pseudo-Fleischer ring, 166*t*
Pseudoguttae, 53
Pseudo-Hurler polydystrophy (ML III), 254, 254*t*
Pseudomembrane inflammation, 50*t*
Pseudomonas aeruginosa, 320, 335–336, 335*f*, 337*t*
Pseudopemphigoid, 370, 371
Pseudophakic corneal edema, 480, 484
Pseudopolycoria, 146
Pseudopterygium, 159
Pterygia, 35, 278
Pterygium, 56*t*, 107–114, 125, 158–160, 158–161*f*
Pterygium excision
  about, 107–108, 108*f*, 161*f*
  bare sclera coverage following, 109*t*, 110–111*f*, 110–113
  cataract extraction following, 160
  complications, 113–114, 113*f*
  indications, 159
  postoperative care, 113
  recurrence rates, 109*t*
  technique, 108–110
PTK. *See* Phototherapeutic keratectomy
PUK. *See* Peripheral ulcerative keratitis
Punctal occlusion
  congenital corneal anesthesia treatment, 153
  dry eye treatment, 368
  exposure keratopathy treatment, 94
  graft-vs-host disease treatment, 374
  limbal stem cell deficiency treatment, 101
  MPM treatment, 373
  neurotrophic keratopathy treatment, 96
  postoperative epithelial defect treatment, 477
  SLK treatment, 91*t*
Punctate epithelial erosions
  of conjunctiva, 48*t*
  of cornea, 49*t*
  differential diagnosis, 53*t*
  epithelial basement membrane dystrophy association, 189
  exposure keratopathy sign, 93
  radiation injury sign, 434
  reactive arthritis association, 376
  seborrheic blepharitis sign, 79
  signs and symptoms, 52, 54*f*
  Thygeson superficial punctate keratitis sign, 376
  vernal keratoconjunctivitis sign, 359–360
Punctate epithelial granularity, 52, 54*f*
Punctate epithelial keratitis (PEK)
  description, 49*t*
  differential diagnosis, 53*t*

of herpes zoster ophthalmicus, 300
marginal keratitis sign, 82–83
OSD sign, 49*t*, 52, 54*f*
viral infection sign, 288, 288*f*
Punctate occlusion, 70–71, 71*f*
Punctate staining patterns, 27, 28*f*
Pupillary block, 45, 501–502, 501*f*
Purkinje images (reflexes), 21
Pyogenic granuloma, 113, 417–418, 418*f*

Rabies (rhabdoviruses), 315–316
Racial melanosis (complexion-associated melanosis), 411*t*, 412, 412*f*
Radial keratoneuritis, 344
Radial perineuritis, 344
Radiation
injuries, 433–435
lymphoid hyperplasia treatment, 419
lymphoma treatment, 421
Raynaud disease, 433
RBCD. *See* Reis-Bücklers corneal dystrophy
Reactive arthritis (Reiter syndrome), 375–376
Reactive lymphoid hyperplasia (lymphoid hyperplasia), 419–420, 420*f*
Rebleeding prevention, 443–446, 444*f*
Rebound anterior uveitis, 439
Rebubbling, 495, 500, 506
Recombinant human nerve growth factor, 96
Reconstruction of ocular surface. *See also* Autologous transplantation
amniotic membrane grafts, 119–120
anterior stromal puncture, 99, 126–127, 127*f*
bandage contact lens use, 128–129
for bare sclera coverage, 109*t*, 110–111*f*, 110–113
conjunctival biopsy evaluation, 118
conjunctival fixation, 119
conjunctival flap, 114–118, 115–117*f*
conjunctival interventions, 107–124
corneal biopsy evaluation, 125
corneal interventions, 125–135
for corneal perforations, 130–132, 131*f*
corneal tattooing, 134–135, 134–135*f*
for corneal thinning/descemetocele, 129–130, 129–130*f*
epithelial debridement, 126
excimer laser ablation, 125–126, 128
limbal stem cell transplantation, 120–123, 120*t*, 122–123*f*
mucous membrane grafts, 123–124
patching, 128
pterygium excision, 107–110, 108*f*, 109*t*, 113–114, 113*f*
resection of conjunctiva, 119
superficial cauterization, 119
superficial keratectomy, 125–126
tarsorrhaphy, 132–133*f*, 132–134
Recurrent erosion syndrome (RES)
Cockayne syndrome sign, 267*t*
diabetes and, 275
differential diagnosis, 98, 153
EBMD association, 98, 98*f*
epithelial basement membrane dystrophy association, 189
pathogenesis, 97–99, 98*f*
signs and symptoms, 97, 97–98*f*
treatment, 99, 126–128, 127*f*, 190
Redundant tissue excision, 92, 93*f*
Reflective amblyopia, 142
Refractive error, 487
Refractive power, 32
Refractive surgery, 35, 36, 38*f*, 43, 44
Reis-Bücklers corneal dystrophy (RBCD; corneal dystrophy of Bowman layer type 1, atypical granular corneal dystrophy), 186*t*, 192–194, 193*f*, 195, 196*t*
Reiter syndrome (reactive arthritis), 375–376
Relaxing keratotomy, 487
Remdesivir, 314
Renal failure (chronic), 168*t*
RES. *See* Recurrent erosion syndrome
Resection, of conjunctiva, 119, 406
Reticular scarring, 220, 222*f*
Retinal degradation, 254
Retinal detachment
Ehlers-Danlos syndrome sign, 266
of herpes zoster ophthalmicus, 301
Peters anomaly association, 139*t*, 147
treatment, 114
Retinal microvasculopathy, 315
Retinitis pigmentosa, 219*t*
Retinoblastoma, 443
Retinopathy, 248
Retinopathy of prematurity, 219*t*
Retrobulbar optic neuritis, 301
Retroillumination reflex, 25, 26*f*
Retroprosthetic membrane formation, 510
Retroviruses, 315
Reverse Marcus Gunn response, 451
Reversible punctal occlusion, 70–71, 71*f*
Rhabdomyosarcoma, 419
Rhabdoviruses (rabies), 315–316
Rheumatoid arthritis
differential diagnosis, 53*t*
peripheral ulcerative keratitis association, 382, 383
scleritis association, 389, 390, 391*f*, 394
signs and symptoms, 53*t*, 259*t*
Rhodopsin, 272–273
Rho kinase inhibitors, 506
Riboflavin (vitamin B_2), 241
Richner-Hanhart syndrome (tyrosinemia type II), 259–260
Rieger anomaly (Axenfeld-Rieger syndrome), 139*t*, 146, 147*f*, 215*t*
Rifabutin, 181
Rifampin, 333
Rigid contact lens, 189, 271
Riley-Day syndrome, 153
Ring infiltrate, 344*f*, 346
Ripasudil, 506
Rituximab (injectable), 421

Rituximab (intravenous), 373*t*, 399, 421
Rizzuti sign, 220
RNA viruses, 313–316, 313*t*
Rosacea (acne rosacea)
dry eye disease association, 56*t*, 76–78, 77*f*
marginal keratitis association, 381
meibomian gland disease association, 65
pathogenesis, 77*f*, 78
signs and symptoms, 76, 77*f*, 78
treatment, 78
Rose bengal stain, 29, 60, 60*f*
Rotational autograft, 509, 509*f*
Rothmund-Thomson syndrome, 268*t*
Rubella, 314
Rubeola (measles), 314, 378
Rubeosis iridis, 441, 443
Rubinstein-Taybi syndrome, 152
Ruptured globe, 485, 490
Rust, 447*f*, 448–449, 449*f*

SAC. *See* Seasonal allergic conjunctivitis
SAFE strategy, for trachoma treatment and prevention, 331
Salivary glands, 63
Salmon patch, 152, 379, 379*f*
Salzmann nodular degeneration
description, 169, 170–171*f*
treatment, 125, 169–170, 469*t*
Sanfilippo syndrome (MPS III), 248, 249*t*
Sarcoid nodules, 418
Sarcoidosis, 168*t*, 277, 292*t*
SARS-CoV-2 (severe acute respiratory syndrome coronavirus 2), 282
Scaling, of eyelid, 79, 278
Scanning-slit technology, 37, 38
Scarring
apical, 220, 222*f*, 226, 228
conjunctival, 105, 265, 367
corneal
corneal tattooing and, 134, 135*f*
dry eye and, 59
evaluation, 35
immune disorder associations, 370, 374, 375*f*
keratoconus sign, 220, 222*f*, 226, 228
meibomian gland disease association, 65
rosacea-associated, 77*f*, 78
systemic disorder associations, 278
treatment, 125
vitamin A deficiency sign, 272
herpetic eye disease complication, 297, 300
limbal, 83
stromal, 220
SCC. *See* Squamous cell carcinoma
SCD. *See* Schnyder corneal dystrophy
Scheie syndrome (MPS IS), 248, 249*t*, 251
Scheimpflug-based corneal tomography, 37, 39, 39*f*, 40, 471
Schirmer tests, 30, 60
Schlichting dystrophy (posterior polymorphous corneal dystrophy), 177*t*, 213–214, 213–214*f*, 215*t*
Schnyder corneal dystrophy (SCD), 171, 199*t*, 204–205, 205*f*, 259*t*
Schwalbe line, 12, 145, 146*f*
Schwannomas, 416
Scissoring of the light reflex, 220
Sclera. *See also* Blue sclera
bare sclera coverage interventions, 109*t*, 110–111*f*, 110–113
degenerations and depositions, 178–179
examination, 26
melting, 113, 432
OSD sign, 48*t*
scleritis, 388–394. *See also* Scleritis
structure and function, 8
trauma to, 440–446, 442–444*f*
Scleral contact lenses
congenital corneal anesthesia treatment, 153
for dry eye symptoms, 69
dry eye treatment, 368
graft-vs-host disease treatment, 375, 375*f*
limbal stem cell deficiency treatment, 101
neurotrophic keratopathy treatment, 96
SJS treatment, 368
Scleral reinforcement, 394
Scleral spur, 45
Scleritis
classification, 388, 388*f*, 389–391, 389*t*
complications, 391–392, 392*f*
differential diagnosis, 382*t*, 387, 392
diffuse, 350
immune disorder associations, 388–394, 389*t*
infectious disease associations, 350, 388
laboratory evaluation, 392–393
microbial, 349–351, 350*f*
nodular, 350
pathogenesis, 388–389
signs and symptoms, 388, 388*f*
treatment, 373*t*, 393–394
viral etiology, 300, 314
Sclerocornea, 100, 138*t*, 139*t*, 143, 144, 144*f*
Sclerokeratitis, 391–392, 392*f*
Sclerokeratoplasty, 151
Scleromalacia perforans, 390, 391*f*
Sclerotic scatter, 23*f*, 25
Screen time, 56*t*, 58
Scurf, of eyelid, 79
Seasonal allergic conjunctivitis (SAC), 356–358, 358*t*
Sebaceous carcinoma, 81, 82, 407, 408*f*
Seborrheic blepharitis, 78–79, 79*f*, 80*t*
Seborrheic dermatitis, 78
Secondary acquired melanosis, 413, 414
Secondary anisometropic amblyopia, 152
Secondary glaucoma, 410, 425, 435
Secondary hyperparathyroidism, 277
Secondary liquid keratopathy, 174, 174*f*
Secondary localized amyloidosis, 262*t*
Secondary Sjögren syndrome, 63, 64*t*, 384
Secondary spheroidal degeneration, 164–165
Secondary systemic amyloidosis, 262*t*
Sectoral iris atrophy, 300

Seidel test, 28, 29*f*, 451
Selenium sulfide shampoos, 79
Senile plaque (Cogan plaque), 179, 179*f*
Seronegative spondyloarthropathies, 389
Serratia spp, 337*t*
Sessile conjunctival papilloma, 400–401, 401*f*
Severe acute respiratory syndrome coronavirus 2 (SARS-CoV-2), 282
Severe superficial keratitis, 168*t*
Shield ulcers, 360, 360*f*, 361
Shingles, 299–303, 299*t*, 300–301*f*
Sickle cell hemoglobinopathies, 445–446, 446*t*
Siderosis, 166*t*, 457, 459*f*
Siepser knot, 458
Silicone punctal plug, 70, 71, 71*f*
Silver depositions, 166*t*, 408
Simple limbal epithelial transplantation (SLET), 101, 112, 432
Single pedicle flap, 116, 117*f*
Sinskey hook, 460*f*
SIS. *See* Surgically induced scleritis
Sjögren's Foundation, 56
Sjögren syndrome
  biomarkers, 30
  classification, 62–63, 62*t*, 64*t*, 384
  dry eye risk factor, 56*t*
  lymphoma risk factor, 420
  signs and symptoms, 62–63, 62*t*
SJS. *See* Stevens-Johnson syndrome
SJS/TEN (Stevens-Johnson syndrome/toxic epidermal necrolysis) overlap, 365–368, 366f
Skeletal and connective tissue disorder manifestations, 266–271, 267–268*t*. *See also specific disorders*
Sleep apnea, 219*t*
SLET. *See* Simple limbal epithelial transplantation
Slit-lamp biomicroscopy
  about, 21–22
  clinical use, 22*f*, 26, 60, 62
  differential diagnosis algorithm, 22*f*
  diffuse illumination, 23, 23*f*
  direct illumination techniques, 22–24, 22–25*f*
  fluorescein stain, 27–29, 27*t*, 28–29*f*
  focal illumination, 23, 24*f*
  indirect illumination techniques, 22*f*, 24–25, 26*f*
  points to remember, 21, 24
  preoperative transplant evaluation with, 471
  proximal illumination, 25
  retroillumination, 23*f*, 25
  sclerotic scatter, 23*f*
  specular reflection, 23–24, 23*f*, 25*f*
SLK. *See* Superior limbic keratoconjunctivitis
Sly syndrome (MPS VII), 248, 250*t*
Smallpox (variola) virus, 311–312
Smooth-muscle tumors, 416
Snell's law of refraction, 32
Snow blindness, 433
Sodium citrate, 384, 431
Sodium hydroxide, 424*t*
Soil, as foreign body, 453
SP. *See* Swelling pressure
Spectinomycin, 327
Specular microscopy, 40–41, 41*f*
Spheroidal degeneration, 163–165, 164*f*, 169, 260
Sphingolipidoses, 251–254, 252*t*, 253*f*
Sphingomyelin, 251, 252*t*
Spindle cell carcinoma, 404
Spontaneous hyphemas, 441–442
Sporotrichosis, 333
Squamous carcinoma in situ, 402
Squamous cell carcinoma (SCC), 312. *See also* Ocular surface squamous neoplasia
Squamous dysplasia, 402
SSPE. *See* Subacute sclerosing panencephalitis
Staphylococcus aureus, 80, 82, 84, 317, 318–319*t*, 324*t*, 325, 337*t*, 362
Staphylococcus epidermidis, 317, 318*t*, 319*t*, 337*t*
Staphylococcus spp
  atopic keratoconjunctivitis association, 362, 363
  blepharitis cause, 65, 78, 80–81, 80*f*, 84*f*, 322, 381, 381*f*
  blepharoconjunctivitis cause, 81–82, 83*f*, 325
  keratitis cause, 337, 337*t*, 338*t*
  methicillin-resistant, 337
  as normal flora, 317, 318*t*
  pathogenesis, 320
  phlyctenulosis cause, 84
Staphyloma, 140*t*, 150–151, 151*f*, 390, 391*f*
Steroids. *See* Corticosteroids (topical)
Steroid-sparing agents. *See* Tacrolimus ointment
Stevens-Johnson syndrome (SJS)
  about, 365
  keratoprosthesis for, 510
  limbal stem cell deficiency cause, 101
  ocular surface disease treatment, 124
  pathogenesis, 366–367
  signs and symptoms, 365–366, 366*f*
  TEN overlap, 365–368, 366*f*
  treatment, 367–368
  trichiasis cause, 89
Stings, from bees and wasps, 435
Stocker-Holt variant, 186*t*, 191
Stocker line (iron line), 159, 160*f*, 165, 165*f*, 166*t*
Strabismus, 114, 270
Streptococcus pneumoniae, 324–325, 337*t*
Streptococcus pyogenes, 323
Streptococcus spp
  infectious crystalline keratopathy etiology, 336
  as normal flora, 317
  pathogenesis, 320
  Stevens-Johnson syndrome cause, 367
Streptokinase drugs, 437
Stroma
  conjunctival, 8, 157
  corneal
    cell morphology, 11, 12*f*
    depositions and degenerations, 163, 166*t*, 170–174, 171–174*f*
    dystrophies of, 185*t*, 202–209
    OSD sign, 52–53, 55*f*
    structure and function, 9*f*, 11–12, 12*f*, 24*f*

infiltrates, 23, 25, 435, 436
melting, 93, 96, 425
scleral, 8
Stromal graft rejection, 53*t*
Stromal keratitis
Cogan syndrome sign, 380
differential diagnosis, 53*t*, 380
Epstein-Barr virus, 303, 304*f*, 305
herpes simplex virus, 284, 286, 291–296, 292–293*f*, 292*t*, 294–295*t*, 438
herpes zoster, 301
microsporidiosis, 347–349, 347–349*f*
mumps as cause of, 314
rosacea-associated, 76, 77*f*
syphilis association, 379
traumatic injury as cause of, 438
treatment, 438
Stromal melting, 93, 96, 425
Sturge-Weber syndrome, 417
Styes (external hordeola), 84
Subacute sclerosing panencephalitis (SSPE), 314
Subconjunctival hemorrhage, 163*t*, 436–437, 436*f*
Subepithelial amyloidosis (gelatinous droplike corneal dystrophy), 191, 192*f*, 261
Subepithelial fibrosis, 362, 374
Subepithelial infiltrates, 49*t*, 380
Subepithelial nevi, 410–411
Subluxation of lens, 269
Substantia propria, 8, 157
Sulfonamides, 366
Sulfuric acid, 424*t*
Sunflower cataract, 265, 273
Sunflower stock, 436
Sunlamps, 433
Superficial cauterization, 119
Superficial corneal epithelial cells, 6
Superficial keratectomy, 125–126
Superior limbic keratoconjunctivitis (SLK), 90–92, 90*f*, 91*t*
Supplements. *See* Dietary supplements
Surgically induced scleritis (SIS), 394
Suture-related problems, 479, 479*f*
Swelling pressure (SP), 12
Symblepharon
atopic keratoconjunctivitis sign, 362
chemical injury sign, 430*f*
description, 48*t*
MPM sign, 369, 370*f*
neoplastic, 408*f*
OSD sign, 48*t*
porphyria sign, 265
Stevens-Johnson syndrome sign, 366, 366*f*
Synechiae, 444, 446*t*
Syphilis
congenital syphilis, 151–152, 378
differential diagnosis, 292*t*
granular conjunctivitis etiology, 333
interstitial keratitis association, 151–152, 377–379, 379*f*
scleritis and, 350, 388
Syphilitic intrauterine keratitis, 151–152
Systane iLUX MGD Thermal Pulsation System, 75–76
Systemic disorder manifestations
amino acid, nucleic acid, protein, and mineral metabolism disorders, 257–266
background, 247–248
dermatologic diseases, 277–279
endocrine diseases, 275–277
hematologic disorders, 273–275
inherited metabolic diseases, 248–266
lysosomal storage diseases, 248, 249–250*t*, 251–256
nutritional disorders, 272–273
skeletal and connective tissue disorders, 266–271, 267–268*t*
Systemic lupus erythematosus, 389
Systemic malignant lymphoma, 420

Tacrolimus ointment
atopic dermatitis treatment, 356
atopic keratoconjunctivitis treatment, 362–363
conjunctivitis (palpebral vernal keratoconjunctivitis) treatment, 359*f*
contact dermatoblepharitis treatment, 355
graft rejection prophylaxis, 484
graft rejection treatment, 483
Thygeson superficial punctate keratitis treatment, 377
vernal keratoconjunctivitis treatment, 361
Tamoxifen, 180
Tangential curvature map, 34, 36*f*
Tangier disease, 255–256
Tanning beds, 433
Taping of eyelids, 88, 94, 133
Tarantula hair keratitis, 435*f*
Tarsal (palpebral) conjunctiva, 7, 8
Tarsorrhaphy
about, 132–133*f*, 132–134
alternatives to, 133
chemical injury treatment, 432
congenital corneal anesthesia treatment, 153
descemetocele treatment, 130
dry eye treatment, 71
exposure keratopathy treatment, 94
mucous membrane grafts combined with, 124
neurotrophic keratopathy treatment, 96
persistent epithelial defect treatment, 129
for postoperative complications, 113
postoperative epithelial defect treatment, 477
radiation injury treatment, 434
thermal burn treatment, 433
Tay-Sachs disease (GM_2 gangliosidosis type I), 251, 252*t*, 253–254
TBCD. *See* Thiel-Behnke corneal dystrophy
TBUT. *See* Tear breakup time
T-cell lymphoma, 420
T cells, 15–16*f*, 16–17, 57–58
Tear breakup time (TBUT), 27–28, 32, 60, 65
Tear deficiencies. *See* Tear production
Tear film
debris or mucus in, ATD sign, 59
defense mechanisms, 7*f*, 15–16, 15–16*f*

dry eye and, 54, 57–58, 57*f*, 65
examination, 26, 27–28, 30–31, 31*f*, 34
instability, 54
refractive power and, 32
structure and function, 6–7, 7*f*, 24*f*
tests, 30–32, 31*f*
Tear Film and Ocular Surface Society Dry Eye Workshop II (TFOS DEWS II) diagnostic classification scheme, 67, 67*f*
Tear film instability, 54, 58
Tear hyperosmolarity, 54, 57, 57*f*
Tear meniscus, 26, 28, 59, 60
Tear production. *See also* Dry eye
decreased, ectodermal dysplasia sign, 278
as defense mechanism, 15
evaluation of, 29, 30–32, 60
function of, 3
medications that decrease, 66*t*
overflow, 8
production of, 3, 6, 10
radiation injuries and, 434
Tea tree oil, 79, 322–323
Teff cells (effector T cells), 15–16*f*
Telangiectasias, 76, 163*t*, 417, 434
TEN. *See* Toxic epidermal necrolysis
Terrien marginal degeneration (TMD), 172–173, 173*f*, 231*t*, 382*t*, 488
Testosterone eyedrops (topical), 69
Tetracycline (oral), 74–75, 78, 96, 166*t*, 332, 431
Textural interface opacity (TIO), 503–504, 503*f*
TFOS DEWS II (Tear Film and Ocular Surface Society Dry Eye Workshop II) diagnostic classification scheme, 67, 67*f*
TGF-β. *See* Transforming growth factor β
TGFBI epithelial-stromal (keratoepithelin-associated) dystrophies, 185–186*t*, 192–202
Therapeutic interventions, for ocular surface disorders
amniotic membrane grafts, 119–120
anterior stromal puncture, 126–127, 127*f*
autologous transplantation, 114, 120*t*. *See also* Autologous transplantation
bandage contact lens use, 128–129
for bare sclera coverage, 110–111*f*, 110–114
biopsy, 118
conjunctival fixation, 119
conjunctival flap, 114–118, 115–117*f*
conjunctival interventions, 107–124
conjunctival resection, 119
for corneal perforations, 130–132, 131*f*
corneal tattooing, 134–135, 134–135*f*
for corneal thinning/descemetocele, 129–130, 129–130*f*
epithelial debridement, 126
excimer laser ablation, 99, 125–126, 128
limbal stem cell transplantation, 120–123, 120*t*, 122–123*f*
mucous membrane grafts, 123–124
patching, 128
pterygium excision, 107–110, 108*f*, 109*t*, 113–114, 113*f*
superficial cauterization, 119
superficial keratectomy, 125–126
tarsorrhaphy, 132–133*f*, 132–134
Therapeutic soft contact lens, 375, 375*f*
Thermal injuries, 432–433, 433*f*
Thiel-Behnke corneal dystrophy (TBCD), 186*t*, 193*f*, 194–195, 195*f*, 196*t*
Thorns, 448
Thrombolytic drugs, 437
Thygeson epithelial keratitis, 52, 54*f*
Thygeson superficial punctate keratitis, 27, 376–377
Thyroid eye disease, 56*t*, 90–91
Thyroid function tests, 91
Tight lens syndrome, 177*t*
Timolol, 370
TIO. *See* Textural interface opacity
Tissue inhibitor of matrix metalloproteinase 1 (TIMP 1), 7
TKPro, 510
TMD. *See* Terrien marginal degeneration
TNF-α. *See* Tumor necrosis factor alpha
Tobramycin, 81, 354
Tomography, 36–39, 38–39*f*, 38*t*
Tonometer tip cleaning, 308
Topical anti-inflammatory agents, 69
Topical ocular medications. *See specific drugs*
Topography, 33–35, 35–37*f*
Total (eight-ball) hyphemas, 441, 443*f*
Toxic epidermal necrolysis (TEN), 365–368, 366*f*
Toxic keratitis, 88, 104
Toxic ocular surface disease, 102–105, 103*t*, 104*f*
Toxic reactions, to ocular medications, 102–105, 103*t*, 104*f*. *See also* Chemical injuries
Toxic ulcerative keratopathy, 103
Trabeculectomy, 470
Trabeculectomy bleb, 28–29
Trabeculitis (endotheliitis), 177*t*, 292, 305, 305*f*
Tranexamic acid, 445
Transepithelial corneal crosslinking, 245
Transforming growth factor β (TGF-β), 7*f*, 15–16*f*
Transparency (corneal clarity), 10, 11, 13, 247
Transplantations. *See* Corneal transplantation; Grafts
Transthyretin *(TTR)* gene, 263
Traumatic hyphema, 440–446, 442–444*f*
Traumatic injuries
blunt trauma, 436–446. *See also* Blunt trauma
evaluation of, 450–451, 451–452*t*
foreign bodies, 447–450, 447–450*f*. *See also* Foreign bodies
as keratitis risk factor, 334, 342
penetrating and perforating, 446–461. *See also* Penetrating and perforating trauma
as RES cause, 97
treatment of, 451–461
Treacher Collins syndrome (mandibulofacial dysostosis), 268*t*
Treponema pallidum, 151, 328*t*, 379
Triamcinolone acetonide, 484
Triazoles, 346
Trichiasis, 81, 88–89, 89*f*, 368, 369, 370, 373

Trifluridine (topical)
  adverse effects, 354
  epithelial (dendritic) keratitis treatment, 291
  herpes simplex viral eye infections, 287*t*, 294*t*
  herpetic interstitial keratitis treatment, 295
  toxic reactions to, 103
  vaccinia treatment, 312
Trigeminal anesthesia, 153
Trigeminal nerve (cranial nerve V), 6*f*, 70, 95, 286, 300, 409, 433
Trisomy 8 mosaicism syndrome, 152
TrueTear (Allergan), 70
Tuberculosis, 53*t*, 292*t*, 333, 350, 388, 393, 394
Tube shunt surgery, 470
Tularemia, 333
Tumor necrosis factor alpha (TNF-α), 16
Tumors. *See* Neoplastic disorders
Tyrosine, 259–260
Tyrosinemia, 257*t*, 259–260, 259*t*, 260*f*
Tyrosinemia type II (Richner-Hanhart syndrome), 259–260

UBM. *See* Ultrasound biomicroscopy
UDVA. *See* Uncorrected distance visual acuity
Ulceration
  of cornea
    bacterial, 334, 335*f*
    description, 49*t*
    differential diagnosis, 50*t*, 438
    fungal keratitis risk factor, 342
    mooren ulcer, 53*t*, 231*t*, 373*t*, 385–386, 385–386*f*
    OSD sign, 49*t*
    vitamin A deficiency sign, 272
  exposure keratopathy sign, 93
  of eyelid, 48*t*
  rosacea association, 78
Ulcerative keratitis, 78, 327
Ultrasound biomicroscopy (UBM), 45, 45*f*, 471
Ultrathin DSEK, 496
Ultraviolet light, 158, 241, 245
Ultraviolet radiation injuries, 433–434
Uncorrected distance visual acuity (UDVA; uncorrected visual acuity), 237
Urate depositions, 167, 168*t*
Uric acid depositions, 264
Uroporphyrinogen decarboxylase deficiency, 266
Urticating hairs, 435
Uveitis, 168*t*, 391, 392, 471. *See also* Anterior uveitis

Vaccinations
  for chickenpox, 298, 299
  for COVID-19, 314
  for shingles, 302
Vaccinia, 311–312
Vaccinia-immune globulin (VIG), 312
Valacyclovir (oral), 287*t*, 291, 295, 302
Valganciclovir (oral), 287*t*, 306
Vancomycin, 453, 458
Varicella-zoster virus (VZV)
  background, 298
  diagnostic techniques, 283*t*
  differential diagnosis, 292*t*
  differentiating features, 298*t*
  disciform keratitis, 292
  herpes zoster ophthalmicus, 300, 300*f*, 315
  keratitis, 52, 53*t*, 54*f*, 300–301
  keratoplasty complications and, 470
  primary infection, 298–299
  recurrent infection, 299–303, 299*t*, 300–301*f*
  risk factors, 299
  scleritis association, 388
  scleritis cause, 350
  trabeculitis, 177*t*
  treatment, 302–304
  vaccination, 302
Variola (smallpox) virus, 311–312
Vascularization. *See* Neovascularization and vascularization
Vascularized pannus, 53, 55*f*, 65, 121, 122*f*, 173, 329, 330*f*
Vascular tumors
  benign, 416–417, 416*t*
  inflammatory, 417–418, 418*f*
  malignant, 418–419
Vasoactive intestinal peptide (VIP), 15–16*f*
Vernal conjunctivitis, 88
Vernal keratitis, 292*t*
Vernal keratoconjunctivitis (VKC), 219*t*, 358–361, 359–360*f*, 362*t*
Verrucae, 312
Vesicle
  description, 48*t*
  differential diagnosis, 300
  herpesvirus sign, 300
  OSD sign, 48*t*
Vidarabine, 287*t*
VIG. *See* Vaccinia-immune globulin
VIP. *See* Vasoactive intestinal peptide
Viral infections
  background, 281–284, 282–283*f*, 283*t*
  classification of viruses, 282, 283*f*
  diagnostic techniques for, 283*t*
  DNA viruses, 284–313. *See also* Adenovirus infections; Cytomegalovirus; Epstein-Barr virus; Herpesviruses; Papillomaviruses; Poxviruses
  dry eye risk factor, 56*t*
  pathogenesis, 318–322, 319*t*
  RNA viruses, 313–316, 313*t*
  specimen collection and evaluation, 320*t*, 322*f*
Vision assessment, preoperative, 470–471, 471*f*
Vitamin A, 101
Vitamin A deficiency, 272–273, 272*f*, 314
Vitamin B_2 (riboflavin), 241
Vitamin C, 260, 431
Vitamin D toxicity, 168*t*, 277
Vitrectomy, 470
Vitreous veils, 261
VKC. *See* Vernal keratoconjunctivitis

Vogt striae, 220, 221*f*
Voriconazole, 343, 346, 348
VZV. *See* Varicella-zoster virus

Waite-Beetham lines, 275
Waldenström macroglobulinemia, 259*t*, 273, 274, 274*f*
Warfarin, 437
Wasp stings, 435
Wegener granulomatosis (granulomatosis with polyangiitis), 389
Weight implants, 94
Welding, 433
Werner syndrome, 268*t*
White lashes (poliosis), 81
White limbal girdle of Vogt, 168, 169*f*
WHO. *See* World Health Organization
Wilson disease (hepatolenticular degeneration), 166*t*, 264–265, 265*f*
With-the-rule astigmatism, 35*f*, 108*f*, 143
World Health Organization (WHO), 331

Xeroderma pigmentosum, 278–279
Xerophthalmia, 58, 272
Xerosis, 272–273
X-linked ichthyosis, 139*t*, 146
XYZ hypothesis, of stem cell differentiation, 14

Zeis, glands of, 4, 4–5*f*, 84
Zoster dermatitis, 300
Zoster Eye Disease Study (ZEDS), 303
Zoster virus. *See* Varicella-zoster virus